The Genetics of Neurological Disorders

Editor: Billy Acord

FOSTER ACADEMICS
www.fosteracademics.com

www.fosteracademics.com

FOSTER ACADEMICS

Cataloging-in-Publication Data

The genetics of neurological disorders / edited by Billy Acord.
p. cm.
Includes bibliographical references and index.
ISBN 978-1-63242-725-0
1. Neurogenetics. 2. Nervous system--Diseases. 3. Neurosciences. I. Acord, Billy.
RC346.4 .G45 2019
616.804 42--dc23

Foster Academics,
118-35 Queens Blvd., Suite 400,
Forest Hills, NY 11375, USA

ISBN 978-1-63242-725-0 (Hardback)

Printed and bound in China.

Contents

Preface

This book was inspired by the evolution of our times; to answer the curiosity of inquisitive minds. Many developments have occurred across the globe in the recent past which has transformed the progress in the field.

The field of neurogenetics explores the role of genetics in neurological disorders. Any structural, electrical and biochemical abnormality in the brain, spinal cord or other nerves can be termed as a neurological disorder. Neurodegenerative diseases such as Parkinson's disease and Alzheimer's disease are a subset of neurological disorders. While the genetic influence on simple neurological diseases have been established, the genetics of complex disorders is a matter of significant research. Using genome wide association studies, the genetic variability within the human population and the associated link with diseases can be investigated. Research in neurogenetics strives to find strategies to reverse the progression of neurodegenerative disorders, which till date have no viable cure. The aim of this book is to present researches pertaining to the genetics of neurological disorders that can advance the understanding of neurological diseases and aid in their clinical management. It presents this complex study in the most comprehensible language. With state-of-the-art inputs by acclaimed experts of this field, this book targets students and professionals.

This book was developed from a mere concept to drafts to chapters and finally compiled together as a complete text to benefit the readers across all nations. To ensure the quality of the content we instilled two significant steps in our procedure. The first was to appoint an editorial team that would verify the data and statistics provided in the book and also select the most appropriate and valuable contributions from the plentiful contributions we received from authors worldwide. The next step was to appoint an expert of the topic as the Editor-in-Chief, who would head the project and finally make the necessary amendments and modifications to make the text reader-friendly. I was then commissioned to examine all the material to present the topics in the most comprehensible and productive format.

I would like to take this opportunity to thank all the contributing authors who were supportive enough to contribute their time and knowledge to this project. I also wish to convey my regards to my family who have been extremely supportive during the entire project.

Editor

Genetic Knock-Down of *Hdac3* Does Not Modify Disease-Related Phenotypes in a Mouse Model of Huntington's Disease

Lara Moumné[1], Ken Campbell[2], David Howland[3], Yingbin Ouyang[2], Gillian P. Bates[1]*

1 Department of Medical and Molecular Genetics, King's College London, London, United Kingdom, **2** Taconic, Cranbury, New Jersey, United States of America, **3** CHDI Management/CHDI Foundation, Princeton, New Jersey, United States of America

Abstract

Huntington's disease (HD) is an autosomal dominant progressive neurodegenerative disorder caused by an expansion of a CAG/polyglutamine repeat for which there are no disease modifying treatments. In recent years, transcriptional dysregulation has emerged as a pathogenic process that appears early in disease progression and has been recapitulated across multiple HD models. Altered histone acetylation has been proposed to underlie this transcriptional dysregulation and histone deacetylase (HDAC) inhibitors, such as suberoylanilide hydroxamic acid (SAHA), have been shown to improve polyglutamine-dependent phenotypes in numerous HD models. However potent pan-HDAC inhibitors such as SAHA display toxic side-effects. To better understand the mechanism underlying this potential therapeutic benefit and to dissociate the beneficial and toxic effects of SAHA, we set out to identify the specific HDAC(s) involved in this process. For this purpose, we are exploring the effect of the genetic reduction of specific HDACs on HD-related phenotypes in the R6/2 mouse model of HD. The study presented here focuses on HDAC3, which, as a class I HDAC, is one of the preferred targets of SAHA and is directly involved in histone deacetylation. To evaluate a potential benefit of *Hdac3* genetic reduction in R6/2, we generated a mouse carrying a critical deletion in the *Hdac3* gene. We confirmed that the complete knock-out of *Hdac3* is embryonic lethal. To test the effects of HDAC3 inhibition, we used *Hdac3*$^{+/-}$ heterozygotes to reduce nuclear HDAC3 levels in R6/2 mice. We found that *Hdac3* knock-down does not ameliorate physiological or behavioural phenotypes and has no effect on molecular changes including dysregulated transcripts. We conclude that HDAC3 should not be considered as the major mediator of the beneficial effect induced by SAHA and other HDAC inhibitors in HD.

Editor: Xiao-Jiang Li, Emory University, United States of America

Funding: This work was funded by CHDI Foundation, a privately-funded non-profit biomedical research organization exclusively dedicated to discovering and developing therapeutics that slow the progression of Huntington's disease. DH was involved in the design and generation of the Hdac3 KO mouse. With the exception of this, the funders had no role in study design, data collection and analysis, decision to publish, or preparation of the manuscript.

Competing Interests: DH is employed by CHDI Management, Inc. and YO and KC are employees of Taconic. There are no patents, products in development or marketed products to declare. This does not alter the authors' adherence to all the PLoS ONE policies on sharing data and materials.

* E-mail: gillian.bates@kcl.ac.uk

Introduction

Huntington's disease (HD) is an autosomal dominant progressive neurodegenerative disorder with a mean age of onset of 40 years. The main clinical manifestations are chorea, cognitive impairment, psychiatric disorders and weight loss. The disease duration is 15–20 years and in the absence of disease modifying treatments, the disease progresses inexorably until death [1]. The mutation responsible for HD is an unstable expansion of a CAG repeat in the *HTT* gene that leads to a polyglutamine expansion in the N-terminus of the huntingtin (HTT) protein [2]. Neuropathologically, HD is characterized by neuronal loss in several brain regions including the striatum and the cortex as well as the deposition of nuclear and cytoplasmic HTT-containing aggregates [3].

A variety of mouse models have been used to study the pathogenic pathways involved in HD [4]. These include the R6/2 model, which is transgenic for a single-copy of exon 1 of human *HTT*, which in our colony carries approximately 200 CAG repeats [5,6] and the *Hdh*Q150 knock-in model in which 150 CAGs have been inserted into the mouse *Htt* gene [7,8]. The R6/2 mouse has an early onset progressive phenotype that recapitulates many features of the human disease. Motor and cognitive impairment appear before 6 weeks, HTT aggregation can clearly be detected from 3 weeks, whereas neuronal cell loss in the striatum occurs at later stages [9,10,11]. Mice with an average 200 CAG repeats are not usually kept beyond 15 weeks. The early and reproducible phenotype of this mouse line has made it an ideal model screening compounds and performing genetic crosses. At late-stage disease, the R6/2 and *Hdh*Q150 models have developed remarkably similar phenotypes [8,12,13,14] supporting the hypothesis that the generation of a toxic fragment is a critical event in HD pathogenesis [15].

In recent years, transcriptional dysregulation has emerged as a pathogenic process that appears early in disease progression and has been recapitulated across multiple HD model systems including the R6/2 and *Hdh*Q150 mouse models [12,16]. Histone acetylation/deacetylation is an important mechanism involved in gene transcriptional regulation and altered histone acetylation has been proposed to underlie transcriptional dysregulation in HD [17]. In general, acetylation of lysines by histone acetyl transferases (HAT) leads to activation of transcription whereas removal of acetyl groups by histone deacetylases (HDAC) leads to gene silencing [18]. There are two evolutionary divergent types of HDACs: the zinc-dependent HDACs (human HDAC1-11) and the NAD^+ dependent HDACs also called sirtuins (human SIRT1-7). Inhibitors of the zinc-dependant HDACs include suberoylanilide hydroxamic acid (SAHA) and trichostatin A (TSA) [19], whereas sirtuins are inhibited by nicotinamide [20]. The human zinc-dependent HDAC family comprises eleven members divided into four classes: I (HDAC1, 2, 3 and 8), IIa (HDAC4, 5, 7 and 9), IIb (HDAC6 and 10) and IV (HDAC11). HDAC inhibition has been shown to improve polyglutamine-dependent phenotypes in several models of HD [21,22,23,24,25,26]. Although administration of SAHA improves HD-related phenotypes in the R6/2 mouse model, therapeutic doses have toxic effects and induce profound weight loss [24].

To better understand the mechanism underlying this potential therapeutic benefit and to dissociate the beneficial and toxic effects of SAHA, we set out to identify the specific HDAC(s) involved in this process. For this purpose, we are exploring the effect of the genetic reduction of specific HDACs on HD-related phenotypes in R6/2 mice. Genetic reduction (knock-down or complete knock-out) of *Hdac5, 6, 7 and 9* failed to induce a phenotypic improvement ([27,28] and unpublished data) whereas knock-down of *Hdac4* induces a significant beneficial effect (unpublished data).

The study presented here focuses on HDAC3, which is the most highly expressed class I HDAC in the brain [29]. This HDAC is of particular interest for several reasons. Class I HDACs are directly involved in histone deacetylation and as a class I HDAC, HDAC3 is one of the main cellular targets of SAHA [30]. A recent study showed that the class I inhibitor HDACi **4b**, which is reported to be more specific for HDAC3 than the other class I HDACs, ameliorated the disease phenotype and reversed many of the transcriptional abnormalities found in the brain of R6/2 mice [26]. Moreover, studies involving genetic reduction of specific HDACs in invertebrate models of HD have implicated class I HDACs in the reduction of polyglutamine-dependent toxicity. In *Drosophila melanosgaster*, knock-down of the class I HDAC *rpd3*, that is homologous to human *HDAC1/2* but also partially homologous to *HDAC3*, suppresses pathogenesis [31]. Similarly, in *C. Elegans*, only the knock-down of the *hda-3*, that shares homology with human class I HDACs, suppressed polyglutamine-dependant toxicity [21]. Finally, the catalytic domain of HDAC4 interacts with HDAC3 via the transcriptional corepressor complex N-CoR/SMRT, and suppression of HDAC4 binding to SMRT/N-CoR and to HDAC3 results in the loss of enzymatic activity associated with HDAC4 [32]. Given the beneficial effect of *Hdac4* knock-down on HD-related phenotypes in R6/2 mice, we might expect that a reduction of *Hdac3* expression would lead a reduced HDAC4 activity and an improvement in R6/2 phenotypes.

To evaluate a potential benefit of *Hdac3* genetic reduction in R6/2, we generated a genetically engineered mouse in which part of the *Hdac3* gene is deleted. We observed that a complete knock-out of *Hdac3* is embryonic lethal. *Hdac3* mRNA levels were reduced to 50% of wild type (WT) in the brains of *Hdac3*$^{+/-}$ heterozygotes (knock-down) with a corresponding reduction in HDAC3 protein in the nucleus but not in the cytoplasm. We found that *Hdac3*$^{+/-}$ heterozygotes are viable and fertile, with no overt phenotype. We performed a genetic cross between R6/2 mice and *Hdac3*$^{+/-}$ heterozygotes and found that *Hdac3* knock-down does not ameliorate physiological or behavioural phenotypes in R6/2 mice, does not modulate HTT aggregation and has no effect on transcriptional dysregulation. We conclude that HDAC3 should not be considered as the major mediator of the beneficial effect induced by SAHA and other HDAC inhibitors in HD.

Results

Conventional heterozygous deletion of *Hdac3*

We generated a conventional null allele of *Hdac3* in order to evaluate whether a reduction in HDAC3 level has beneficial effects in the R6/2 mice. For this purpose, loxP sites were introduced upstream of exon 11 and within exon 15 by homologous recombination inducing a deletion covering exon 11 to 14 and the 5′ end of exon 15 (Fig. 1A). This mutation removes a part of the nuclear localization signal and a C-terminal region necessary for both deacetylase activity and transcriptional repression [33,34]. Heterozygous F1 mice were generated and deletion of *Hdac3* was confirmed at the genomic level by PCR and sequencing (Fig. 1B). We intercrossed *Hdac3*$^{+/-}$ mice in order to generate nullizygotes, but did not obtain any *Hdac3* knock-out offspring at birth or between embryonic stages E8.5 and E15.5. This result reveals that a complete lack of *Hdac3* induces an embryonic lethality prior to E8.5 and confirms previous studies showing that *Hdac3*$^{-/-}$ mice die before E9.5 [35,36]. Given this embryonic lethality we used *Hdac3*$^{+/-}$ heterozygotes for our study. These mice are viable and fertile, with no overt phenotype.

It was important first to confirm that the *Hdac3* expression level was reduced in *Hdac3*$^{+/-}$ mice as it has been previously shown that *Hdac1*, another class I HDAC, autoregulates its expression to wild-type (WT) levels in *Hdac1*$^{+/-}$ heterozygous mice [37]. It was also important to determine whether *Hdac3* levels might be regulated by the R6/2 transprotein. Therefore, we crossed R6/2 males to *Hdac3*$^{+/-}$ heterozygous females to generate WT, *Hdac3*$^{+/-}$, R6/2 and R6/2::*Hdac3*$^{+/-}$ double mutant (Dbl) mice and performed RT-qPCR on cDNA prepared from cortex, cerebellum and striatum of 15-week old mice. The RT-qPCR primer sequences were located within the deletion (at the junction between exon 14 and 15) so that only the WT allele can be detected. We observed a significant reduction of *Hdac3* mRNA to 50% of the WT level in all the brain regions irrespective of the presence of the R6/2 transprotein (Fig. 2A). In order to verify the specificity of *Hdac3* reduction we analyzed the expression level of the other *Hdacs* by RT-qPCR and showed that these were not changed in *Hdac3*$^{+/-}$ mice compared to WT (Fig. S1).

In order to see whether this mRNA reduction translates into a reduction at the protein level, we performed western blotting on whole brain lysates using an HDAC3 specific antibody. Surprisingly, the protein level was only reduced to 80% of the WT level (Fig. S2). As HDAC3 is present in both the nucleus and the cytoplasm in mammalian cells [33], we investigated whether HDAC3 levels might differ between these two intracellular compartments. For this purpose, we performed nuclear and cytoplasmic fractionation of whole brains from 4 week old mice. We first confirmed that HDAC3 is present in both the nucleus and cytoplasm in WT mouse brain (Fig. 2B). Analysis of brains from WT, *Hdac3*$^{+/-}$, R6/2 and Dbl mice revealed that cytoplasmic HDAC3 is not reduced in *Hdac3*$^{+/-}$ and Dbl brains as compared to WT and R6/2. In contrast, its expression is reduced to 60% of the WT level in *Hdac3*$^{+/-}$ heterozygotes irrespective of the presence of the R6/2 transgene (Fig. 2C and D). As we are primarily interested in the involvement of HDAC3 in transcriptional repression through histone deacetylation, a specific reduction of HDAC3 in the nucleus would be expected to be

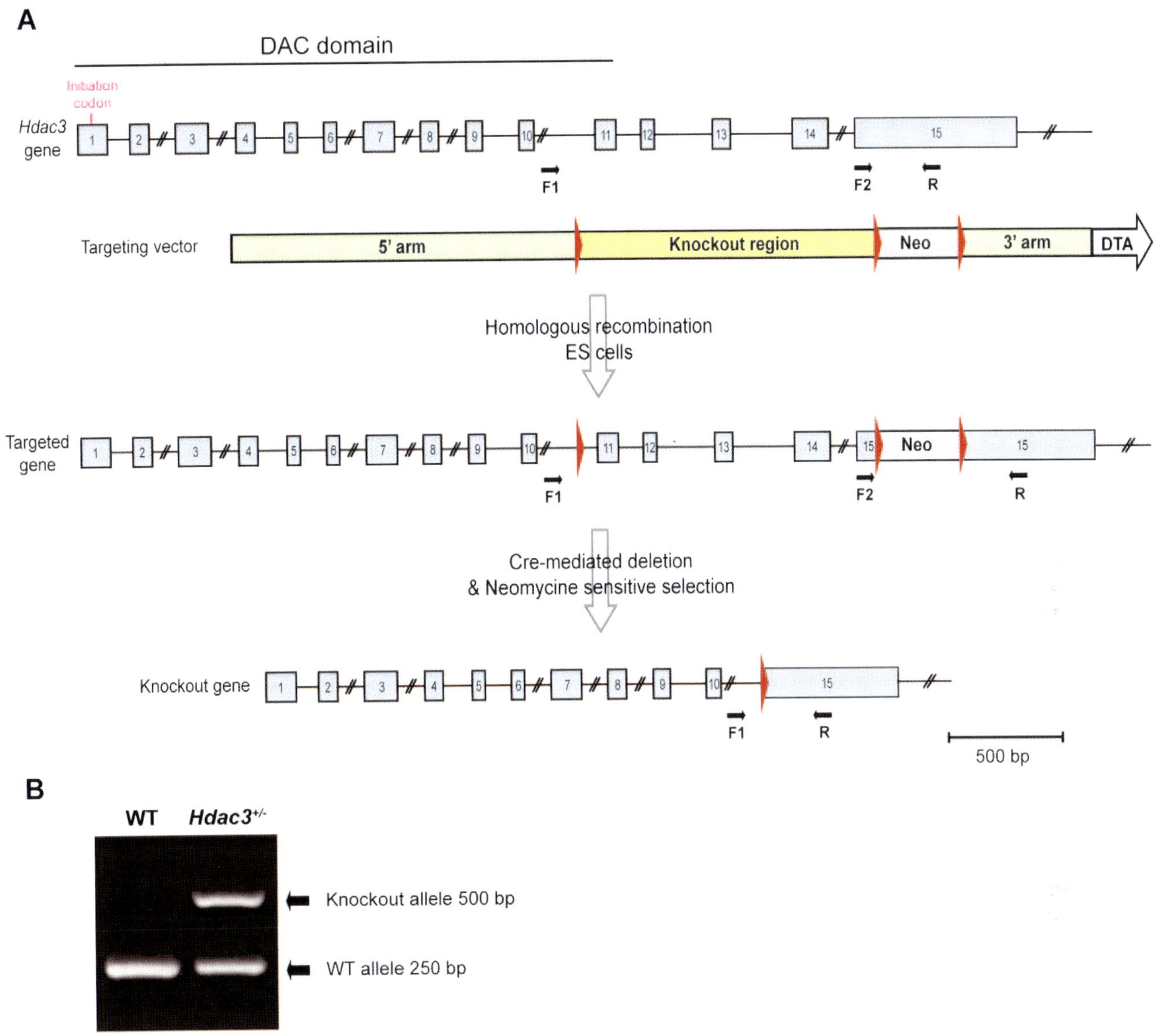

Figure 1. Generation of an *Hdac3* convention knock-out allele. (A) Strategy to generate an *Hdac3* conventional knock-out allele. The genomic structure and the targeting vector are shown. The *Hdac*3 gene contains 15 exons (blue rectangles). LoxP sites (red triangles) were introduced upstream exon 11 and within exon 15. The vector contains a 5′ homology arm covering the exonic and intronic region from intron 3–4 to intron 10–11 and a 3′ homology arm covering a part of exon 15 and the 3′UTR (green rectangle). The conditional knock-out region (yellow rectangle) covers exon 11 to 14 and 5′ end of exon 15. This conditional allele was introduced by homologous recombination in ES cells. The neomycine cassette (pink rectangle) flanked by 2 LoxP sites was removed by electroporation of Cre recombinase in ES cells and the cells containing the allele corresponding to a complete deletion of exon 11 to 14 were selected. Primers used for genotyping are represented as black arrows. F1 = forward 1; F2 = forward 2; R = Reverse. (B) Representative genotyping PCR on mouse genomic DNA. Duplex PCR with F1, F2 and R primers detects both the WT (250 bp band with primers F2/R) and the knock-out (500 bp with primers F1/R) allele.

sufficient to mimic inhibition of HDAC3 histone deacetylase activity and explore its potential benefit in HD.

Genetic reduction of *Hdac3* does not modify the R6/2 phenotype

A set of previously established quantitative tests was used to evaluate whether a genetic reduction of *Hdac3* had an effect on HD-related phenotypes in R6/2 mice. In order to generate mice for this analysis, R6/2 males were bred with *Hdac3*$^{+/-}$ females to generate at least 12 mice per genotype (males and females, WT n = 16, *Hdac3*$^{+/-}$ n = 14, R6/2 n = 12, Dbl n = 15). The mice were born over a period of 5 days and the 4 genotypes were recovered in a Mendelian ratio. The average CAG repeat size did not differ between the R6/2 group and the Dbl group (204±3.16 vs 205±0.91; p = 0.11). Body weight, RotaRod performance, grip strength and exploratory activity were monitored from 4 to 15 weeks of age, and in each case, a specific test was performed by the same operator, on the same day and at the same time during the weeks in which measurements were taken.

Mice were weighed weekly from 4 to 15 weeks of age. As expected, R6/2 mice weighed less overall than WT mice [$F_{(1,49)} = 32.657$, $p<0.001$] and gained weight at a slower rate [$F_{(4,539)} = 38.086$, $p<0.001$] (Fig. 3A). No significant differences in the overall weight [$F_{(1,49)} = 3.267$, $p = 0.077$] or in weight gain

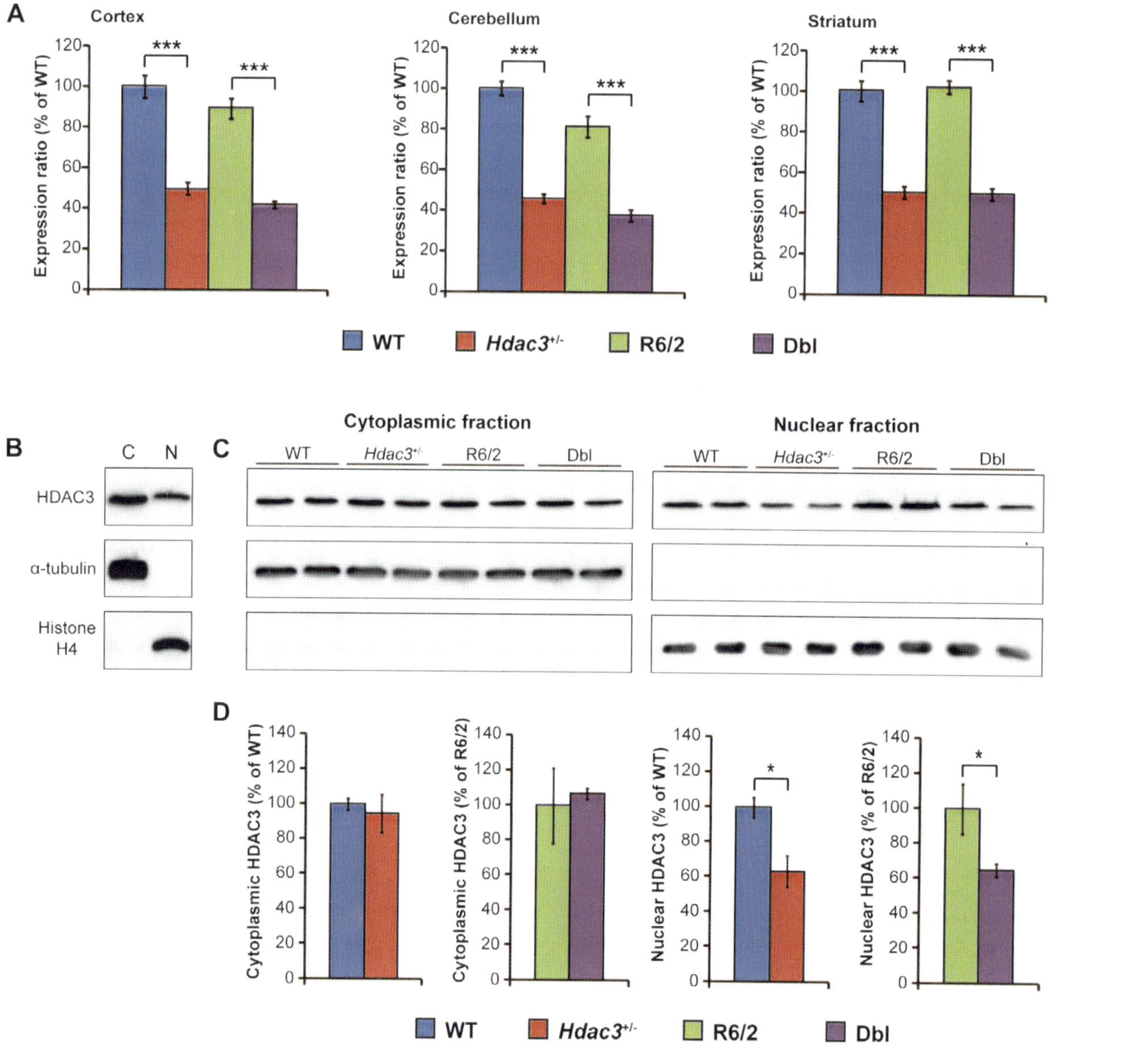

Figure 2. *Hdac3* mRNA and protein expression in *Hdac3+/−* heterozygous mouse brain. (A) *Hdac3* mRNA expression levels in 15 week old mouse cortex, cerebellum and striatum are shown as a relative expression ratio to the WT level. *Hdac3*$^{+/-}$ (red) and Dbl (purple) mice express the mRNA at 50% of the WT (blue) and R6/2 (green) levels in all brain regions. Error bars correspond to S.E.M. (n = 8) ***p<0.001. (B) Western blot showing the expression of HDAC3 protein in the cytoplasmic (C) and the nuclear (N) fraction of WT mouse whole brain. Antibodies to α-tubulin (cytoplasmic) and histone H4 (nuclear) were used to control for the purity of the fractions. (C) Representative western blot and (D) quantification of cytoplasmic and nuclear fraction prepared from WT (blue), *Hdac3*$^{+/-}$ (red), R6/2 (green) and Dbl (purple) 15 week old-mouse whole brains. Antibodies to α-tubulin (cytoplasmic) and histone H4 (nuclear) were used as both purity and loading controls. Cytoplasmic HDAC3 was not affected by *Hdac3* deletion whereas nuclear HDAC3 was reduced to 60% of the WT level. Error bars correspond S.E.M. (n = 3) *p<0.05.

[$F_{(4,539)}$ = 0.254, p = 0.887] between WT and *Hdac3*$^{+/-}$ mice were observed. However, there was a trend for *Hdac3*$^{+/-}$ mice to weigh more than WT (p = 0.077). Genetic reduction of *Hdac3* had no effect on R6/2 weight [$F_{(1,49)}$ = 0.218, p = 0.643] and did not attenuate the rate of R6/2 weight loss [$F_{(4,539)}$ = 1.458, p = 0.222]. Therefore, genetic reduction of *Hdac3*$^{+/-}$ does not improve the weight loss phenotype in the R6/2 mice.

RotaRod performance is a sensitive indicator of balance and motor coordination, which has been reliably shown to decline in R6/2 mice. RotaRod was assessed at 4, 8, 10, 12 and 14 weeks of age. Consistent with previous data, R6/2 mice displayed a significant decline in overall RotaRod performance [$F_{(1,49)}$ = 75.523, p<0.001] and this worsened with age [$F_{(3,980)}$ = 23.764, p<0.001] (Fig. 3B). *Hdac3* knock-down had no effect on overall RotaRod performance of *Hdac3*$^{+/-}$ mice [$F_{(1,49)}$ = 0.386, p = 0.537] and did not significantly change the overall performance of R6/2 mice [$F_{(1,49)}$ = 0.478, p = 0.493]. Furthermore, *Hdac3* knock-down had no effect on the deterioration of R6/2 RotaRod performance with age [$F_{(3,980)}$ = 0.344, p = 0.792].

Forelimb grip strength was assessed at 4 weeks of age and then weekly when the mice were 11 to 14 weeks old. Consistent with previous data, R6/2 mice performance was significantly decreased compared to WT [$F_{(1,49)}$ = 105.705, p<0.001] and deteriorated with age [$F_{(3,392)}$ = 25.804, p<0.001] (Fig. 3C). The grip strength

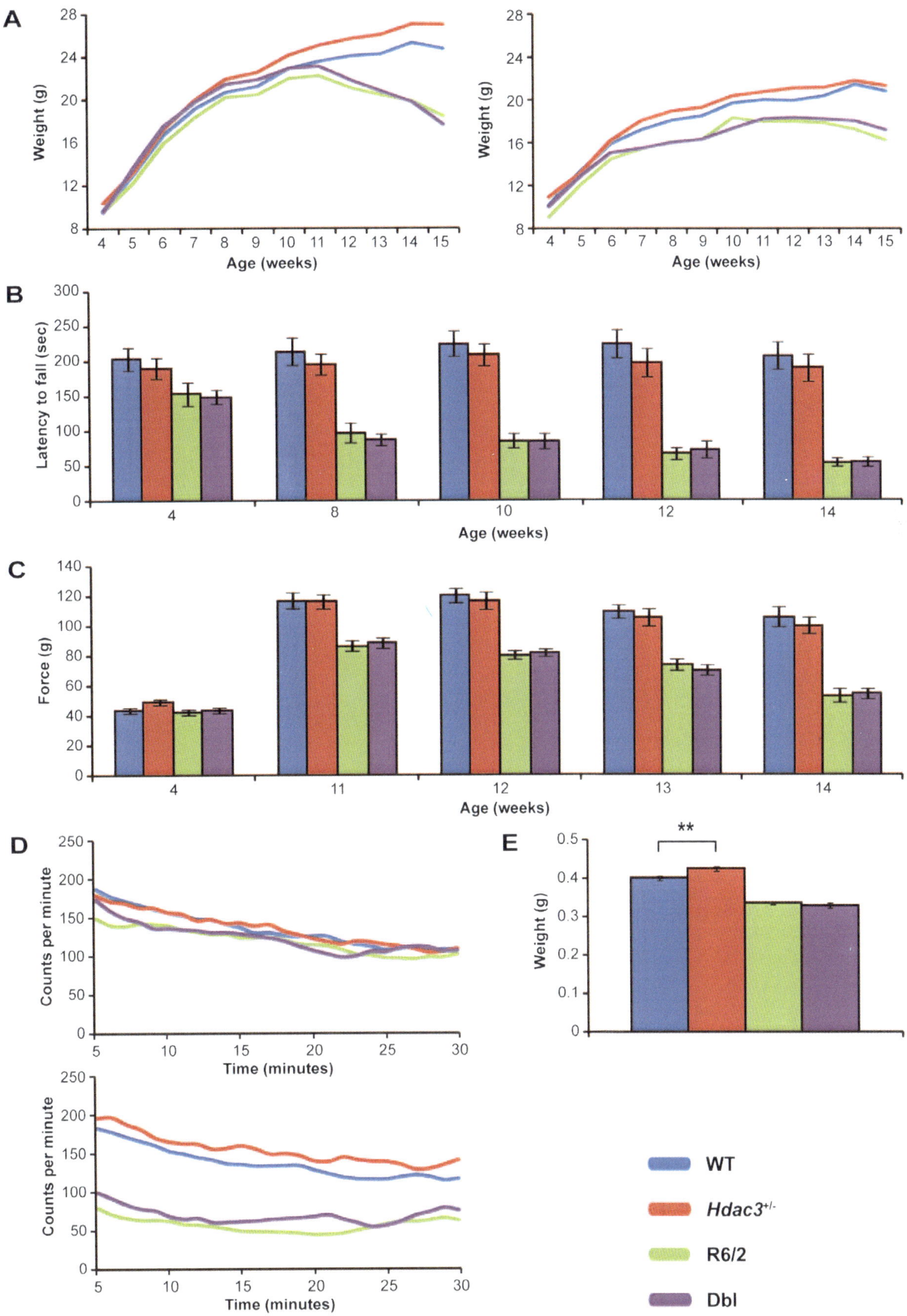

Figure 3. *Hdac3* genetic reduction does not modify R6/2 phenotypes. (A) Weight loss in males (left panel) and females (right panel) are shown between 4 and 15 weeks of age. *Hdac3* genetic reduction did not induce a significant increase of the body weight in R6/2 (B) RotaRod performance is represented as the average latency to fall in each group at 4, 8, 10, 12 and 14 weeks. *Hdac3* genetic reduction did not ameliorate the

impairment in RotaRod performance in R6/2 (C) Average grip strength in each group is represented at 4, 11, 12, 13 and 14 weeks. *Hdac3* genetic reduction did not induce a significant improvement in the grip strength in R6/2 mice (D) Average activity for each genotype is shown at 5 (upper panel) and 13 (lower panel) weeks of age. *Hdac3* genetic reduction did not reverse the hypoactivity observed in R6/2 mice (E) Average brain weight for each group was measured at 15 weeks of age. *Hdac3* genetic reduction did not modify the brain weight loss in R6/2 but a slight increase in brain weight was observed in WT animals **p<0.01. Error bars correspond to SEM (n>12). The same color code (blue = WT; red = Hdac3; green = R6/2 and purple = Dbl) was used for all measured parameters.

of *Hdac3*$^{+/-}$ mice was comparable to WT mice, both overall [$F_{(1,49)} = 0.230$, $p = 0.634$] and over the course of the experiment [$F_{(3,392)} = 0.675$, $p = 0.586$]. Furthermore, genetic reduction of *Hdac3* did not improve R6/2 overall grip strength performance [$F_{(1,49)} = 0.603$, $p = 0.441$] or deterioration with age [$F_{(3,392)} = 0.846$, $p = 0.483$].

Exploratory activity was assessed fortnightly from 5 to 13 weeks of age as described previously and analyzed by repeated measures general linear model (GLM) ANOVA. Mice were assessed for a period of 30 min for total activity, rearing, centre rearing and mobility. The *p*-values obtained for each parameter are displayed in Table S1. For all genotypes, the mice are highly active and mobile during the first part of the assessment period and this decreased over the course of the 30 min (Fig. 3D and Fig. S3). R6/2 mice show an overall hypoactivity and decreased mobility relative to WT mice from 7 weeks onwards. Rearing and centre rearing are also significantly decreased in R6/2 mice from 9 and 11 weeks of age respectively. *Hdac3*$^{+/-}$ mice were indistinguishable from WT mice for all of the parameters. Furthermore, *Hdac3* genetic reduction does not improve hypoactivity in the R6/2 mice.

Finally, we evaluated whether *Hdac3* genetic reduction had an effect on brain weight. Loss of brain weight has been observed in R6/2 mice in previous studies [6]. Brains were harvested from mice at 15 weeks of age, at the end of the trial. As expected, R6/2 mice displayed a significant decrease in brain weight [$F_{(1,49)} = 182.333$, $p<0.001$] (Fig. 3E). ANOVA analysis failed to detect any significant change in brain weight as a result of *Hdac3* genetic reduction [$F_{(1,49)} = 1.865$, $p = 0.178$]. Analysis of the results by Student's *t*-test revealed that *Hdac3* knock-down induces a significant increase in brain weight in the WT context ($p = 0.0074$) but no significant change was observed in the transgenic context (Fig. 3E). The brain weight of the Dbl mice is not significantly different from R6/2 ($p = 0.3857$). This result suggests that *Hdac3* knock-down has no effect on R6/2 mice brain weight loss.

Hdac3 genetic reduction does not ameliorate the dysregulated expression of genes of interest in R6/2 mouse brains

HDAC inhibitors have been shown to reverse transcriptional dysregulation in wide variety of HD models [17,26,38]. In order to evaluate whether a genetic reduction of *Hdac3* might modulate the transcriptional changes observed in HD, we used RT-qPCR to analyze the expression level of a set of 'genes of interest' in different brain regions. This included cortical *Bdnf* as well as cerebellar and striatal genes that are dysregulated in HD mouse models [8,12]. This analysis was performed on brain regions taken from 15 week old WT, *Hdac3*$^{+/-}$, R6/2 and Dbl mice. Changes in gene expression induced by the transgene were consistent with previous results for all the genes that were tested (Fig. 4A, B, C). Genetic reduction of *Hdac3* had no effect on the levels of the dysregulated transcripts in R6/2 brain regions except for *Bdnf* V (decreased expression, $p = 0.037$) and *Cnr1* (increased expression, $p = 0.028$) for which very mild but statistically significant changes were observed in the cortex and in striatum respectively (Fig. 4A and C). Similarly *Hdac3* genetic reduction had no effect on the expression of these genes in non-transgenic animals except for *Cnr1* for which a significant decrease in expression was observed in *Hdac3*$^{+/-}$ compared to WT striata ($p = 0.012$; Fig. 4C). We also found that *Hdac3* reduction does not affect the expression of the R6/2 transgene in the cortex (Fig. 4D), cerebellum (Fig. 4E) and striatum (Fig. 4F).

Hdac3 genetic reduction does not reduce Huntingtin aggregation in R6/2 mouse brains

HTT aggregation is a hallmark of brain pathology in HD and has been consistently observed in all HD models including the R6/2 mouse. Aggregation can be detected in several R6/2 brain regions from 3–4 weeks of age and increases with age [11]. In order to evaluate whether *Hdac3* reduction has an effect on this aggregation, we used a SEPRION ligand-based ELISA that provides a highly quantitative assay for measuring HTT aggregation in mouse brains [14]. Aggregates were captured from proteins extracted from the cortex, hippocampus and brain stem of 4, 9 and 15 week-old mice and detected with the MW8 antibody [39]. As expected, HTT aggregation was detectable at 4 weeks in all three brain regions, increased with age and this was not modified by *Hdac3* reduction. Levels of soluble HTT in these lysates can be quantified by western blot using the HTT specific antibody S830 [40]. The soluble trans-protein migrates at around 95 kDa whereas the aggregated protein remains in the stacking gel. Fig. 5B shows the results that we obtained for hippocampi from mice of 4, 9 and 15 weeks of age. The soluble fraction decreased with age in both R6/2 and Dbl mice and did not differ significantly between these genotypes at any time point (Fig. 5C). Similarly, a qualitative difference of the aggregated fraction was not detected. Taken together, the data obtained from the ELISA and western blotting revealed that *Hdac3* genetic reduction has no effect on HTT aggregation.

Discussion

HDAC inhibitors were first investigated as therapeutics in the context of HD to counteract transcriptional dysregulation, thought to contribute to the molecular pathogenesis of HD. They were first shown to be protective in a *Drosophila melanogaster* model [25] and following on from the demonstration that SAHA, a potent HDAC inhibitor, improves HD-related phenotypes in the R6/2 mouse, (Hockly et al., 2003), protective effects of the butyrates in HD mouse models were also reported [22,23]. However, therapeutic doses of SAHA were not well tolerated, leading to a marked weight loss in both WT and R6/2 animal. Therefore, if HDAC inhibitors are to be further developed as therapeutics for HD, it is essential that efficacy can be uncoupled from toxicity as far as is possible. As a pan-HDAC inhibitor, SAHA targets the eleven zinc-dependant HDACs with a preference for class I HDACs (1, 2, 3 and 8) and the class IIb HDAC, HDAC6 [30]. Identifying more specific inhibitors that target the HDAC(s) responsible for the beneficial effects observed in HD mouse models might be one mechanism by which the toxic effects could be diminished. Toward this aim, we are systematically investigating the effects of genetically reducing the levels of individual HDAC enzymes in the R6/2 mouse. In this study, we focus on HDAC3 and show that the

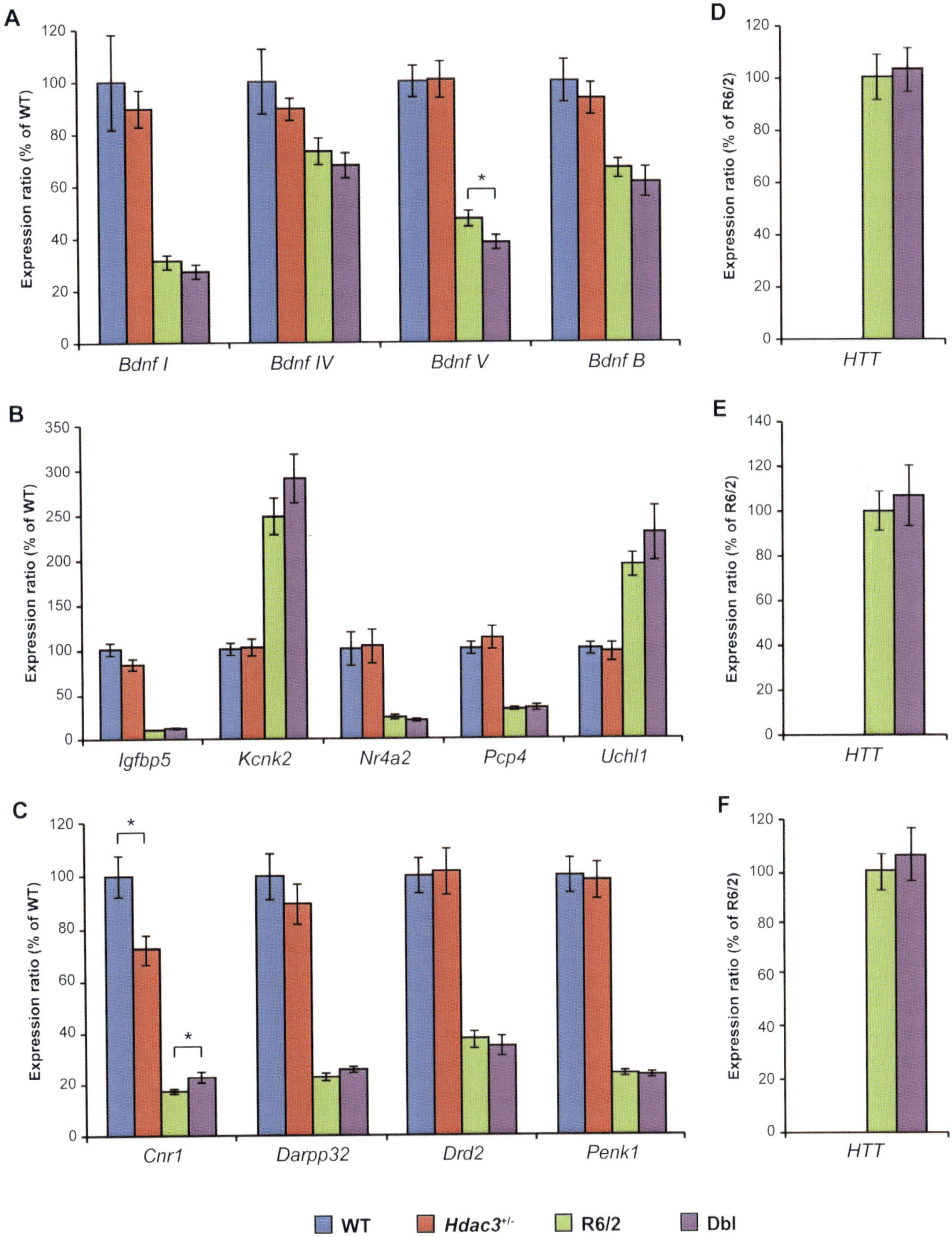

Figure 4. ***Hdac3*** **genetic reduction does not reverse transcriptional dysregulation in R6/2.** (A) Expression of *Bdnf* transcripts from different promoters (*Bdnf I, IV* and *V*) and the coding region (*Bdnf B*) in the cortex are represented as a percent of WT expression levels. With the exception of a slight decrease in *Bdnf* V, *Hdac3* reduction did not affect *Bdnf* expression. (B) Expression levels of genes specifically altered in the cerebellum of R6/2

mice are represented as a percent of WT expression. No significant difference was induced by *Hdac3* genetic reduction. (C) Expression levels of genes specifically altered in the striatum of R6/2 mice are represented as a percent of WT expression. A significant decrease in the expression of *Cnr1* in non-transgenic animals was observed as well as a slightly significant increase in *Cnr1* expression in R6/2 striata. Expression of the R6/2 transgene in Dbl brains is represented as a percent of that in R6/2 brains for cortex (D), cerebellum (E) and striatum (F). *Hdac3* reduction did not induce a significant change in transgene expression. Error bars correspond to S.E.M. (n = 8) *p<0.05. The same color code (blue = WT; red = Hdac3; green = R6/2 and purple = Dbl) was used for all the graphs. *Bdnf I, IV V*, brain derived neurotrophic factor promoter I, IV, V; *Bdnf B*, brain derived neurotrophic factor coding exon B; *Igfbp5*, insulin-like growth factor binding protein 5; *Kcnk2*, potassium channel subfamily K, member 2; *Nr4a2*, nuclear receptor subfamily 4, group A, member 2; *Pcp4*, Purkinje cell protein 4; *Uchl1*, ubiquitin C-terminal hydrolase L1; *Cnr1*, cannabinoid receptor 1; *Darpp32*, dopamine and cAMP regulated neuronal phosphoprotein; *Drd2*, dopamine D2 receptor; *Penk1*, proenkephalin.

reduction of nuclear HDAC3 to approximately 60% of WT levels has no effect on HD-related behavioral and physiological phenotypes or HTT aggregation. Importantly, the expression levels of a specific set of dysregulated gene transcripts were not restored.

HDAC3 was an interesting candidate for a number of reasons. The specific HDACs involved in the therapeutic benefits observed in invertebrate models of HD have also been explored by systematic genetic invalidation-based studies. Although a direct comparison with the mammalian enzymes cannot be made, as there are only four HDACs in *Drosophila melanogaster* and eight in *Caenorhabditis elegans* [21,31] both studies pointed to the class I HDACs as being the critical mediators of the beneficial effects. In *Drosophila melanogaster*, *rpd3* knock-down suppressed neurodegeneration and extended the survival of transgenic flies [31]. *Rpd3* is a class I HDAC that shares amino-acid sequence similarities with human *HDAC1*, *2* and *3* at 82%, 76% and 57% respectively. In *Caenorhabditis elegans*, of the eight HDAC enzymes, it was only knock-down of *Hda-3* that induced a neuroprotective effect, whereas knock-down of other HDACs, including the other class I orthologues *Hda-1* and *Hda-2*, exacerbated toxicity [21]. However, it was a pharmacological study in the R6/2 mouse model of HD that indicated that HDAC3 rather than the other class I HDACs might be the most relevant in a mammalian system. HDACi **4b** is one of a series of inhibitors for which the preferred cellular target has been reported to be HDAC3 [41]. HDACi **4b** was shown to improve motor performance and body weight of R6/2 mice, associated with a reversal of histone H3 hypoacetylation and the correction of specific brain mRNA levels [26]. Given that we have found that the genetic reduction of HDAC4 has beneficial effects in the R6/2 mouse (unpublished data) and that the enzyme activity of HDAC4 is dependent on its presence in the multi-protein complex that contains HDAC3 and the SMRT/N-CoR transcriptional repressors [32], HDAC3 was a therapeutic target that merited further investigation.

Although HDAC3 is the most highly expressed HDAC in the brain [29] little is known about its function in the central nervous system. Specific silencing of *Hdac3* in the hippocampus has been shown to lead to long-term memory enhancement [42]. The overexpression of *Hdac3* in rat cerebellar neurons induces neuronal death whereas suppression of its expression by shRNA protects against low-potassium-induced neuronal death [43]. Unlike HDAC1 and 2, which are predominantly nuclear proteins, HDAC3 contains a nuclear export signal and is present in both the nucleus and the cytoplasm in mammalian cells [33,44]. Investigations into the functions of the class I HDACs have been confined to their roles in the nucleus: HDACs 1 and 2 are part of the CoREST/mSin3a/NuRD repressor complex whereas HDAC3 interacts with NCoR/SMRT to repress gene expression [44], and in cortical neurons, HDAC3 is likely to be important for SMRT nuclear retention [45]. We were surprised to find that the cytoplasmic levels of HDAC3 in the brains of $Hdac3^{+/-}$ heterozygous mice were equivalent to that in WT brains, whereas nuclear levels were reduced to approximately 60% of WT. The fact that cytoplasmic HDAC3 levels are maintained in the $Hdac3^{+/-}$ heterozygous state suggests that cytoplasmic HDAC3 may be tightly bound in a protein complex that sequesters HDAC3 and prevents it from migrating to the nucleus.

Our inability to detect any beneficial consequences of reducing nuclear HDAC3 levels in R6/2 mice was disappointing. The fact that $Hdac3^{-/-}$ nullizygous mice die early in embryogenesis indicates that another protein cannot compensate for HDAC3 function. We might expect that reduction of nuclear HDAC3 to approximately 60% of WT levels could be similar to the level of inhibition achieved by pharmacological approaches. Therefore, the $Hdac3^{+/-}$ heterozygous mice present a suitable model with which to further investigate the therapeutic potential of reducing HDAC3 nuclear function. Our negative results would appear to contradict the report that the administration of HDACi **4b** to R6/2 mice improves transcriptional dysregulation as well as behavioural phenotypes [26]. However these previously reported beneficial effects are surprising in the light of the physical stability and metabolic issues concerning HDACi **4b** that have recently been highlighted (Beconi et al. unpublished data). Taken together, the current data raise doubts as to the validation of HDAC3 inhibition as a therapeutic target for HD.

Materials and Methods

Generation of an *Hdac3* null allele

The *Hdac3*-targeting vector was generated by PCR and standard cloning. The 5′ homology arm (4.7 kb), the 3′ homology arm (4.9 kb) and the knock-out region (4.5 kb) were generated by PCR using high fidelity Prime Star HS DNA polymerase (Takara) and RP23-24H23 BAC clone as a template. Aside from the homologous arms, the final vector (HighQ1B-mHdac3) also contains loxP sequences flanking the knock-out region (4.5 kb), a neomycine resistance cassette (Neo, for positive selection of the ES cells), and a diphtheria toxin gene cassette (DTA, for negative selection of the ES cells). The targeting vector was linearized with NotI and electroporated into C57BL/6NTac ES cells (an ES cell line derived from C57BL/6 Taconic mice). The cells were selected with 200 ug/ml G418 and 192 neo resistant ES clones were screened for homologous recombination by Southern blot analysis. Targeted ES cells were electroporated with the Cre-recombinase and G418 sensitive clones were picked and analyzed by Southern blot. Clones carrying a deletion of Exon 11 to 14 were identified and microinjected into the blastocysts of C57BL/6 females to generate chimeric mice. Chimeras were bred to C57BL/6 females to achieve germ-line transmission and generate heterozygotes. The deletion was confirmed at the genomic level by PCR and sequencing.

Mouse maintenance and breeding

All animal work was approved by the King's College London Ethical Review Panel and experimental procedures were performed in accordance with the UK Home Office regulations.

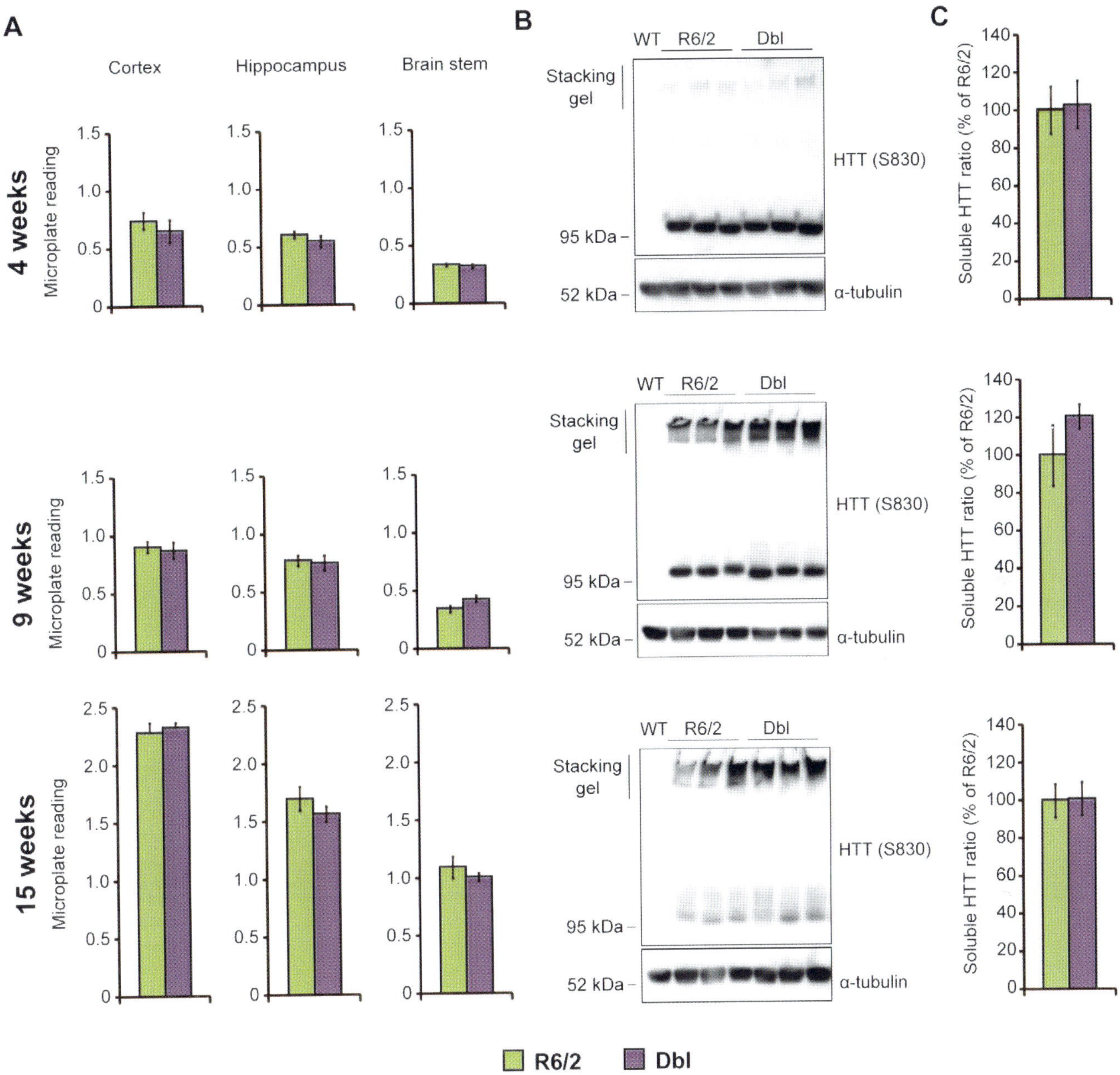

Figure 5. Hdac3 genetic reduction does not reduce HTT aggregation in R6/2 mouse brain. (A) The SEPRION ligand based ELISA assay was used to quantify HTT aggregation in the cortex, hippocampus and brain stem of 4, 9 and 15 week-old mice. The graphs represent the microtitre-plate reading of R6/2 (green) and Dbl (purple) lysates. Background readings obtained with WT and *Hdac3* lysates were comparable to water. Aggregation levels augment with age but are not modified by *Hdac3* reduction. Error bars correspond to S.E.M. (n>6). (B) Representative western blot of hippocampal lysates at 4, 9 and 15 weeks of age. The aggregated HTT fraction (stacking gel) augments with age whereas the soluble fraction decreases with age. α-tubulin was used as a loading control. (C) Quantification of (B). Soluble HTT is represented as a percentage of the soluble fraction in R6/2. Error bars correspond to S.E.M. (n = 6). The same color code (R6/2 = green; Dbl = purple) is used in (A) and (C).

Hemizygous R6/2 mice were bred and reared in our colony by backcrossing R6/2 males to (CBA×C57Bl/6) F1 (CBF) females (B6CBAF1/OlaHsd, Harlan Olac). *Hdac3*$^{+/-}$ heterozygotes originated in a C57Bl/6 background and were backcrossed once to CBF females before breeding to R6/2 males. All animals had unlimited access to water and breeding chow (Special Diet Services, Witham, UK). Housing conditions and environmental enrichment were used as previously described [46]. *Hdac3*$^{+/-}$ females were crossed to R6/2 males to generate WT, *Hdac3*$^{+/-}$, R6/2 and Dbl mice. All cages contained at least one mouse of each genotype and mice were additionally given mash that consist of powdered chow mixed with water from 4 to 15 weeks. Mice were subject to a 12 h light/12 h dark cycle.

Genotyping of R6/2 and *Hdac3*$^{+/-}$ mice and CAG repeat sizing

R6/2 mice were genotyped by PCR of tail-tip genomic DNA. PCR was performed using 1× Thermo-start master mix (Thermo scientific), 10% DMSO, 10 ng/ul forward primer 33727 (5′-CGCAGGCTAGGGCTGTCAATCATGCT-3′), 10 ng/ul reverse primer 32252 (5′-TCATCAGCTTTTCCAGGGTCGC-CAT-3′) and 100 ng genomic DNA. Amplification conditions were: 15 min at 94°C, 35× (30 s at 94°C; 30 s at 60°C; 60 s at 72°C), 10 min at 72°C. The amplicon for the R6/2 transgene is 272 bp. The CAG repeat size was determined as follow: amplification of the CAG repeat from R6/2 mouse DNA was performed with a FAM labelled forward primer (5′-GA-GTCCCTCAAGTCCTTCCAGCA-3′) and reverse primer (5′-GCCCAAACTCACGGTCGGT-3′) with 0.2 mM dNTPs; 10% DMSO; AM buffer (67 mM TrisHCL pH 8.8; 16.6 mM $(NH_4)SO_4$; 2 mM $MgCl_2$; 0.17 mg/ml BSA) and 0.5 U AmpliTaq DNA polymerase (Applied Biosystems). Amplification conditions were: 90 s at 94°C, 24× (30 s at 94°C; 30 s at 65°C; 90 s at 72°C), 10 min at 72°C. All instruments and materials were obtained from Applied Biosystems unless indicated. The FAM-tagged PCR product (1 ul) together with MegaBACETM ET900 (AmershamBioscience) internal size standard (0.04 ul) were denatured for 5 min at 94°C in 9 ul of HiDi-formamide and analysed using an ABI3730 sequencer. Data analysis was performed using platemanager application GeneMapper v5.2- 3730XL. *Hdac3*$^{+/-}$ mice were genotyped by duplex PCR in a 10 ul reaction containing 100 ug gDNA, 2 ul of 5× Promega buffer, 1.2 ul of 25 mM MgCl2, 1 ul of 10× PCR Enhancer (Invitrogen), 1 ul of 2 mM dNTP, 1 ul of 10 uM forward 1 (F1) primer (5′- GCTTAGCCTACTTGGCAAGTGCCAG-3′), 1 ul of 10 uM forward 2 (F2) primer (5′-GGCCAGAAGCACCCAAT-GAGTTCTA-3′), 1 ul of 10 uM reverse (R) primer (5′- ACAAT-CATCAGGCCGTGAGAGTTTG-3′), 0.2 ul of Promega Taq DNA polymerase and 4.4 ul H_2O. Amplification conditions were: 10 min at 94°C, 40× (30 s at 94°C; 30 s at 58°C; 60 s at 72°C) 10 min at 72°C. The WT allele product is 250 bp and the *Hdac3* knock-out allele is 500 bp.

Phenotypic analysis

The phenotypic analysis was performed on mice from 4 weeks to 15 weeks of age (WT males n = 9, females n = 7; *Hdac3*$^{+/-}$ males n = 7, females n = 7; R6/2 males n = 5, females n = 7; Dbl males n = 10, females n = 5). Mice were weaned 4 days before the beginning of the analysis. Mice were weighed weekly to the nearest 0.1 g. Motor coordination was assessed using an Ugo Basile 7650 accelerating RotaRod with an acceleration set to run from 4 to 40 RPM in 300 seconds (Linton Instrumentation, UK). At 4 weeks of age, mice were tested on four consecutive days, with three trials per day. At 8, 10, 12 and 14 weeks of age, mice were tested on three consecutive days with three trials per day. Forelimb grip strength was measured once a week at 4 and from 11 to 14 weeks using a San Diego Instruments Grip Strength Meter (San Diego, CA, USA) as described in [24]. Exploratory spontaneous motor activity was recorded and assessed fortnightly at 5, 7, 9, 11 and 13 weeks of age for 30 min during the day using infra-red activity monitoring cages (Linton Instruments, AM1053) as described in [47]. Briefly, activity (total number of beam breaks in the lower level), mobility (at least two consecutive beam breaks in the lower level) and rearing (number of rearing beam breaks) were measured. The data were collected and analyzed as described in [47]. At 15 weeks of age mice were sacrificed, brains were extracted and weighed to the nearest 0.01 g.

RNA extraction and gene expression analysis

Brain regions were dissected, snap-frozen in liquid nitrogen and stored at −80°C until required. Cortices, cerebella and striata were homogenized in Qiazol reagent and extracted using Qiagen RNeasy Mini kit (Qiagen). After quantification with a Nanodrop 1000 spectrophotometer (Labtech international), 1 ug of total RNA was reverse transcribed in 20 ul RT reaction using MMLV-RT kit (Invitrogen) and P21 random hexamers as described in Benn et al, 2008. RT reaction was diluted 10 times in nuclease-free Sigma water and 5 ul was used in 25 ul reaction containing Precision MasterMix (PrimerDesign), 300 nM gene-specific primers and 200 nM fluorescent reporting probe (FAM labelled and TAMRA quenched) specific to each target gene of interest using the Opticon2 Real Time PCR detection system (MJ research). Housekeeping genes previously identified [48] were used as ready-mixed PerfectProbe sets containing primers and probe (PrimerDesign). The geometric mean of three housekeeping genes for each brain region (*Atp5b*, *Canx*, and *Ubc* for cortex; *Atp5b*, *Eif4a2*, and *Ubc* for cerebellum, *Atp5b*, *Ubc* and *Ywhaz* for striatum) was used as a reference in order to determine relative expression ratio of the genes of interest using $2^{-\Delta\Delta Ct}$ method. For *Hdac3* expression analysis, primers and probe were designed using Primer3 software at the junction between exon 14 and 15 so only the WT allele can be detected (forward primer 5′- CGACGCTGAAGAGAGA-GGTC -3′, reverse primer 5′- TTTCCTTGTCGTTGTC-ATGG-3′; probe 5′- CCGAGGAGAACTACAGCAGG-3′). The amplicon was sequence-verified. For the other target genes, primers and probes were used as in previous studies [28,48,49] and their sequences are available in Table S2.

Isolation of nuclear and cytoplasmic fractions from mouse brains

Brains were extracted from mice, snap-frozen in −50°C isopenthane and stored at −80°C until required. All procedures were performed on ice. Each brain was homogenized in 2 ml ice-cold buffer 1 (575 mM sucrose; 25 mM KCl; 50 mM Triethanolamine; 5 mM MgCl2; 5 mM DTT; 0.5 mM PMSF; 1 tablet complete protease inhibitor cocktail from Roche) with 5–10 strokes in a 5 ml ice-cold homogenizer. The homogenate was then centrifuged at 800 g for 15 min at 4°C. The supernatant corresponds to the cytoplasmic fraction. The pellet was then homogenized in 3 ml buffer 1 and 2 volumes (6 ml) of Buffer 2 (2.3 M sucrose; 24.8 mM KCl; 50 mM Triethanolamine; 5 mM MgCl2; 1 mM DTT; 0.5 mM PMSF; 1 tablet complete protease inhibitor cocktail from Roche) were added and mixed to the homogenate. The mix was then centrifuged at 124000 g for 1 hour at 4°C (SW40 rotor in Beckman ultracentrifuge). The pellet (nuclear fraction) was washed twice in Buffer 1 and finally resuspended in 100 ul of Buffer 1.

Seprion ligand ELISA assay

Brain regions were dissected, snap-frozen in liquid nitrogen and stored at −80°C until required. A 2.5% lysate was prepared by ribolysing tissues for 3×30 sec in Lysing matrix tubes (Lysing matrix D; MP Biomedicals) in ice-cold RIPA buffer (50 mM Tris-HCl pH 8.0; 120 mM NaCl; 1% Igepal; 3.125% sodium deoxycholate; 0.01% SDS; 1 mM β-mercaptoethanol; 1 uM PMSF; 1 mM DTT; 1 tablet complete protease inhibitor cocktail from Roche). Lysates were then stored at −80°C and used within 12 h. Fifteen microliters of homogenate was mixed to 3 ul 10% SDS, 62 ul H_2O and 20 ul 5× capture buffer (Microsens Biotechnologies). A total of 100 ul was transferred to the well of a Seprion ligand-coated ELISA plate, and incubated with shaking for 1 h at room temperature (RT). The well was then washed 5× in PBS-T (PBS; 0.1% Tween) and incubated shaking for 1 h at RT with 100 ul MW8 primary antibody (mouse monoclonal antibody [39]) diluted 1:3000 in conjugate buffer (150 mM NaCl; 4% BSA; 1% non-fat dried milk; 0.1% Tween 20 in PBS). After 5 washes with PBS-T, the well was incubated shaking for 45 min at RT with 100 ul horse radish peroxidase (HRP)-conjugated anti-mouse secondary antibody (DAKO) diluted 1:2000 in conjugate buffer. The well was then washed 5× in PBS-T and

100 ul of RT TMB substrate (SerTec) was added and incubated in the dark at RT for 5 min. Reactions were terminated by adding 100 ul 0.5 M HCl and the absorption at 450 nm was measured using a plate reader (Biorad).

Western blotting and antibodies

The protein concentration of the whole brain cytoplasmic fraction and RIPA extracted brain regions (ELISA) were determined using the BCA assay kit (Thermo scientific). Twenty micrograms of proteins were denatured in one volume of 2× sample buffer (125 mM Tris-HCl pH 6.8, 4% SDS, 20% Glycerol, 10% β-mercaptoethanol, 0.004% bromophenol blue) for 10 min at 95°C. Four microliters of the total 100 ul nuclear fraction was also denatured in one volume of 2× sample buffer for 10 min at 95°C. Lysates were then fractionated on 12% (nuclear and cytoplasmic fraction) or 10% (RIPA-extracted protein lysates) SDS-PAGE gels and electro-transferred into nitrocellulose membranes (Whatman) by submerged transfer apparatus (Bio-Rad) in (25 mM Tris, 192 mM glycine, 20% v/v methanol). Membranes were blocked for 1 h at RT in 5% non-fat dried milk in PBS-T (PBS; 0.2% Tween). Membranes containing nuclear and cytoplasmic fractions were then incubated with gentle agitation over night at 4°C with an HDAC3 antibody (rabbit polyclonal Abcam, 1/1000) or 20 min RT with a mouse monoclonal α-tubulin antibody (1/30000, Sigma) or rabbit polyclonal histone H4 antibody (1/5000, Millipore) in PBS-T, 5% non-fat dried milk. Membranes containing RIPA-extracted protein lysates were incubated 1 h RT with the sheep polyclonal S830 huntingtin antibody [40] diluted 1:2000 in PBS-T, 5% non-fat dried milk or α-tubulin antibody (20 min). For chemiluminescent detection, membranes were washed 3× in PBS-T probed with HRP-linked secondary antibodies (HRP conjugated anti-rabbit mouse or sheep antibody (1:10000, Dako) in PBS-T, 5% non-fat dried milk for 45 min at RT and washed 3× in PBS-T. Protein was detected by chemiluminescense (ECL reagent GE healthcare) according to the manufacturer's instructions. The signals were quantified using a GS-800 calibrated densitometer (Bio-Rad).

Statistical analysis

Statistical analysis was performed by Student's *t*-test (Excel or SPSS), one-way ANOVA, two-way ANOVA and repeated measures GLM ANOVA, with the Greenhouse Geisser correction for non-sphericity using SPSS.

Supporting Information

Figure S1 *Hdac3* genetic reduction does not affect the expression of the other *Hdacs*. Expression of *Hdac1-11* transcripts are represented as a percent of WT expression levels in the cortex (A), the cerebellum (B) and the striatum (C) of 6 week old WT and *Hdac3*$^{+/-}$ mice. The level of *Hdac3* is the only significant difference between WT and *Hdac3*$^{+/-}$ brain regions. Error bars correspond to S.E.M. (n = 6) ***p<0.001. The same color code (blue = WT; red = Hdac3) was used for all the graphs.

Figure S2 HDAC3 protein expression in *Hdac3+/−* heterozygous mouse brain. (A) Representative western blot showing the expression of the HDAC3 protein in 4 week old mouse whole brains extracted with RIPA buffer. α-tubulin was used as a loading control (B) Quantification of (A). A slight significant decrease (≈20%) was induced by *Hdac3* genetic reduction. Error bars correspond to S.E.M. (n = 3) *p<0.05. Blue = WT; red = Hdac3.

Figure S3 *Hdac3* genetic reduction does not modify R6/2 exploratory activity. Average activity (left) rearing (middle) and mobility (right) for each genotype is shown at 5, 7, 9, 11 and 13 weeks of age. The same color code (blue = WT; red = *Hdac3*$^{+/-}$; green = R6/2 and purple = Dbl) was used for all the graphs. R6/2 mice show an overall hypoactivity and decreased mobility relative to WT mice from 7 weeks onwards and rearing is significantly decreased in R6/2 mice from 9 weeks of age. *Hdac3*$^{+/-}$ mice were indistinguishable from WT mice for all of the parameters. Genetic reduction of *Hdac3* failed to induce any improvement for these parameters in R6/2 mice.

Table S1 *Hdac3* genetic reduction does not modify R6/2 exploratory activity. The numbers displayed in Table S1 indicate the *p*-values for each of the parameters analysed (R6/2 genotype, *Hdac3* genotype, time in the activity cages) at 5, 7, 9, 11 and 13 weeks of age. Significant *p*-values are highlighted in yellow for *p*<0.05, orange for *p*<0.01 and pink for *p*<0.001. Mice in activity cages are shown to behave differently with respect to measures of exploratory behaviour (as determined by measuring activity, mobility and rearing) over a period of 30 min (Time). R6/2 mice exhibit an overall hypoactivity and a reduced mobility from 7 weeks and rearing is significantly reduced from 9 weeks (R6/2 genotype) and (Time*R6/2 genotype). *Hdac3* genetic reduction does not influence the behaviour of mice for any parameter assessed (*Hdac3* genotype) and (Time**Hdac3* genotype) and furthermore, there appears to be no interaction between *Hdac3* and R6/2 genotypes (R6/2**Hdac3*) and (R6/2**Hdac3**time).

Table S2 Sequences of primers and Taqman probes used in real-time PCR assays. *Bdnf I, IV V*, brain derived neurotrophic factor promoter I, IV, V; *Bdnf B*, brain derived neurotrophic factor coding exon B; *Cnr1*, cannabinoid receptor 1; *Darpp32*, dopamine and cAMP regulated neuronal phosphoprotein; *Drd2*, dopamine D2 receptor; *Hdac1-11*, histone deacetylase 1–11; *Htt*, huntingtin gene; *Igfbp5*, insulin-like growth factor binding protein 5; *Kcnk2*, potassium channel subfamily K, member 2; *Nr4a2*, nuclear receptor subfamily 4, group A, member 2; *Pcp4*, Purkinje cell protein 4; *Penk1*, proenkephalin; *Uchl1*, ubiquitin C-terminal hydrolase L1.

Acknowledgments

We thank Donna Groom and members of the Neurogenetics Laboratory for the provision of R6/2 males for breeding.

Author Contributions

Conceived and designed the experiments: LM KC DH YO GB. Performed the experiments: LM KC YO. Analyzed the data: LM KC YO GB. Contributed reagents/materials/analysis tools: DH. Wrote the paper: LM GB.

References

1. Bates G, Harper PS, Jones L (2002) Huntington's disease. Oxford: Oxford University Press.
2. The Huntington's Disease Collaborative Research Group (1993) A novel gene containing a trinucleotide repeat that is expanded and unstable on Huntington's

disease chromosomes. The Huntington's Disease Collaborative Research Group. Cell 72: 971–983.

3. DiFiglia M, Sapp E, Chase KO, Davies SW, Bates GP, et al. (1997) Aggregation of huntingtin in neuronal intranuclear inclusions and dystrophic neurites in brain. Science 277: 1990–1993.
4. Crook ZR, Housman D. Huntington's disease: can mice lead the way to treatment? Neuron 69: 423–435.
5. Mangiarini L, Sathasivam K, Seller M, Cozens B, Harper A, et al. (1996) Exon 1 of the HD gene with an expanded CAG repeat is sufficient to cause a progressive neurological phenotype in transgenic mice. Cell 87: 493–506.
6. Davies SW, Turmaine M, Cozens BA, DiFiglia M, Sharp AH, et al. (1997) Formation of neuronal intranuclear inclusions underlies the neurological dysfunction in mice transgenic for the HD mutation. Cell 90: 537–548.
7. Lin CH, Tallaksen-Greene S, Chien WM, Cearley JA, Jackson WS, et al. (2001) Neurological abnormalities in a knock-in mouse model of Huntington's disease. Hum Mol Genet 10: 137–144.
8. Woodman B, Butler R, Landles C, Lupton MK, Tse J, et al. (2007) The Hdh(Q150/Q150) knock-in mouse model of HD and the R6/2 exon 1 model develop comparable and widespread molecular phenotypes. Brain Res Bull 72: 83–97.
9. Carter RJ, Lione LA, Humby T, Mangiarini L, Mahal A, et al. (1999) Characterization of progressive motor deficits in mice transgenic for the human Huntington's disease mutation. J Neurosci 19: 3248–3257.
10. Lione LA, Carter RJ, Hunt MJ, Bates GP, Morton AJ, et al. (1999) Selective discrimination learning impairments in mice expressing the human Huntington's disease mutation. J Neurosci 19: 10428–10437.
11. Stack EC, Kubilus JK, Smith K, Cormier K, Del Signore SJ, et al. (2005) Chronology of behavioral symptoms and neuropathological sequela in R6/2 Huntington's disease transgenic mice. J Comp Neurol 490: 354–370.
12. Kuhn A, Goldstein DR, Hodges A, Strand AD, Sengstag T, et al. (2007) Mutant huntingtin's effects on striatal gene expression in mice recapitulate changes observed in human Huntington's disease brain and do not differ with mutant huntingtin length or wild-type huntingtin dosage. Hum Mol Genet 16: 1845–1861.
13. Moffitt H, McPhail GD, Woodman B, Hobbs C, Bates GP (2009) Formation of polyglutamine inclusions in a wide range of non-CNS tissues in the HdhQ150 knock-in mouse model of Huntington's disease. PLoS One 4: e8025.
14. Sathasivam K, Lane A, Legleiter J, Warley A, Woodman B, et al. (2010) Identical oligomeric and fibrillar structures captured from the brains of R6/2 and knock-in mouse models of Huntington's disease. Hum Mol Genet 19: 65–78.
15. Landles C, Sathasivam K, Weiss A, Woodman B, Moffitt H, et al. Proteolysis of mutant huntingtin produces an exon 1 fragment that accumulates as an aggregated protein in neuronal nuclei in Huntington disease. J Biol Chem 285: 8808–8823.
16. Cha JH (2007) Transcriptional signatures in Huntington's disease. Prog Neurobiol 83: 228–248.
17. Sadri-Vakili G, Bouzou B, Benn CL, Kim MO, Chawla P, et al. (2007) Histones associated with downregulated genes are hypo-acetylated in Huntington's disease models. Hum Mol Genet 16: 1293–1306.
18. Kuo MH, Allis CD (1998) Roles of histone acetyltransferases and deacetylases in gene regulation. Bioessays 20: 615–626.
19. Codd R, Braich N, Liu J, Soe CZ, Pakchung AA (2009) Zn(II)-dependent histone deacetylase inhibitors: suberoylanilide hydroxamic acid and trichostatin A. Int J Biochem Cell Biol 41: 736–739.
20. Avalos JL, Bever KM, Wolberger C (2005) Mechanism of sirtuin inhibition by nicotinamide: altering the NAD(+) cosubstrate specificity of a Sir2 enzyme. Mol Cell 17: 855–868.
21. Bates EA, Victor M, Jones AK, Shi Y, Hart AC (2006) Differential contributions of Caenorhabditis elegans histone deacetylases to Huntingtin polyglutamine toxicity. J Neurosci 26: 2830–2838.
22. Ferrante RJ, Kubilus JK, Lee J, Ryu H, Beesen A, et al. (2003) Histone deacetylase inhibition by sodium butyrate chemotherapy ameliorates the neurodegenerative phenotype in Huntington's disease mice. J Neurosci 23: 9418–9427.
23. Gardian G, Browne SE, Choi DK, Klivenyi P, Gregorio J, et al. (2005) Neuroprotective effects of phenylbutyrate in the N171-82Q transgenic mouse model of Huntington's disease. J Biol Chem 280: 556–563.
24. Hockly E, Richon VM, Woodman B, Smith DL, Zhou X, et al. (2003) Suberoylanilide hydroxamic acid, a histone deacetylase inhibitor, ameliorates motor deficits in a mouse model of Huntington's disease. Proc Natl Acad Sci U S A 100: 2041–2046.
25. Steffan JS, Bodai L, Pallos J, Poelman M, McCampbell A, et al. (2001) Histone deacetylase inhibitors arrest polyglutamine-dependent neurodegeneration in Drosophila. Nature 413: 739–743.
26. Thomas EA, Coppola G, Desplats PA, Tang B, Soragni E, et al. (2008) The HDAC inhibitor 4b ameliorates the disease phenotype and transcriptional abnormalities in Huntington's disease transgenic mice. Proc Natl Acad Sci U S A.
27. Bobrowska A, Paganetti P, Matthias P, Bates GP (2011) Hdac6 knock-out increases tubulin acetylation but does not modify disease progression in the R6/2 mouse model of Huntington's disease. PLoS One 6: e20696.
28. Benn CL, Butler R, Mariner L, Nixon J, Moffitt H, et al. (2009) Genetic knock-down of HDAC7 does not ameliorate disease pathogenesis in the R6/2 mouse model of Huntington's disease. PLoS One 4: e5747.
29. Broide RS, Redwine JM, Aftahi N, Young W, Bloom FE, et al. (2007) Distribution of histone deacetylases 1–11 in the rat brain. J Mol Neurosci 31: 47–58.
30. Salisbury CM, Cravatt BF (2007) Activity-based probes for proteomic profiling of histone deacetylase complexes. Proc Natl Acad Sci U S A 104: 1171–1176.
31. Pallos J, Bodai L, Lukacsovich T, Purcell JM, Steffan JS, et al. (2008) Inhibition of specific HDACs and sirtuins suppresses pathogenesis in a Drosophila model of Huntington's disease. Hum Mol Genet 17: 3767–3775.
32. Fischle W, Dequiedt F, Hendzel MJ, Guenther MG, Lazar MA, et al. (2002) Enzymatic activity associated with class II HDACs is dependent on a multiprotein complex containing HDAC3 and SMRT/N-CoR. Mol Cell 9: 45–57.
33. Yang WM, Tsai SC, Wen YD, Fejer G, Seto E (2002) Functional domains of histone deacetylase-3. J Biol Chem 277: 9447–9454.
34. Guenther MG, Barak O, Lazar MA (2001) The SMRT and N-CoR corepressors are activating cofactors for histone deacetylase 3. Mol Cell Biol 21: 6091–6101.
35. Bhaskara S, Knutson SK, Jiang G, Chandrasekharan MB, Wilson AJ, et al. Hdac3 is essential for the maintenance of chromatin structure and genome stability. Cancer Cell 18: 436–447.
36. Montgomery RL, Potthoff MJ, Haberland M, Qi X, Matsuzaki S, et al. (2008) Maintenance of cardiac energy metabolism by histone deacetylase 3 in mice. J Clin Invest 118: 3588–3597.
37. Schuettengruber B, Simboeck E, Khier H, Seiser C (2003) Autoregulation of mouse histone deacetylase 1 expression. Mol Cell Biol 23: 6993–7004.
38. Ryu H, Lee J, Olofsson BA, Mwidau A, Dedeoglu A, et al. (2003) Histone deacetylase inhibitors prevent oxidative neuronal death independent of expanded polyglutamine repeats via an Sp1-dependent pathway. Proc Natl Acad Sci U S A 100: 4281–4286.
39. Ko J, Ou S, Patterson PH (2001) New anti-huntingtin monoclonal antibodies: implications for huntingtin conformation and its binding proteins. Brain Res Bull 56: 319–329.
40. Sathasivam K, Woodman B, Mahal A, Bertaux F, Wanker EE, et al. (2001) Centrosome disorganization in fibroblast cultures derived from R6/2 Huntington's disease (HD) transgenic mice and HD patients. Hum Mol Genet 10: 2425–2435.
41. Xu C, Soragni E, Chou CJ, Herman D, Plasterer HL, et al. (2009) Chemical probes identify a role for histone deacetylase 3 in Friedreich's ataxia gene silencing. Chem Biol 16: 980–989.
42. McQuown SC, Barrett RM, Matheos DP, Post RJ, Rogge GA, et al. HDAC3 is a critical negative regulator of long-term memory formation. J Neurosci 31: 764–774.
43. Bardai FH, D'Mello SR. Selective toxicity by HDAC3 in neurons: regulation by Akt and GSK3beta. J Neurosci 31: 1746–1751.
44. Yang XJ, Seto E (2008) The Rpd3/Hda1 family of lysine deacetylases: from bacteria and yeast to mice and men. Nat Rev Mol Cell Biol 9: 206–218.
45. Soriano FX, Hardingham GE (2011) In cortical neurons HDAC3 activity suppresses RD4-dependent SMRT export. PLoS One 6: e21056.
46. Hockly E, Woodman B, Mahal A, Lewis CM, Bates G (2003) Standardization and statistical approaches to therapeutic trials in the R6/2 mouse. Brain Res Bull 61: 469–479.
47. Hockly E, Tse J, Barker AL, Moolman DL, Beunard JL, et al. (2006) Evaluation of the benzothiazole aggregation inhibitors riluzole and PGL-135 as therapeutics for Huntington's disease. Neurobiol Dis 21: 228–236.
48. Benn CL, Fox H, Bates GP (2008) Optimisation of region-specific reference gene selection and relative gene expression analysis methods for pre-clinical trials of Huntington's disease. Mol Neurodegener 3: 17.
49. Mielcarek M, Benn CL, Franklin SA, Smith DL, Woodman B, et al. (2011) SAHA decreases HDAC 2 and 4 levels in vivo and improves molecular phenotypes in the R6/2 mouse model of Huntington's disease. PLoS One in press.

Mechanisms of Hearing Loss in Neurofibromatosis Type 2

Ashok R. Asthagiri[1]*, Raul A. Vasquez[1,2], John A. Butman[3], Tianxia Wu[4], Keaton Morgan[1], Carmen C. Brewer[5], Kelly King[5], Chris Zalewski[5], H. Jeffrey Kim[6], Russell R. Lonser[1]

1 Surgical Neurology Branch, National Institute of Neurological Disorders and Stroke, National Institutes of Health, Bethesda, Maryland, United States of America, **2** Department of Neurological Surgery, University of Florida, Gainesville, Gainesville, Florida, United States of America, **3** Radiology and Imaging Sciences, The Clinical Center at the National Institutes of Health, National Institutes of Health, Bethesda, Maryland, United States of America, **4** Clinical Neurosciences Program, National Institute of Neurological Disorders and Stroke, National Institutes of Health, Bethesda, Maryland, United States of America, **5** Audiology Unit, Otolaryngology Branch, National Institute on Deafness and Other Communication Disorders, National Institutes of Health, Bethesda, Maryland, United States of America, **6** Office of the Clinical Director, National Institute on Deafness and Other Communication Disorders, National Institutes of Health, Bethesda, Maryland, United States of America

Abstract

Introduction: Patients with neurofibromatosis type 2 (NF2) develop bilateral cochleovestibular schwannomas (CVSs) that cause binaural deafness in most individuals. Hearing loss occurs in an unpredictable manner and the underlying mechanisms are not known. To gain insight into the pathophysiologic basis for hearing loss in NF2, we performed a prospective cross-sectional study of untreated ears in NF2 patients.

Methods: One hundred consecutive NF2 patients in a prospective natural history study were included. Clinical and audiometric data were analyzed for treatment naïve ears. In addition to standard MR-imaging sequences, alterations in intralabyrinthine protein content were determined utilizing high resolution FLAIR, the presence of cochlear aperture obstruction was determined by examining 3D T2 sequences, and endolymphatic hydrops was identified on delayed post-contrast FLAIR sequences.

Results: Eighty-nine ears harboring 84 untreated CVSs in 56 consecutive NF2 patients (age 30±16 years) were analyzed. Thirty-four (38%) ears had varying degrees of hearing loss. Elevated intralabyrinthine protein was identified in 70 (75%) ears by FLAIR MR-imaging and was strongly associated with the presence of hearing loss (32/34 hearing loss ears; 94%)(Fisher's exact test; P = .005). Elevated intralabyrinthine protein was associated with the presence of CVS-associated cochlear aperture obstruction (64 of 67 ears with elevated protein; 96%)(Fisher's exact test; P<0.0001) in both normal and hearing loss ears. Elevated intralabyrinthine protein was not identified in ears without CVS (5 ears). While larger tumor size was associated with hearing loss (P = 0.006), 16 hearing loss ears (47%) harbored CVSs less than 0.5 cm^3, including 14 ears (88%) with block of the cochlear aperture and elevated protein.

Discussion: These findings are consistent with a model in which hearing loss develops as a result of cochlear aperture obstruction and accumulation of intralabyrinthine protein. MRI based identification of elevated intralabyrinthine protein may help identify the ear at-risk for developing hearing loss.

Editor: Mike Chen, City of Hope, United States of America

Funding: This research was supported by the Intramural Research Program of the National Institute of Neurologic Disorders and Stroke, National Institute on Deafness and Other Communication Disorders and the Clinical Center at the National Institutes of Health. The funders had no role in study design, data collection and analysis, decision to publish, or preparation of the manuscript.

Competing Interests: The authors have declared that no competing interests exist.

* E-mail: asthagiria@ninds.nih.gov

Introduction

Neurofibromatosis type 2 (NF2) is an autosomal dominant heritable neoplasia syndrome. It results from a germline mutation of the *NF2* tumor suppressor gene located on the long arm of chromosome 22 [1]. NF2 has an incidence of 1 in 25,000 persons and a penetrance of nearly 100% by age 60 years [2,3]. While the clinical manifestations of NF2 include central and peripheral nervous system tumors (nerve sheath tumors, meningiomas and ependymomas), cutaneous lesions, ocular pathology and peripheral neuropathy [4], the hallmark of NF2 is the development of bilateral cochleovestibular schwannomas (CVSs) [5]. Bilateral CVSs are present in 90 to 95% of NF2 patients [5]. Although CVSs are benign tumors, they cause significant audiovestibular morbidity, including deafness. While binaural hearing loss occurs in nearly all NF2 patients, its course remains unpredictable and therefore management paradigms have remained inconsistent.

Despite the significant audiologic morbidity identified in patients with NF2, the mechanisms by which the CVS causes hearing loss are not understood. The most frequently cited hypothesis is the enlarging CVS causes hearing loss through direct compression and stretching of the cochlear nerve. Several phenomena, including the unpredictable onset of hearing loss, frequent association of hearing loss with small tumors and progressive hearing loss in patients with non-growing CVS specifically suggest that such a simple association between tumor size and/or growth rate with hearing loss does not exist [6,7,8,9]. Further, in addition to gradual hearing loss, progression of hearing loss may be stepwise, relapsing and remitting, or sudden. These variable patterns of hearing loss suggest that additional mechanisms of hearing loss such as intralabyrinthine hemorrhage, development of endolymphatic hydrops, disruption of cochlear vascular supply and alteration in the biochemical milieu of inner ear fluids that result in cochlear hair cell degeneration and dysfunction may play a more critical role in the pathophysiology of hearing loss in patients with NF2. Because of the incomplete understanding of the pathophysiologic mechanisms underlying onset and variable progression of hearing loss in NF2 (even between ears in the same patient), the optimal management of CVSs in NF2 has not been determined. To identify markers for hearing loss and underlying pathophysiological mechanisms, we prospectively analyzed the clinical, imaging, and audiologic findings in a large cohort of NF2 patients.

Methods

Patients

Patients enrolled in a National Institute of Neurological Disorders and Stroke (NINDS) institutional review board (IRB)-approved prospective NF2 natural history study (NIH#08-N-0044) were included. Informed written consent was obtained from all adult participants. Informed written consent from the next of kin, carers or guardians on behalf of minors participating in this study was obtained. Both written consent and assent forms were approved for the consenting procedure by the NINDS IRB. Treatment naïve ears with no evidence of conductive hearing loss were used for analysis. Patients had NF2 diagnosed by clinical and/or genetic criteria [10].

Patient Evaluation

Clinical and audiologic evaluation. Detailed histories were obtained and comprehensive otologic and neurologic examinations were conducted in all patients to exclude the presence of middle ear disease. Concurrent audiometric evaluations were performed that included air- and bone- conduction thresholds from 250–8000 Hz and 250–4000 Hz, respectively. Hearing was stratified utilizing the four frequency pure-tone average (PTA) as normal [PTA≤20 dB], mild hearing loss [PTA 21–40 dB], moderate [PTA 41–70 dB], severe [PTA 71–95 dB], or profound [PTA>95 dB] [11]. _ Ears with a conductive hearing loss component (>10 dB difference between the air and bone PTA) were excluded from the study. For statistical analysis, hearing status was simplified to a binary score based on the presence (mild, moderate, severe, profound) or absence (normal) of hearing loss.

Imaging evaluation. Patients underwent magnetic resonance (MR)-imaging with and without contrast (T1 weighted) of the craniospinal axis. A neuroradiologist, blind to the hearing status of individual patients and ears, interpreted all imaging findings. Inner ear MR-imaging was performed with less than 1 mm in plane resolution utilizing a 3T-MR-scanner (Phillips; Andover, MA). Non-contrast enhanced fluid attenuated inversion recovery (FLAIR) sequences were performed to assess for the presence of elevated protein within the inner ear. Because saline-based solutions become hyperintense relative to brain parenchyma at defined protein concentration thresholds, identification of elevated intralabyrinthine protein by pre-contrast FLAIR MR-imaging is dependable and was reported as either being "elevated" or "normal" [12]. Co-registered T2-VISTA MR-images were performed to assess for the presence of cochlear aperture obstruction, as defined by the absence of a patent cerebrospinal fluid (CSF) pathway between the posterior fossa and the cochlear aperture (cochlear nerve entry point into the osseous spiral ligament). The presence or absence of intralabyrinthine hemorrhage was assessed on precontrast T1-weighted MR-images [13]. To assess for endolymphatic hydrops, delayed FLAIR and matching T2-weighted images were obtained in a plane parallel to that of the horizontal semicircular canal 6 to 18 hours after contrast injection MR-imaging [14,15]. On the delayed FLAIR, marked distension of the scala media (normally not visible) due to the differential elimination of contrast from the endolymphatic compartment relative to the retention of contrast material within the perilymph was noted as direct visualization of endolymphatic hydrops.

Volume of the CVS was determined utilizing post-contrast T1-weighted images [16] and the following formula: volume = maximum anteroposterior dimension X maximal mediolateral dimension X maximum craniocaudal dimension / 2) [17]. Volumetric measurements for CVSs were divided into posterior fossa and canalicular components if portions of the tumor [16] were present in both anatomic areas. The multilobulated posterior fossa component of tumors was further divided into individual compartments to improve accuracy of volumetric measurement (compartmental volume determined by equation defined above). Total CVS volume was determined by summing the volumes of the individual compartments. Identification of small discrete intralabyrinthine tumors by post-contrast images was confirmed by the presence of a negative outline on T2 VISTA sequences in co-registered images.

Statistical Analysis

Statistical analyses were performed as defined in text. A P-value less than or equal to 0.05 was considered significant.

Results

Patient Characteristics

Of 100 consecutive patients (200 ears) enrolled into the NF2 natural history study, ears that underwent surgery (84 ears in 58 patients) and/or received radiation therapy (26 ears in 20 patients) for management of cochleovestibular schwannomas were excluded from this study. Additionally, 5 patients (10 ears) receiving chemotherapeutics at the time of this study and 1 patient (2 ears) unable to complete audiometric examination (English second language) were also excluded from evaluation. Three ears with mild hearing loss were also excluded from analysis due to the presence of a conductive hearing loss component by otologic and audiologic evaluation. Therefore, 89 treatment naïve ears (43 right, 46 left) in 56 consecutive patients (17 male, 39 female) were included. In 23 patients (41%), one ear met criteria for inclusion and in 33 patients (59%) both ears met inclusion criteria. MR-imaging evidence of CVS was present in 84 of the 89 ears; 5 ears had no MR-imaging evidence of CVS. Mean patient age at evaluation was 30±16 years (range, 8 to 68 years). Forty-nine patients (88%) had audiovestibular symptoms associated with a CVS (Table 1). Mean age at onset of any disease related symptom was 21.7±14.5 years (range, 0.3 to 57 years).

Audiologic Findings

Fifty-five ears (62% of all evaluated ears) had normal hearing (PTA≤20 dB), including 5 (6%) ears without a CVS. Thirty-four ears (38%) had associated hearing loss (mild, 14 ears, 16%; moderate, 12 ears, 13%; severe, 4 ears, 4%; profound, 4 ears, 4%). Mean PTA was 54±29 dB (range, 22.5 to 118.75 dB) in the ears with associated hearing loss. Hearing loss occurred gradually over

Table 1. Audiovestibular and MR-imaging findings in the 56 study patients (89 ears).

Findings	**Number of patients/ears (%)***		
None	7 patients (12.5%)		
Hearing loss	34 ears (38.2%)		
Tinnitus	48 ears (53.9%)		
Vertigo	8 patients (14.2%)		
Aural fullness	9 ears (10.1%)		
MR-imaging characteristic	**Normal Hearing ears**	**Hearing Loss ears**	**Total (n = 89)**
Elevated protein	35	32	67 (75%)
Cochlear aperture block	36	31	67 (75%)
Intralabyrinthine tumor	5	8	13 (14.6%)
Discrete	*2*	*3*	*5 (5.6%)*
Direct invasion	*3*	*5*	*8 (9.0%)*
Endolymphatic hydrops	4	3	7 (7.9%)
Intralabyrinthine hemorrhage	0	0	0
Brainstem stroke	0	0	0

*Specific to the ear analyzed in the current study.

months to years (12 ears; 35% of ears with hearing loss), in a stepwise manner characterized by periodic decrements in hearing associated with intervening periods of stable hearing (10; 29%), in a relapsing-remitting pattern defined by periodic decrements in hearing coupled with partial recovery of hearing during intervening periods (4; 12%), or in a sudden and complete fashion (sudden profound sensorineural hearing loss) (5; 15%). Subjective hearing loss was not reported in 3 ears (9%) in 3 patients with audiometric evidence of mild hearing loss.

Imaging Correlates in Hearing Loss Ears

Imaging and audiologic findings. Radiographic and audiologic analysis in the 34 hearing loss ears revealed that 32 ears (94% of ears with hearing loss) had elevated intralabyrinthine protein on FLAIR MR-imaging (Figure 1). The 2 hearing loss ears without elevated intralabyrinthine protein had auditory brainstem responses that suggested central nervous system dysfunction or were associated with a large CVS (greater than 2.5 cm^3). Other imaging findings and audiovestibular symptoms in the 56 study patients (89 ears) are detailed in Table 1.

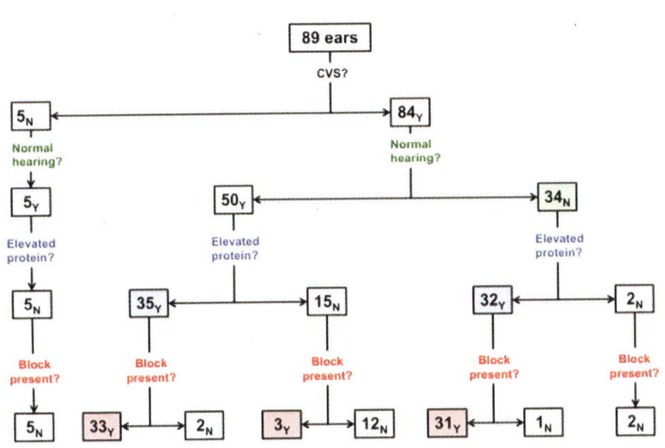

Figure 1. Features of normal hearing and hearing loss ears.

Mechanism of elevated intralabyrinthine protein. Cochlear aperture obstruction by a CVS was closely associated with identification of elevated intralabyrinthine protein in hearing loss ears (Fisher's exact test; $P = 0.005$). While 31 hearing loss ears (91%) with elevated protein in the labyrinth had cochlear aperture obstruction by a CVS, only 1 ear (3%) with elevated intralabyrinthine protein did not have evidence of cochlear aperture obstruction (Figure 1, 2). Ears with hearing loss without elevated intralabyrinthine protein (2 ears, 6%) did not demonstrate cochlear aperture obstruction.

Twenty-three ears (out of 31 hearing loss ears with elevated protein and cochlear aperture obstruction; 74%) had isolated cochlear aperture obstruction and 8 (26%) had cochlear aperture obstruction associated with either a discrete intralabyrinthine tumor (3 ears) (Figure 2) or direct invasion of the labyrinth by a CVS (5 ears). Three ears with elevated intralabyrinthine protein, cochlear aperture obstruction and discrete intralabyrinthine tumors (1 ear) or direct invasion of the labyrinth by a CVS (2 ears) also had endolymphatic hydrops based on MRI findings.

Imaging Correlates in Normal Hearing Ears

Imaging findings. Fifty normal hearing ears (91%) harbored a CVS and 5 ears (9%) did not have an associated CVS. Radiographic and audiologic analysis of the 50 normal hearing ears with a CVS demonstrated elevated intralabyrinthine protein in 35 ears (70% of all normal hearing ears with a CVS) and normal intralabyrinthine protein in 15 ears (30%) on FLAIR MR-imaging. The 5 normal hearing ears without CVS did not have evidence of elevated intralabyrinthine protein (Figure 1).

Mechanism of elevated intralabyrinthine protein. Similar to hearing loss ears, cochlear aperture obstruction by a CVS was associated with elevated intralabyrinthine protein in normal hearing ears (Fisher's exact test; $P<0.0001$). While 33 normal hearing ears (94% of normal hearing ears with elevated intralabyrinthine protein) with elevated intralabyrinthine protein had cochlear aperture obstruction by a CVS, only 2 ears (6%) with elevated intralabyrinthine protein did not have evidence of cochlear aperture obstruction.

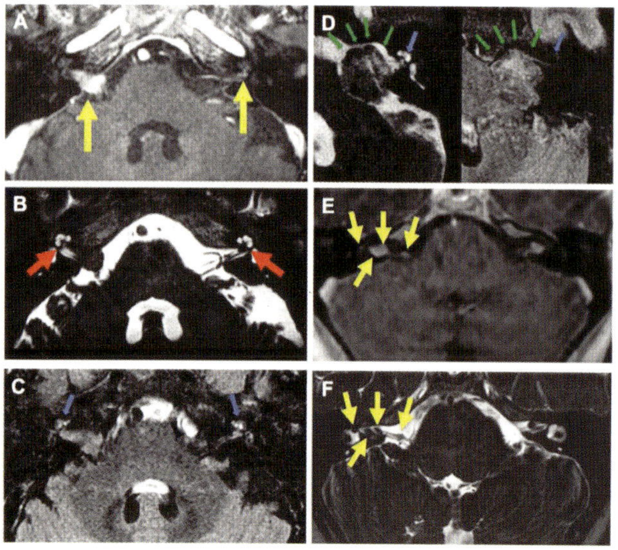

Figure 2. Magnetic resonance imaging in patients with neurofibromatosis type 2. Magnetic resonance (MR) imaging performed in a 47-year old patient with neurofibromatosis type 2 (NF2): (A) Axial, contrast enhanced, T1-weighted, magnetic resonance imaging demonstrates bilateral cochleovestibular schwannomas (CVS) (yellow arrows). (B) T2-VISTA sequence identifies the presence of a cerebrospinal fluid obstruction between the posterior fossa and the cochlear aperture (red arrows) bilaterally, independent of tumor size. (C) Pre-contrast fluid attenuated inversion recovery (FLAIR) sequence demonstrates the presence of elevated protein within the labyrinth (blue arrows). MR-imaging performed in a 48-year old patient with NF2: (D) Axial T2-VISTA and pre-contrast FLAIR sequences demonstrate the presence of normal labyrinthine protein (blue arrow) in the setting of a large CVS with an open CSF pathway (green arrows) between the posterior fossa and the cochlear aperture. MR-imaging performed in a 8-year old patient with NF2. (E) Axial, contrast enhanced, T1-weighted, magnetic resonance imaging demonstrates bilateral cochleovestibular schwannomas (CVS) with multiple tumors present on the right (yellow arrows). (F) T2-VISTA sequence identifies 4 discrete tumors, including a discrete intralabyrinthine tumor (yellow arrows).

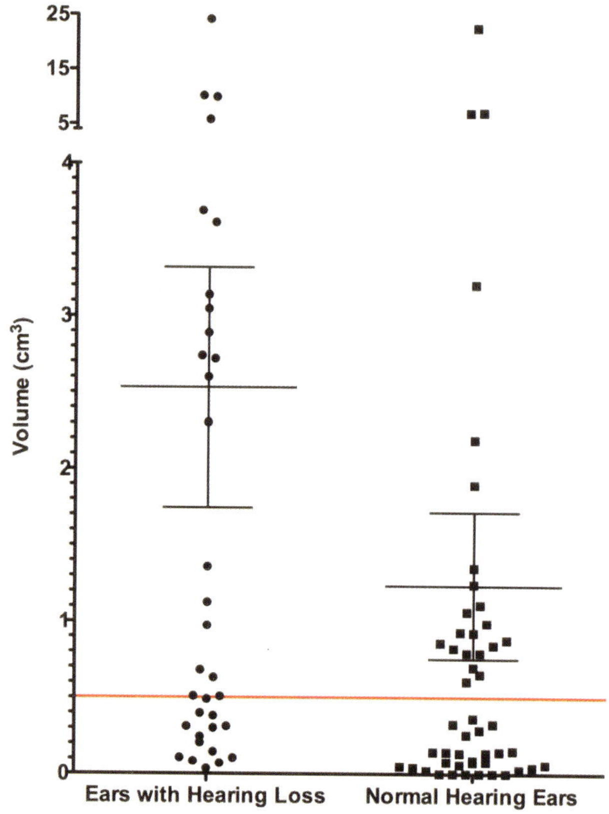

Figure 3. Graph demonstrating volume of tumors identified in ears with and without evidence of hearing loss.

Specific factors associated with elevated intralabyrinthine protein included isolated cochlear aperture obstruction by CVS (28 ears; 80%), cochlear aperture obstruction with direct labyrinthine invasion by CVS (3 ears; 9%), cochlear aperture obstruction with a discrete intralabyrinthine tumor (2 ears; 6%) or unknown mechanism (2 ears, 6%). Endolymphatic hydrops was also detected by MR-imaging in 3 normal hearing ears with elevated protein and block of the cochlear aperture.

Twelve normal hearing ears harboring a CVS (80% of all normal hearing ears without elevated labyrinthine protein) without elevated intralabyrinthine protein did not have block of the cochlear aperture, including 1 ear (8%) with associated hydrops. Three normal hearing ears (20%) had evidence of cochlear aperture block by CVS without elevated protein.

Tumor Volume and Hearing Loss

CVSs were identified in 84 ears (94%) and were purely intracanalicular in 38 ears (45%). Mean tumor volume (in 84 ears) was 1.8 ± 4.0 cm^3 (approximately 1.5 cm in maximum linear dimension). While the presence of hearing loss was correlated with larger CVS volume in hearing loss ears (mean volume in normal hearing ears, 1.2 ± 3.4 cm^3 versus hearing-loss ears, 2.5 ± 4.6 cm^3)(Mann-Whitney; $P = 0.007$), 16 (47%) hearing loss ears had a CVS that was less than approximately 0.5 cm^3 (Figure 3). Among 38 ears with a purely intracanalicular CVS, hearing loss was evident in 12 ears (32%) with a mean volume of 0.2 ± 0.2 cm^3 (range, 0.03 cm^3 to 0.7 cm^3).

Discussion

NF2-Associated Hearing Loss

Previous studies have demonstrated that CVS-associated binaural hearing loss will occur in an unpredictable manner over the lifetime of most NF2 patients [6,7,8]. Moreover, hearing loss patterns in one ear do not predict the clinical course of the contralateral ear in the same individual with NF2 [7]. Because of the uncertain clinical course associated with CVSs and because of the lack of understanding of the mechanisms that underlie hearing loss associated with CVSs in NF2, the management of these tumors has not been consistent or optimized. Here, we examined radiographic and audiometric findings associated with hearing loss in NF2 to better understand the pathophysiologic mechanisms underlying onset and progression of hearing loss in this hereditary neoplastic disorder.

Current Study

Elevated intralabyrinthine protein. The most common imaging findings identified in CVS-associated hearing loss in NF2 was the presence of elevated intralabyrinthine perilymphatic protein and the presence of cochlear aperture obstruction on MR-imaging. Elevated intralabyrinthine protein was found in 94% of hearing loss ears (32 of 34 ears) and in 70% of normal hearing ears (35 of 50 ears). Blockage of the cochlear aperture by an associated CVS was found in 96% of ears (64 of 67 ears) with elevated protein and only in 14% of ears (3 of 22 ears) without evidence of elevated intralabrynthine protein. These findings are consistent with the findings by Silverstein and colleagues [18] that demonstrated that a 2.5-fold increase in intralabyrinthine protein obtained from perilymph aspirates could accurately identify the presence of CVSs in patients in the era before MR-imaging was available for non-invasive diagnosis.

The importance that elevated intralabyrinthine protein plays in hearing loss is underscored by previous clinical-imaging studies of the inner ear in other conditions, including sporadic vestibular schwannomas and sudden sensorineural hearing loss (SNHL) [19,20]. Recent findings indicate that increased protein within the perilymph visualized on FLAIR MR-imaging can be correlated with hearing loss associated with sporadic acoustic schwannomas [20]. Elevated intralabyrinthine protein on FLAIR MR-imaging in patients with SNHL has also been correlated with hearing prognosis and extent of hearing loss that will persist [19].

Mechanisms of intralabyrinthine protein elevation. The findings of the current study indicate that cochlear aperture block underlies elevation of intralabyrinthine protein. The sensitivity and specificity of cochlear aperture obstruction in identifying elevated perilymphatic protein within the labyrinth was 96% and 87%, respectively. This indicates a pathophysiologic association between cochlear aperture obstruction and the presence of elevated intralabyrinthine protein may exist in NF2-associated CVSs. Based on the results from this study and previous studies examining elevated intralabyrinthine protein in other hearing loss syndromes, NF2-associated tumors may lead to elevated intralabyrinthine protein levels in several ways related to cochlear aperture obstruction that causes abnormal protein clearance and deposition.

Elevated intralabyrinthine protein could be the result of cochlear aperture obstruction and disruption of the blood-CSF/labyrinthine barrier caused by permeable tumor vessels [20]. CVSs cause increased protein content within the circulating cerebrospinal fluid compartment due to permeable tumor vessels, and this may be further concentrated in the lateral internal auditory canal in cases where CSF is trapped due to cochlear aperture obstruction [21,22]. Concentrated proteins can rapidly diffuse into the perilymphatic space across the porous canaliculi located within the modiolar region of the osseous spiral lamina [23]. Previous studies have shown gadolinium accumulation in the perilymphatic compartment within 10 minutes after intravenous administration in ears with CVS compared to contralateral unaffected ears, supporting the presence of a breach in the blood-CSF/labyrinthine barrier and rapid diffusion into the perilymphatic spaces in ears with CVSs [20].

Another mechanism by which protein can accumulate within the perilymph associated with cochlear aperture obstruction involves impaired clearance caused by the CVS. It has been shown that the cochlear nerve is integral in the rapid transport of proteins from the cochlea to the cochlear nucleus [24]. Although large CVSs may impact the cochlear nerve through compression within the internal auditory canal disrupting axonal transport, small tumors situated within the cochlear nerve itself may also lead to cochlear aperture obstruction and disruption of axonal transport. Therefore, when CVSs cause obstruction of the cochlear aperture, independent of size, it is likely that this results in impaired cochlear nerve axonal transport that can, in turn, underlie perilymphatic protein accumulation due to impaired clearance [25].

Elevated intralabyrinthine protein could also be the result of increased protein production or deposition. Analogous to cerebellopontine angle CVSs that are known to cause increased protein content within the circulating cerebrospinal fluid compartment [21], increased protein secretion of a plasma ultrafiltrate by permeable tumor vessels of tumors within the labyrinth (both distinct and due to CVS invasion) may permit direct extravasation of plasma proteins into the inner ear perilymph. This process could potentially underlie (in part) the protein elevation and endolymphatic hydrops seen with these tumors. Similarly, increased tumor vessel permeability with leakage of plasma ultrafiltrate and plasma proteins into the surrounding anatomic region has been described in hemangioblastomas and endolymphatic sac tumors in von Hippel-Lindau disease and may underlie peritumoral cyst formation and inner ear hydrops [26].

Mechanisms of hearing loss associated with elevated protein. Elevated intralabyrinthine protein on MR-imaging was closely associated with the presence of hearing loss. The importance of elevated intralabyrinthine protein underlying hearing loss is supported by previous studies examining unique perilymphatic proteins that are elevated in CVSs, including μ-Crystallin (CRYM) and low density lipoprotein-related protein 2 (LRP2) [27]. Mutations of these proteins are associated with genetic syndromes that present with deafness not related to tumors. Further, previous studies have utilized histopathological evaluation to indirectly support biochemical degradation of the cochlea is caused by increased protein [28,29,30,31]. Finally, multiple studies have revealed that hearing loss may progress in the absence of CVS growth [32,33], confirming that an unknown factor underlies hearing loss in these ears. Although causality cannot be directly determined by the intimate association between elevated intralabyrinthine protein and hearing loss observed in our cohort, the high sensitivity of elevated protein in identifying hearing loss ears (94%) and the high negative predictive value of normal protein content in identifying a normal hearing ear (91%) presented in this study coupled with previous studies delineating the functional and degenerative sequelae of unique perilymphatic proteins that are elevated in the setting of vestibular schwannoma indicate that the increased protein content evident by labyrinthine FLAIR MR-signal may not only be an imaging marker of hearing loss, but contribute to the pathophysiology of hearing loss and cochlear degeneration.

Tumor size and hearing loss. A simple association between tumor size and hearing loss does not explain several phenomena. For instance, hearing loss in NF2 has an unpredictable onset and variable progression, which may be gradual, stepwise, relapsing and remitting, or sudden and complete. While previous studies have attempted to link increasing tumor size with hearing loss in patients with NF2, this association has not been established because of the ubiquitous presence of small tumors within all series that are associated with hearing loss. Because hearing loss in NF2 may be caused by end organ degeneration [34] (cochlea) from accumulated protein, the functional consequences of tumor location as it relates to the cochlear aperture appears to play an important role in the pathogenesis of hearing loss. This may also explain why schwannomas of various sizes in other cranial and peripheral nerves are often not associated with neurologic deficit in patients with NF2.

Alternative mechanisms of hearing loss in NF2. Other pathophysiologic processes of the inner ear structures have been implicated with hearing loss, including the development of endolymphatic hydrops and intralabyrinthine hemorrhage [13]. Although endolymphatic hydrops was identified in 7 ears (7.6%) with CVS in this study, the MR-based identification of endolymphatic hydrops did not correlate with hearing status (Table 1). Furthermore, the infrequent identification of endolymphatic hydrops and intralabyrinthine hemorrhage (0 ears), suggests these processes are not a significant underlying mechanism of hearing loss in this patient population.

Bevacizumab induced hearing response. Bevacizumab, initially utilized in NF2 clinical trials for the treatment of growing vestibular schwannomas was associated with hearing improvement in a subset of patients (4/7 patients, 57%) [35]. While this improvement in hearing was initially thought to be due to a reduction in intraneural edema and tumor shrinkage, a subsequent larger scale follow-up study confirmed a lack of correlation between radiographic response (tumor shrinkage) and hearing response, suggesting that a stochastic mechanism underlies the rapid hearing improvement (usually within 3 months) that is observed in approximately 50% of patients [36]. Because vascular endothelial growth factor (VEGF) is a known mediator of vessel permeability, bevacizumab (a VEGF-neutralizing antibody) may be affecting hearing response through restoration of protein homeostasis within the inner ear by decreasing production of protein rich plasma ultrafiltrate from both CPA and intralabyrinthine tumors.

Identification of the at-risk ear. The appropriate stratification of benefit to risk ratio for hearing preservation attempts in NF2 requires delineation of at-risk ears for hearing loss. Because hearing loss is currently the most likely outcome in NF2 ears, it becomes imperative to avoid risk when hearing loss is unlikely to occur. Despite the variable presentation of hearing loss in NF2, most ears with normal perilymphatic protein signal had normal hearing (20/22 ears, 91%) and most ears with hearing loss had elevated perilymphatic protein (35/37 ears, 95%).

Based on the available body of evidence and the current findings that indicate elevated perilymphatic proteins may underlie the final common pathway leading to hearing loss, MR-identification of labyrinthine hyperintensity in normal hearing ears (35 of 50 ears in this study) may serve as a potent imaging biomarker of ears at-risk for developing hearing loss.

Author Contributions

Conceived and designed the experiments: ARA JAB RRL. Performed the experiments: ARA RAV JAB KM CCB KK CZ HJK. Analyzed the data: ARA RAV JAB TW CCB KK CZ HJK RRL. Contributed reagents/materials/analysis tools: ARA JAB TW CCB HJK RRL. Wrote the paper: ARA RAV RRL.

References

1. Trofatter JA, MacCollin MM, Rutter JL, Murrell JR, Duyao MP, et al. (1993) A novel moesin-, ezrin-, radixin-like gene is a candidate for the neurofibromatosis 2 tumor suppressor. Cell 75: 826.
2. Evans DG, Huson SM, Donnai D, Neary W, Blair V, et al. (1992) A genetic study of type 2 neurofibromatosis in the United Kingdom. I. Prevalence, mutation rate, fitness, and confirmation of maternal transmission effect on severity. J Med Genet 29: 841–846.
3. Evans DG, Moran A, King A, Saeed S, Gurusinghe N, et al. (2005) Incidence of vestibular schwannoma and neurofibromatosis 2 in the North West of England over a 10-year period: higher incidence than previously thought. Otol Neurotol 26: 93–97.
4. Asthagiri AR, Parry DM, Butman JA, Kim HJ, Tsilou ET, et al. (2009) Neurofibromatosis type 2. Lancet 373: 1974–1986.
5. Evans DG, Huson SM, Donnai D, Neary W, Blair V, et al. (1992) A clinical study of type 2 neurofibromatosis. Q J Med 84: 603–618.
6. Abaza MM, Makariou E, Armstrong M, Lalwani AK (1996) Growth rate characteristics of acoustic neuromas associated with neurofibromatosis type 2. The Laryngoscope 106: 694–699.
7. Fisher LM, Doherty JK, Lev MH, Slattery WH (2009) Concordance of bilateral vestibular schwannoma growth and hearing changes in neurofibromatosis 2: neurofibromatosis 2 natural history consortium. Otol Neurotol 30: 835–841.
8. Masuda A, Fisher LM, Oppenheimer ML, Iqbal Z, Slattery WH (2004) Hearing changes after diagnosis in neurofibromatosis type 2. Otol Neurotol 25: 150–154.
9. Graamans K, Van Dijk JE, Janssen LW (2003) Hearing deterioration in patients with a non-growing vestibular schwannoma. Acta oto-laryngologica 123: 51–54.
10. Baser ME, Friedman JM, Wallace AJ, Ramsden RT, Joe H, et al. (2002) Evaluation of clinical diagnostic criteria for neurofibromatosis 2. Neurology 59: 1759–1765.
11. King KA, Makishima T, Zalewski CK, Bakalov VK, Griffith AJ, et al. (2007) Analysis of auditory phenotype and karyotype in 200 females with Turner syndrome. Ear and hearing 28: 831–841.
12. Melhem ER, Jara H, Eustace S (1997) Fluid-attenuated inversion recovery MR imaging: identification of protein concentration thresholds for CSF hyperintensity. AJR Am J Roentgenol 169: 859–862.
13. Butman JA, Kim HJ, Baggenstos M, Ammerman JM, Dambrosia J, et al. (2007) Mechanisms of morbid hearing loss associated with tumors of the endolymphatic sac in von Hippel-Lindau disease. JAMA 298: 41–48.
14. Tagaya M, Yamazaki M, Teranishi M, Naganawa S, Yoshida T, et al. (2011) Endolymphatic hydrops and blood-labyrinth barrier in Meniere's disease. Acta Otolaryngol 131: 474–479.
15. Nakashima T, Naganawa S, Teranishi M, Tagaya M, Nakata S, et al. (2010) Endolymphatic hydrops revealed by intravenous gadolinium injection in patients with Meniere's disease. Acta Otolaryngol 130: 338–343.
16. Slattery WH, Lev MH, Fisher LM, Connell SS, Iqbal Z, et al. (2005) MRI evaluation of neurofibromatosis 2 patients: a standardized approach for accuracy in interpretation. Otol Neurotol 26: 733–740.
17. Lundin P, Pedersen F (1992) Volume of pituitary macroadenomas: assessment by MRI. J Comput Assist Tomogr 16: 519–528.
18. Silverstein H (1973) Labyrinthine tap as a diagnostic test for acoustic neurinoma. OTOLARYNGCLINNAMER 6: 229–244.
19. Yoshida T, Sugiura M, Naganawa S, Teranishi M, Nakata S, et al. (2008) Three-dimensional fluid-attenuated inversion recovery magnetic resonance imaging findings and prognosis in sudden sensorineural hearing loss. The Laryngoscope 118: 1433–1437.
20. Yamazaki M, Naganawa S, Kawai H, Nihashi T, Fukatsu H, et al. (2009) Increased signal intensity of the cochlea on pre- and post-contrast enhanced 3D-FLAIR in patients with vestibular schwannoma. Neuroradiology 51: 855–863.
21. Gardner WJ, Spitler DK, Whitten C (1954) Increased intracranial pressure caused by increased protein content in the cerebrospinal fluid; an explanation of papilledema in certain cases of small intracranial and intraspinal tumors, and in the Guillain-Barre syndrome. The New England journal of medicine 250: 932–936.
22. Froin G (1903) Inflammations méningées avec reaction chromatique, fibrineuse et cytologique du liquide céphalo-rachidien. Gaz d hop 76.
23. Shepherd RK, Colreavy MP (2004) Surface microstructure of the perilymphatic space: implications for cochlear implants and cell- or drug-based therapies. Archives of otolaryngology–head & neck surgery 130: 518–523.
24. Wenthold RJ, McGarvey ML (1982) Changes in rapidly transported proteins in the auditory nerve after hair cell loss. Brain research 253: 263–269.
25. Thomsen J, Saxtrup O, Tos M (1982) Quantitated determination of proteins in perilymph in patients with acoustic neuromas. ORL; journal for oto-rhino-laryngology and its related specialties 44: 61–65.
26. Butman JA, Linehan WM, Lonser RR (2008) Neurologic manifestations of von Hippel-Lindau disease. JAMA : the journal of the American Medical Association 300: 1334–1342.
27. Lysaght AC, Kao SY, Paulo JA, Merchant SN, Steen H, et al. (2011) Proteome of human perilymph. Journal of proteome research 10: 3845–3851.
28. Eckermeier L, Pirsig W, Mueller D (1979) Histopathology of 30 non-operated acoustic schwannomas. Archives of oto-rhino-laryngology 222: 1–9.
29. Schuknecht HF, Ishii T (1966) Hearing loss caused by atrophy of the stria vascularis. Nihon Jibiinkoka Gakkai kaiho 69: 1825–1833.
30. Silverstein H, Schuknecht HF (1966) Biochemical studies of inner ear fluid in man. Changes in otosclerosis, Meniere's disease, and acoustic neuroma. Archives of otolaryngology 84: 395–402.
31. Dix MR, Hallpike CS (1950) Observations on the pathological mechanism of conductive deafness in certain cases of neuroma of the VIIIth nerve. The Journal of laryngology and otology 64: 658–666.
32. Graamans K, Van Dijk JE, Janssen LW (2003) Hearing deterioration in patients with a non-growing vestibular schwannoma. Acta oto-laryngologica 123: 51–54.
33. Pennings RJE, Morris DP, Clarke L, Allen S, Walling S, et al. (2011) Natural history of hearing deterioration in intracanalicular vestibular schwannoma. Neurosurgery 68: 68–77.
34. Roosli C, Linthicum FH, Jr., Cureoglu S, Merchant SN (2012) Dysfunction of the cochlea contributing to hearing loss in acoustic neuromas: an underappreciated entity. Otology & neurotology : official publication of the American Otological Society, American Neurotology Society [and] European Academy of Otology and Neurotology 33: 473–480.
35. Plotkin SR, Stemmer-Rachamimov AO, Barker FG, 2nd, Halpin C, Padera TP, et al. (2009) Hearing improvement after bevacizumab in patients with neurofibromatosis type 2. The New England journal of medicine 361: 358–367.
36. Plotkin SR, Merker VL, Halpin C, Jennings D, McKenna MJ, et al. (2012) Bevacizumab for progressive vestibular schwannoma in neurofibromatosis type 2: a retrospective review of 31 patients. Otology & neurotology : official publication of the American Otological Society, American Neurotology Society [and] European Academy of Otology and Neurotology 33: 1046–1052.

3

A Direct Comparison of Local-Global Integration in Autism and other Developmental Disorders: Implications for the Central Coherence Hypothesis

Inês Bernardino[1], Susana Mouga[1,2], Joana Almeida[2], Marieke van Asselen[1], Guiomar Oliveira[1,2,3], Miguel Castelo-Branco[1]*

1 Visual Neuroscience Laboratory, IBILI, Faculty of Medicine, Coimbra, Portugal, **2** Neurodevelopment and Autism Department from Child Center of Pediatric Hospital of Coimbra, Coimbra, Portugal, **3** Research and Clinical Training Department from Pediatric Hospital of Coimbra, Coimbra, Portugal

Abstract

The weak central coherence hypothesis represents one of the current explanatory models in Autism Spectrum Disorders (ASD). Several experimental paradigms based on hierarchical figures have been used to test this controversial account. We addressed this hypothesis by testing central coherence in ASD (n = 19 with intellectual disability and n = 20 without intellectual disability), Williams syndrome (WS, n = 18), matched controls with intellectual disability (n = 20) and chronological age-matched controls (n = 20). We predicted that central coherence should be most impaired in ASD for the weak central coherence account to hold true. An alternative account includes dorsal stream dysfunction which dominates in WS. Central coherence was first measured by requiring subjects to perform local/global preference judgments using hierarchical figures under 6 different experimental settings (memory and perception tasks with 3 distinct geometries with and without local/global manipulations). We replicated these experiments under 4 additional conditions (memory/perception*local/global) in which subjects reported the correct local or global configurations. Finally, we used a visuoconstructive task to measure local/global perceptual interference. WS participants were the most impaired in central coherence whereas ASD participants showed a pattern of coherence loss found in other studies only in four task conditions favoring local analysis but it tended to disappear when matching for intellectual disability. We conclude that abnormal central coherence does not provide a comprehensive explanation of ASD deficits and is more prominent in populations, namely WS, characterized by strongly impaired dorsal stream functioning and other phenotypic traits that contrast with the autistic phenotype. Taken together these findings suggest that other mechanisms such as dorsal stream deficits (largest in WS) may underlie impaired central coherence.

Editor: Michael J. Proulx, Queen Mary University of London, United Kingdom

Funding: This research was supported by the Portuguese Foundation for Science and Technology [grant numbers: PTDC/SAU-NEU/68483/2006 and PIC/IC/82986/2007 to SM and MCB (PI); PTDC/PSI-PCO/108208/2008 to MvA and an individual scholarship - SRFH/BD/41401/2007 to IB]. The funders had no role in study design, data collection and analysis, decision to publish, or preparation of the manuscript.

Competing Interests: The authors have declared that no competing interests exist.

* E-mail: mcbranco@fmed.uc.pt

Introduction

A cognitive theory - the Weak Central Coherence (WCC) account [1] - has been proposed to address cognitive weaknesses and strengths in Autism Spectrum Disorder (ASD). ASD is characterized by a symptomatic triad including severely impaired social interaction, deficits in communication and restricted/stereotyped patterns of behavior, interests and activities [2,3]. Superior visuospatial skills have been described in ASD, particularly in which concerns visual search [4,5,6] and puzzle assembly tasks [7,8]. Nevertheless, there is some evidence of a distinctive visual perceptual style in this disorder that has been considered to account for high level deficits particularly in the face processing domain [9,10,11].

The WCC account describes the perceptual and cognitive biases in ASD according to the claim that these patients perceive visual scenes as a sparse set of details rather than as a congruent and meaningful unit, failing in the extraction of the global configuration [1,12]. This hypothesis explains the cognitive phenotype of ASD in terms of dissociation between local and global information processing that has been mostly analyzed in the visual domain.

An extensive range of experimental paradigms have been used to measure WCC in ASD, namely the block design subtest [7,13], the embedded-figure test [14,15], the copying impossible-figure [16] and visual illusion tasks [17,18]. However, the main paradigm in this domain has been the study of coherent visual processing using hierarchical figures, such as Navon stimuli [15,19,20,21]. This stimulus type provides an explicit separation of both local and global levels of visual processing. The pattern of findings has been inconsistent suggesting the need for controlled experiments in multiple clinical populations directly testing the main statement of that hypothesis [22,23,24,25,26]. Plaisted et al. [20] reported this pattern of mixed findings by showing that ASD patients exhibited local advantage and local interference effects in a divided attention task while they showed a global precedence effect (as typically developing participants did) in a selective attention task. The authors explain these differences based on the different task demands by suggesting that there is an intact global processing in ASD patients alongside with a voluntarily selective attention bias to local information in the absence of overt instructions. This is in line with the enhanced perceptual functioning model (EPF) which postulates an autistic perceptual endophenotype characterized by locally-oriented processing in ASD without disrupting global information processing aspects [27,28]. This model is consistent with the observation that tasks with high perceptual load conduct to superior performance in ASD patients in contrast with typically developing controls [29].

Although the WCC account has been formulated to explain the distinctive cognitive phenotype of ASD, the detailed-focused cognitive style has been described in other developmental disorders, such as Williams syndrome (WS), although a distinct behavioral phenotype is observed in this condition. This leads to a question about the distinctiveness of the WCC in ASD and renders the direct comparison between the ASD and WS phenotypes important for the elucidation of this debate.

WS is a genetic neurodevelopmental disorder characterized by predominant visuospatial impairment [30,31] contrasting with relatively spared verbal processing [32,33,34]. Visual dorsal stream deficits are the hallmark of this disorder [35]. These visuospatial deficits have been explored in terms of local-global visual processing and a local processing bias in this disorder is particularly evident in the visuoconstructive domain [36,37].

The mixed findings particularly found in ASD emphasize the notion that global processing in these disorders seems to be affected under some task conditions and spared under others. Therefore, it is crucial to test the central coherence abilities in ASD (and other neurodevelopmental conditions) under the same task requirements in order to clarify their pattern of visual processing. In this domain, there are several important methodological issues that should be addressed to better understand the pattern of visual perception of these developmental disorders. Accordingly, it is important to separate the ability to perceive global information from the detailed focused cognitive style characterized by the preferential use of local approaches when analyzing a visual scene in the absence of overt instructions. Indeed, some studies focused on attention tasks giving direct instructions to attend to either local or global levels of information [16,20,36] while others only required free viewing to assess preference [21,37]. So far, this crucial distinction remains to be done, in the same study, under the same task conditions, and with different clinical populations and control groups. In the current study, we explicitly separated perceptual bias and cognitive style from global processing impairment by using multiple measures of central coherence based on the classical Navon paradigm [19]. In addition, we also attempted a separation between perceptual and visuoconstructive components of local-global processing, which has not been addressed before in ASD (in contrast with WS).

In sum, the WCC account proposes that detailed-focused cognitive style in ASD is a contributory cause of some characteristics of this disorder, in particular defective face processing [10]. However, the fact that WCC is a common denominator of both ASD and WS is at odds with their substantially distinct cognitive profile. Therefore, we predict that if WCC is distinctive in ASD and underlies its pathophysiology the coherence deficits should dominate in ASD patients. Although we believe that such deficits may emerge under certain conditions (as also found in this study), this would also mean that they do not provide a full account of the phenotype and that complementary mechanisms, such as dorsal stream deficits, should also be considered. Our main goal was to test the hypothesis that WCC is unique and distinctive to ASD by using classical paradigms of central coherence in clinical populations with clear categorical differences concerning intellectual disability and cognitive phenotype. This would allow us to understand if these conditions share the same underlying cognitive mechanisms of integration or if this perceptual feature can alternatively be considered specific to the pathophysiology of ASD. The understanding of the neurobehavioral relevance of central coherence in ASD requires addressing both perceptual bias and performance levels as well as the impact of intellectual disability in central coherence measures. In the current study, intellectual disability was controlled for by selecting appropriate matched clinical and control groups. Participants were tested under three experimental tasks: a Preference task without a priori "correct" response to assess spontaneous visual processing preferences, a Correct Choice task to evaluate the accuracy in perceiving both global and local information and a Drawing task to explore visuoconstructive integrative abilities. We further explored the effect of the physical presence of the stimulus on the visual processing of hierarchical stimuli by introducing both perceptual and memory conditions. Furthermore, in the preference task, we addressed the invariance of the processing bias to local and global rotation manipulations that were introduced to increase task sensitivity in the detection of mild perceptual bias.

Methods

Ethics Statement

This study and all the procedures were reviewed and approved by the Ethics Commissions of the Faculty of Medicine of the University of Coimbra (Comissão de Ética da Faculdade de Medicina da Universidade de Coimbra) and of the Pediatric Hospital of Coimbra (Comissão de Ética do Hospital Pediátrico de Coimbra) and was conducted in accordance with the declaration of Helsinki. Written informed consent was obtained from participants older than 18 years of age and from the parents/guardians in the case of participants younger than 18 years of age. Children and adolescents younger than 18 years of age gave oral informed consent.

Participants

Ninety-seven participants were included in this study: 18 WS patients, 19 ASD patients with intellectual disability (ASD_ID) (Intelligence Quotient (IQ) <80), 20 ASD patients without intellectual disability (ASD_noID) (IQ ≥90), 20 typically developing participants matched for chronological age (C_TD) and 20 control participants with intellectual disability matched for IQ (C_ID). The characteristics of clinical and control groups are summarized in Table 1.

ASD participants were recruited from the Neurodevelopment and Autism Department from the Child Center of Pediatric Hospital of Coimbra. ASD diagnoses were assigned on the basis of gold standard instruments such as: parental or caregiver interview (Autism Diagnostic Interview Revised, ADI-R [38]), direct structured proband assessment (Autism Diagnostic Observation Schedule, ADOS [39]), and clinical examination performed by an experienced neurodevelopmental Pediatrician, based on the diagnostic criteria for autistic disorder from Diagnostic and Statistical Manual of Mental Disorders IV, DSM-IV-TR [2]. All ASD patients had positive results in the ADI-R and ADOS for autism or ASD, and met the criteria for autistic disorder from the DSM-IV-TR. Only idiopathic cases were included (negative kariotypic results in, fluorescence in situ hybridization - FISH ch 15 q11-13 - and FMR1 mutation). In this group, 7 patients were medicated with Risperidone and 2

Table 1. Characteristics of clinical and control groups.

	Chronological Age (years)		Education (years)		IQ (WISC-III or WAIS-III)		Gender
	Mean (SE)	**Range**	**Mean (SE)**	**Range**	**Mean (SE)**	**Range**	**(m:f)**
WS (n = 18)	17.33 (1.81)	8–34	5.00 (1.00)	0–12	53.94 (2.01)	42–75	11:7
ASD_ID (n = 19)	13.26 (0.58)	10–18	6.74 (0.43)	4–9	64.47 (1.76)	52–79	15:4
ASD_noID (n = 20)	12.10 (0.46)	10–17	6.55 (0.48)	4–11	103.40 (2.41)	90–129	20:0
C_TD (n = 20)	15.70 (1.81)	7–34	6.80 (0.79)	2–14	107.94 (1.73)	95–119	11:9
C_ID (n = 20)	15.35 (0.96)	10–29	7.15 (0.46)	3–9	58.60 (1.95)	40–74	15:5

Note. WS = Williams Syndrome group; ASD_ID = Autism Spectrum Disorders group with intellectual disability; ASD_noID = Autism Spectrum Disorders group without intellectual disability; C_TD = typically developing control group; C_ID = control group with intellectual disability; WISC-III = Wechsler Intelligence Scale for Children, 3rd. ed.; WAIS-III = Wechsler Adult Intelligence Scale, 3rd ed.

were medicated with Methylphenidate. However, parents of these children were requested not to give their children the medication on the days of the testing.

WS participants were recruited from a database used in previous studies [30,31]. All patients were diagnosed based on clinical and genetic examinations confirmed by FISH analysis, which demonstrated the hemyzigous Elastin deletion. Additional genetic analysis sequenced the breakpoint regions and revealed the same deletion size (~1.55 Mb) in all WS participants.

Control participants matched for IQ were recruited from the same department and from local special education institutes. None of these participants were taking selective serotonin reuptake inhibitor or neuroleptic medications. Co-morbid conditions were explicitly excluded (epilepsy, brain injury, sensory deficits, associated genetic syndromes, and motor deficits that could interfere with task response).

Control participants matched for chronological age were healthy, with no history of psychiatric, neurologic and ophthalmologic illnesses and naïve concerning to the testing procedures. They were recruited from local schools and were individually tested at their own schools.

The parents of participants included in WS and C_ID groups completed the Social Communication Questionnaire to exclude co-morbidity with ASD [40]. The scores were below 15, which is the positive cut-off for ASD. All participants included in the study received the Portuguese adapted version of the Wechsler Intelligence Scale for Children – 3rd edition (WISC-III) [41] or the Wechsler Adult Intelligence Scale – 3rd edition (WAIS-III) [42], according to the participant's age. The ASD_ID group only includes subjects with IQ inferior to 80 while the ASD_noID group includes subjects with IQ superior or equal to 90, which is consistent with Wechsler definition of intellectual disability [41,42].

The three clinical groups (WS, ASD_ID and ASD_noID) were matched for chronological age and education level with both C_TD-matched (Mann-Whitney test, $p>0.05$) and C_ID-matched (Mann-Whitney test, $p>0.05$) control groups. Additionally, the clinical groups with intellectual disability (WS and ASD_ID) were matched for IQ (Mann-Whitney test, $p>0.05$) with the C_ID-matched control group.

Procedure

We used Navon's hierarchical stimuli [19], which consisted of global geometrical figures made up of 18 smaller geometrical figures. In each hierarchical form, the shape of the local level differed from the shape of the global level. The stimuli were shown on a 33,8 cm×27,1 cm computer screen (1280×1024 pixels) using the software package Presentation (Neurobehavioral systems). The size of the local shapes was 0.57° horizontally and 0.57° vertically and the distance between them was 0.57°. The horizontal and vertical sizes of the global shapes differed accordingly to the figure configuration. The color of the stimuli was black and they were shown on a white background at high contrast (95%).

Participants were individually tested in a quiet and darkened room, seated at a distance of 50 cm from the computer screen. They were asked to perform three experimental tasks: a Preference task, a Correct Choice task and, finally, a Drawing task.

PreferenceTasks. On each trial, participants performed a match to sample similarity task by comparing two figures with one target figure. This task was performed under different task conditions, in which task requirements (visual perception and visual memory tasks) and the geometric configuration of the stimuli (non-inversion, local-inversion, and global-inversion conditions) were manipulated. For the visual perception preference task, the participants viewed a display containing a target figure at the top of the screen and two comparison figures at the bottom (Figure 1A). One of the comparison figures shared only the global shape with the target figure and the other had the same local elements as the target but had different global configuration. That is, each comparison figure shared only one level (local or global) with the target figure and appeared randomly and equally often on the left and right positions. For the visual memory preference task, each trial comprehended a presentation phase, in which the target figure was shown during 2500 ms, followed by the appearance, without delay, of the two comparison figures (Figure 1B). For both perceptual judgment and memory tasks, participants were asked to indicate which of the two bottom figures was more similar to the target, thereby reporting their visual processing preferences (bias). The instructions for the perceptual preference task were as follows (translated from Portuguese): "In this screen, you have three figures, one up here (pointing) and two below (pointing). You should look closely at all these pictures and indicate, in your opinion, which of the two figures down here (pointing), is more similar to the figure above". It is important to note that, in this task, there is no correct response and the subjects' answers reflect only the preferred pattern of visual analysis when analyzing a hierarchical figure.

In both perception and visual memory preference tasks, we included a no-rotation condition in which the local and global information of the comparison figures were presented in the same orientation of the target figure. Additionally, two control conditions (with different geometrical configurations) were also administered, namely local-rotation and global-rotation conditions, in which the orientation of either the local or global elements

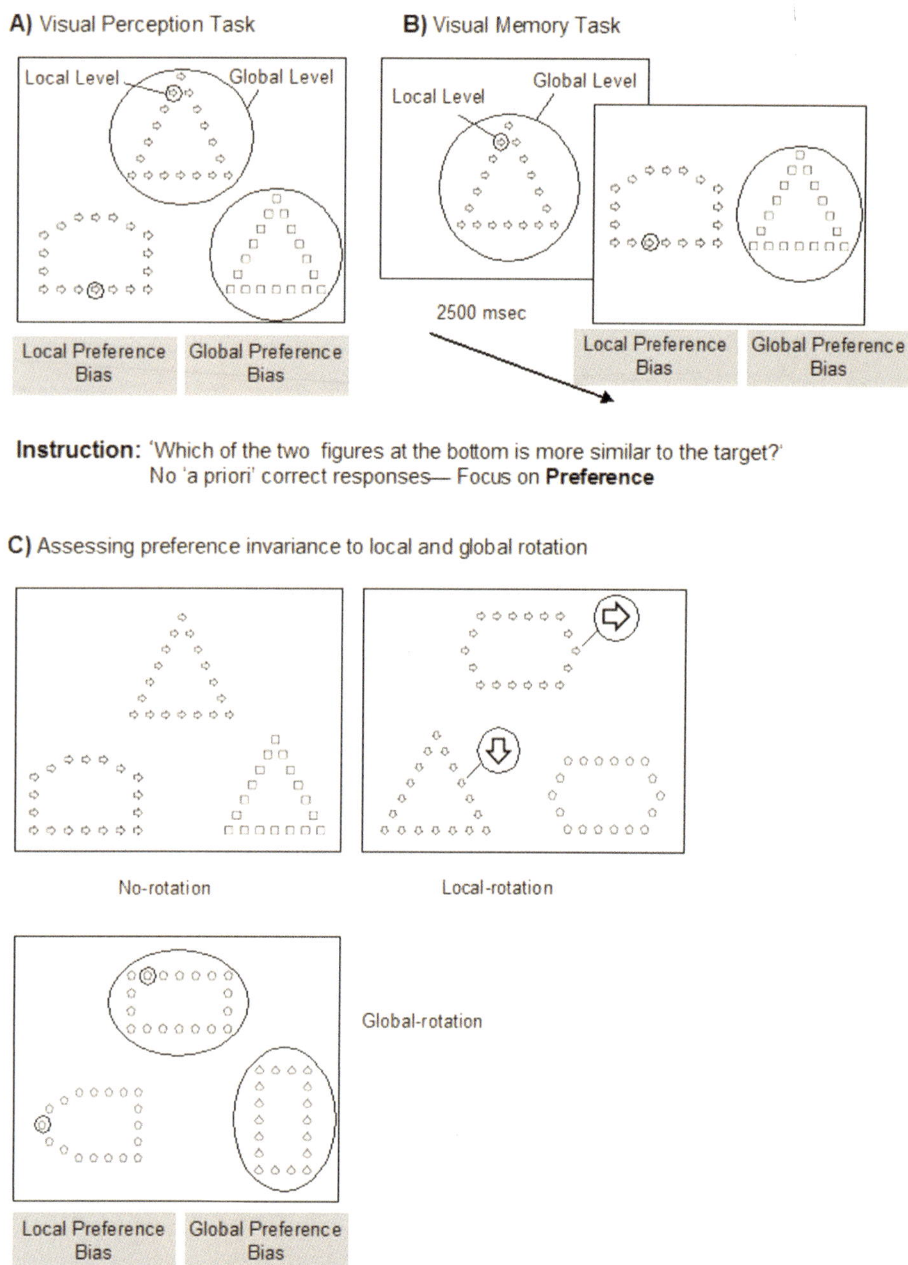

Figure 1. Illustration of the Visual Preference Tasks. Example of the configurations used in A) visual perception preference tasks and B) visual memory preference tasks. C) Illustration of the non-inversion, local-inversion and global-inversion conditions used on visual perception preference and visual memory preference tasks to assess preference invariance to global and local rotation. Note. Figures are presented according to the real scale (not real size) and, therefore, visibility was higher in the experimental task.

of the stimulus was manipulated to provide generalization and further, enhance the likelihood of detecting subtle forms of perceptual bias (Figure 1C). The local elements or the global shape were rotated 90 or 180 degrees to ensure that the figures exhibited different orientations of those presented in the target figure. In the local-rotation condition we rotated the local elements of the comparison figure matched for local level with the target figure. This approach favoured a change to a more global bias. In the global-rotation condition, we rotated the global shape of the comparison figure matched for global configuration with the target figure in order to explicitly increase the local similarity. This strategy favoured a change to a local bias.

Participant underwent 20 test trials in each task condition performing a total of 60 test trials. Eight familiarization trials were administered for each task. The familiarization phase was repeated whenever the subjects did not understand the instructions or had difficulties coordinating the motor response. All participants included in the task understood the task instructions. The visual perception task was provided before the visual memory task for all participants.

Correct choice tasks. Two different task conditions were included, namely a match-to-local choice task and a match-to-global choice task, differing only on the instruction given to the participants (but both requiring a correct response, unlike the

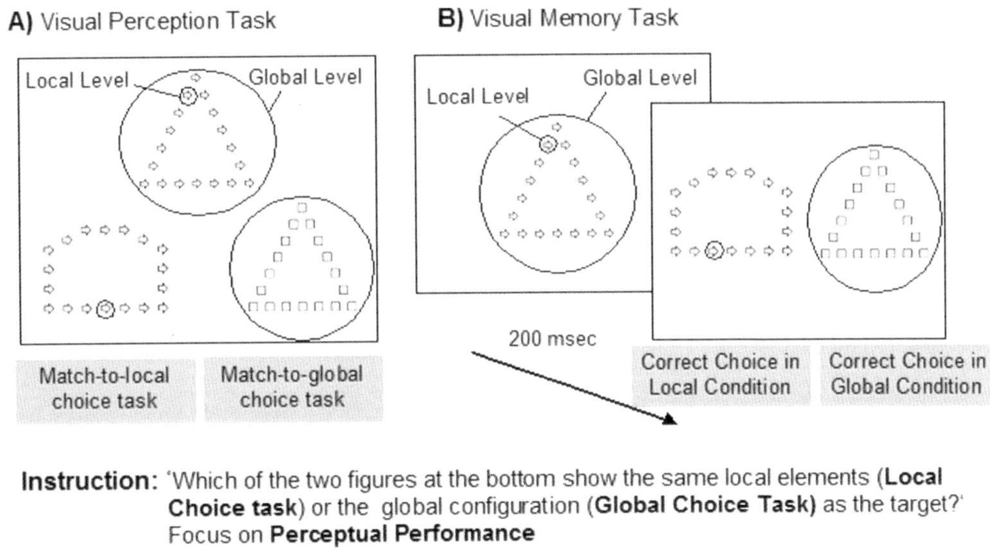

Figure 2. Illustration of the Correct Choice Tasks. Example of the configuration used in A) visual perception correct choice tasks and B) visual memory correct choice tasks. Note. Figures are presented according to the real scale (not real size) and, therefore, visibility was higher in the experimental task. Note that questions posed to participants were in simple Portuguese.

Preference Tasks). In the match-to-local choice task, participants indicated which of the two comparison figures had the same local shapes as the target, while in the match-to-global choice task participants indicated which of the two comparison figures was matched with the target in terms of the global configuration. Additionally, as occurred in the Preference task, participants were performed visual judgments under visual perception and visual memory conditions. In the visual perception correct choice task, participants viewed a display containing one target figure and two comparison figures (Figure 2A). In the visual memory correct choice task, the target figure was presented during 200 ms, followed by the appearance of two comparison figures (Figure 2B). For both experimental tasks, we presented six blocks of eight trials each, alternating between match-to-local and match–to-global conditions (three blocks for each condition). Participants performed a total of 48 trials for each perception and memory conditions. Five consecutive correct practice trials were administered for all conditions to ensure that all participants understood the task instructions.

Drawing task. A Drawing (visuoconstructive) task was included, in which participants copied two hierarchical figures (a large triangle made of smaller arrows and a large 'P' made of smaller 'A's') (Figure 3). Designs were shown in an A5 paper until participants finished the copy. There was no time limit for completion of the task. A rating scale, similar to that used by Porter & Coltheart [23], was created to rate visuoconstructive integrative ability. Three scores were carried out for each drawing task, namely a local score, a global score and an integration score. For local and global scores, ratings were between 0 ("totally absent") and 3 ("perfect reproduction"). We computed the local and global scores for each participant by summing the score of the two drawings produced by each participant. In sum, local and global scores had a minimum score of zero and a maximum of six. For the integration score, ratings were 0 (if the local and global shapes were drawn independently) or 1 (if the local and global configurations were accurately integrated as a whole). Two WS participants were not able to draw the triangle and one refused to draw the hierarchical letter resulting in a total of 191 drawings produced by the clinical and control groups which were rated by two independent raters. The raters were not aware that the drawings had been produced by different groups. Inter-rater reliability scores were 0.912 for local score, 0.880 for global score and 0.878 for integration score (Spearman's rho correlations, $p<0.05$).

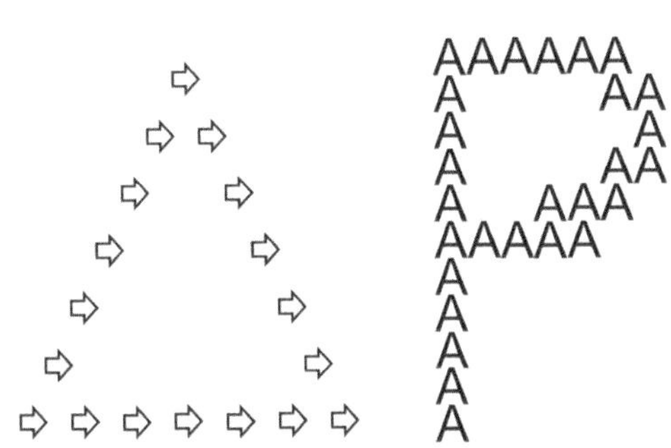

Figure 3. Stimuli used in the drawing task. A simple geometric figure and a letter used in the drawing task.

Statistical Analysis

Nonparametric statistics (Mann-Whitney U tests, Fisher's Exact Tests and Spearman's Rho correlations) were carried out for all statistical analyses to avoid biases due to deviations from normality and variance heterogeneity. All statistical analyses were performed with the IBM SPSS Statistics 19.0 software package.

Results

Preference (bias) Tasks

Visual perception preference task. Group analyses revealed that both ASD clinical groups with or without intellectual disability (ASD_ID and ASD_noID) have a relative preference for global configurations in all no-rotation, local-rotation and global-rotation conditions. Surprisingly, their choice behavior was similar to both C_TD and C_ID control groups. Thus, no significant

Table 2. Group comparison analyses for Preference Tasks considering visual perception and visual memory preference tasks as well as no-rotation, local-rotation and global-rotation task conditions.

	Visual Perception Preference Task			Visual Memory Preference Task		
	No-rotation	Local-rotation	Global-rotation	No-rotation	Local-rotation	Global-rotation
ASD_ID vs. C_TD	p = 0.080	p = 0.623	p = 0.715	p = 0.112	p = 0.122	p = 0.013*
ASD_ID vs. C_ID	p = 0.852	p = 0.314	p = 0.143	p = 0.763	p = 0.852	p = 0.550
ASD_noID vs. C_TD	p = 0.585	p = 0.988	p = 0.322	p = 0.483	p = 0.797	p = 0.560
WS_local vs. C_TD	p = 0.000**	p = 0.001*	p = 0.002*	p = 0.001*	p = 0.001*	p = 0.035*
WS_local vs. C_ID	p = 0.002*	p = 0.003*	p = 0.002*	p = 0.000**	p = 0.003*	p = 0.090
WS_global vs. C_TD	p = 0.018*	p = 0.182	p = 0.087	p = 0.006*	p = 0.022*	p = 0.009*
WS_global vs. C_ID	p = 0.541	p = 0.915	p = 0.884	p = 0.149	p = 0.586	p = 0.487

All comparisons signaled in red are significant and related to increased local bias.
Mann-Whitney U tests; * $p<0.05$, ** $p<0.001$.
WS_local = Williams Syndrome subgroup with local bias; WS_global = Williams Syndrome subgroup with global bias; ASD_ID = Autism Spectrum Disorders group with intellectual disability; ASD_noID = Autism Spectrum Disorders group without intellectual disability; C_TD = typically developing control group; C_ID = control group with intellectual disability.

differences were found between the ASD clinical groups and respective control groups in all task conditions (Mann-Whitney U test, $p>0.05$, see Table 2 for details on exact p-values and specific comparisons).

Conversely, in the WS group we found a bimodal distribution specifically for this task, with a subgroup showing a clear preference for local strategies (with more than 80% of local choices) while the other subgroup showed a clear global visual bias (with more than 80% of global choices). The WS subgroup who preferred local bias showed significantly more local choices than both C_TD and C_ID controls groups on all task conditions (Mann-Whitney U test, $p<0.05$). Concerning the WS subgroup who preferred global choices, no significant differences were found when comparing with the C_ID control group for all task conditions (Mann-Whitney U test, $p>0.05$), however, significant differences were found when comparing with the C_TD group but only for the local-rotation condition (Mann-Whitney U test, $p<0.05$) and the global-rotation condition (Mann-Whitney U test, $p<0.05$).

Visual memory preference task. Similar results were found for the visual memory preference task with group analyses revealing no significant differences between the ASD_ID group

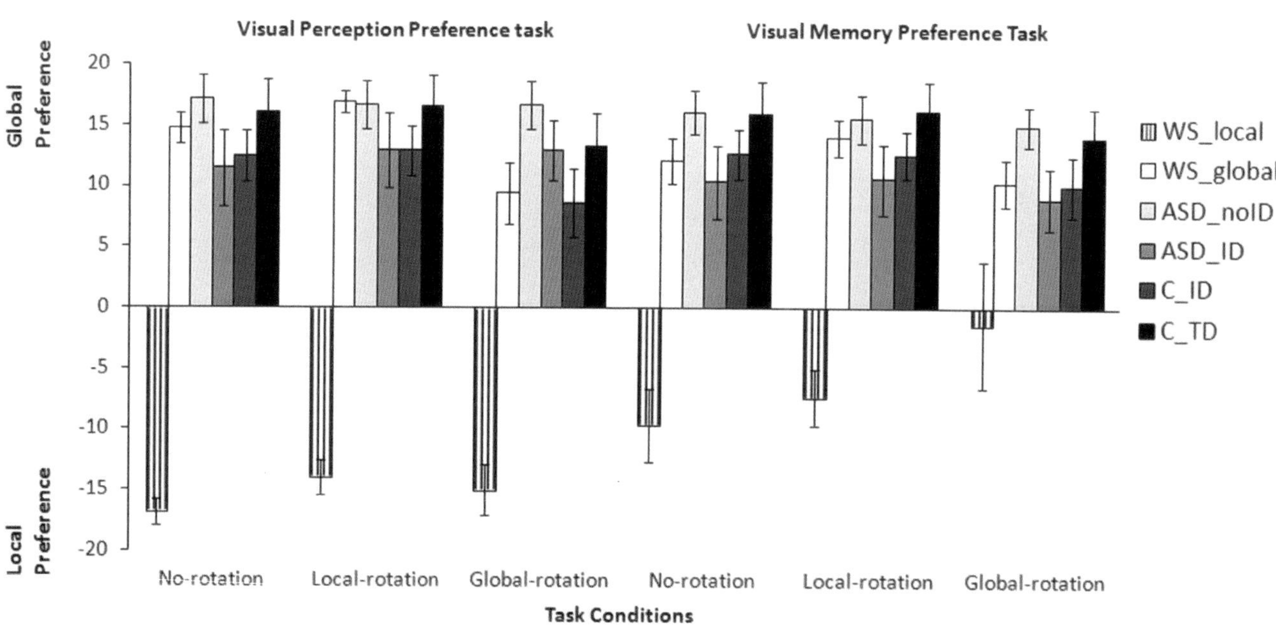

Figure 4. Mean percentage of global responses for all clinical and control groups for the visual perception preference task conditions and the visual memory preference task conditions. Given the bimodal pattern found in WS only for this task, and for sake of clarity we plot two WS subgroups, according to dominantly local or global preference (see text). WS_local = Williams Syndrome subgroup with local bias; WS_global = Williams Syndrome subgroup with global bias; ASD_ID = Autism Spectrum Disorders group with intellectual disability; ASD_noID = Autism Spectrum Disorders group without intellectual disability; C_TD = typically developing control group; C_ID = control group with intellectual disability.

Table 3. Group comparison analyses for Correct Choice Tasks considering visual perception and visual memory correct choice tasks as well as match-to-global and match-to-local task conditions.

	Visual Perception Correct Choice Task		Visual Memory Correct Choice Task	
	Global condition	**Local condition**	**Global condition**	**Local condition**
ASD_ID vs. C_TD	p = 0.012*	p = 0.131	p = 0.020*	p = 0.012*
ASD_ID vs. C_ID	p = 0.479	p = 0.162	p = 0.282	p = 0.283
ASD_noID vs. C_TD	p = 0.223	p = 0.171	p = 0.452	p = 0.659
WS vs. C_TD	p = 0.002*	p = 0.000**	p = 0.000**	p = 0.000**
WS vs. C_ID	p = 0.158	p = 0.024*	p = 0.001*	p = 0.037*

All comparisons signaled in red are significant and related to increased number of errors.
Mann-Whitney U tests; * $p<0.05$, ** $p<0.001$.
WS = Williams Syndrome group; ASD_ID = Autism Spectrum Disorders group with intellectual disability; ASD_noID = Autism Spectrum Disorders group without intellectual disability; C_TD = typically developing control group; C_ID = control group with intellectual disability.

and the C_ID across no-rotation, local-rotation and global-rotation conditions (Mann-Whitney U test, $p>0.05$, for details on exact p-values see Table 2). When comparing the ASD_ID group with the C_TD group no significant differences were found for no-rotation (Mann-Whitney U test, $p>0.05$) and local-rotation (Mann-Whitney U test, $p>0.05$) conditions but significant differences emerged for the global-condition (Mann-Whitney U test, $p<0.05$), as expected from the fact that global stimulus rotation induces a local bias. Likewise, no significant differences were found between the ASD_noID and the C_TD (Mann-Whitney U test, $p>0.005$) group, both evidencing a preference for using global strategies when analyzing hierarchical geometric figures irrespective of the control manipulations introduced in the task. In the WS group we replicated the bimodal pattern found in the perception preference task. Significant differences were found between the WS subgroup who preferred local choices and both C_TD and C_ID control groups for all task conditions (Mann-Whitney U test, $p<0.05$), showing a clear preference for using local strategies when performing a match to sample similarity task with no a priori correct responses. Concerning the WS subgroup who preferred global choices, significant differences were found when comparing with the C_TD control group for all task conditions (Mann-Whitney U test, $p<0.05$) but no significant differences were found when comparing with the C_ID control group for all task conditions (Mann-Whitney U test, $p>0.05$). Results are summarized in Table 2 and Figure 4.

Correct Choice (performance) Tasks

Visual perception correct choice task. Group analyses revealed no significant differences when comparing the ASD_ID group with the C_ID group in both match-to-local and match-to-global conditions (Mann-Whitney U tests; $p>0.05$; see Table 3 for details on exact p-values and specific comparisons). However, when comparing the ASD_ID and the C_TD groups, results indicated that the clinical group made significantly more errors than the control group for the match-to-global condition (Mann-Whitney U test; $p<0.05$), but not for the local-to-match condition (Mann-Whitney U test; $p>0.05$). No significant differences were found when comparing ASD_noID group with the matched C_TD control group concerning the identification of local and

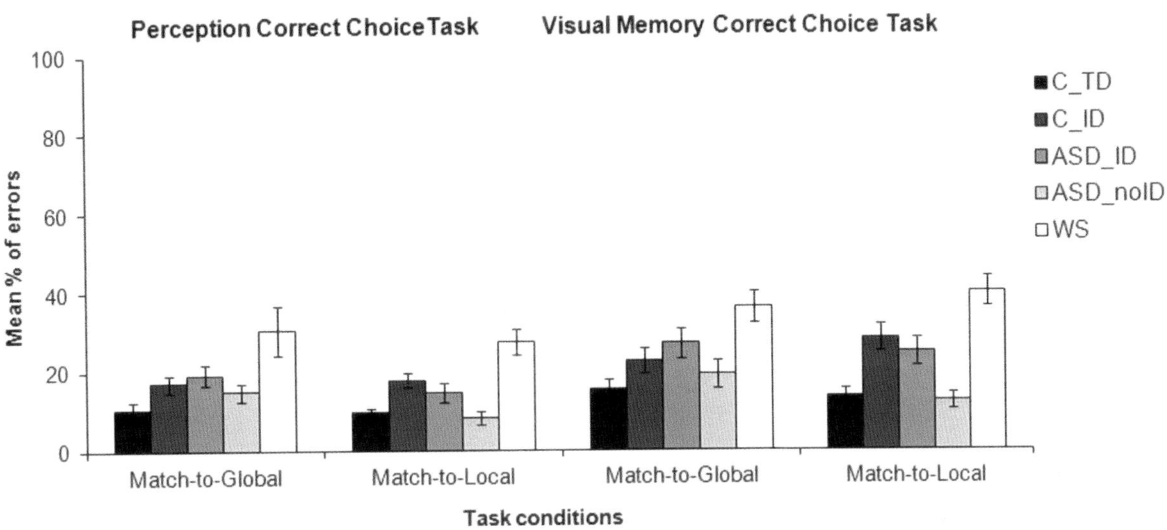

Figure 5. Mean percentage of errors for all clinical and control groups for the visual perception and visual memory "correct choice" task conditions. WS = Williams Syndrome group; ASD_ID = Autism Spectrum Disorders group with intellectual disability; ASD_noID = Autism Spectrum Disorders group without intellectual disability; C_TD = typically developing control group; C_ID = control group with intellectual disability.

Table 4. Comparison of blinded Local and Global scores obtained from two independent raters of the visuoconstructive drawing task.

	Drawing Task	
	Global score	Local score
ASD_ID vs. C_TD	p = 0.092	p = 0.051
ASD_ID vs. C_ID	p = 0.567	p = 0.396
ASD_noID vs. C_TD	p = 0.721	p = 0.222
WS vs. C_TD	p = 0.000**	p = 0.000**
WS vs. C_ID	p = 0.000**	p = 0.000**

All comparisons signaled in red are significant and related to lower global and local scores.
Mann-Whitney U tests; **p<0.001.
WS = Williams Syndrome group; ASD_ID = Autism Spectrum Disorders group with intellectual disability; ASD_noID = Autism Spectrum Disorders group without intellectual disability; C_TD = typically developing control group; C_ID = control group with intellectual disability.

Table 5. Comparison of blinded Integration score obtained from two independent raters.

	Drawing Task: Integration Score	
	'P' Drawing	Triangle Drawing
ASD_ID vs. C_TD	p = 0.106	p = 0.155
ASD_ID vs. C_ID	p = 0.283	p = 0.305
ASD_noID vs. C_TD	p = 0.500	p = 0.500
WS vs. C_TD	p = 0.000**	p = 0.004*
WS vs. C_ID	p = 0.000**	p = 0.001*

All comparisons signaled in red are significant and related to lower integration scores.
Fisher's Exact Test; * p<0.05, **p<0.001.
WS = Williams Syndrome group; ASD_ID = Autism Spectrum Disorders group with intellectual disability; ASD_noID = Autism Spectrum Disorders group without intellectual disability; C_TD = typically developing control group; C_ID = control group with intellectual disability.

global similarities (Mann-Whitney U tests; $p>0.05$). Significant differences were found when comparing WS group with the C_TD group in all conditions (Mann-Whitney U tests; $p<0.05$), but when comparing with the C_ID group significant differences were specifically found for the local condition (Mann-Whitney U tests; $p<0.05$).

Visual memory correct choice task. Similar results were found as in the perception task. The ASD_ID group performed in a similar way as the C_ID group in all task conditions (Mann-Whitney U tests; $p>0.05$; see Table 3 for further details), but made significantly more errors than the (non IQ-matched) C_TD group on both match-to-local (Mann-Whitney U test; $p<0.05$) and match-to-global (Mann-Whitney U tests; $p<0.05$) task conditions. The WS group made significantly more errors than both C_TD and C_ID control groups in all conditions (Mann-Whitney U tests; $p<0.05$). Results are summarized in Table 3 and Figure 5.

Visuoconstructive Task Requiring Integration of Local and Global Elements

Drawing task. For global and local scores, between-group comparisons revealed that both ASD groups (ASD_ID and ASD_noID) did not differ significantly from the C_TD and the C_ID control groups on both local and global scores (Mann-Whitney U tests; $p>0.05$; see Table 4 for details on exact p-values). Therefore, the ASD groups were able to draw the global and local configuration in a similar way when compared with control participants (see examples in Figure 6). Conversely, significant differences were found when comparing WS group with both control groups regarding local and global scores, which indicates that WS participants were worse at copying global and local shapes (Mann-Whitney U tests; $p<0.001$).

Concerning the integration score, ASD participants as well as their matched control groups were able to integrate the local elements in order to correctly construct the global configuration. Thus, group comparison analyses revealed that the number of subjects who were able to integrate both triangle and 'P' drawing did not differ between the ASD groups and the control

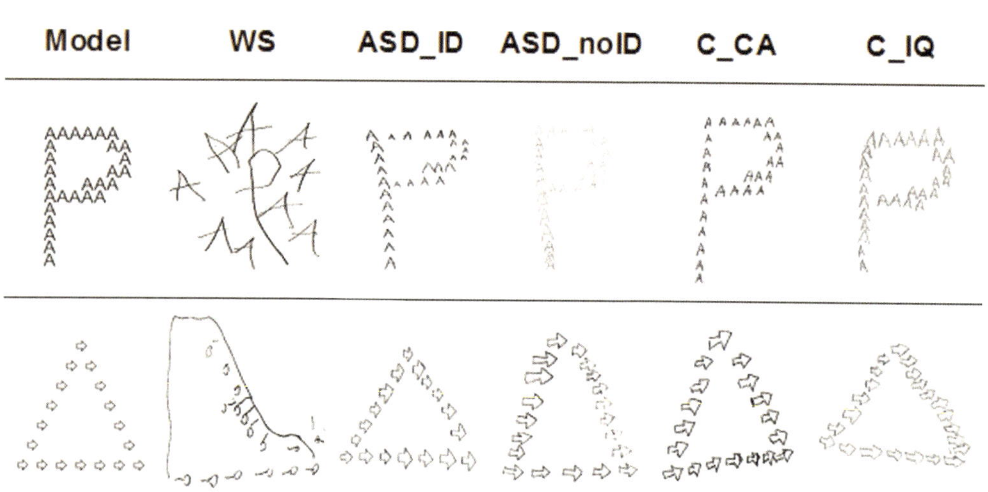

Figure 6. Examples of drawings produced by clinical and control groups. WS = Williams Syndrome group; ASD_ID = Autism Spectrum Disorders group with intellectual disability; ASD_noID = Autism Spectrum Disorders group without intellectual disability; C_TD = typically developing control group; C_ID = control group with intellectual disability.

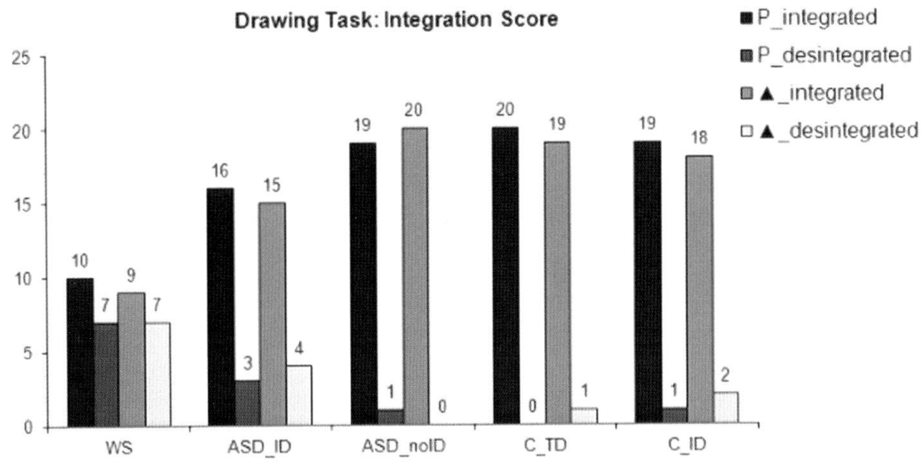

Figure 7. Visuoconstructive integrative abilities. Integration score for all groups indicating the number of subjects who were able to integrate the local elements in order to correctly reproduce the global configuration regarding the geometric hierarchical figure (Triangle) and the hierarchical letter ('P'). WS = Williams Syndrome group; ASD_ID = Autism Spectrum Disorders group with intellectual disability; ASD_noID = Autism Spectrum Disorders group without intellectual disability; C_TD = typical developing control group; C_ID = control group with intellectual disability.

participants (Fisher's Exact Test; $p>0.05$; see Table 5 for details on exact p-values). However, considering the WS group, results indicated that they were significantly worse at integrating local and global levels of analysis when compared with C_TD and C_ID control groups (Fisher's Exact Test; $p<0.05$). Results are summarized in Figure 7.

Discussion

In this study we tested the hypothesis that WCC is unique and distinctive to ASD. In order to assess this model we used classical markers of central coherence under distinct task constraints in several clinical populations (with categorical distinctions in intellectual disability and cognitive phenotype). Tasks were performed in the perceptual, memory and visuoconstructive domains, with explicit manipulations of levels of bias to better understand the distinction between cognitive style and performance.

ASD participants showed a surprising global preference pattern that is at odds with previous claims [1], although we also replicated local preference under particular conditions (see below). On the other hand, a significant bias towards local information was in general found in the WS group (a model of dorsal stream dysfunction), regardless of IQ. In other words, weakest central coherence was not found in the autistic group but in the WS (with explicitly excluded autistic co-morbidity). Therefore, we found a gradient of central coherence impairment (WS>ASD>‴ C_ID = C_TD) that is not consistent with the pattern derived from the WCC account (ASD>WS>C_ID = C_TD). Interestingly we could experimentally manipulate the preference level, in agreement with the task dependence and clinical heterogeneity found in previous studies [43].

Our study demonstrated that the global bias in ASD patients is accompanied by the presence of a global visual processing adequate to their intellectual level. Conversely, in WS the local bias co-exists with a deficit in correctly perceiving local and global visual information and with clear visuoconstructive integration impairment. It is important to note that ASD patients also showed tendency towards a local bias when experimental manipulations emphasized local processing as occurred in the global-rotation condition in the preference task. In other words, we could replicate the local pattern found in other studies, showing that it can indeed emerge under particular conditions, but that it is not general. Physical properties of the hierarchical stimulus have been described to influence the pattern of global-local processing [44]. Although there is evidence that ASD patients are not vulnerable to changes in visual angle and exposure time [28], it is known that perceptual sensitivity of ASD patients can be modulated by the level of the perceptual task load [29]. The manipulation of levels of stimulus rotation, in our task, may have contributed to the increase of local processing in ASD under these conditions. Moreover, ASD patients were, in general, able to process global information when the level of intellectual disability was controlled for, which agrees with previous claims [13,15,24,25].

Thus, ASD patients may oscillate between a local versus a global mode depending on task requirements and stimulus configuration. A different pattern was detected in WS with consistent local perceptual bias irrespective of task manipulations. Therefore, our findings provide a novel perspective on the WCC debate, without disputing previous findings.

The presence of a stronger detailed-focused perception as well as pronounced coherence deficits in WS may suggest a determinant link between weak central coherence and specific deficits within the dorsal visual stream. WS has been widely referred as involving deficits in tasks subserved by the visual dorsal stream (motion, 2D/3D object coherence and visuoconstructive ability), such as in perceiving 2D form-from-motion stimuli [45], discriminating 2D coherent motion [46] and visuomotor planning [47]. Additionally, Mendes et al. [30] found a 3D coherence deficit, larger than the 2D deficit suggesting that dorsal stream coherence deficits build up in the processing hierarchy. Accordingly, WS patients exhibit a considerable visual coherence and visuoconstructive impairment in particular when they are required to integrate local and global information, which was confirmed by our results. These findings are consistent with identified anatomical abnormalities in the superior parietal sulcus [48], and functional neuroimaging data [49,50].

Deficits along the dorsal visual stream have also been suggested in ASD, although the results indicate subtle [51,52] or even inexistent [53,54] general dorsal stream impairment. This led to the prediction that if central coherence is subserved by dorsal stream processing then it should be weaker in WS than ASD. Our results support this notion. In accordance with this prediction, recently, Poirel et al. [55], studied the shift from local to global visual processing in 6 year-old children and found that the global visual processing is associated to the loss of grey matter in areas along the dorsal visual stream (occipital and parietal visuospatial areas).

In sum, we conclude that abnormal central coherence is not a unique and distinctive characteristic in ASD but may be a marker of dorsal stream dysfunction. Largest dorsal stream deficits are present in populations (WS) with most impaired central coherence and with phenotypic traits (such as hypersociability) that contrast with the autistic phenotype.

Acknowledgments

We are grateful to the participants and their families, "Rumo ao Futuro" School, "Associação Portuguesa de Pais e Amigos do Cidadão com Deficiência Mental" (APPACDM) of Coimbra and "Associação Paralisia Cerebral Coimbra (APCC)/Quinta da Conraria" for their participation and support.

Author Contributions

Conceived and designed the experiments: IB MvA GO MCB. Performed the experiments: IB SM JA. Analyzed the data: IB SM MvA MCB. Contributed reagents/materials/analysis tools: SM JA GO MCB. Wrote the paper: IB SM MvA GO MCB.

References

1. Frith U (1989) Autism: explaining the enigma. Oxford, UK; Cambridge, MA, USA: Basil Blackwell. x, 204 p.
2. Association AP (1994) Diagnostic and Statistical Manual of mental Disorders. Washington DC: American Psychiatric Press.
3. Kanner L (1943) Autistic Disturbances of Affective Contact. Nervous Child 2: 217–250.
4. Plaisted K, O'Riordan M, Baron-Cohen S (1998) Enhanced visual search for a conjunctive target in autism: a research note. J Child Psychol Psychiatry 39: 777–783.
5. Keehn B, Brenner L, Palmer E, Lincoln AJ, Muller RA (2008) Functional brain organization for visual search in ASD. J Int Neuropsychol Soc 14: 990–1003.
6. Joseph RM, Keehn B, Connolly C, Wolfe JM, Horowitz TS (2009) Why is visual search superior in autism spectrum disorder? Dev Sci 12: 1083–1096.
7. Shah A, Frith U (1993) Why do autistic individuals show superior performance on the block design task? J Child Psychol Psychiatry 34: 1351–1364.
8. Happe FG (1994) Wechsler IQ profile and theory of mind in autism: a research note. J Child Psychol Psychiatry 35: 1461–1471.
9. Deruelle C, Rondan C, Salle-Collemiche X, Bastard-Rosset D, Da Fonseca D (2008) Attention to low- and high-spatial frequencies in categorizing facial identities, emotions and gender in children with autism. Brain Cogn 66: 115–123.
10. Dakin S, Frith U (2005) Vagaries of visual perception in autism. Neuron 48: 497–507.
11. Deruelle C, Rondan C, Gepner B, Tardif C (2004) Spatial frequency and face processing in children with autism and Asperger syndrome. J Autism Dev Disord 34: 199–210.
12. Frith U, Happe F (1994) Autism: beyond "theory of mind". Cognition 50: 115–132.
13. Caron MJ, Mottron L, Berthiaume C, Dawson M (2006) Cognitive mechanisms, specificity and neural underpinnings of visuospatial peaks in autism. Brain 129: 1789–1802.
14. Shah A, Frith U (1983) An islet of ability in autistic children: a research note. J Child Psychol Psychiatry 24: 613–620.
15. Mottron L, Burack JA, Iarocci G, Belleville S, Enns JT (2003) Locally oriented perception with intact global processing among adolescents with high-functioning autism: evidence from multiple paradigms. J Child Psychol Psychiatry 44: 904–913.
16. Mottron L, Belleville S, Menard E (1999) Local bias in autistic subjects as evidenced by graphic tasks: perceptual hierarchization or working memory deficit? J Child Psychol Psychiatry 40: 743–755.
17. Happe FG (1996) Studying weak central coherence at low levels: children with autism do not succumb to visual illusions. A research note. J Child Psychol Psychiatry 37: 873–877.
18. Ropar D, Mitchell P (1999) Are individuals with autism and Asperger's syndrome susceptible to visual illusions? J Child Psychol Psychiatry 40: 1283–1293.
19. Navon D (1977) Forest before trees: the precedence of global features in the visual perception. Cognitive Psychology 9: 253–383.
20. Plaisted K, Swettenham J, Rees L (1999) Children with autism show local precedence in a divided attention task and global precedence in a selective attention task. J Child Psychol Psychiatry 40: 733–742.
21. Rondan C, Deruelle C (2007) Global and configural visual processing in adults with autism and Asperger syndrome. Res Dev Disabil 28: 197–206.
22. Rinehart NJ, Bradshaw JL, Moss SA, Brereton AV, Tonge BJ (2000) Atypical interference of local detail on global processing in high-functioning autism and Asperger's disorder. J Child Psychol Psychiatry 41: 769–778.
23. Porter MA, Coltheart M (2006) Global and local processing in Williams syndrome, autism, and Down syndrome: perception, attention, and construction. Dev Neuropsychol 30: 771–789.
24. Ozonoff S, Strayer DL, McMahon WM, Filloux F (1994) Executive function abilities in autism and Tourette syndrome: an information processing approach. J Child Psychol Psychiatry 35: 1015–1032.
25. Mottron L, Burack JA, Stauder JE, Robaey P (1999) Perceptual processing among high-functioning persons with autism. J Child Psychol Psychiatry 40: 203–211.
26. Perreault A, Gurnsey R, Dawson M, Mottron L, Bertone A (2011) Increased sensitivity to mirror symmetry in autism. PLoS One 6: e19519.
27. Mottron L, Dawson M, Soulieres I, Hubert B, Burack J (2006) Enhanced perceptual functioning in autism: an update, and eight principles of autistic perception. J Autism Dev Disord 36: 27–43.
28. Wang L, Mottron L, Peng D, Berthiaume C, Dawson M (2007) Local bias and local-to-global interference without global deficit: a robust finding in autism under various conditions of attention, exposure time, and visual angle. Cogn Neuropsychol 24: 550–574.
29. Remington AM, Swettenham JG, Lavie N (2012) Lightening the Load: Perceptual Load Impairs Visual Detection in Typical Adults but Not in Autism. J Abnorm Psychol. In Press.
30. Mendes M, Silva F, Simoes L, Jorge M, Saraiva J, et al. (2005) Visual magnocellular and structure from motion perceptual deficits in a neurodevelopmental model of dorsal stream function. Brain Res Cogn Brain Res 25: 788–798.
31. Castelo-Branco M, Mendes M, Sebastiao AR, Reis A, Soares M, et al. (2007) Visual phenotype in Williams-Beuren syndrome challenges magnocellular theories explaining human neurodevelopmental visual cortical disorders. J Clin Invest 117: 3720–3729.
32. Mervis CB, Robinson BF, Bertrand J, Morris CA, Klein-Tasman BP, et al. (2000) The Williams syndrome cognitive profile. Brain Cogn 44: 604–628.
33. Wang PP, Doherty S, Rourke SB, Bellugi U (1995) Unique profile of visuo-perceptual skills in a genetic syndrome. Brain Cogn 29: 54–65.
34. Bellugi U, Lichtenberger L, Jones W, Lai Z, St George M (2000) I. The neurocognitive profile of Williams Syndrome: a complex pattern of strengths and weaknesses. J Cogn Neurosci 12 Suppl 1: 7–29.
35. Meyer-Lindenberg A, Mervis CB, Berman KF (2006) Neural mechanisms in Williams syndrome: a unique window to genetic influences on cognition and behaviour. Nat Rev Neurosci 7: 380–393.
36. Farran EK, Jarrold C, Gathercole SE (2003) Divided attention, selective attention and drawing: processing preferences in Williams syndrome are dependent on the task administered. Neuropsychologia 41: 676–687.
37. Rondan C, Santos A, Mancini J, Livet MO, Deruelle C (2008) Global and local processing in Williams syndrome: drawing versus perceiving. Child Neuropsychol 14: 237–248.
38. Lord C, Rutter M, Le Couteur A (1994) Autism Diagnostic Interview-Revised: a revised version of a diagnostic interview for caregivers of individuals with possible pervasive developmental disorders. J Autism Dev Disord 24: 659–685.
39. Lord C, Rutter M, DiLavore P, Risis S (1999) Autism Diagnostic Observation Schedule (ADOS). Los Angeles: Western Psychological Services.
40. Rutter M, Bailey A, Lord C (2003) Social Communication Questionnaire. Los Angeles: Western Psychological Services.
41. Wechsler D (2003) Manual for intelligence scale for children. Lisbon: Cegoc-Tea.
42. Wechsler D (2008) Manual for intelligence scale for adults. Lisbon: Cegoc-Tea.
43. Porter MA, Coltheart M (2005) Cognitive heterogeneity in Williams syndrome. Dev Neuropsychol 27: 275–306.
44. Navon D (2003) What does a compound letter tell the psychologist's mind? Acta Psychol (Amst) 114: 273–309.
45. Reiss JE, Hoffman JE, Landau B (2005) Motion processing specialization in Williams syndrome. Vision Res 45: 3379–3390.
46. Atkinson J, Braddick O, Anker S, Curran W, Andrew R, et al. (2003) Neurobiological models of visuospatial cognition in children with Williams syndrome: measures of dorsal-stream and frontal function. Dev Neuropsychol 23: 139–172.
47. Atkinson J, Braddick O, Rose FE, Searcy YM, Wattam-Bell J, et al. (2006) Dorsal-stream motion processing deficits persist into adulthood in Williams syndrome. Neuropsychologia 44: 828–833.
48. Jackowski AP, Rando K, Maria de Araujo C, Del Cole CG, Silva I, et al. (2009) Brain abnormalities in Williams syndrome: a review of structural and functional magnetic resonance imaging findings. Eur J Paediatr Neurol 13: 305–316.
49. Meyer-Lindenberg A, Kohn P, Mervis CB, Kippenhan JS, Olsen RK, et al. (2004) Neural basis of genetically determined visuospatial construction deficit in Williams syndrome. Neuron 43: 623–631.

50. Mobbs D, Eckert MA, Menon V, Mills D, Korenberg J, et al. (2007) Reduced parietal and visual cortical activation during global processing in Williams syndrome. Dev Med Child Neurol 49: 433–438.
51. Spencer J, O'Brien J, Riggs K, Braddick O, Atkinson J, et al. (2000) Motion processing in autism: evidence for a dorsal stream deficiency. Neuroreport 11: 2765–2767.
52. Bertone A, Mottron L, Jelenic P, Faubert J (2003) Motion perception in autism: a "complex" issue. J Cogn Neurosci 15: 218–225.
53. Koldewyn K, Whitney D, Rivera SM (2010) The psychophysics of visual motion and global form processing in autism. Brain 133: 599–610.
54. Koldewyn K, Whitney D, Rivera SM (2011) Neural correlates of coherent and biological motion perception in autism. Dev Sci 14: 1075–1088.
55. Poirel N, Simon G, Cassotti M, Leroux G, Perchey G, et al. (2011) The shift from local to global visual processing in 6-year-old children is associated with grey matter loss. PLoS One 6: e20879.

4

Genome-Wide Histone Acetylation Is Altered in a Transgenic Mouse Model of Huntington's Disease

Karen N. McFarland[1¤a], Sudeshna Das[2], Ting Ting Sun[1], Dmitri Leyfer[2¤b], Eva Xia[1], Gavin R. Sangrey[1], Alexandre Kuhn[3], Ruth Luthi-Carter[3], Timothy W. Clark[2], Ghazaleh Sadri-Vakili[1], Jang-Ho J. Cha[1]*

1 Department of Neurology, MassGeneral Institute for Neurodegenerative Disease, Massachusetts General Hospital, Charlestown, Massachusetts, United States of America, **2** MIND Informatics, MassGeneral Institute for Neurodegenerative Disease, Massachusetts General Hospital, Cambridge, Massachusetts, United States of America, **3** Brain Mind Institute, Ecole Polytechnique Fédérale de Lausanne, Lausanne, Switzerland

Abstract

In Huntington's disease (HD; MIM ID #143100), a fatal neurodegenerative disorder, transcriptional dysregulation is a key pathogenic feature. Histone modifications are altered in multiple cellular and animal models of HD suggesting a potential mechanism for the observed changes in transcriptional levels. In particular, previous work has suggested an important link between decreased histone acetylation, particularly acetylated histone H3 (AcH3; H3K9K14ac), and downregulated gene expression. However, the question remains whether changes in histone modifications correlate with transcriptional abnormalities across the entire transcriptome. Using chromatin immunoprecipitation paired with microarray hybridization (ChIP-chip), we interrogated AcH3-gene interactions genome-wide in striata of 12-week old wild-type (WT) and transgenic (TG) R6/2 mice, an HD mouse model, and correlated these interactions with gene expression levels. At the level of the individual gene, we found decreases in the number of sites occupied by AcH3 in the TG striatum. In addition, the total number of genes bound by AcH3 was decreased. Surprisingly, the loss of AcH3 binding sites occurred within the coding regions of the genes rather than at the promoter region. We also found that the presence of AcH3 at any location within a gene strongly correlated with the presence of its transcript in both WT and TG striatum. In the TG striatum, treatment with histone deacetylase (HDAC) inhibitors increased global AcH3 levels with concomitant increases in transcript levels; however, AcH3 binding at select gene loci increased only slightly. This study demonstrates that histone H3 acetylation at lysine residues 9 and 14 and active gene expression are intimately tied in the rodent brain, and that this fundamental relationship remains unchanged in an HD mouse model despite genome-wide decreases in histone H3 acetylation.

Editor: Judith Homberg, Radboud University, The Netherlands

Funding: This work was supported by the Huntington's Disease Society of America Coalition for the Cure, the Glendorn Foundation, the National Institutes of Health (NIH NS38106, NS45242) and the Massachusetts General Hospital Fund for Medical Discovery. The funders had no role in study design, data collection and analysis, decision to publish, or preparation of the manuscript.

Competing Interests: The authors have declared that no competing interests exist.

* E-mail: j.cha@merck.com

¤a Current address: Department of Neurology, McKnight Brain Institute, University of Florida, Gainesville, Florida, United States of America
¤b Current address: The Broad Institute, Cambridge, Massachusetts, United States of America

Introduction

Huntington's disease (HD) is a progressive neurodegenerative disorder resulting from a trinucleotide CAG repeat expansion in the *Huntingtin* gene [1]. Pathologically, HD is characterized by a preponderance of neuronal death in the striatum (caudate-putamen). HD patients suffer a triad of movement, cognitive and behavioral issues which steadily worsen throughout the course of the disease [2]. There are currently no effective treatments and the key pathogenic mechanisms that are responsible for the striatal vulnerability leading to the progressive neurodegeneration are unknown.

Transcriptional dysregulation is a characteristic of the disease process in human patients and is faithfully recapitulated in multiple animal and cellular models [3]. Abnormalities in transcription occur prior to the onset of symptoms and are accompanied by changes in histone acetylation, ubiquitylation and methylation [4–9]. However, whether changes in histone modifications result in the transcriptional abnormalities remains a largely unanswered question.

In particular, acetylation of the N-terminal tail of histone H3 is an activating mark for gene expression [10,11], and increases in histone acetylation precede and facilitate increased transcriptional activity [12,13]. In HD, levels of acetylated histone H3 (AcH3) associated with downregulated genes are decreased [6]. In an HD cell line and transgenic HD mouse model, mRNA abnormalities were reversed by treatment with inhibitors of histone deacetylases (HDAC), the family of enzymes that remove acetyl groups from histone tails, with concomitant increases in global histone H3 acetylation [6]. Furthermore, decreases in histone acetylation and mRNA levels in the HD cell line can be mimicked in wild-type cells by inhibiting histone acetyltransferases (HATs), enzymes that catalyze the removal of acetyl groups from histone proteins [6]. These results, though limited to a few genes, suggest that decreasing histone acetylation at gene loci is necessary and sufficient for concomitant decreases in mRNA levels. Subsequently, HDAC inhibition is currently being investigated as potential therapeutic intervention for HD as well as other neurodegenerative disorders [14,15]. However, the relationship between histone acetylation and gene expression has not been studied at the level of the whole genome in the mammalian brain. Furthermore, it is not currently known whether this relationship is altered in the HD brain. While we do know that global levels of histone acetylation do not correspond to histones at specific gene loci [6], it is unknown if the genome-wide distribution of histone acetylation is altered in HD or if the genomic distribution of histone acetylation accounts for gene expression abnormalities.

We used a genome-wide approach to capture acetylated histone H3 K9/K14 (AcH3)-DNA interactions and interrogated the chromatin immunoprecipitation products on DNA microarrays (ChIP-chip) to determine genomic locations of AcH3 in the striatum of wild-type (WT) and transgenic (TG) R6/2 mice, a mouse model for HD [16]. This analysis allowed us to examine AcH3-binding events at gene loci in WT and TG brain and then to draw comparisons of differential binding states. Using a previously published gene expression microarray dataset of R6/2 mice at the same age [17], we then correlated AcH3-bound gene loci with steady-state gene expression levels in the striatum.

We find that AcH3-gene associations are decreased genome-wide in the TG R6/2 striatum. In both WT and TG striata, AcH3 is predominately located within the coding region of the gene as opposed to the upstream promoter region. Additionally, AcH3 association at gene loci strongly correlates with genes that are actively expressed in both WT and TG striatum, suggesting that the fundamental relationship between histone H3 acetylation and gene transcription is not altered in transgenic mice. Furthermore, HDAC inhibitor treatment of TG R6/2 mice reverses transcriptional abnormalities of individual gene and increases global levels of histone H3 acetylation but AcH3 levels at specific gene loci are increased for only a handful of the tested genes. Thus, these data indicate that the overall chromatin environment surrounding a gene is more influential for the transcriptional activity of that gene. These data reveal for the first time the strong correlation between transcription and histone H3 acetylation in the brain and demonstrate that this fundamental relationship is unchanged in an HD mouse model.

Results

DNA products of acetylated histone H3 K9/K14 (AcH3) chromatin immunoprecipitations (ChIP) from WT and TG striatum were labeled and hybridized on promoter microarrays consisting of 60-mer oligonucleotide probes that comprise over 18,000 genes, each of which is represented across multiple probes. Though the microarray used was a genomic promoter microarray, thus representing only a fraction of the entire genome as a tiling microarray would, probes were distributed across the entire gene region and were not restricted to the upstream region of the core promoter immediately near the transcriptional start site of the gene.

AcH3 levels are decreased at gene loci in R6/2 TG striatum

In the wild-type (WT) striatum, we find that AcH3 is present at 10,187 probes or 2.1% of total probes (Figure 1A). These AcH3-bound probes are distributed across 5,606 genes representing 29.6% of genes on the microarray (Figure 1B). At a single gene locus, AcH3 binds at a maximum of 14 individual probes (Figure 2A).

In the transgenic (TG) R6/2 striatum, we find that AcH3 is bound to 5,542 probes representing 1.2% of total probes, a level that is 54.4% of that seen in WT littermates (Figure 1A). In the TG striatum, these AcH3-bound probes are distributed across 4,011 genes (21.2% of total genes, 71.5% of WT littermates, Figure 1B) and bind a maximum of 7 probes per gene (Figure 2A).

AcH3 binding is distributed evenly amongst and along chromosomes

To determine the genome-wide distribution of AcH3 bound genes, we first determined the total number of annotated genes represented on the microarray for each chromosome. We then calculated the percentage of AcH3-bound genes per chromosome. As seen in Figure 2B, AcH3 binding events in the WT striatum are distributed relatively evenly across all chromosomes. In the TG striatum, decreases in histone H3 acetylation were seen across all chromosomes and averaged to approximately 70% of WT levels with the exclusion of chromosome Y which is represented by only 9 genes on the Agilent array. The largest decreases were seen on chromosome 8 where AcH3-gene associations were 54% of WT and the smallest were on chromosome 3 where associations in TG is 87% of WT levels.

Visualization of AcH3 binding events along each chromosome clearly demonstrates that AcH3-gene associations are evenly distributed in WT (Figure 3A). Any clustering of AcH3 binding is primarily due to the high density of genes in these regions (note the clustering of black lines representing gene locations, in Figure 3). Acetylated histone H3 distribution patterns are similar between chromosomes and are not in highly isolated patches along each individual chromosome. In the TG striatum, we see a similar pattern as well in spite of reduced AcH3 levels (Figure 3B). Thus, despite overall decreases in AcH3 levels in the TG striatum, this decrease does not appear to be biased towards any chromosome region.

AcH3 is localized within the coding region of the gene

To determine where AcH3-bound probes are located within the gene, we examined the bound probes by probe type as defined by Agilent's annotation—Promoter, Inside, Downstream, Divergent Promoter and Unknown (see Figure 4A). Here, we examined the number of bound probes as a percentage of total probe type as the promoter and inside probes were predominately represented on the microarray. In the WT striatum, we find that of the 10,187 AcH3-bound probes, AcH3 localization within the gene is unevenly distributed and is found primarily bound to inside probes, which encompasses the coding region of the gene, as well as a smaller percentage of promoter probes (Figure 4B). AcH3-bound probes in the TG striatum follow a similar pattern as in the WT striatum but are decreased with levels ranging from 45% to 67% percent of WT (Figure 4B).

Individual genes can have unique AcH3 binding signatures with AcH3 present only at one region (i.e., exclusively at promoter regions) or a combination of regions (i.e., promoter and inside regions together). Accordingly, we analyzed AcH3-bound genes for these binding signatures and find that the majority of AcH3-bound genes have AcH3 exclusively within the inside coding region (Figure 4C). A smaller number of genes have AcH3 bound solely at the promoter region and an even smaller group of genes have AcH3 bound at both the promoter and inside region together or in the divergent promoter only. In this analysis, we unexpectedly found that decreases in AcH3-bound genes in the TG striatum did not occur evenly for all categories. AcH3-gene associations within "Promoter Only", "Downstream Only" as well as "Inside & Downstream" categories remained at levels similar to WT. AcH3 bound at "Promoter & Inside" regions in addition to "Promoter & Downstream" regions were dramatically reduced to

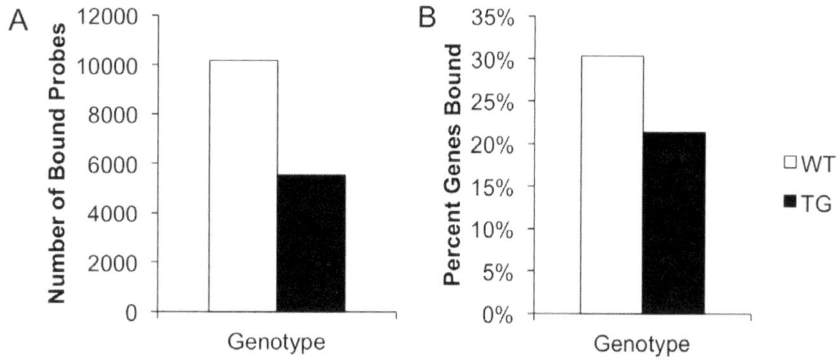

Figure 1. AcH3 interactions at gene loci are decreased in TG striata. (A) The number of AcH3-bound probes in WT (white bars) and TG (black bars) striata. (B) Percent of total genes bound by AcH3 in WT and TG striata.

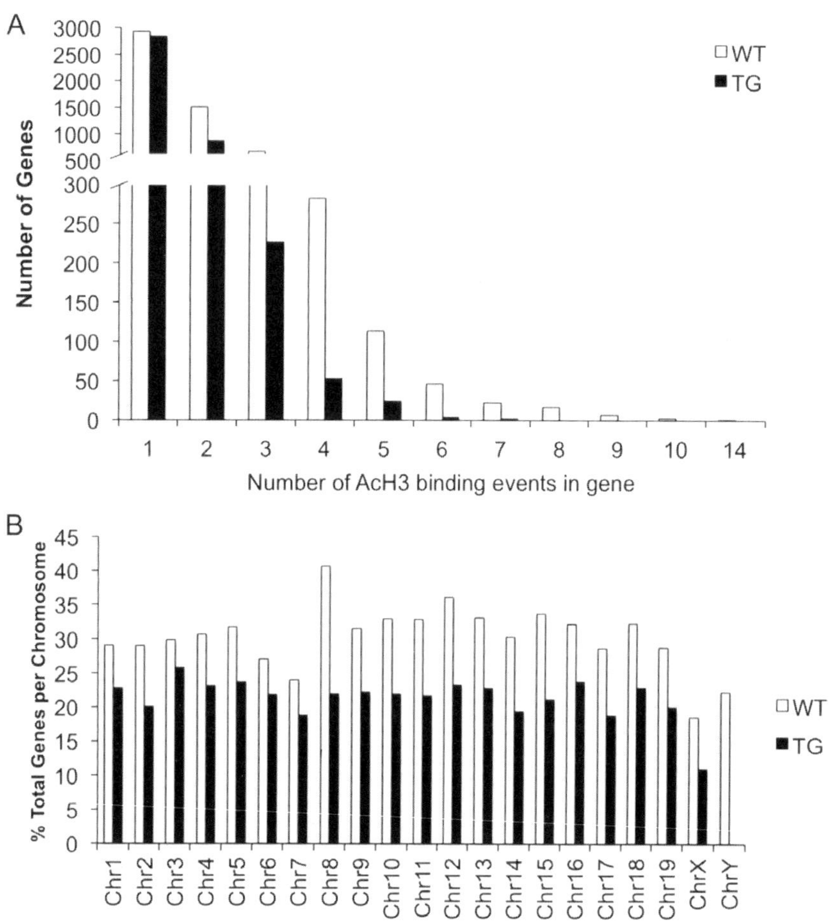

Figure 2. AcH3 binding patterns within a gene and across chromosomes are diminished in TG striata. (A) Distribution of the number of AcH3 binding events in WT and TG striata expressed as probes bound per gene. (B) Distribution of AcH3-gene associations for each chromosome in WT and TG striata expressed as a percentage of AcH3-bound genes per total genes on each chromosome. White bars, WT; black bars, TG.

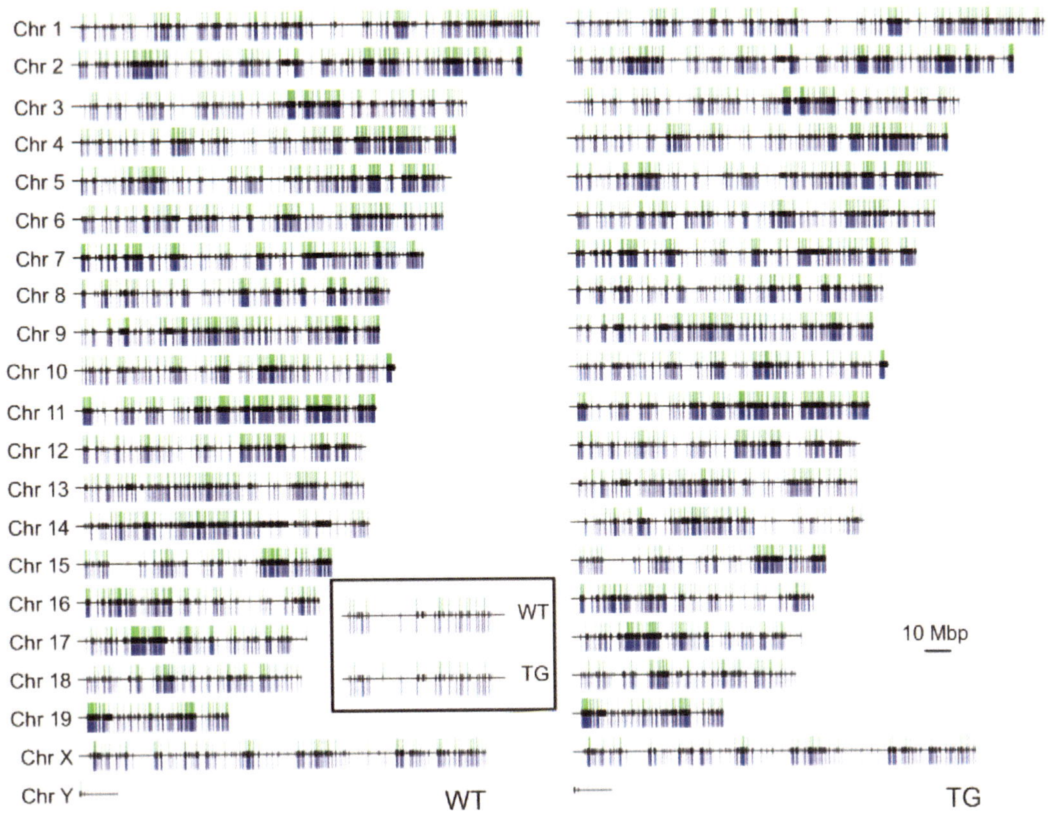

Figure 3. AcH3-gene associations are distributed across the genome and correlate with expressed genes. Localization of AcH3-gene interactions (green) along each chromosome and are co-localized with steady-state gene expression (blue) in WT (left) and TG striata (right). Horizontal black line, length of chromosome; Vertical black lines, locations of genes. Inset, a closer view of Chromosome 1 from 90574275 bp–93452450 bp.

45% and 30% of WT levels, respectively. The remaining categories of AcH3-bound genes were reduced to levels ranging from 66 to 70% of WT.

Individual genes are differentially acetylated between WT and TG striatum

We next examined differential histone H3 acetylation patterns between WT and TG striata at individual genes. Here, we utilized the results from our composite score analysis. This score allows us to quantitatively determine levels of AcH3 levels at gene loci by accounting for the number of probes bound at the gene but also the signal intensity of these probes. With this method we identified genes with decreased histone H3 acetylation in TG (Table 1) as well as a lesser number of genes with increased histone H3 acetylation in TG (Table 2).

Using the composite score, we further categorized four types of differential AcH3-gene binding: 1) "Not acetylated in TG", where AcH3 is bound at the gene in WT, but not in TG; 2) "Hypoacetylated in TG", where AcH3 is bound at the gene in both WT and TG but to a lesser degree in TG; 3) "Ectopically acetylated in TG", where AcH3 is bound at the gene in TG, but not in WT; and 4) "Hyperacetylated in TG", where AcH3 is bound at the gene in both WT and TG, but to a greater degree in TG (Figure 5). A large number of genes fell into a fifth category where AcH3 was not present at the gene in either WT or TG striata. In this comparison between WT and TG striata, we find differential AcH3 levels are predominately decreased with "Hypoacetylated in TG" and "Not acetylated in TG" categories accounting for greater than 85% of the changes seen. Surprisingly, in spite of globally decreased levels of AcH3-gene interactions in TG striatum, we also found genes with increased histone acetylation at specific gene loci in TG striatum which accounted for the remaining 13.2% differentially acetylated genes.

We analyzed the genes within these four categories ("Hypoacetylated in TG", "Not acetylated in TG", "Hyperacetylated in TG" and "Ectopically acetylated in TG") for gene ontology (GO) functional annotation term clustering to identify similar GO terms associated with these gene lists (Tables S3, S4, S5, S6). Annotation clustering ranks groups of functionally related annotations [18]. For our analysis, we included functional groups with enrichment scores of greater than 1.3 as this corresponds to a non-log value of 0.05. Not surprisingly as it was the most numerous list, "hypoacetylated in TG" genes were the most densely populated list of annotation clusters. "Not acetylated in TG" genes also had a number of annotation clusters and only a handful of these clusters were shared between these two gene lists (e.g., protein localization or mRNA processing). "Hyperacetylated in TG" and "ectopically acetylated in TG" gene lists each had only two annotation clusters with an enrichment score of 1.3 or greater. These clusters included genes involved in transcription (cluster 1, hyperacetylated in TG) and protein localization (cluster 2, hyperacetylated in TG) as well as gonad development and reproductive processes (cluster 1, ectopically acetylated in TG) and cell motility and migration (cluster 2, ectopically acetylated in TG).

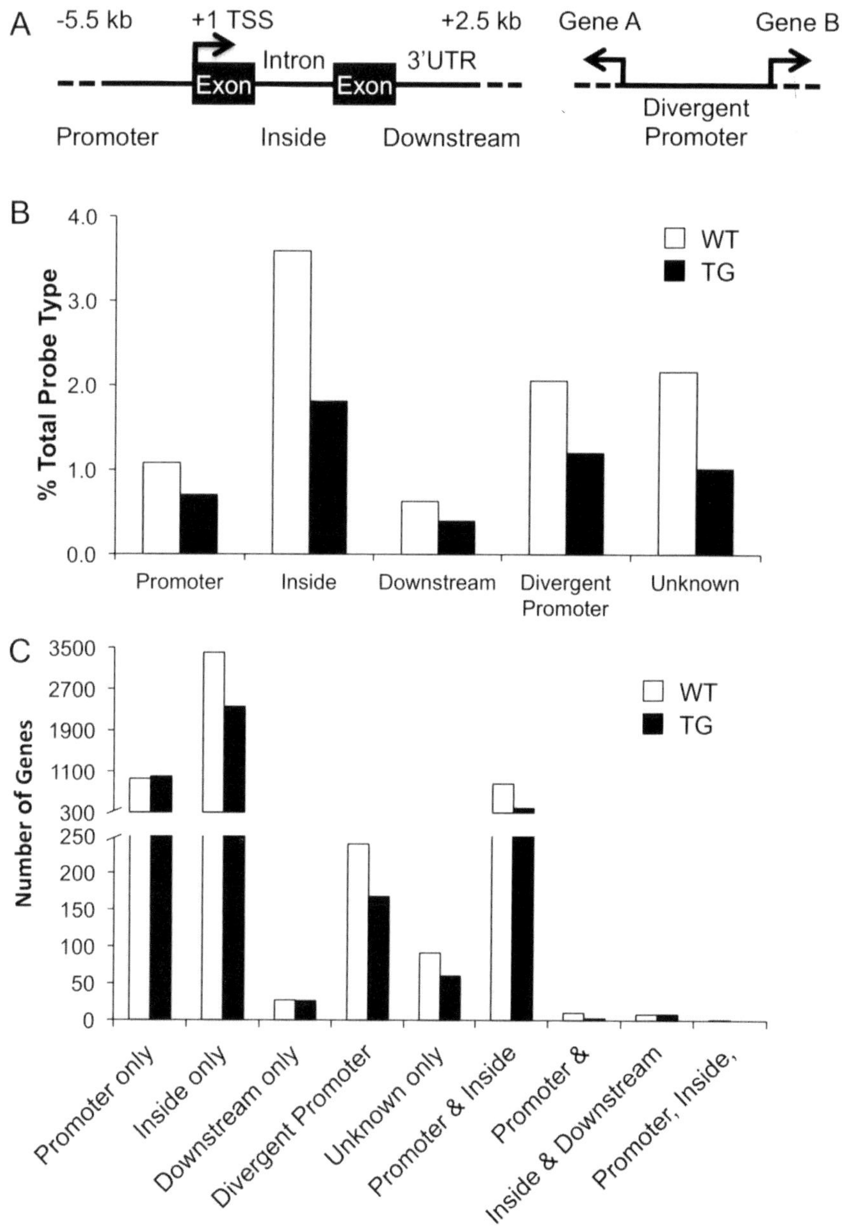

Figure 4. AcH3 localization is found downstream of transcriptional start sites within the gene. (A) Schematic indicating the location of probes as defined by Agilent annotation. Promoter = upstream of transcriptional start site; Inside = within coding region of gene; Downstream = downstream of coding region; Divergent promoter = located within the upstream region of two genes transcribed in opposite directions; Unknown = unannotated. (B) Locations of probes within the gene expressed as percent bound of total probe type within the microarray. (C) Numbers of genes bound as expressed by AcH3-bound locationsWhite bars, WT; black bars, TG.

Single Gene ChIP confirmation

We then ranked genes using the composite score to determine those with the greatest changes in histone H3 acetylation levels between WT and TG. Genes with the greatest decreases in histone H3 acetylation are listed in Table 1. Within this table, the majority of these genes are classified as hypoacetylated given that the probes for these gene are bound in both WT and TG with a reduced number of probes and reduced signal (data not shown) for that gene bound in TG striata. Using the same approach, we ranked genes whose acetylation levels are increased in TG striata (Table 2).

We then designed gene-specific primers for single-gene ChIP testing of hypoacetylated gene loci. The primer pairs were based on the microarray annotation supplied by Agilent and amplified genomic sequences surrounding differentially bound probes within the gene loci. Of those genes tested, we confirmed that there is a decrease in AcH3-association at these gene loci in TG striata (Figure 6A). We performed a similar analysis of hyperacetylated genes—AcH3 association was increased in the TG striatum at only a few of the genes tested (Figure 6B); however, these increases did not reach a level of significance.

Table 1. The top genes with decreased histone H3 acetylation in TG striata.

Rank	Gene Symbol	Gene Name	Chromosome	No of WT Probes	No of TG Probes	Composite Score
1	*Zfp469/Tnrc18*	*zinc finger protein 469; trinucleotide repeat containing protein 18*	chr5	14	6	−11.33
2	*Per1*	*period homolog 1 (Drosophila)*	chr11	8	2	−10.60
3	*BC057627/Zc3h4*	*zinc finger CCCH-type containing type 4*	chr7	10	2	−10.53
4	*Pik3r1*	*phosphatidylinositol 3-kinase, regulatory subunit, polypeptide 1 (p85 alpha)*	chr13	9	3	−9.17
5	*Homer1*	*homer homolog 1 (Drosophila)*	chr13	9	2	−8.59
6	*mmu-mir-124a-2*	*microRNA*	chr3	9	1	−8.53
7	*Lrrtm2*	*leucine rich repeat transmembrane neuronal 2*	chr18	9	4	−8.02
8	*Cpeb4*	*cytoplasmic polyadenylation element binding protein 4*	chr11	10	5	−7.90
9	*Gpm6a*	*glycoprotein m6a*	chr8	8	1	−7.81
10	*Chn1*	*chimerin (chimaerin) 1*	chr2	9	3	−7.67
11	*Elmod1*	*ELMO domain containing 1*	chr9	7	1	−7.65
12	*Epc1*	*enhancer of polycomb homolog 1*	chr18	10	5	−7.49
13	*Stmn4*	*stathmin-like 4*	chr14	6	0	−7.41
14	*Cacna2d3*	*calcium channel, voltage-dependent, alpha2/delta subunit 3*	chr14	6	0	−7.39
15	*Rtn1*	*reticulon 1*	chr12	8	2	−7.32
16	*Negr1*	*neuronal growth regulator 1*	chr3	8	3	−7.12
17	*Sec14l1*	*SEC14-like 1 (S. cerevisiae)*	chr11	6	1	−7.03
18	*Mgrn1*	*mahogunin, ring finger 1*	chr16	7	2	−7.00
19	*Neto1*	*neuropilin (NRP) and tolloid (TLL)-like 1*	chr18	7	3	−6.97
20	*Eif3s7/Eif3d*	*eukaryotic translation initiation factor 3, subunit D*	chr15	8	2	−6.95
21	*Grik2*	*glutamate receptor, ionotropic, kainate 2 (beta 2)*	chr10	7	3	−6.91
22	*Bat2*	*HLA-B associated transcript 2*	chr17	8	5	−6.89
23	*Kcnj2*	*potassium inwardly-rectifying channel, subfamily J, member 2*	chr11	8	4	−6.81
24	*Zfhx2*	*zinc finger homeobox 2*	chr14	7	3	−6.75
25	*9430023L20Rik*	*RIKEN cDNA 9430023L20 gene*	chr15	7	1	−6.74
26	*Rab30*	*RAB30, member RAS oncogene family*	chr7	8	4	−6.63
27	*mmu-mir-124a-1*	*microRNA*	chr14	8	5	−6.61
28	*Mark2*	*MAP/microtubule affinity-regulating kinase 2*	chr19	6	2	−6.58
29	*Cugbp2*	*CUGBP, Elav-like family member 2*	chr2	8	2	−6.55
30	*Rgs9*	*regulator of G-protein signaling 9*	chr11	5	1	−6.50

Gene symbol annotation for these genes was checked with NCBI's Entrez Gene database (http://www.ncbi.nlm.nih.gov/sites/entrez). In the instances where gene annotation has been updated, we have left the original Agilent annotation intact and added the updated information subsequent to this in the form of Original Gene Symbol/Updated Gene Symbol.

Histone H3 acetylation at gene loci predicts active gene transcription

We further investigated the relationship between histone H3 acetylation at the gene and expression of that gene. Here, we wanted to determine whether the presence of histone H3 acetylation at the gene loci correlates to the presence of the gene's transcript upon analysis of gene expression microarrays. For this, we confined our analysis to the subset of nearly 13,000 genes that are common to both the Agilent ChIP-chip microarrays as well as the Affymetrix expression microarrays.

We examined the association between histone H3 acetylation at gene loci and the presence of the gene transcript in WT and TG striatum (Tables 3 & 4, respectively). We simplified this analysis by qualitatively categorizing each gene as bound or not bound by AcH3 and its transcript as expressed or not expressed. We find that in both WT and TG striatum, the majority of AcH3-associated genes also have a gene transcript present indicating active gene transcription. In the WT striatum, 93% of genes associated with acetylated histone H3 are transcribed (Table 3) revealing a significant association between the presence of histone

Table 2. The top genes with increased histone H3 acetylation in TG striata.

Rank	Gene Symbol	Gene Name	Chromosome	No of WT Probes	No of TG Probes	Composite Score
1	*Olfr1446*	*olfactory receptor 1446*	chr19	0	2	4.03
2	*A430060F13Rik*	*RIKEN cDNA A430060F13 gene*	chr11	0	1	3.63
3	*Slc26a6*	*solute carrier family 26, member 6*	chr9	0	1	3.13
4	*Wif1*	*Wnt inhibitory factor 1*	chr10	0	1	3.05
5	*Zfp367*	*zinc finger protein 367*	chr13	1	2	2.99
6	*A130007F10Rik/Dcaf12l2*	*DDB1 and CUL4 associated factor 12-like 2*	chrX	0	3	2.67
7	*Ankrd54/C730048E16Rik-Eif3s6ip/ Eif3l*	*ankyrin repeat domain 54- eukaryotic translation initiation factor 3, subunit L*	chr15	0	1	2.30
8	*A730017C20Rik*	*RIKEN cDNA A730017C20 gene*	chr18	0	1	2.14
9	*Gprc6a*	*G protein-coupled receptor, family C, group 6, member A*	chr10	0	1	2.06
10	*BC089469/2210408I21Rik*	*RIKEN cDNA 2210408I21 gene*	chr13	0	1	1.77
11	*Olfr1500*	*olfactory receptor 1500*	chr19	0	1	1.75
12	*Tbc1d5*	*TBC1 domain family, member 5*	chr17	1	1	1.73
13	*Mrpl16*	*mitochondrial ribosomal protein L16*	chr19	0	1	1.71
14	*9230117N10Rik/Il33*	*interleukin 33*	chr19	0	1	1.60
15	*Tmem16a/Ano1*	*anoctamin 1, calcium activated chloride channel*	chr7	0	2	1.58
16	*Vkorc1l1*	*vitamin K epoxide reductase complex, subunit 1-like 1*	chr5	0	2	1.53
17	*Xrn1*	*5′-3′ exoribonuclease 1*	chr9	1	2	1.50
18	*Slc25a37*	*solute carrier family 25, member 37*	chr14	0	2	1.50
19	*Fgf9*	*fibroblast growth factor 9*	chr14	0	2	1.49
20	*Trim42*	*tripartite motif-containing 42*	chr9	0	1	1.47
21	*Olfr735*	*olfactory receptor 735*	chr14	0	1	1.42
22	*Kcnh6*	*potassium voltage-gated channel, subfamily H (eag-related), member 6*	chr11	0	2	1.41
23	*1110051M20Rik*	*RIKEN cDNA 1110051M20 gene*	chr2	0	2	1.39
24	*ENSMUST00000078552*	*Ensembl gene BX119986.8-201*	chrX	0	2	1.39
25	*Arhgap17*	*Rho GTPase activating protein 17*	chr7	0	2	1.37
26	*Chuk*	*conserved helix-loop-helix ubiquitous kinase*	chr19	2	4	1.37
27	*BC042698/Dennd1b*	*DENN/MADD domain containing 1B*	chr1	0	2	1.37
28	*Map3k3*	*mitogen-activated protein kinase kinase kinase 3*	chr11	0	2	1.37
29	*Terf2*	*telomeric repeat binding factor 2*	chr8	0	2	1.34
30	*Pisd*	*phosphatidylserine decarboxylase*	chr5	0	2	1.33

Gene symbol annotation for these genes was checked with NCBI's Entrez Gene database (http://www.ncbi.nlm.nih.gov/sites/entrez). In the instances where gene annotation has been updated, we have left the original Agilent annotation intact and added the updated information subsequent to this in the form of Original Gene Symbol/Updated Gene Symbol.

H3 acetylation at the gene locus and the presence of its transcript (odds ratio = 11.8, 99% confidence interval = 10.0, 13.9, $p<2.2e-16$). Similarly in TG striatum, 91% of AcH3-associated genes also have a gene transcript present (Table 4; odds ratio = 7.3, 99% confidence interval = 6.2, 7.3, $p<2.2e-16$). Visualizing AcH3 association at a gene locus along with the presence of its transcripts along each chromosome highlights this association in both WT and TG striata (Figure 3). Here, the coincidence of histone H3 acetylation at the gene and the presence of the gene's transcript are easily seen (see insets in Figure 3). From this analysis, we conclude that the presence of acetylated histone H3 at a gene locus is sufficient to predict its expression and that this basic relationship between histone H3 acetylation and gene expression are unaffected in the R6/2 TG striatum.

AcH3 localization within the gene region differs on gene transcription

We furthered this analysis by examining the location of AcH3 bound probes within the gene locus itself. We divided genes by their expression pattern (expressed or not expressed) and then

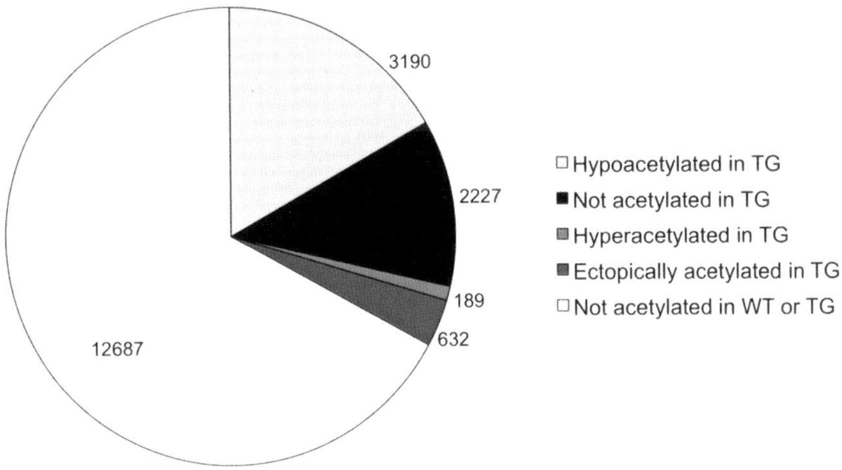

Figure 5. Differential histone H3 acetylation within WT and TG striata. Hypoacetyled in Tg (light grey), gene is bound by AcH3 in both WT and TG but binding is decreased in TG; **Not acetylated in TG** (black), AcH3 is associated with the gene only in the WT state; **Hyperacetylated in TG** (medium grey), gene is bound by AcH3 in both WT and TG but binding is increased in TG; **Ectopically acetylated in TG** (dark grey), AcH3 is associated with the gene only in the TG state; **Not acetylated**, gene does not have AcH3 associated in either WT or TG states.

categorized them by the location of AcH3 binding (Figure 7). For expressed genes, we find the AcH3 is mostly associated at the inside coding regions and these numbers are decreased numbers in the TG striatum (Figure 7). A smaller number of AcH3-expressed gene associations occur at the promoter region and at both the promoter and inside regions, a pattern identical to the previous analysis that looked at all genes regardless of their transcriptional status. However, surprisingly, a similar number of genes were bound only at the promoter between WT and TG striata (Figure 7).

For genes that are not expressed, a similar trend was seen although the overall number of AcH3 bound genes was decreased. In this case, an unexpected pattern seen in the TG striatum was the increase over WT in the number of genes bound by AcH3 at the promoter (Figure 7). Of note, AcH3 binding appeared nearly equally distributed between binding at promoter and binding at inside regions for non-expressed genes.

Differential histone H3 acetylation does not correlate well with differential gene expression

Throughout the course of our analysis, we noted that within our list of the top hypoacetylated genes, that the expression levels of five of these genes were downregulated—*Homer1*; *Cacna2d3*; *Sec14l1*; *Grik2* and *Rgs9*. To further investigate whether changes in histone H3 acetylation are associated with changes in gene expression between WT and TG striata, we examined which genes are differentially expressed and then interrogated their pattern of differential histone H3 acetylation. If we postulate that decreases in histone H3 acetylation correspond to decreases in the transcriptional activity of the associated gene, then we would expect to find that the majority of genes with decreased expression in the TG striatum also have decreases in histone H3 acetylation at the gene.

However, we find that the majority of genes with decreased expression in TG striata have no AcH3 associated at their genes in either WT or TG striata (Figure 8). Only 38% of downregulated genes have decreased levels of histone H3 acetylation at their gene loci. Unexpectedly, a similar pattern of differential histone H3 acetylation is also seen for genes with increased levels of expression in TG strata (Figure 8). Furthermore, an overwhelming majority of genes with both increases and decreases in expression levels do not have histone H3 acetylation association. Taken together, these data indicate that changes in histone H3 acetylation alone are not sufficient to account for changes in gene expression in the R6/2 HD model.

HDAC inhibitor treatment does not act at specific gene loci

Another surprising result from our study reveals that global levels of AcH3 do not predict the degree of genomic binding of AcH3. In fact, globally, AcH3 levels are marginally increased in the livers and cerebella of TG mice, as compared to WT littermates (Figure 9). Therefore, in order to determine if global HDAC inhibitor treatment changes histone H3 acetylation at individual gene loci, we treated 12-week R6/2 TG and WT littermates with phenylbutyrate or vehicle and examined changes in global histone H3 acetylation levels, gene expression and histone H3 acetylation at specfic gene loci. As expected, we find that phenylbutyrate treatment increases global histone H3 acetylation in the histone extracts from WT and TG liver (Figure 9A, B) and cerebella (Figure 9C, D). At the same time, transcript levels of downregulated genes are increased in TG striata following phenylbutyrate treatment (Figure 10A). However, at specific gene loci, only two, *Homer1* and *Cacna2d3*, of the five genes tested have increased histone H3 acetylation in the TG striatum following phenylbutyrate treatment (Figure 10B). These results suggest that changes in the global chromatin environment rather than at specific gene loci may be more important for causing transcriptional changes as a result of HDAC inhibitor treatment.

Discussion

Genome-wide histone H3 acetylation in the normal and HD mammalian striatum

This study is the first to analyze histone H3 K9/K14 acetylation (AcH3) at gene loci and gene expression across the entire genome in the mammalian brain. In the R6/2 mouse model for Huntington's disease (HD) and the corresponding control littermates, we analyzed genome-wide histone H3 acetylation at gene

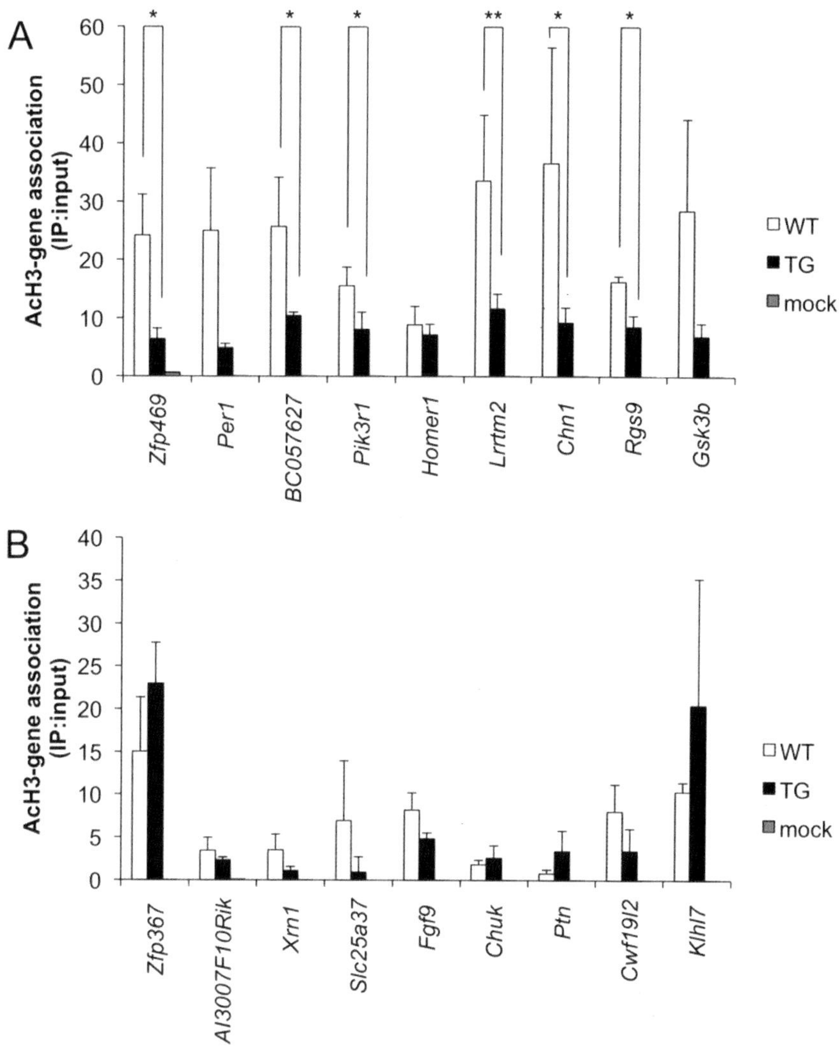

Figure 6. Single gene ChIP confirmation of differentially acetylated genes. (A) Genes with decreased acetylation as predicted by their composite score. (B) Genes with increased acetylation as predicted by their composite score. The order of the genes from left-right indicates their relative ranking by composite score. *, p-value<0.05; **, p-value<0.01. White bars, WT; black bars, TG; grey bars, mock condition. Error bars are standard deviation.

loci. An important point to note from our study is that global levels of acetylated histone H3 do not predict its levels at the genome. Though global levels were similar if not slightly elevated in TG animals, overall histone H3 K9/K14 acetylation at gene loci was decreased in the TG striatum. Furthermore, we observed in both WT and TG striatum that AcH3 localization within the gene locus was unevenly distributed and was more likely to occur within the coding region—downstream of the transcriptional start site rather than the region of the core promoter which is upstream of the transcriptional start site.

Histone H3 acetylation at gene loci predicts gene expression in WT and TG striata

Another novel result from our study comes with correlating AcH3 at gene loci with gene expression data. It is well known that increases in histone H3 acetylation precede increases in transcriptional activity [10–13] and similar correlations between histone H3 acetylation and gene expression have been made at the single gene level in multiple studies of human cell lines [19–23]. Our data are the first to demonstrate this important relationship in a normal mammalian brain as well as in a transgenic model for HD.

Table 3. Histone H3 acetylation and gene expression in WT striata.

	Gene is expressed in WT (8655)	Gene is not expressed in WT (4164)
AcH3 present at gene in WT (4475 genes)	4171	304
AcH3 is not present at gene in WT (8344 genes)	4484	3860

Table 4. Histone H3 acetylation and gene expression in TG striata.

	Gene is expressed in TG (8582)	Gene is not expressed in TG (4237)
AcH3 present at gene in TG (3158 genes)	2883	275
AcH3 is not present at gene in TG (9661 genes)	5669	3962

We found a strong correlation between the presence of acetylated K9/K14 histone H3 at a gene locus and the presence of the gene's transcript. While this finding demonstrates that histone acetylation is sufficient for gene transcription, our data do not support the notion that it is also necessary as a large number of expressed genes do not have acetylated histone H3 present at their gene locus.

Differential histone H3 acetylation does not predict transcriptional changes in HD

Furthermore, we did not find a clear pattern between differential changes in histone H3 K9/K14 acetylation with changes in gene expression between WT and TG striata. Therefore, as changes in histone H3 acetylation alone are not adequate to explain changes in gene expression, some additional mechanism must account for the downstream transcriptional changes seen in HD. This may not be too surprising given that we find fewer than half of expressed genes in the normal WT brain (and even fewer in the TG, see Tables 3 and 4) actually have associated AcH3 at their loci. These data together indicate that while histone H3 acetylation at specific gene loci is sufficient to cause increases in gene expression, there may be other mechanisms at play requiring other factors or histone modifications. One such factor may be Huntingtin (Htt) itself. Htt interactions with genomic DNA could influence transcription as we have demonstrated that Htt can interact with genomic DNA *in vivo* and *in vitro* with both wild-type and mutant forms of Htt interacting at different locations within the genome [24].

Mechanisms of systemic HDAC inhibitor treatments?

Results from our study suggest that global levels of histone H3 K9/K14 acetylation levels do not predict the levels of AcH3 present at chromatin. And despite increased global acetylated histone H3 levels and increased transcript levels of downregulated genes following HDAC inhibitor treatments, AcH3 levels at the gene were not significantly altered.

However, broad-spectrum HDAC inhibitors clearly have beneficial effects in animal models of various neurodegenerative diseases and dramatically improve multiple phenotypes. Broad-spectrum HDAC inhibitors, such as sodium butyrate, result in increased global levels of acetylated histone H3 and H4 [25–28]. Furthermore, HDAC inhibitors improve molecular, cellular and

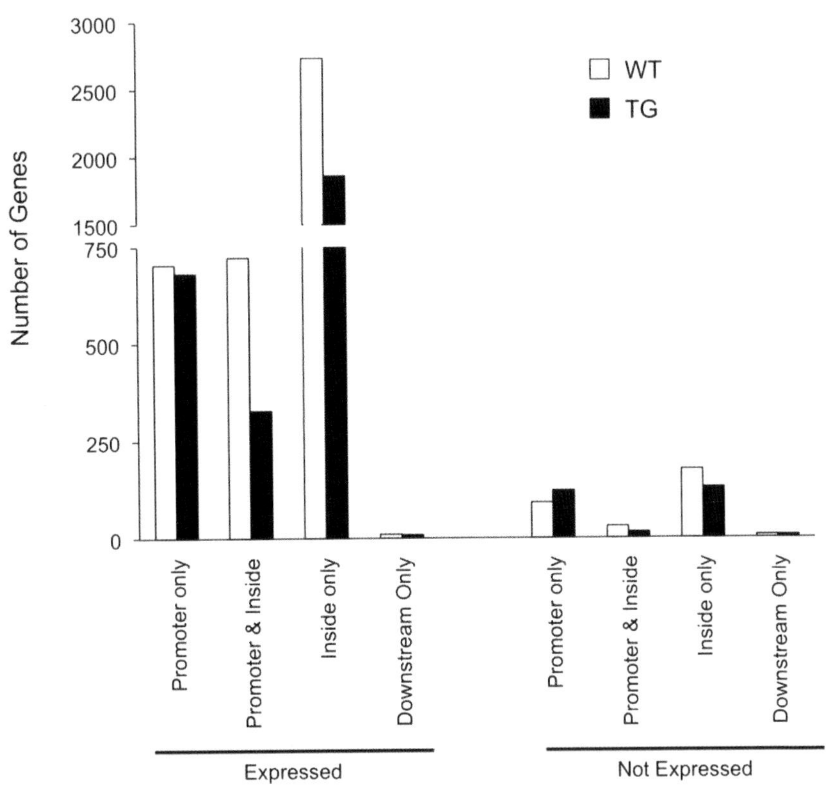

Figure 7. AcH3-localization within the gene changes upon gene expression. AcH3-localization within the gene changes on transcriptional status of the gene. White bars, WT; black bars, TG.

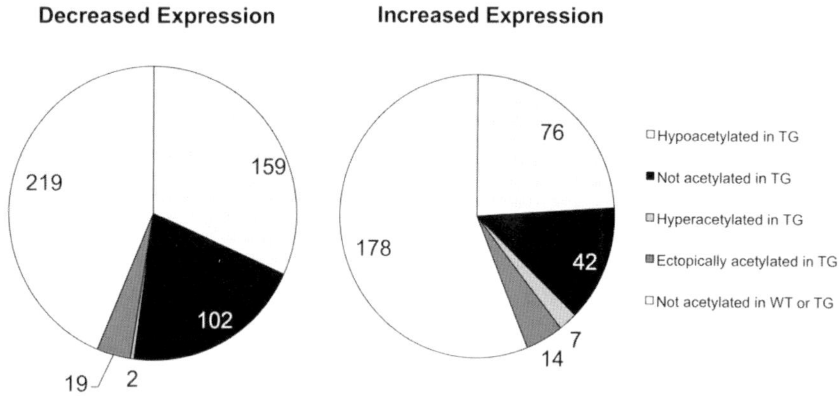

Figure 8. Gene expression changes are not strongly associated with changes in histone H3 acetylation in the R6/2 TG striatum. (A) Classification of differentially acetylated histone H3 genes whose expression are decreased in the TG striatum. (B) Classification of differentially acetylated histone H3 genes whose expression are increased in the TG striatum.

behavioral phenotypes in animal models for a number of neurodegenerative diseases including HD [6,29–34], Parkinson's disease [35], spinal and bulbar muscular atrophy [36], Alzheimer's disease [37,38], dentatorubral-pallidoluysian atrophy [39], amyotrophic lateral sclerosis [40,41] and Friedreich's ataxia [42].

If their effects are not directly on histone acetylation, how could they convey such a beneficial action? Acetylation is a relatively transient form of histone modification and may not correlate well with steady-state mRNA measurements. Thus, simply reversing decreases in AcH3 by HDAC inhibitor treatment in the TG striatum may have a beneficial impact on overall chromatin structure and the epigenetic environment. Such increases in overall acetylation levels by HDAC inhibitor treatment could then lead to changes of other histone modifications, such as ubiquitylation or methylation. Such trans-histone crosstalk is well documented for activating as well as repressive histone modifications, is predicted by the histone code [10,43] and has the potential to consolidate a transient modification such as acetylation into more stable, long-lived modifications such as ubiquitylation or methylation. For example, crosstalk between acetylation and phosphorylation plays a role in transcriptional elongation [44]. Coordination of acetylation on histone H3 and trimethylation of lysine residue 4 of histone H3 (H3K4me3), both of which are associated with active transcription, occurs through subunits of histone acetylatransferase complexes [45,46] allowing for binding of TFIID of the RNA polymerase complex to H3K4me3 [47]. Furthermore, HDAC inhibitor treatment of human cell lines increases histone acetylation with concomitant decreases in DNA methylation, a well-known indicator of silenced genes [48].

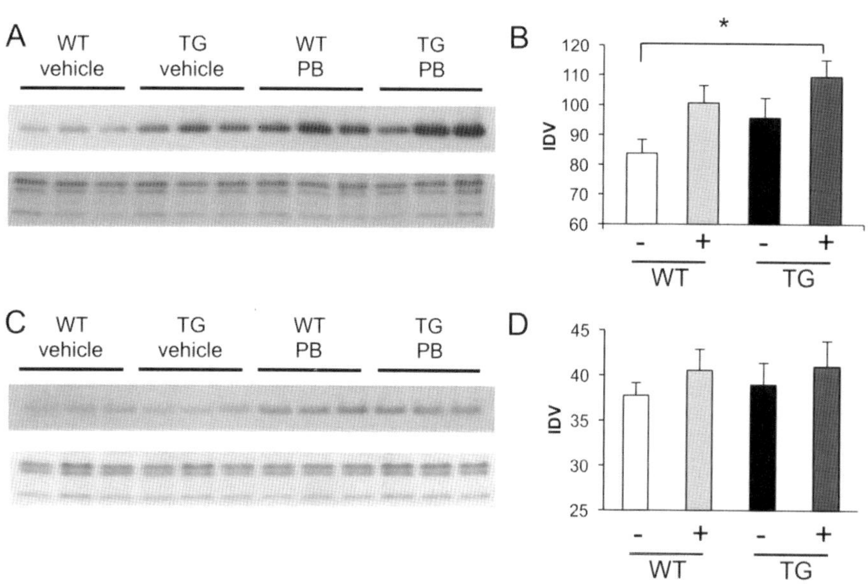

Figure 9. Phenylbutyrate treatment increases global histone H3 acetylation in R6/2 liver and cerebellum. (A) Western blot demonstrating AcH3 levels in histone extracts from WT and TG R6/2 livers (top), Coomassie blue gel staining demonstrates equal loading (bottom). (B) Integrated densitometry values (IDV) for AcH3 levels in A. (C) Western blot demonstrating AcH3 levels in histone extracts from WT and TG R6/2 cerebellum (top). Coomassie blue gel staining demonstrates equal loading (bottom). (D) Integrated densitometry values (IDV) for AcH3 levels in C. White bars, WT, vehicle (veh) treated (n = 9); Light grey bars, WT, phenylbutyrate (PB) treated (n = 8); Black bars, Tg, vehicle (veh) treated (n = 7); Dark grey bars, Tg, phenylbutyrate (PB) treated (n = 11). *, p-value<0.05. Error bars are standard deviation.

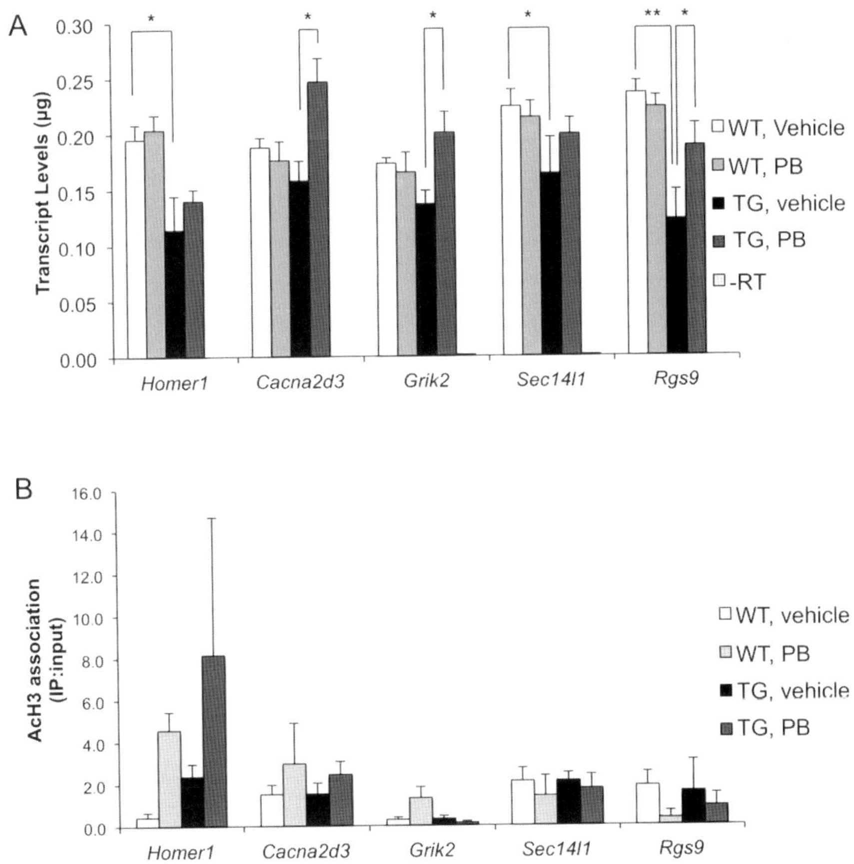

Figure 10. Phenylbutyrate treatment increases transcript levels of downregulated gene in TG striata but does not increase acetylation levels at gene loci. (A) Transcript levels of downregulated genes in the Tg striata. (B) Single-gene ChIP for the enrichment of AcH3 at gene regions. White bars, WT, vehicle treated; Light grey bars, WT, phenylbutyrate treated; Black bars, Tg, vehicle treated; Dark grey bars, Tg, phenylbutyrate treated. *, $p<0.05$; **, $p<0.01$. Error bars are standard deviation.

Additionally, HDAC inhibitor therapy may also exert effects on the non-transcriptional and nuclear, non-histone targets of HDACs as well. Disrupting HDAC1 and HDAC2 function alters their interactions with members of the Wnt signaling pathway [49]. HDACs also target non-nuclear proteins such as alpha-tubulin [50], the acetylation of which is thought to play a role in HD progression [51]. Mutant forms of Htt (mHtt) can themselves be acetylated which facilitates their clearance from the cell while inhibiting HDAC1 increases acetylated forms of mHtt and improved mHtt clearance from the cell [52].

In summary, this is the first study to demonstrate a strong link between histone acetylation and gene expression in the normal brain as well as an HD model. Global levels of AcH3 are not predictive of the degree of genomic binding of AcH3. We find that histone H3 acetylation strongly correlates with gene expression in both WT and TG R6/2 striata. AcH3 levels at gene loci are decreased in the TG striatum; however, these decreases do not correlate with changes in transcript levels of individual genes in HD. These observations suggest that gene expression changes may be related to the overall chromatin environment, part of which is determined by histone H3 K9/K14 acetylation. Furthermore, our data reveal that the mechanistic relationship between histone H3 K9/K14 acetylation at gene loci and active gene expression is unchanged in an HD model, shedding light onto other potential mechanisms for the action of HDAC inhibitor therapy in the treatment of HD and other neurodegenerative disorders.

Materials and Methods

Animals

Ethics Statement. All animal care, husbandry and experimentation were performed with the approval of and according to the guidelines set by the Massachusetts General Hospital Subcommittee on Research Animal Care.

Mouse Husbandry & Tissue Procurement. Transgenic (TG) and wild-type (WT) littermate controls from the R6/2 mouse line were used for these experiments. The TG R6/2 mouse contains the exon 1 portion of the human *Huntingtin* gene containing the CAG repeat expanded to 110 to 150 repeats and is expressed under the control of the human *Huntingtin* promoter [16]. The R6/2 line was maintained by backcrossing genotyped R6/2 TG males to F1 hybrid females from a C57BL/6 male x CBA female cross (B6CBAF1/J; The Jackson Laboratory, Bar Harbor, ME) as described [16]. In our R6/2 colony, the CAG repeat size expanded to approximately 200 repeats. 12-week old R6/2 wild-type animals were sacrificed by the administration of carbon dioxide and their brains were quickly removed and regionally dissected over ice before snap-freezing in liquid isopentane cooled with dry ice. Brains were stored at −80°C until needed.

Phenyl Butryate treatment. Twelve week old R6/2 TG and WT littermates were injected with phenylbutyrate daily by intraperitoneal injection (400 mg/kg/day, SPB11, Scandinavian Formula, Sellersville, PA) or vehicle (phosphate buffered saline) for seven consecutive days and sacrificed on the eighth day as described above. Each treatment group contained a minimum of six animals. Livers and cerebella were dissected to determine global acetylated histone H3 levels while the striata were used for ChIP assays. Analyses were performed on the dissected tissue from each animal individually.

Chromatin immunoprecipitation (ChIP) assay

ChIP homogenates were prepared from the dissected striata of R6/2 TG and WT animals according to published protocols [53,54]. For ChIP-chip experiments, each biological replicate contained striata from 8 animals (16 striata total). Each experiment contained two biological replicates. For single gene, confirmatory ChIP, a total of 4–6 biological replicates were used. Protein-DNA interactions were captured by formaldehyde crosslinking and genomic DNA was sheared to lengths of ~500 bp using a probe sonicator (Fisher Scientific, Pittsburgh, PA, Sonic Dismembrenator Model 500). Prior to ChIP, a sample of each homogenate representing 1% of the total volume was removed and set aside as input, i.e. whole-cell extract (WCE). Antibodies directed against di-acetylated histone H3 on K9 and K14 (AcH3; Millipore, Billerica, MA; catalog number 06-599) were used in ChIP reactions. Negative controls included IgG (Jackson ImmunoResearch, West Grove, PA) or no antibody conditions.

IP and WCE products from ChIP were quantified using the luciferase- and T4 DNA polymerase-based DNA Quantitation System (Promega, Madison, WI) according to manufacturer's instructions. The light output was immediately measured in a luminometer (TD-20/20 Luminometer, Turner Designs, Sunnyvale, CA). ChIP products were also quantified using Quant-iT PicoGreen dsDNA reagent (Invitrogen, Carlsbad, CA) and assayed on the Wallac Victor 1420 Multilabel Counter (PerkinElmer, Waltham, MA) with excitation and emission wavelengths of 485 nm and 535 nm, respectively.

ChIP-chip

Whole Genomic Amplification. Recovered IP and WCE DNA products were amplified using the GenomePlex Whole Genome Amplification kit (Sigma, St. Louis, MO). Ten ng of WCE or ChIP DNA was used in each reaction and the manufacturer's procotol was followed with the exception of skipping the initial random fragmentation step. The resulting product was purified using the QIAquick-PCR purification kit (Qiagen, Valencia, CA) and DNA yields were measured using a NanoDrop (ThermoScientific, Waltham, MA).

Labeling. IP and WCE amplified products were fluorescently labeled with Cy5- and Cy3-dUTP (GE Healthcare, Piscataway, NJ), respectively, using the Klenow-based BioPrime Array CGH Genomic Labeling kit (Invitrogen). 2 ug of amplified DNA was used in each reaction. Unincorporated fluorescent nucleotides were removed from DNA products using the purification columns included in the kit. Labeled products were quantified on a NanoDrop (ThermoScientific).

Hybridization and Washing. Amplified and labeled IP (Cy5) and WCE (Cy3) DNA products were hybridized to Agilent Technologies (Santa Clara, CA) mouse promoter arrays (G4490A; UCSC mm7/NCBI release 35, August 2005). These promoter arrays cover approximately 18,000 mouse transcripts with an average of 25 probes per gene. The 60-mer oligonucleotide probes are spaced every ~100–300 bp and cover −5.5 kb to +2.5 kb for a typical gene (transcriptional start site is denoted as +1).

IP and WCE-labeled DNA products (5 ug each) were combined and co-hybridized in hybridization buffer in the presence of blocking agent and mouse cot-1 DNA at a final concentration of 0.1 mg/ml. All hybridization, washing and drying buffers as well as the blocking agent were supplied as part of the Agilent aCGH hybridization kit. Arrays were placed in the Agilent hybridization chambers and hybridized in a rotisserie hybridization oven set at 20 rpm for 40 h at 65°C. Arrays were washed as follows: hybridization chamber disassembly in Oligo aCGH Wash Buffer 1 at room temperature, Oligo aCGH Wash Buffer 1 at room temperature for 5 min, Oligo aCGH Wash Buffer 2 at 37°C for 1 min, acetonitrile wash at room temp for 1 min and a final incubation in the Stabilization and Drying Solution (Agilent) for 1 min. Microarray slides were scanned at a 5 μm resolution using the Agilent scanner. Raw fluorescence intensities were obtained from scanned images using Agilent's Feature Extraction Software. Background and noise were removed from the data and the feature extractions were monitored. Fluorescent intensities of Cy5/Cy3 (IP/WCE ratios) were calculated for each individual feature on the array and represent the binding events of the amplified ChIP product.

Data Analysis. Pre-processed data were normalized and analyzed using the ChIP Analytics Software 1.3 (Agilent). Replicates were normalized together using the intra-array LOWESS intensity dependent normalization and the results were averaged using the replicate support extended Whitehead error model v1.0 and the peak detection and evaluation was computed using the Whitehead per-array Neighbourhood Model v1.0. Results of the combined analyses were used to generate spreadsheet reports for the probes, segments and gene levels results, UCSC track files, Ensembl DAS files and quality control reports. Probe intensity values were calculated by:

$$\log_2\left(\frac{normalized\quad IP\quad signal}{normalized\quad WCE\quad signal}\right)$$

For qualitative analyses, we analyzed the ChIP-chip data at the probe and gene levels in a binary bound/not bound fashion. An individual probe was defined as bound if $p \leq 0.005$, while a gene was defined as bound if at least one probe representing that gene is bound.

For quantitative analyses, we determined differentially bound genes between WT and TG samples by calculating a composite score for each gene by subtracting the summation of all WT bound probes from the summation of all TG bound probes as follows:

$$composite\ score = \left(\sum_{\substack{of\quad bound\\ probes\quad only}} \log_2\left(\frac{IP\quad signal\quad TG}{WCE\quad signal\quad TG}\right)\right) - \left(\sum_{\substack{of\quad bound\\ probes\quad only}} \log_2\left(\frac{IP\quad signal\quad WT}{WCE\quad signal\quad WT}\right)\right)$$

Gene Expression Analysis. Using a previously published gene expression microarray dataset [17] from 12-week old R6/2 TG and WT littermates, we used Affymetrix MAS5 analysis to normalize probe intensities and monitor present/absent calls. Since a single gene can be represented across multiple probesets, we calculated the expression value for each gene as the mean for all probesets representative for that gene. We defined genes as expressed in WT or TG striata when the average expression value was greater than 100. To determine differentially expressed genes, tests were computed with two-tailed unpaired t-test for unknown variance and unpaired two classes analysis using the Significance Analysis of Microarrays (SAM) algorithm using Bioconductor and R [55]. We defined genes as up- or down-regulated when the differential expression ratio was at least 1.5-fold and the difference between the two groups was statistically significant ($p \leq 0.05$).

Combined Gene Expression and ChIP-chip datasets. Since the ChIP-chip (containing >18,000 genes) and Affymetrix gene expression (containing >20,000 genes) microarray datasets do not contain the same set of genes, we defined the common gene set present on both microarrays as the union of each individual microarray gene list. Within this common list, information for each gene was extracted from the microarray dataset as well as the ChIP-chip dataset and were combined into a common spreadsheet. This combined ChIP-chip/expression dataset was used for further analysis using Microsoft Excel.

GO functional annotation. Gene lists for "Hypoacetylated in TG," "Not acetylated in TG," "Hyperacetylated in TG," and "Ectopically acetylated in TG" categories were analyzed using DAVID 6.7 (http://david.abcc.ncifcrf.gov/home.jsp) for functional annotation clustering [18]. Annotation clusters with enrichment scores greater than 1.3 are reported.

Primer design for single-gene ChIP and RT-qPCR validation assays

To determine differentially acetylated genes, we ranked the genes by composite score. Gene-specific primers for single-gene ChIP were designed based on differentially bound probes. Using the genomic location of differentially bound probes based on the annotation provided by Agilent, sequences from each region were obtained from the UCSC mm7 browser (http://genome.ucsc.edu/cgi-bin/hgGateway?db=mm7) and used to design gene-specific primers for single-gene ChIP. Gene-specific primers for RT-qPCR were designed to the region containing the 5′UTR and the start codon as described by the annotation provided in NCBI's accession record for the mRNA of each gene (found at http://www.ncbi.nlm.nih.gov/nuccore/). Primer-BLAST [56] at the NCBI website (http://www.ncbi.nlm.nih.gov/tools/primer-blast/index.cgi?LINK_LOC=BlastHome) was used to design primers. Prior to their use in qPCR reactions, primers were tested in a conventional PCR reaction using genomic DNA as template and checked on an agarose gel to ensure the primers resulted in a single band of expected size. Primer sequences for single-gene ChIP and RT-qPCR are provided in Tables S1 and S2, respectively.

Single-gene ChIP assays

Input and IP samples were interrogated with gene-specific primers in replicate reactions in real-time PCR analysis as previously described [53,54]. Using iCycler software (BioRad, Hercules, CA), threshold amplification cycle numbers (C_T) were used to calculate IP DNA quantities as ratios of corresponding inputs. IP to input ratios of AcH3-gene associations were calculated as follows: $\log_2$ (C_t of IP/C_t of input).

Histone extractions

Cerebella and livers from phenylbutyrate- and vehicle-treated R6/2 TG and WT littermates were used. In order to minimize the number of mice for these experiments, cerebellar tissues were used as "in-brain" controls in order to assess the efficacy of phenyl butyrate treatments, reserving the striatal tissue for ChIP experiments. Histones were acid-extracted as follows. Tissues were homogenized in ice-cold 5% Triton buffer (5% Triton, 3 mM DTT, 1 mM sodium orthovanadate, 5 mM sodium fluoride, 1 mM PMSF, 5 mM sodium butyrate in 1× PBS containing a protease inhibitor cocktail). Cells were lysed on ice and nuclei were collected by gentle centrifugation. Nuclei were washed 3× in ice cold 5% Triton buffer and proteins were extracted in 0.2 M HCl with vigorous shaking at 4°C for 3 hrs. Supernatants were cleared by centrifugation and neutralized with 1 M NaOH to a neutral pH. Protein concentrations were determined using the Bradford reagent (BioRad).

Western blots

Histone extracts were diluted in 2× Tricine SDS sample buffer (Invitrogen) and boiled for 5 min. Proteins were fractionated on a 10–20% Tricine gel (Invitrogen) at 120 V until the dye front reached the bottom of the gel. Proteins were then transferred to PVDF using the iBlot transfer system (Invitrogen) according to the manufacturer's instructions. Coomassie blue staining of the gels after transfer was used to ensure equal loading across wells. Membranes were blocked in 5% non-fat dry milk in TBST (50 mM Tris, 150 mM NaCl, 0.1% Tween 20) for 1 h at room temperature before incubation with primary antibodies. Following primary antibody (AcH3; 05-699, Millipore) incubation, blots were washed in TBST and then incubated in secondary antibody of HRP-conjugated goat anti-rabbit IgG (Jackson ImmunoResearch). Immunocomplexes were visualized with the Western Lightning Plus enhanced chemiluminescent (ECL) detection system (PerkinElmer) and exposed to film (GE Healthcare).

RNA extractions and RT-qPCR

Total RNA was extracted from a single striatum of phenylbutyrate- or vehicle-treated R6/2 TG and WT littermates using the RNeasy Mini kit (Qiagen) following the manufacturer's instructions. Total RNA was quantified using a spectrophotometer and cDNA was generated using equal amounts of total RNA, random hexamers and the SuperScript First Strand reaction kit (Invitrogen). Transcript levels were quantified as described [7]. Briefly, cDNA was used as template with gene specific primers in a PCR reaction using the SYBR Green PCR Master Mix (Applied Biosystems, Foster City, CA). Real-time thermal cycling was performed using an iCycler thermal cycler (Bio-Rad, Hercules, CA), with continuous SYBR Green monitoring according to the manufacturer's specifications.

Supporting Information

Table S1 Gene-specific primer sequences for single-gene ChIP confirmation experiments.

Table S2 Gene-specific primer sequences for RT-qPCR analysis.

Table S3 Gene Ontology (GO)-Biological Process (GO-TERM_BP_FAT) Functional Annotation Clustering of "Hypoacetylated in TG" genes.

Table S4 Gene Ontology (GO)-Biological Process (GO-TERM_BP_FAT) Functional Annotation Clustering of "Not acetylated in TG" genes.

Table S5 Gene Ontology (GO)-Biological Process(GO-TERM_BP_FAT) Functional Annotation Clustering of "Hyperacetylated in TG" genes.

Table S6 Gene Ontology (GO)-Biological Process (GOTERM_BP_FAT) Functional Annotation Clustering of "Ectopically acetylated in TG" genes.

Author Contributions

Conceived and designed the experiments: JHJC GSV TTS KNM. Performed the experiments: KNM TTS EX GRS. Analyzed the data: KNM SD DL. Contributed reagents/materials/analysis tools: AK RLC SD DL TC KNM. Wrote the paper: KNM GSV JHJC.

References

1. Huntington's Disease Collaborative Research Group (1993) A novel gene containing a trinucleotide repeat that is expanded and unstable on Huntington's disease chromosomes. Cell 72: 971–983.
2. Bates G, Harper PS, Jones L (2002) Huntington's Disease.
3. Cha JH (2007) Transcriptional signatures in Huntington's disease. Prog Neurobiol 83: 228–248.
4. Stack EC, Del Signore SJ, Luthi-Carter R, Soh BY, Goldstein DR, et al. (2007) Modulation of nucleosome dynamics in Huntington's disease. Hum Mol Genet 16: 1164–1175.
5. Ryu H, Lee J, Hagerty SW, Soh BY, McAlpin SE, et al. (2006) ESET/SETDB1 gene expression and histone H3 (K9) trimethylation in Huntington's disease. Proc Natl Acad Sci U S A 103: 19176–19181.
6. Sadri-Vakili G, Bouzou B, Benn CL, Kim MO, Chawla P, et al. (2007) Histones associated with downregulated genes are hypo-acetylated in Huntington's disease models. Hum Mol Genet 16: 1293–1306.
7. Kim MO, Chawla P, Overland RP, Xia E, Sadri-Vakili G, et al. (2008) Altered histone monoubiquitylation mediated by mutant huntingtin induces transcriptional dysregulation. J Neurosci 28: 3947–3957.
8. Igarashi S, Morita H, Bennett KM, Tanaka Y, Engelender S, et al. (2003) Inducible PC12 cell model of Huntington's disease shows toxicity and decreased histone acetylation. Neuroreport 14: 565–568.
9. Sadri-Vakili G, Cha JH (2006) Mechanisms of disease: Histone modifications in Huntington's disease. Nat Clin Pract Neurol 2: 330–338.
10. Kouzarides T (2007) Chromatin modifications and their function. Cell 128: 693–705.
11. Li B, Carey M, Workman JL (2007) The role of chromatin during transcription. Cell 128: 707–719.
12. VG A, Faulkner R, Mirsky AE (1964) Acetylation and methylation of histones and their possible role in the regulation of RNA synthesis. Proc Natl Acad Sci U S A 51: 786–794.
13. Marushige K (1976) Activation of chromatin by acetylation of histone side chains. Proc Natl Acad Sci U S A 73: 3937–3941.
14. Kazantsev AG (2009) New therapeutic strategies for treatment of neurodegenerative diseases. Curr Pharm Des 15: 3917–3918.
15. Gottesfeld JM, Pandolfo M (2009) Development of histone deacetylase inhibitors as therapeutics for neurological disease. Future Neurol 4: 775–784.
16. Mangiarini L, Sathasivam K, Seller M, Cozens B, Harper A, et al. (1996) Exon 1 of the HD gene with an expanded CAG repeat is sufficient to cause a progressive neurological phenotype in transgenic mice. Cell 87: 493–506.
17. Kuhn A, Goldstein DR, Hodges A, Strand AD, Sengstag T, et al. (2007) Mutant huntingtin's effects on striatal gene expression in mice recapitulate changes observed in human Huntington's disease brain and do not differ with mutant huntingtin length or wild-type huntingtin dosage. Hum Mol Genet 16: 1845–1861.
18. Huang DW, Sherman BT, Lempicki RA (2009) Systematic and integrative analysis of large gene lists using DAVID bioinformatics resources. Nat Protoc 4: 44–57.
19. Koch CM, Andrews RM, Flicek P, Dillon SC, Karaoz U, et al. (2007) The landscape of histone modifications across 1% of the human genome in five human cell lines. Genome Res 17: 691–707.
20. Heintzman ND, Stuart RK, Hon G, Fu Y, Ching CW, et al. (2007) Distinct and predictive chromatin signatures of transcriptional promoters and enhancers in the human genome. Nat Genet 39: 311–318.
21. Wang Z, Zang C, Rosenfeld JA, Schones DE, Barski A, et al. (2008) Combinatorial patterns of histone acetylations and methylations in the human genome. Nat Genet 40: 897–903.
22. Roh TY, Cuddapah S, Cui K, Zhao K (2006) The genomic landscape of histone modifications in human T cells. Proc Natl Acad Sci U S A 103: 15782–15787.
23. Roh TY, Cuddapah S, Zhao K (2005) Active chromatin domains are defined by acetylation islands revealed by genome-wide mapping. Genes Dev 19: 542–552.
24. Benn CL, Sun T, Sadri-Vakili G, McFarland KN, DiRocco DP, et al. (2008) Huntingtin modulates transcription, occupies gene promoters in vivo, and binds directly to DNA in a polyglutamine-dependent manner. J Neurosci 28: 10720–10733.
25. Riggs MG, Whittaker RG, Neumann JR, Ingram VM (1977) n-Butyrate causes histone modification in HeLa and Friend erythroleukaemia cells. Nature 268: 462–464.
26. Vidali G, Boffa LC, Bradbury EM, Allfrey VG (1978) Butyrate suppression of histone deacetylation leads to accumulation of multiacetylated forms of histones H3 and H4 and increased DNase I sensitivity of the associated DNA sequences. Proc Natl Acad Sci U S A 75: 2239–2243.
27. Vidali G, Boffa LC, Mann RS, Allfrey VG (1978) Reversible effects of Na-butyrate on histone acetylation. Biochem Biophys Res Commun 82: 223–227.
28. Boffa LC, Vidali G, Mann RS, Allfrey VG (1978) Suppression of histone deacetylation in vivo and in vitro by sodium butyrate. J Biol Chem 253: 3364–3366.
29. Ferrante RJ, Kubilus JK, Lee J, Ryu H, Beesen A, et al. (2003) Histone deacetylase inhibition by sodium butyrate chemotherapy ameliorates the neurodegenerative phenotype in Huntington's disease mice. J Neurosci 23: 9418–9427.
30. Steffan JS, Bodai L, Pallos J, Poelman M, McCampbell A, et al. (2001) Histone deacetylase inhibitors arrest polyglutamine-dependent neurodegeneration in Drosophila. Nature 413: 739–743.
31. Hockly E, Richon VM, Woodman B, Smith DL, Zhou X, et al. (2003) Suberoylanilide hydroxamic acid, a histone deacetylase inhibitor, ameliorates motor deficits in a mouse model of Huntington's disease. Proc Natl Acad Sci U S A 100: 2041–2046.
32. Pallos J, Bodai L, Lukacsovich T, Purcell JM, Steffan JS, et al. (2008) Inhibition of specific HDACs and sirtuins suppresses pathogenesis in a Drosophila model of Huntington's disease. Hum Mol Genet 17: 3767–3775.
33. Gardian G, Browne SE, Choi DK, Klivenyi P, Gregorio J, et al. (2005) Neuroprotective effects of phenylbutyrate in the N171-82Q transgenic mouse model of Huntington's disease. J Biol Chem 280: 556–563.
34. Zadori D, Geisz A, Vamos E, Vecsei L, Klivenyi P (2009) Valproate ameliorates the survival and the motor performance in a transgenic mouse model of Huntington's disease. Pharmacol Biochem Behav 94: 148–153.
35. Monti B, Gatta V, Piretti F, Raffaelli SS, Virgili M, et al. (2010) Valproic acid is neuroprotective in the rotenone rat model of Parkinson's disease: involvement of alpha-synuclein. Neurotox Res 17: 130–141.
36. Minamiyama M, Katsuno M, Adachi H, Waza M, Sang C, et al. (2004) Sodium butyrate ameliorates phenotypic expression in a transgenic mouse model of spinal and bulbar muscular atrophy. Hum Mol Genet 13: 1183–1192.
37. Kilgore M, Miller CA, Fass DM, Hennig KM, Haggarty SJ, et al. (2010) Inhibitors of class 1 histone deacetylases reverse contextual memory deficits in a mouse model of Alzheimer's disease. Neuropsychopharmacology 35: 870–880.
38. Ricobaraza A, Cuadrado-Tejedor M, Perez-Mediavilla A, Frechilla D, Del Rio J, et al. (2009) Phenylbutyrate ameliorates cognitive deficit and reduces tau pathology in an Alzheimer's disease mouse model. Neuropsychopharmacology 34: 1721–1732.
39. Ying M, Xu R, Wu X, Zhu H, Zhuang Y, et al. (2006) Sodium butyrate ameliorates histone hypoacetylation and neurodegenerative phenotypes in a mouse model for DRPLA. J Biol Chem 281: 12580–12586.
40. Ryu H, Smith K, Camelo SI, Carreras I, Lee J, et al. (2005) Sodium phenylbutyrate prolongs survival and regulates expression of anti-apoptotic genes in transgenic amyotrophic lateral sclerosis mice. J Neurochem 93: 1087–1098.
41. Petri S, Kiaei M, Kipiani K, Chen J, Calingasan NY, et al. (2006) Additive neuroprotective effects of a histone deacetylase inhibitor and a catalytic antioxidant in a transgenic mouse model of amyotrophic lateral sclerosis. Neurobiol Dis 22: 40–49.
42. Rai M, Soragni E, Jenssen K, Burnett R, Herman D, et al. (2008) HDAC inhibitors correct frataxin deficiency in a Friedreich ataxia mouse model. PLoS One 3: e1958.
43. Jenuwein T, Allis CD (2001) Translating the histone code. Science 293: 1074–1080.
44. Zippo A, Serafini R, Rocchigiani M, Pennacchini S, Krepelova A, et al. (2009) Histone crosstalk between H3S10ph and H4K16ac generates a histone code that mediates transcription elongation. Cell 138: 1122–1136.
45. Hung T, Binda O, Champagne KS, Kuo AJ, Johnson K, et al. (2009) ING4 mediates crosstalk between histone H3 K4 trimethylation and H3 acetylation to attenuate cellular transformation. Mol Cell 33: 248–256.
46. Saksouk N, Avvakumov N, Champagne KS, Hung T, Doyon Y, et al. (2009) HBO1 HAT complexes target chromatin throughout gene coding regions via multiple PHD finger interactions with histone H3 tail. Mol Cell 33: 257–265.
47. Vermeulen M, Mulder KW, Denissov S, Pijnappel WW, van Schaik FM, et al. (2007) Selective anchoring of TFIID to nucleosomes by trimethylation of histone H3 lysine 4. Cell 131: 58–69.
48. Ou JN, Torrisani J, Unterberger A, Provencal N, Shikimi K, et al. (2007) Histone deacetylase inhibitor Trichostatin A induces global and gene-specific DNA demethylation in human cancer cell lines. Biochem Pharmacol 73: 1297–1307.
49. Ye F, Chen Y, Hoang T, Montgomery RL, Zhao XH, et al. (2009) HDAC1 and HDAC2 regulate oligodendrocyte differentiation by disrupting the beta-catenin-TCF interaction. Nat Neurosci 12: 829–838.
50. Hubbert C, Guardiola A, Shao R, Kawaguchi Y, Ito A, et al. (2002) HDAC6 is a microtubule-associated deacetylase. Nature 417: 455–458.

51. Dompierre JP, Godin JD, Charrin BC, Cordelieres FP, King SJ, et al. (2007) Histone deacetylase 6 inhibition compensates for the transport deficit in Huntington's disease by increasing tubulin acetylation. J Neurosci 27: 3571–3583.
52. Jeong H, Then F, Melia TJJ, Mazzulli JR, Cui L, et al. (2009) Acetylation targets mutant huntingtin to autophagosomes for degradation. Cell 137: 60–72.
53. Braveman MW, Chen-Plotkin AS, Yohrling GJ, Cha JH (2004) Chromatin immunoprecipitation technique for study of transcriptional dysregulation in intact mouse brain. Methods Mol Biol 277: 261–276.
54. Chen-Plotkin AS, Sadri-Vakili G, Yohrling GJ, Braveman MW, Benn CL, et al. (2006) Decreased association of the transcription factor Sp1 with genes downregulated in Huntington's disease. Neurobiol Dis 22: 233–241.
55. Tusher VG, Tibshirani R, Chu G (2001) Significance analysis of microarrays applied to the ionizing radiation response. Proc Natl Acad Sci U S A 98: 5116–5121.
56. Rozen S, Skaletsky HJ (2000) Primer3 on the WWW for general users and for biologist programmers. In: Krawetz S, Misener S, editors. Bioinformatics Methods and Protocols: Methods in Molecular Biology. Totowa, NJ: Humana Press. pp. 365–386.

5

Fragments of *Hdh*Q150 Mutant Huntingtin Form a Soluble Oligomer Pool That Declines with Aggregate Deposition upon Aging

David Marcellin[1], Dorothee Abramowski[1], Douglas Young[1], Jens Richter[1], Andreas Weiss[1], Audrey Marcel[1], Julia Maassen[1], Muriel Kauffmann[1], Miriam Bibel[1], Derya R. Shimshek[1], Richard L. M. Faull[2], Gillian P. Bates[3], Rainer R. Kuhn[1], P. Herman Van der Putten[1], Peter Schmid[1], Gregor P. Lotz[1]*

1 Novartis Institutes for BioMedical Research, Novartis Pharma AG, Basel, Switzerland, **2** Centre for Brain Research, Auckland University, Auckland, New Zealand, **3** Department of Medical and Molecular Genetics, King's College London, London, United Kingdom

Abstract

Cleavage of the full-length mutant huntingtin (mhtt) protein into smaller, soluble aggregation-prone mhtt fragments appears to be a key process in the neuropathophysiology of Huntington's Disease (HD). Recent quantification studies using TR-FRET-based immunoassays showed decreasing levels of soluble mhtt correlating with an increased load of aggregated mhtt in the aging *Hdh*Q150 mouse brain. To better characterize the nature of these changes at the level of native mhtt species, we developed a detection method that combines size exclusion chromatography (SEC) and time-resolved fluorescence resonance energy transfer (TR-FRET) that allowed us to resolve and define the formation, aggregation and temporal dynamics of native soluble mhtt species and insoluble aggregates in the brain of the *Hdh*Q150 knock-in mouse. We found that mhtt fragments and not full-length mhtt form oligomers in the brains of one month-old mice long before disease phenotypes and mhtt aggregate histopathology occur. As the *Hdh*Q150 mice age, brain levels of soluble full-length mhtt protein remain similar. In contrast, the soluble oligomeric pool of mhtt fragments slightly increases during the first two months before it declines between 3 and 8 months of age. This decline inversely correlates with the formation of insoluble mhtt aggregates. We also found that the pool-size of soluble mhtt oligomers is similar in age-matched heterozygous and homozygous *Hdh*Q150 mouse brains whereas insoluble aggregate formation is greatly accelerated in the homozygous mutant brain. The capacity of the soluble mhtt oligomer pool therefore seems exhausted already in the heterozygous state and likely kept constant by changes in flux and, as a consequence, increased rate of insoluble aggregate formation. We demonstrate that our novel findings in mice translate to human HD brain but not HD patient fibroblasts.

Editor: David R. Borchelt, University of Florida, United States of America

Funding: The authors have no funding or support to report.

Competing Interests: DM, DA, DY, JR, AW, AM, JM, MK, MB, DRS, RRK, HvdP, PS and GPL are employees of Novartis Pharma AG. There are no patents, products in development or marketed products to declare. This does not alter the authors' adherence to all the PloS ONE policies on sharing data and materials, as detailed online in the guide for authors.

* E-mail: gregor.lotz@novartis.com

Introduction

A major hypothesis in Huntingtoǹs Disease (HD) is that misfolding of mutant huntingtin (mhtt) protein leads to aggregation and causes neurodegeneration. Consistent with this idea, neurons in HD brains form intracellular inclusion bodies (IBs) composed mainly of aggregated mhtt protein. The mhtt protein present in IBs cross-reacts only with antibodies to N- but not C-terminal epitopes suggesting that mainly N-terminal mhtt fragments form IBs [1]. This is also supported by findings showing that mhtt N-terminal fragments, as compared to full-length mhtt, aggregate much more readily *in vitro* [2] and when expressed inside living cells [3]. Furthermore, intracellular proteolytic cleavage of the full-length mhtt protein [4,5] gives rise to shorter aggregation-prone mhtt fragments while the expression of mhtt resistent to cleavage by caspase 6 is sufficient to preserve the detrimental effects of the protein on striatal volume and behavior in a YAC mouse HD model [6,7]. Altogether, these findings strengthen the hypothesis that cleavage of full-length mhtt results in a pool of soluble toxic protein fragments that aggregate and are implicated in the pathophysiology of HD.

Quantification studies using time-resolved fluorescence resonance energy transfer (TR-FRET)-based immunoassays have revealed decreasing levels of soluble mhtt correlating with an increased load of aggregated mhtt in the aging HD mouse brain [8]. To better understand the nature of these changes at the level of native mhtt species, we developed a detection method that combines size exclusion chromatography (SEC) and TR-FRET immunoassay. Full-length and mhtt fragment complexes are separated according to size and shape and the fractions collected are further characterized using a TR-FRET based immunoassay that specifically detects soluble mhtt [8]. This TR-FRET assay uses two different fluorophore labeled-monoclonal antibodies, a terbium-labeled 2B7 antibody (2B7-Tb) that recognizes an epitope in the first N-terminal 17 aa of mhtt and a D2-labeled MW1 antibody (MW1-D2) that binds specifically to the polyQ region of mhtt [8]. A second TR-FRET assay (MW8-Tb/MW8-D2) was used to detect specifically insoluble aggregates [8]. In our previous study we used both TR-FRET assays to establish an inverse correlation between soluble and aggregated mhtt in *HdhQ*150 brains [8]. However, we were not able to discriminate mhtt species in larger protein complexes containing either fragments and/or full-length mhtt. In this study the combination of SEC and TR-FRET (SEC-FRET) allowed us to unmask previously unrecognized age- and gene-dosage dependent changes in abundance and heterogeneity of native soluble mhtt complexes.

Here, we demonstrate that the *HdhQ*150 mouse brain harbors a pool of mhtt fragment-oligomers whereas full-length htt remains monomeric. The mhtt fragment-oligomer pool is already present in the brain of one month-old *HdhQ*150 mice, long before disease phenotypes and mhtt aggregate histopathology appear. We demonstrate, that the pool-size changes of soluble mhtt fragment-oligomers correlate inversely with the accumulation of insoluble aggregates in an age-dependent manner whereas the levels of soluble full-length mhtt protein remain stable as the mice age. The formation of insoluble aggregates is most prominent in the striatum and markedly accelerated in a dose-dependent fashion in homozygous as compared to heterozygous *HdhQ*150 mice. In contrast, the pool-size of soluble mhtt oligomers seems mhtt allele-dose independent which seems in line with the hypothesis that flux-rate of mhtt fragments through this pool but not its size might be rate-limiting in the formation of insoluble IBs [9]. The importance of our findings with respect to the disease in humans is further emphasized by showing the existence of a mhtt fragment-oligomer pool in a human HD brain. Therefore, applying SEC-FRET analysis may become a novel and important cornerstone methodology to identify disease-modifying targets in HD that directly affects mhtt fragmentation or aggregation.

Materials and Methods

Ethic Statement

All experiments were carried out in accordance with authorization guidelines of the Swiss Federal and Cantonal veterinary offices for the care and use of laboratory animals. Studies described in this report were approved by the Swiss Cantonal veterinary offices (Basel-City) and preformed according to Novartis animal license number BS-1858.

Animals

Heterozygous *HdhQ*150 knock-in mice [10] were obtained from the laboratory of G. P. Bates. *The HdhQ*150 mice were maintained on a C57BL/6J background. The offspring were genotyped by polymerase chain reaction (PCR) using DNA obtained from ear punches. The animals were housed in a temperature-controlled room that was maintained on a 12 h light/dark cycle. Food and water were available *ad libitum*. Animals were sacrificed by decapitation in deep isoflurane narcosis. Tissues were then collected immediately and were snap-frozen on a metal plate placed on dry ice.

Cell Lines

Mouse embryonic stem (ES) cells expressing human exon1 or full-length mhtt (Q145) from the ROSA26 locus were cultivated in 3i–medium [11,12]. Neurons were derived from ES cells as described [13]. These cells differentiated to glutamatergic pyramidal neurons and were kept in culture for 21 days.

SV 40 Immortalized Human HD Fibroblasts and Human HD Brain

Fibroblasts were received from Coriell Institute for medical research, New Jersey, USA [Code GM04729 and GM04723]. Fibroblast cells expressing wildtype Q17 or mutant Q68 were cultured in MEME - medium (Sigma, cat# M-5650) +15% FCS (Gibco, cat# 10270) +5 ml Glutamax (Gibco, cat# 35050) +5 ml PenStrep (Gibco, cat# 15140) and were grown on 15 cm dishes (1.5×10^6) until confluence. Human brain tissue was obtained from the Neurological Foundation of New Zealand Human Brain Bank.

Western Blotting Analysis

Cells were harvested and lysed in ice-cooled lysis buffer (phosphate buffered saline, Invitrogen #14190; 1% Triton X-100), containing anti-proteases (Roche, cOmplete, Mini Protease Inhibitor Cocktail Tablets, 04693124001) and anti-phosphatases (Roche, PhosStop Phosphatase Inhibitor Tablets, 04906845001). Lysates were kept on ice for 15 min before to be completely homogenized by sonication for 5 seconds. A BCA assay (Thermo Scientific, 23227) was used for protein quantification. Samples were diluted in NuPAGE loading buffer (Invitrogen, NP0007; NP0009) and heated 10 min at 95°C. The samples were loaded onto 4–12% NuPAGE Bis-Tris gels or 3–8% Tris-acetate gels (Invitrogen, NP0335, EA03752). Proteins were transfered to PVDF membranes for 10 minutes with the iBlot Dry Blotting System (Invitrogen, IB-4010-01) according to manufacturer instructions. The membrane was then incubated for one hour in phosphate buffered saline, 0.1% Tween 20, 5% (w/v) dried milk. Incubation with primary antibodies was done over-night (O/N) at 4°C; before secondary horseradish peroxidase conjugated goat anti-mouse (GE Healthcare, RPN4201) were applied for one hour. Protein bands were detected with chemiluminescent substrate (ECL, GE Healthcare).

Antibodies

MW1 and MW8 antibodies were developed by Paul Patterson [14] and obtained from the Developmental Studies Hybridoma Bank, developed under the auspices of the NICHD and maintained by The University of Iowa, Department of Biological Sciences, Iowa City, IA 52242. Generation and characterization of 2B7 was described previously [15].

Immunostaining

10 µm frozen sagittal sections were prepared from snap frozen brain hemispheres, placed onto SuperFrost plus glass slides (Menzel) and air dried for 10 minutes. Sections were then fixed for 30 minutes at room temperature with 4% paraformaldehyd/PBS pH 7.4, rinsed 3 times for 5 minutes in PBS, incubated for 1 hour with PBS containing 2% goat serum, reacted over night at 4°C with 3 µg/ml Alexa 488-labeled MW8 diluted in PBS containing 2% goat serum, washed 3 times in PBS and mounted with Prolong Gold containing DAPI nucleic acid counterstain (Invitrogen). To increase staining intensity, some slides were reacted over night with 3 µg/ml unlabeld MW8, rinsed in PBS and incubated for 1 hour at room temperature with Alexa 594-labeled secondary antibody (Invitrogen) before beeing mounted. Quantitative evaluation of aggregate size was performed with CellF (Olympus Soft Imaging Solutions) software.

Size Exclusion Chromatography (SEC): Analysis of Soluble mhtt by SEC-FRET

All samples were prepared in 500 µl of complete ice-cooled lysis buffer [phosphate buffered saline, (Invitrogen #14190), 1% Triton

X-100, anti-proteases (Roche, cOmplete, Mini Protease Inhibitor Cocktail Tablets, 04693124001) and anti-phosphatases (Roche, PhosStop Phosphatase Inhibitor Tablets, 04906845001)]. *Hdh*Q150 brain tissues (forebrain, striata pool) were homogenized with ceramic beads (Precellys, Bertin Technologies) according to the manufacturer instructions and finally sonicated for 10 seconds. Cells (ES lines and human fibroblasts) were resuspended in complete ice-cooled lysis buffer and sonicated for 10 seconds. Human post-mortem brain cortices were provided already homogenized in complete lysis buffer. Extracts were then clarified by ultra-centrifugation for 30 min at 100,000 g. Supernatants were filtered through a 0.45 µm membrane (Millipore, Millex PTFE) and protein concentrations were determined by BCA. Proteins were injected and fractionated by SEC on a Superdex 200 10/300 column. The total protein loaded on the column in a sample volume of 500 µl were respectively, 300 µg for the ES cell lines, 3.0 mg for the *Hdh*Q150 forebrain and striata pool, 4.0 mg for the human fibroblasts and 1.0 mg for human post-mortem brain cortices. The separation was performed at 4°C with a flow rate of 0.5 ml/min in PBS 0.05% Triton X-100. The elution was done with one column volume and fractions (250 µl per fraction) were collected in 96-well plate format and 10µl from each were applied for TR-FRET measurement with indicated antibody combinations. Protein standards were used to estimate size of htt peaks (**Fig. S1A**).

Analysis of Insoluble mhtt Aggregates by TR-FRET

Pellet from *HdhQ150* brain homogenate obtained by ultra-centrifugation at 100000 g (density separation) were washed once with PBS +1%Triton X-100 and resuspended in the same buffer and sonicated. 10 µl of the pellet suspension were assayed for TR-FRET measurement with MW8-Tb/MW-8-D2 as previous described (8). Protein concentration was determined for normalization.

Time-resolved Förster Resonance Energy Transfer (TR-FRET)

Assays were performed as described previously [16,17,18]. Briefly, 10 µl of sample (lysate or SEC fractions) was transferred to a low-volume plate (Greiner Bio-one, #784080) and 1 µl of antibody mix added. Soluble mhtt was measured with 2B7-Tb/MW1-D2. Aggregated mhtt was measured with MW8-Tb/MW8-D2. Fluorophore labeling of antibodies was performed by CisBio Bioassays (Parc Marcel Boiteux, France). TR-FRET measurements were done after over night incubation at 4°C using an EnVision Reader (Perkin Elmer, excitation 320 nm, time delay 100 msec; integration time 400 msec). Values are expressed as the ratio between the emission at 665 nm and 620 nm. Each ratio was then expressed in Delta F: the sample ratio was first reduced with the background signal ratio (antibodies in lysis buffer), then divided by the background signal ratio and finally multiplied by 100. Delta F values were then normalized to protein concentration in the case of brain tissues.

Results

Detection of Soluble mhtt Protein Fragments in Embryonic Stem Cell-derived Neurons Expressing Full-length mhtt

To determine the existence, the size and the relative abundance of different soluble mhtt protein fragments in cells expressing a full-length mhtt protein, we first analyzed cell lysates of mouse ES cell-derived neurons that over-express a human full-length mhtt protein with a polyQ length of 145 (145Q). The mhtt gene is inserted into the ROSA26 locus [11,12]. Western Blot analysis of these cell lysates identified several mhtt protein fragments ranging in size between 90 and 250 kDa and indicating that cleavage of the full-length mhtt protein occurs in these neurons (**Fig. 1B**). To characterize in more depth the native biochemical and molecular features of these mhtt protein fragments in solution, we separated them from mhtt full-length proteins by size-exclusion-chromatography followed by TR-FRET-based analysis of the different fractions (**Fig. 1A**). The TR-FRET- immunoassay we used, specifically detects soluble mhtt and not wildtype htt or insoluble mhtt [8] (**Fig. 1A**). After injection of 300 µg total soluble protein into the size exclusion column, full-length mhtt protein is detected in fractions of molecular weights around 1000 kDa (peak1 in **Fig. 1C, E**). Interestingly, another fraction containing soluble mhtt appeared around 160 kDa (peak 2b in **Fig. 1C,E**) suggesting it might contain oligomerized mhtt fragments. Analysis of wildtype ES cell extracts which contain only endogenous mouse wildtype htt protein revealed no FRET signals above background confirming the specificity of the 2B7-Tb/MW1-D2 TR-FRET assay detecting only mhtt but not wild-type htt species (**Fig.1 C and D**) [**8**].

Next, we ran SEC-FRET assays also on extracts of neurons derived from mouse ES cells that over-express mhtt human exon1 (Q145) located in the ROSA26 locus. A key question we wanted to address was whether exon1-derived mhtt protein species differ in their biochemical nature and size from mhtt fragments generated by cleavage of full-length mhtt. As shown in **Fig. 1C and 1F**, the peak profile of the 250 kDa fractions of the exon1 cell extract only partially overlaps with that of the 160 kDa fractions in the ES-derived neurons expressing full-length mhtt. Western blot analysis revealed that the exon1-derived mhtt fragments differ from those generated in the cells expressing full-length mhtt (**Fig. 1B**). We also noted that the 2B7-Tb/MW1-D2 TR-FRET assay detects fragments with much greater sensitivity (about 10 fold) than mhtt full-length (**Fig. 1B and C**). Note, total mhtt protein expression levels in the two ES-derived neuronal cell types were similar (**Fig. 1B**). Altogether, the findings in these two ES-derived neuronal cell populations suggest that mhtt fragments and the soluble complexes they form, differ when derived from full-length cleavage as compared to exon-1 mhtt. Interestingly, the formation of mhtt-containing aggregates is only observed in the exon-1 mouse ES cell model but not in its counterpart expressing full-length mhtt (data not shown). Whether this relates to different intracellular fragment concentrations achieved in the two cellular systems and/or to their biochemical nature requires further clarification. Taken together, the results in these two cellular models demonstrate that SEC-FRET is a valid and useful methodology to further characterize the size, biochemical nature and relative abundance of soluble complexes of mhtt fragments in different HD-relevant biological systems.

An Invariant Soluble Pool of mhtt Oligomers in the *Hdh*Q150 Mouse Brain is Rate-limiting to IB Formation

SEC-FRET was used to characterize mhtt protein products in forebrain extracts of 8 month-old *Hdh*Q150 knock-in mice expressing endogenous full-length mhtt protein that is known to generate multiple proteolytic cleavage-products [19]. In heterozygous mice, SEC-FRET analysis using the 2B7-Tb/MW1-D2 antibody pair revealed a full-length mhtt species in the 1000 kDa fraction (peak1) and one major lower molecular weight peak at around 200 kDa (peak2) (**Fig. 2B**), indicating that in these mice mhtt oligomeric fragment assemblies exist similar to those we detected in ES-derived neurons that over-express full-length mhtt.

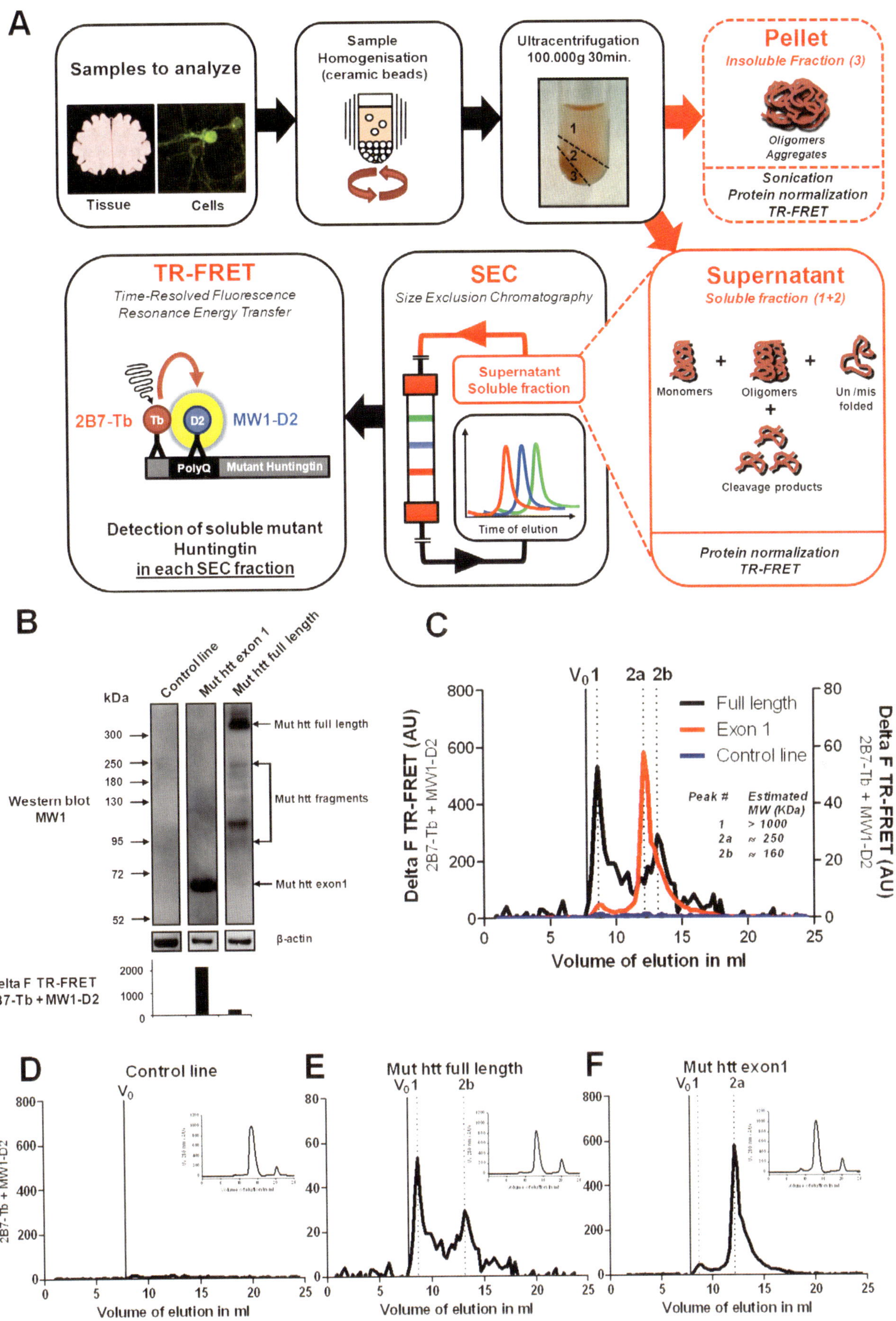

A
Samples to analyze
Tissue
Cells
Sample Homogenisation (ceramic beads)
Ultracentrifugation 100.000g 30min.
Pellet
Insoluble Fraction (3)
Oligomers
Aggregates
Sonication
Protein normalization
TR-FRET
Supernatant
Soluble fraction (1+2)
Monomers
Oligomers
Un /mis folded
Cleavage products
Protein normalization
TR-FRET
SEC
Size Exclusion Chromatography
Supernatant Soluble fraction
Time of elution
TR-FRET
Time-Resolved Fluorescence Resonance Energy Transfer
2B7-Tb
MW1-D2
PolyQ
Mutant Huntingtin
Detection of soluble mutant Huntingtin in each SEC fraction
B
Control line
Mut htt exon 1
Mut htt full length
kDa
Western blot MW1
Mut htt full length
Mut htt fragments
Mut htt exon1
β-actin
Delta F TR-FRET 2B7-Tb + MW1-D2
C
Full length
Exon 1
Control line
Peak # Estimated MW (KDa)
1 > 1000
2a ≈ 250
2b ≈ 160
Delta F TR-FRET (AU) 2B7-Tb + MW1-D2
Volume of elution in ml
D
Control line
E
Mut htt full length
F
Mut htt exon1
Volume of elution in ml

Figure 1. The SEC-FRET technology is a useful tool to detect multiple mhtt species in cell lysate. (A) Schematic overview of the SEC-FRET methodology. (B) Detection of multiple mhtt fragments in lysate of neurons derived from mouse ES cells by Western blot analysis with MW1 antibodies (C) Overlap of all TR-FRET-based detection profiles after SEC (full-length in black, exon1 in red and wt in blue) Estimated MW of TR-FRET peaks (1, 2a and 2b) based on standard marker in Fig. S1. AU: arbitary units. (D, E, F), Individual TR-FRET based detection profiles after SEC with the UV absorbance, as an indicator of protein concentration, in the upper right corner for stem cell derived neurons at 21 days *in-vitro* (D) control line, (E) mhtt full length (Q145) and (F) mhtt Exon1 (Q145).

Western Blot analysis confirmed the presence of full-length mhtt in the 1000 kDa peak 1 fractions and mhtt fragments in the 200 kDa (peak 2) fractions (**Fig. 2D**). Note, Western blot analysis with the 2B7 antibody did not enable the detection of mhtt fragments in the peak 2 SEC-fractions because the concentration of 2B7 cross-reacting fragments is too low. In contrast, Western blot analysis of the total supernatant fraction (100.000 g) before it was loaded onto the SEC column did show mhtt fragments of around 80 kDa (**Fig. S1B**). Note, these were slightly different in size from the mhtt fragments detected in peak 2 with MW1 demonstrating that heteromeric mhtt complexes with monomers of different lengths exist in the peak 2 fractions (**Fig. S1B**). Wild-type mice did not show any signals (**Fig. 2A**).

Unlike longer CAG repeats, homozygosity for the HD mutation in patients appears not to lower significantly the age at onset of symptoms [20]. Rather, doubling the dose of the mhtt allele appears to influence result mainly in a more severe clinical course with the note of caution that the number of homozygous patients analyzed remains low [20]. In mouse models, increasing the expression of transgenes has been shown to accelerate both the onset and the progression of phenotypes [6,21,22,23]. Thus, we compared mhtt (fragments *vs* full-length and soluble oligomers *vs* insoluble aggregates) in age-matched heterozygous and homozygous *Hdh*Q150 mouse brains using immunohistochemistry, TR-FRET, SEC-FRET and Western Blot analysis. The formation of neuronal MW8-positive IBs in the striatum is markedly exacerbated in homozygous as compared to heterozygous *Hdh*Q150 mice as shown in brain sections of 4 month-old mice (**Fig. 2G**). Analysis of forebrain extract using TR-FRET to detect soluble mhtt species: (2B7-Tb/MW1-D2 forebrain extract supernatant, 100,000 g) and insoluble mhtt aggregates (MW8-Tb/MW8-D2: sonicated pellet), revealed no significant differences in the levels of soluble mhtt in hetero- versus homozygous mice. However, homozygous mice showed a highly significant increase in insoluble aggregates (**Fig. 2E**) in line with our immunohistochemical observations (**Fig. 2G**). Most importantly, these results demonstrate that increased gene-dosage of mhtt in homozygous mice greatly accelerates insoluble aggregate formation *in vivo* (**Fig. 2E, G**).

SEC-FRET analysis comparing hetero- and homozygous mice revealed that the relative abundance and heterogeneity of soluble mhtt fragments did not change but, as expected, the amount of full-length mhtt increased in the homozygous brain (**Fig. 2B, C, F**). Western Blot analysis confirmed that mhtt full length protein elutes at 1000 kda (peak1) and mhtt fragments at around 200 kda (peak2) (**Fig. 2D**). Remarkably, the profile of oligomeric mhtt fragments in the 200 kDa fractions of hetero- and homozygous mice did not significantly differ despite the two-fold higher levels of full-length mhtt expressed in the homozygotes, the earlier onset and more numerous formation of IBs (**Fig. 2B, C, F, G, E**). These results suggest that the pool of mhtt fragment-oligomers is remarkably constant with respect to size and profile and largely mhtt gene-dosage independent. On the other hand, gene-dosage is rate-limiting to IB formation in the mouse *in vivo* as it was in cultured cells [**9**]. Altogether, these results seem to fit best with a mhtt cleavage pathway model in which the maximal capacity of an oligomeric mhtt fragment pool is reached and kept constant by dynamics in flux-rate.

Age-dependent Inverse Correlation between Soluble and Aggregated mhtt Fragment-pools

To determine age-dependent changes in SEC-FRET profiles, we analyzed forebrain extracts of heterozygous *Hdh*Q150 mice at the age of 3, 8 and 12 months (**Fig. 3A-D**). Identical protein concentrations (confirmed by UV absorption) were loaded. Accordingly, we could show that the pool size of oligomeric mhtt fragments in the 200 kDa peak fractions decreased over time as the mice aged (**Fig. 3 A, B, D**). In contrast, the levels of full-length mhtt in the 1000 kDa fractions remained constant (**Fig. 2B; Fig. 3A, B, D**) whereas the amounts of insoluble aggregates increased dramatically with age (MW8-Tb/MW8-D2 TR-FRET; **Fig. 3C**).

Using supernatant of forebrain extract (100000 g), soluble mhtt levels were determined by 2B7-Tb/MW1-D2 TR-FRET assay (**Fig. 3C**). The TR-FRET analysis revealed a significant decrease of soluble mhtt occurring between 3 and 8 months of age but no further significant decline between 8 and 12 months (**Fig. 3C**). Strikingly, peak-specific SEC-FRET analysis of the 1000 kDa and 200 kDa fractions confirmed a significant age-dependent decrease between 3 and 8 months in the amounts of soluble mhtt fragments (200 kDa fraction/peak 2) but not in the amount of full-length mhtt (1000 kDa fraction/peak 1) (**Fig. 3D**). Altogether, these findings indicate that the pool of mhtt oligomerized soluble fragments but not the pool of full-length mhtt protein correlates inversely with the formation of insoluble mhtt protein aggregates in *Hdh*150Q mouse forebrain. The inverse correlation is most pronounced in the 3–8 month age interval after which the size of the 200 kDa soluble pool remained at a steady state.

Inverse Correlation of Soluble and Aggregated mhtt Fragments is Most Prominent in the Striatum

The striatum is the most severely affected brain region in HD patients [24,25] and also the earliest and most profoundly affected brain region in *Hdh*Q150 mice [10]. Thus, we analyzed striata of heterozygous *Hdh*Q150 mice at the ages of 2, 4, 6, 8 and 10 months by immunohistochemistry and at 1, 2, 3, 4, 6 and 8 months using the SEC-FRET method (**Fig. 4 and 5**). Immunohistochemical analysis using the MW8 antibody showed that the number and size of intranuclear IBs in the striatum gradually increased with age (**Fig. 4**). Note, that after the age of 8 months, mainly aggregate size but not their number increased significantly (see 8 as compared to 10 month-old immunostaining quantification; **Fig. 4 and Fig. S2**). To conduct SEC-FRET analysis on the striatum, we pooled the striata of five mice into each single age group sample to reach sufficient quantities (3 mg) of total soluble protein for separation on the SEC column. Interestingly, full-length mhtt protein eluted in the 750 kDa fractions (peak 1; **Fig. 5A**) instead of the 1000 kDa fractions as observed in forebrain profiles suggesting a different composition of full-length mhtt protein complexes in the striatum. Western Blot analysis confirmed that full-length mhtt eluted at 750 kDa (**Fig. 5B**). Another observation is that the level of full-length mhtt protein did

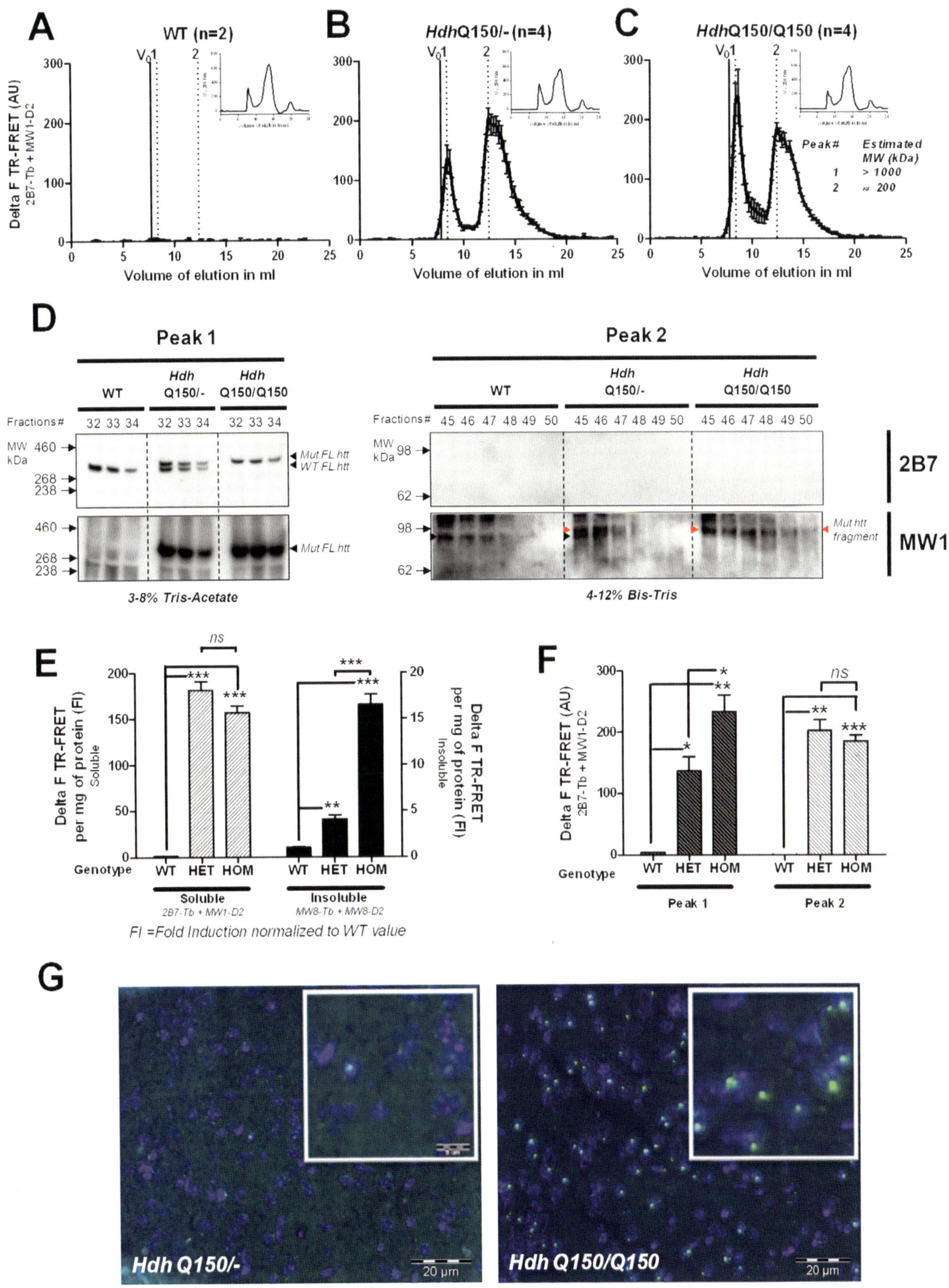
A
WT (n=2)
B
HdhQ150/- (n=4)
C
HdhQ150/Q150 (n=4)
Delta F TR-FRET (AU)
2B7-Tb + MW1-D2
Volume of elution in ml
Peak# Estimated MW (kDa)
1 > 1000
2 ≈ 200
D
Peak 1
Peak 2
WT
Hdh Q150/-
Hdh Q150/Q150
Fractions#
MW kDa
Mut FL htt
WT FL htt
3-8% Tris-Acetate
4-12% Bis-Tris
Mut htt fragment
2B7
MW1
E
Delta F TR-FRET per mg of protein (FI) Soluble
Delta F TR-FRET per mg of protein (FI) Insoluble
Genotype
WT HET HOM
Soluble
2B7-Tb + MW1-D2
Insoluble
MW8-Tb + MW8-D2
FI =Fold Induction normalized to WT value
F
Delta F TR-FRET (AU)
2B7-Tb + MW1-D2
Peak 1
Peak 2
G
Hdh Q150/-
Hdh Q150/Q150
20 μm

Figure 2. Analysis of 8 months *Hdh*Q150 forebrain identified invariant, soluble oligomeric pool of mhtt fragments. (A), (B), (C), Individual TR-FRET based detection profiles after SEC with the UV absorbance in the upper right corner for A: Wild type, B: Heterozygote *Hdh*Q150, C: Homozygote *Hdh*Q150 forebrain samples at 8 months. Molecular weight of TR-FRET peaks are indicated in (C). (D) Western Blot analysis to detect htt full-length in the fractions 32, 33, 34 for peak1 and mhtt fragments at kDa (red arrow) in fractions 45, 46, 47, 48, 49, 50 for peak 2 using either 2B7 or MW1 antibodies. Note, black arrow in wt (peak2) for MW1 detection is non-specific background and below the specific mhtt fragment band in *Hdh Q150/−* and *Hdh Q150/Q150* (E) Quantification of soluble mhtt by 2B7-Tb/MW1-D2 TR-FRET detection in supernatant fraction and of insoluble mhtt by MW8-Tb and MW8-D2 detection in resuspended and sonicated pellet fraction taken from wild type, *Hdh Q150/−* and *Hdh Q150/Q150* forebrain tissue. Delta F values (see experimental procedure) are mean of 4 independent measurements ± SEM. Delta F values are adjusted to protein concentration and then normalized to wild-type. The t-test was used to assess significance (ns $P>0.05$; * $P<0.05$; ** $P<0.01$, *** $P<0.001$) (F) Quantification of soluble mhtt in peak1 and peak 2 by 2B7-Tb/MW1-D2 TR-FRET detection for wild type, *Hdh Q150/−* and *Hdh Q150/Q150*. Delta F values (mean of 4 independent measurements ± SEM) are expressed as the maximal peak value. The t-test was used to assess significance (G) Immunostaining of aggregated mhtt in the striatum of 4 months old heterozygote (left) and 4 months old homozygote *Hdh*Q150 mice (right). Frozen sections were stained with Alexa 488-labeled MW8 and counterstained with DAPI to visualize cell nuclei (blue fluorescence).

not significantly change with age (peak1, **Fig. 5A, Fig. S3A**). Fragments of mhtt eluted as two separate size pools at 250 kDa (peak 2a) and 160 kDa (peak 2b) and both pool sizes first slighlty increased during the first two months followed by their significant decrease starting at the age of 3 months (**Fig. 5A, Fig. S3A**). As compared to the age-dependent decrease of the 200 kDa pool in forebrain tissue (**Fig. 2B and Fig. 3A, B, C**), the age-dependent decrease of the two striatal mhtt fragment pools was much more profound (**Fig. 5A**). In accordance with the immunocytochemical data (**Fig. 4**), insoluble mhtt levels (MW8-Tb/MW8-D2 TR-FRET) showed very significant age-dependent increases in the striatum (**Fig. 5D**). Western blot analysis of the 250 kDa fractions (peak 2) revealed MW1-reactive mhtt fragments of around 85 kDa that were not detected with the 2B7 antibody (see comment for

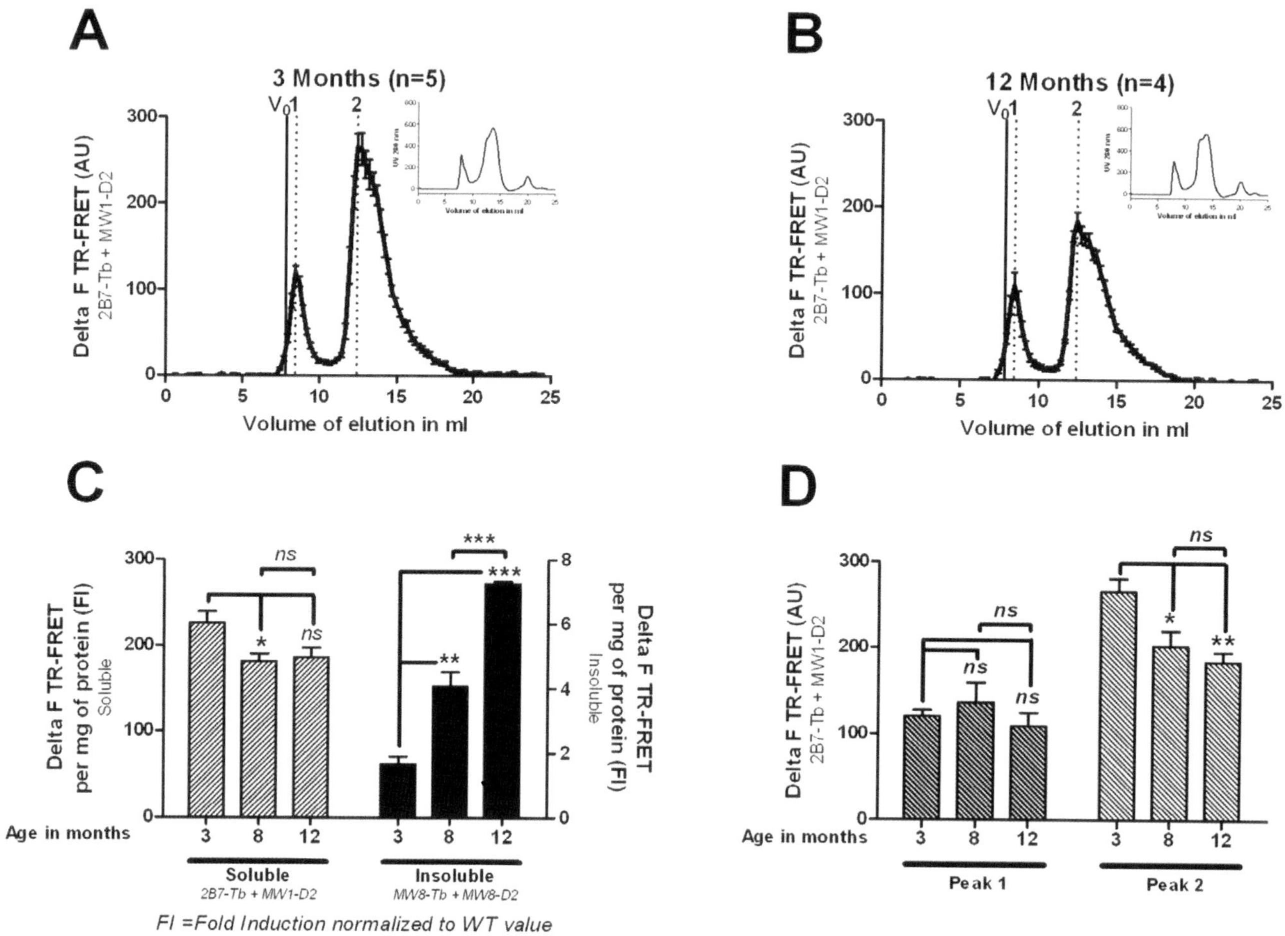

Figure 3. Inverse correlation of soluble and aggregated mhtt fragments analyzed by *Hdh*Q150/− forebrain tissue. SEC-FRET profiles with the UV absorbance in the upper right corner for (A) 3 months and (B) 12 months heterozygote *Hdh Q150/−* forebrain tissue. (C) Quantification of soluble mhtt by 2B7-Tb and MW1-D2 TR-FRET detection in supernatant fraction and of insoluble mhtt by MW8-Tb and MW8-D2 detection in resuspended pellet fraction of *Hdh Q150/−* mice at 3, 8 and 12 months. Delta F values (see experimental procedure) are mean of 4 independent measurements ± SEM. Delta F values are adjusted to protein concentration and then normalized to wild-type. The t-test was used to assess significance (D) Quantification of SEC fractions of peak 1 and of peak 2 by 2B7-Tb and MW1-D2 TR-FRET taken from *Hdh Q150/−* mice at 3, 8 and 12 months. Delta F values (mean of 4 independent measurements ± SEM) are expressed as the maximal peak value; The t-test was used to assess significance.

Fig.2D) (**Fig. 5B**). In addition, these mhtt fragments at around 85 kDa seem to undergo further processing with increased age and generate further fragments at 85 and 60 kDa (**Fig. 5C**). These results demonstrate that the nature of mhtt oligomeric fragments present in forebrain and striatum differs. Also, the inverse relationship between soluble oligomeric mhtt fragments and insoluble aggregates is far more dramatic in striatum as compared to the forebrain (**Fig. 5A, D and Fig. 2B, Fig. 3**).

Next, we used the antibody combination 2B7-Tb and MW8-D2 for the TR-FRET assay. This combination might be more specific for mhtt Exon1 fragments given the specificity of MW8 for a *de novo* generated C-terminal exon-1 epitope [8]. We did see a weak signal that overlapped with oligomers detected by the 2B7-Tb/MW1-D2 TR-FRET (**Fig. 5E and Fig. S3B**). Interestingly, the level of these 2B7-Tb/MW8-D2 soluble fragments increased slightly between 1 and 2 months of age before dramatically decreasing until 6 months of age when it reached a steady-state (**Fig. 5E and Fig. S3B**). Western blot analysis of soluble and insoluble brain protein fractions of 3, 8 and 12 month-old mice demonstrated that indeed, the mhtt fragments accumulate in insoluble aggregates (**Fig. 5F**). These findings support the idea that exon1 fragments rapidly form heteromeric oligomers containing different N-terminal fragments and that later-on, these are sequestered into IBs.

Human Brain but not Fibroblasts Contain Soluble mhtt Fragments

To assess whether our findings may have clinical relevance for human HD, we first compared the SEC-FRET profiles of human fibroblasts from an HD donor with a polyQ stretch of 68Qs in the mhtt allele, with fibroblasts from a healthy donor carrying wildtype htt alleles. As expected, the HD but not the healthy donor-derived fibroblasts contained soluble mhtt species (**Fig. 6.1A, B**). The SEC-FRET profile of HD fibroblasts indicated the presence of full-length mhtt protein (peak at approximately 500 kDa) (**Fig. 6.1B**) but mhtt fragments were absent as confirmed also by Western blot (**Fig. 6.1.C**). These results in HD fibroblasts contrast with the SEC-FRET profile we obtained from human post mortem HD brain tissue of a grade 1 HD patient. This brain tissue revealed several soluble mhtt oligomeric species in 300 kDa size-fractions and that were not found in a healthy control (**Fig. 6.2A, B, C**). These findings demonstrate the presence of mhtt fragment-oligomers in the human HD brain that can be resolved using SEC-FRET.

Discussion

In this study we combined SEC and TR-FRET to better resolve and define the formation, aggregation and age-dependent changes of endogenous mhtt protein complexes in HD cell and animal models. We found that endogenous full-length mhtt in ES-cell derived neurons, mice and human brain gives rise to mhtt N-terminal protein fragments that are present as soluble oligomers. We also found that the oligomers in the *Hdh*Q150 mouse brain can be detected at one month of age long before pathology is observed. In the *Hdh*Q150 mouse brain, the pool size of these soluble oligomers declines with age until about 8 months, from which time point onwards the pool-size seems to remain at steady-state. The decline of the soluble oligomer pool but not the levels of soluble full-length mhtt, inversely correlates with the formation and accumulation of insoluble mhtt aggregates. Finally, we demonstrated that the pool size of soluble mhtt oligomers is little or not influenced by mhtt gene dosage suggesting that the maximal size is reached and flux of mhtt molecules through this pool might be a key rate-limiting step in the formation of insoluble mhtt aggregates.

Our work provides, to our knowledge, for the first time an adequate and sensitive method under non-denaturing conditions for the detection and discrimination of populations of soluble mhtt oligomerized fragments and protein complexes generated by endogenous proteolytic cleavage of full-length mhtt in native settings in cells, mice and the HD patient brain. This is a new approach to our previous publications because its add a new biochemical dimension of oligomer vs aggregated and fragment vs full length relation of htt that may help to identify novel molecular pathways and molecules that are able to modify mhtt proteostasis and change disease course. The methodology we employed here may also facilitate the identification of brain region, species and cell-type specific mhtt protein interactions that may provide entry points for new HD therapies.

Relevant with respect to the use of clinical biopsy material and translational aspects related to measuring changes in mhtt protein in patients, we did not detect soluble mhtt oligomers or aggregates in human HD patient fibroblasts. This is in sharp contrast to their presence in all other samples we analyzed including mouse ES-derived neurons and *Hdh*Q150 mouse forebrain and striatum. This is also in sharp contrast with the analysis of human HD brain that also revealed striking signal of soluble mhtt oligomer formation compared to human brain control although future validation with more samples is here needed. One obvious explanation is that unlike the other specimens that mainly comprise non-mitotic cells, fibroblasts are mitotic cells. In proliferating cells, dilution of the soluble mhtt fragment-based oligomer pool may cause a drop in levels such that they no longer remain detectable using the TR-FRET assay. Note also that aggregation of mhtt in HD fibroblasts has not been observed and similar findings apply to many peripheral HD tissues with high contents of proliferating cells [8,26]. Whether the lack of a soluble mhtt oligomer pool is mainly explained by the proliferative nature of fibroblasts or by cell-type specific processing will require additional experiments. Possibilities to address this question is to use mitotic-arrested fibroblasts, HD patient fibroblast-derived iPS cells, iPS-derived neurons and/or biopsies from human HD tissues including those with a high content of non-proliferating cells such as muscle. One goal of such studies would be to determine whether SEC-FRET analysis can identify oligomer pools in peripherial tissue that are suitable for biomarker studies and determine if these pools correlate with the soluble pool in the brain. Ultimately, this could lead to the identification of a relevant biomarker for HD.

The *Hdh*150Q mouse we used in this study closely geno- and phenocopies pathophysiological changes seen in the human HD brain [10]. Using immuno-precipitation, a recent study identified 14 different mhtt proteolytic N-terminal fragments in the brain of these mice [19]. The authors also provided evidence for MW8 detecting mainly a neo-epitope at the C-terminus of exon-1 and the formation of aggregates by such fragments [19]. Here, we confirmed that IBs in the *Hdh*Q150 mouse brain are detected by the MW8 TR-FRET assay and by MW8 immunostaining. Given the heterogeneous collection of N-terminal mhtt fragments generated in *Hdh*Q150 brains [19] it is perhaps surprising that the heterogeneity in size of soluble mhtt fragment-containing oligomers as detected by SEC-FRET analysis is low because most of the fragments elute in size-fractions of around 200 kDa. This seems to suggest that multiple mhtt fragments of different sizes form soluble heteromeric oligomers or insoluble aggregates.

The existence of exon-1 fragments has previously been described in *Hdh*150Q mice [19]. However, the levels of monomeric exon1 fragments in solution must be very low or

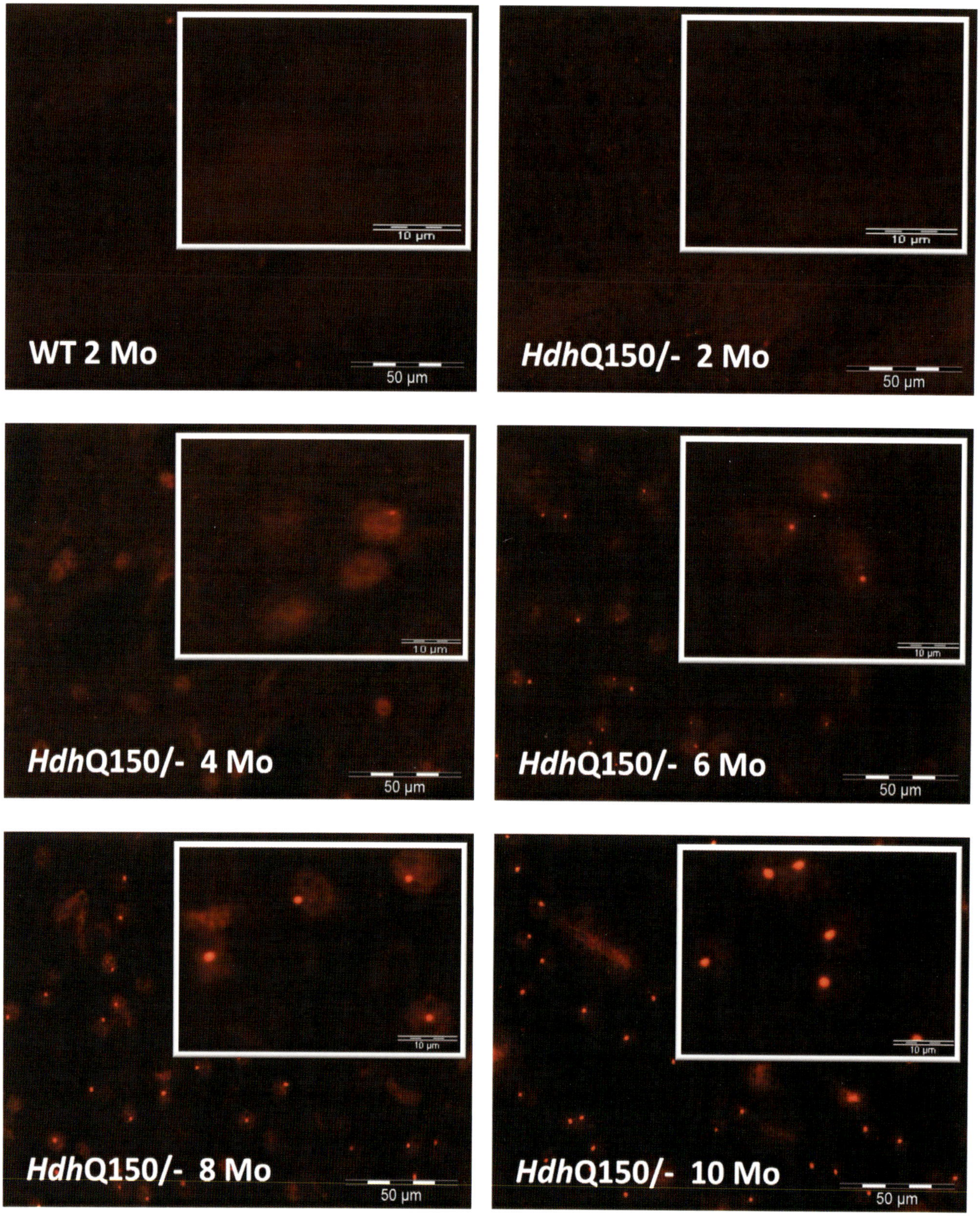

Figure 4. Immunostaining of aggregated mhtt in the striatum of *Hdh*Q150/− mice. Frozen sections were stained with unlabeled MW8 and Alexa 594-labeled secondary antibody. In wt control and at 2 months of age only non-specific background fluorescence is visible. At 4 months of age diffuse granular staining is detectable, predominantly in the nucleus. At 6 months of age the diffuse nuclear staining is less pronounced and small nuclear inclusions are visible. At later stages the nuclear inclusions are significantly larger and the granular staining is strongly diminished at 10 months of age. Note, the large elongated and irregular shaped fluorescent structures visible in images taken from *Hdh*Q150/− mice at 8 and 10 months of age are blood vessels (non-specific staining of mouse IgG by the secondary antibody).

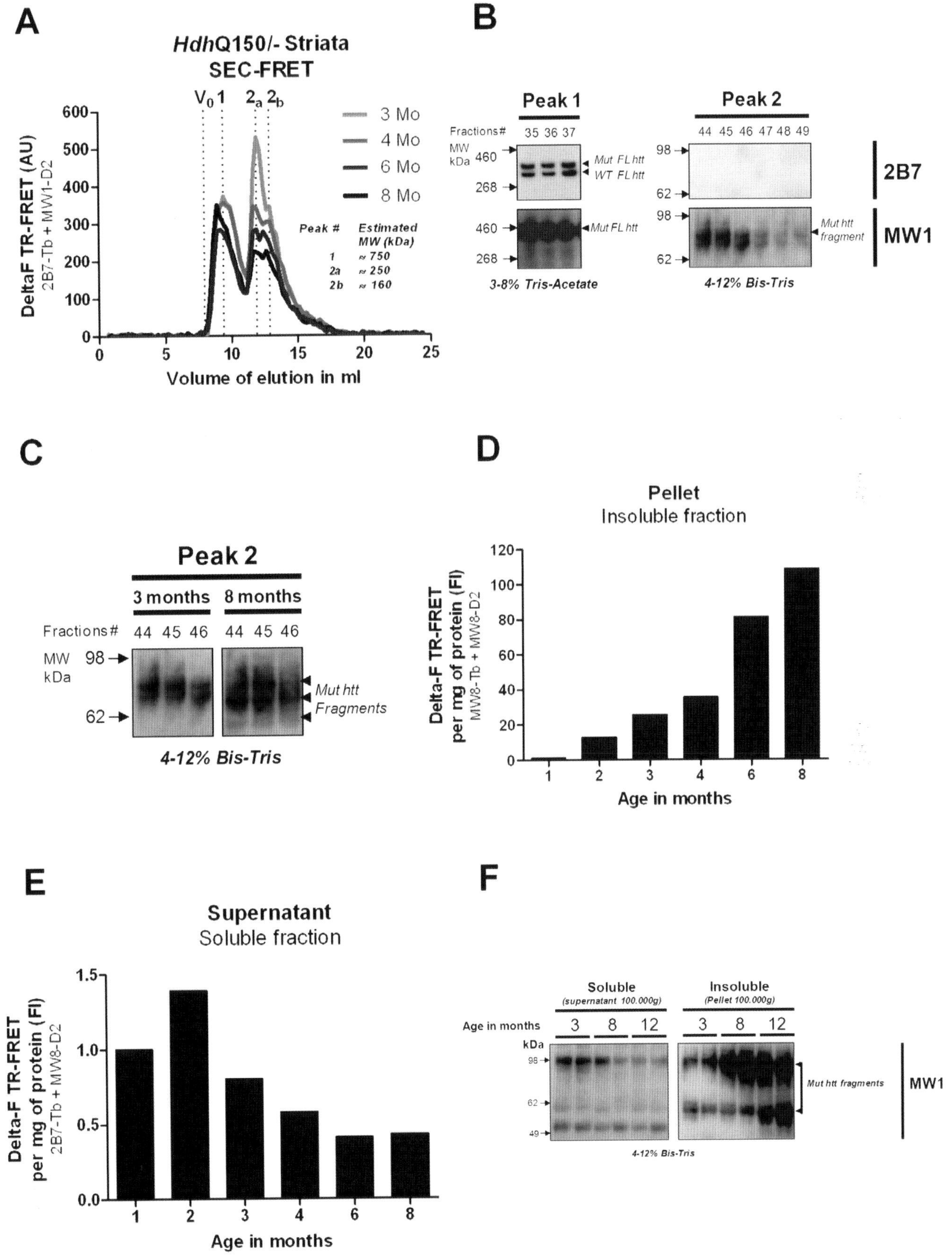

Figure 5. Analysis of *Hdh*Q150/− striatum. (A) Overlapped SEC-FRET profiles at 3, 4, 6 and 8 months of *Hdh*Q150/− striatum samples. (B) Detection of htt full-length protein (FL) by Western blot analysis in fractions 35–37 (peaks 1) and of mhtt fragments in fractions 44–49 (peak 2) using

either 2B7 or MW1 antibodies. (C). Detection of mhtt fragments by Western Blot analysis of fractions 44, 45, 46 of *Hdh*Q150/− striatum samples at 3 and 8 months (D) Quantification of the insoluble mhtt by TR-FRET MW8-Tb and MW8-D2 detection. (E) Quantification of the soluble mhtt by TR-FRET 2B7-Tb and MW8-D2 detection. (F) Detection of mhtt fragments by Western Blot analysis of soluble (supernatant, 100000 g) and insoluble (pellet) brain extracts of *Hdh*Q150/− mice at 3, 8 and 12 months.

absent at least in concentrations in the SEC fractions that no longer can be detected by the 2B7-MW1 TR-FRET. Note, even though this assay is about 10- fold more sensitive in detecting exon1 as compared to longer mhtt fragments or full length mhtt (**Fig1B**). Therefore, it seems likely that the aggregation-prone monomeric exon-1 fragments form very rapidly soluble oligomers or, alternatively, become sequestered into insoluble aggregates. The similar size of the soluble oligomer pool in homozygous and heterozygous mice is intriguing. One explanation for this observation could be that the flux rate of fragments sequestered into and out-of this pool is increased. Alternatively, newly generated mhtt fragments may escape this pool altogether because of its limited capacity and therefore instead flux straight into the insoluble aggregate pool.

One striking finding is that full-length mhtt-containing protein complexes in the striatum eluted at a different size as compared to those in forebrain suggesting that such soluble complexes have different brain region-specific and possibly also cell-type dependent compositions. Why such striking differences exist remains to be determined and awaits a further characterization of possibly variant mhtt N-terminal fragments and associated proteins in these complexes.

The classic model proposed for mhtt aggregation is based on a polyQ region-dependent nucleation and seeding leading to the formation of rigid, stable and fibrillar aggregates with atypical beta-sheet amyloid structure [27,28,29]. This model is proposed and mainly based on results obtained from *in-vitro* studies [27,28,29]. Analysis of HD brains has however provided little evidence for staining with specific amyloid dyes such as Congo Red or Thioflavin T [1] suggesting that mhtt aggregation in cells likely deviates from such a classical amyloid aggregation pathway model. Indeed, a recent study did point out that the aggregation pathway of mhtt fragments might be different *in-vivo* as compared to *in-vitro* [9,30]. Using an elegant sedimentation velocity method to detect mhtt aggregates in cell lysates, these authors described an oligomeric mhtt pool that appeared to be at steady-state and rate-limiting to IB formation [10]. Consistent with these results, our SEC-FRET analysis revealed a broad peak fraction around 200 kDa that contains at least two different mhtt fragments in the same fractions and thus supports the hypothesis that heteromeric complexes form *in-vivo*. Already mentioned before, we can not exclude the possibility that soluble mhtt fragment oligomers are not intermediates in IB formation but rather represent off-pathway species that are directly sequestered in IBs [10,28,31]. However, in our longitudinal SEC-FRET profiling study of heterozygous mice we showed that an inverse correlation exists between the pool-size of soluble mhtt fragment- oligomers and the increase in insoluble aggregates. This seems to suggest that aggregate formation is directly linked to the pool of soluble mhtt fragment-oligomers.

The question arises whether the mhtt species we detected using the 2B7-Tb MW1-D2 TR-FRET assay indeed represent mhtt fragment-oligomers? This TR-FRET assay detects only mutant and not wildtype htt molecules and only mhtt with conformations that expose simultaneously the 2B7 and the MW1 epitope (i.e. the first 17aa residues and the polyQ stretch) [8]. Other mhtt conformations in which one of these epitopes is buried are not detected by this TR-FRET assay [8]. It is likely that both epitopes are exposed in mhtt monomers that may adopt different misfolded conformations [8,32,33,34]. Nonetheless, the SEC-FRET profiles provided little or no evidence for the presence of soluble monomers. In contrast, the identification, detection and co-elution of multiple N-terminal mhtt fragments in single 200 kDa fractions clearly indicates that the 2B7-MW1 TR-FRET does detect mhtt fragments that are part of larger oligomeric complexes in which these mhtt molecules expose both the polyQ and the N-terminal 17 amino acid 2B7 epitope. Support for oligomers that expose polyQ-epitopes comes from a study where gold-labeled MW1-antibodies captured mhtt oligomers from *Hdh*Q150 cortices shown by immuno-electron microscopy [35]. These oligomers likely do not have amyloid character because the polyQ epitope is not buried and inaccessible to the Abs as it is in classical beta-sheet conformations. Therefore, it seems that soluble mhtt complexes contain also other factors, e.g. chaperones, that might prevent beta-sheet formation and stabilize different mhtt conformational states [10,34,36,37].

Previous studies including our recent publication have provided evidence of inverse correlations between the amount of aggregated and soluble mhtt [8,35,38] but they did not provide clues as to which soluble mhtt protein species is prone and a possible precursor to aggregates. Our study provides strong hints that specifically a pool of soluble mhtt fragments and not full-length mhtt protein are causally linked to aggregate formation thereby further strengthening the hypothesis that N-terminal fragments are directly responsible for the formation of IBs rather than full-length mhtt protein undergoing post-aggregation cleavage [3–7].

Our SEC-FRET analysis of homozygous *vs* heterozygous mice suggested that the pool size capacity of soluble oligomers may be limited. Our results also indicate that a chronic saturation of the soluble oligomer pool happens at a much younger age in homozygous as opposed to heterozygous *Hdh*Q150 mice. Therefore, the increased mhtt gene dosage in homozygous *Hdh*Q150 mice likely increases the flux of mhtt fragments into and out of the soluble oligomer pool and into insoluble aggregates. Perhaps this mechanism is a coping strategy that cells have to prevent mhtt fragments from impairing cellular function. In this study we did not address the issue of oligomer toxicity per se. The fact that the oligomer pool is detected already in brains of one month-old *Hdh*Q150 mice, long before any histopathophysiological phenotypes appear, certainly seems in line with the hypothesis that this fragment-oligomer pool may have a protective role preventing misfolded oligomers from exerting cellular toxicity. We therefore propose a working hypothesis (**Fig. 7**) that is based on a limited capacity of the pool size of soluble oligomers as suggested by our SEC-FRET analysis of homozygous versus heterozygous mice. The size of the soluble oligomer pool might depend on the availability of stabilization-factors (SF) of the protein quality control machinery including chaperones and components of the autophagy and proteosome pathways. Chronic saturation of the soluble oligomer pool, something that likely happens at a much younger age in homozygous as opposed to heterozygous *Hdh*Q150 mice, would likely increase the flux of mhtt fragments into and out of the soluble oligomer pool into insoluble aggregates. The latter are perhaps the last resort cells have as coping strategies to prevent mhtt fragments from impairing cell function (**Fig. 7**). During aging, the capacity to form protective soluble oligomeric

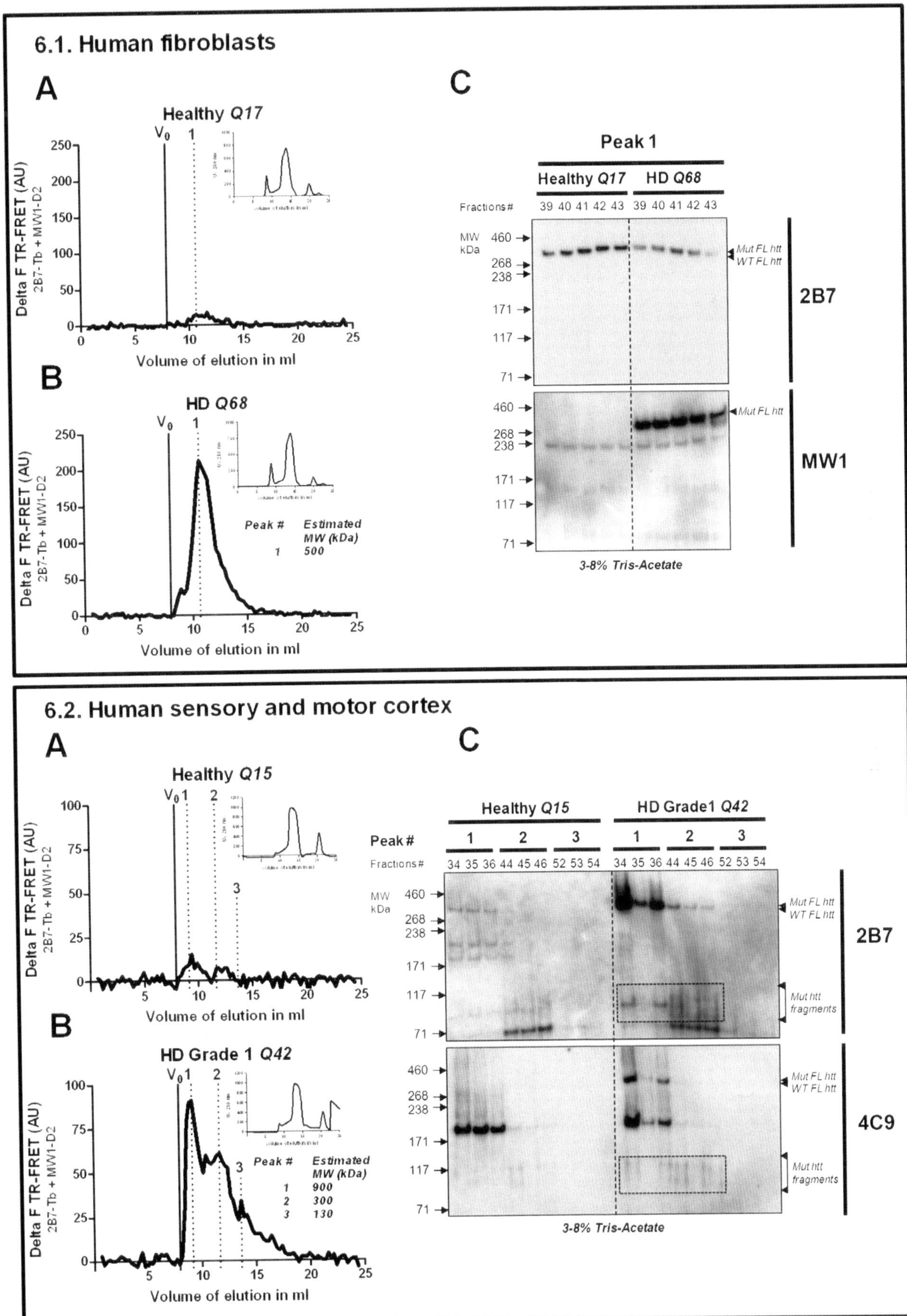
6.1. Human fibroblasts
A
Healthy Q17
Delta F TR-FRET (AU)
2B7-Tb + MW1-D2
Volume of elution in ml
B
HD Q68
Peak # Estimated MW (kDa)
1 500
C
Peak 1
Healthy Q17
HD Q68
Fractions #
39 40 41 42 43 39 40 41 42 43
MW kDa
Mut FL htt
WT FL htt
2B7
MW1
3-8% Tris-Acetate
6.2. Human sensory and motor cortex
A
Healthy Q15
B
HD Grade 1 Q42
Peak # Estimated MW (kDa)
1 900
2 300
3 130
C
Healthy Q15
HD Grade1 Q42
Peak #
Fractions #
34 35 36 44 45 46 52 53 54 34 35 36 44 45 46 52 53 54
Mut htt fragments
4C9
3-8% Tris-Acetate

Figure 6. Detection of mhtt species in human samples using SEC-FRET technology. 6.1. SEC-FRET profiles with the UV absorbance in the upper right corner in human fibroblasts (A) Healthy (Q7), (B) HD (Q68) (C) Detection of mhtt full length protein (FL) in HD fibroblast by Western blot analysis using MW1 or 2B7antibodies 6.2. SEC-FRET profiles with the UV absorbance in the upper right corner in human *post mortem* sensory and motor cortex (A) Healthy, (B) HD grade1. (C) Detection of mhtt full length (peak1) and mhtt fragments (peak2) protein in HD human post mortem brain by Western blot analysis using 4C9 (human poly-proline) or 2B7antibodies.

complexes seems to decline as our analysis in *Hdh*Q150 heterozygote mice have shown. This decline might be the result of age-dependent reductions observed for example in chaperone expression [39] or the activity of degradation systems [40,41]. If the generation of mhtt fragments does not decline, the soluble oligomer pool will gradually have less buffering capacity to capture newly generated mhtt fragments. At the same time, this likely increases the risk of undesirable protein-protein interactions that compromise cell function and viability (**Fig. 7**). From a therapeutic point of view it will be highly interesting to see if modulators such as macroautophagy-inducers or pharmacological chaperones that might increase or decrease the size of the soluble oligomer pool will indeed slow or exacerbate disease progression.

In conclusion, we presented a SEC-FRET based analysis that provided novel insights into the formation of soluble oligomers of mhtt fragments under native conditions. Most striking, mhtt fragments form a soluble oligomer pool which precedes and inversely correlates with the deposition of insoluble aggregates. We believe that the SEC-FRET technology will be useful to address multiple unanswered questions regarding mhtt proteostasis and perhaps it opens new routes to finding modulators of disease in HD and other neurodegenerative protein misfolding diseases [42,43].

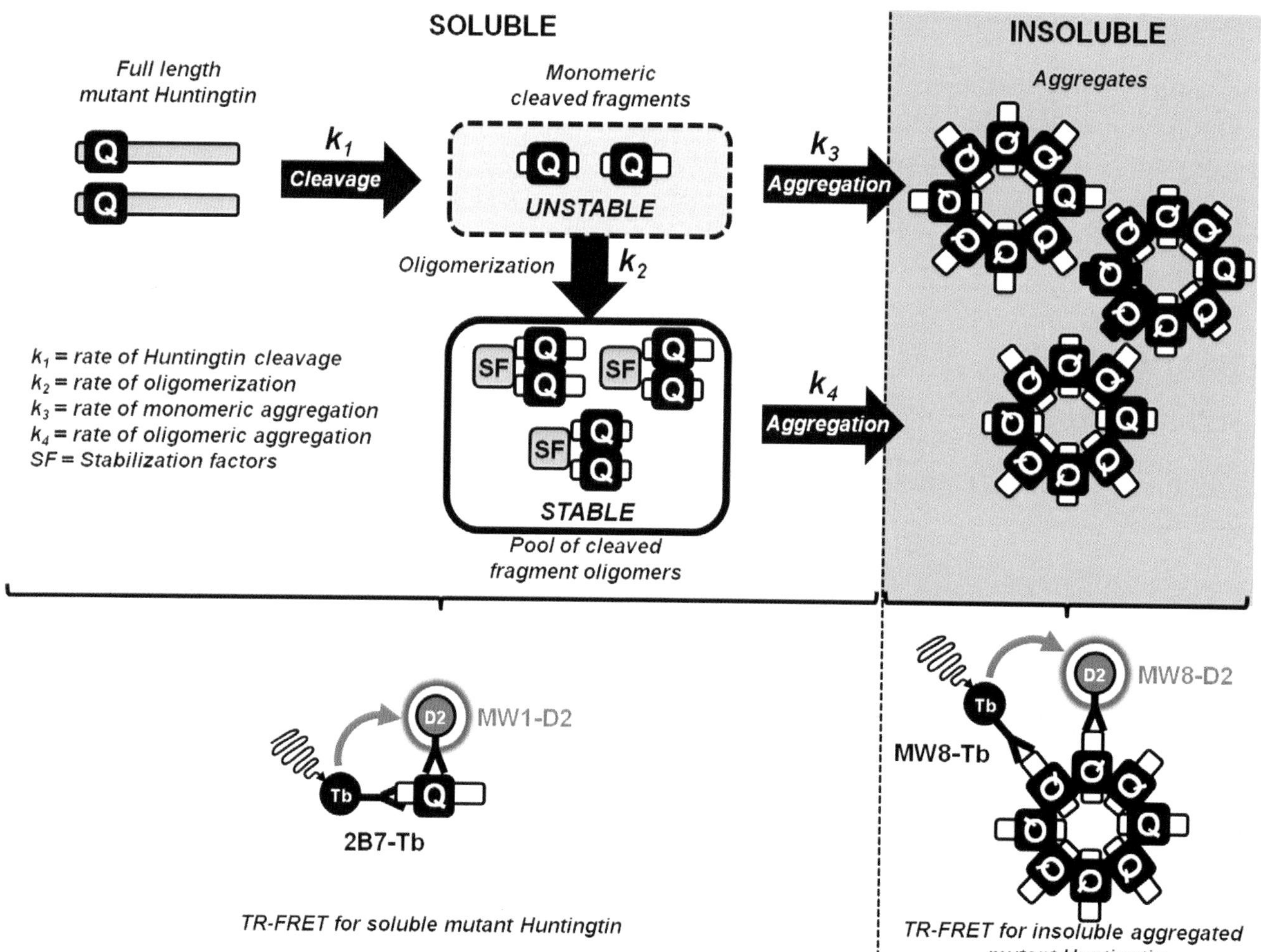

Figure 7. A model of how mutant htt aggregates in cells. After proteolytic cleavage of the full-length mutant htt protein, free monomeric N-terminal fragments are extremely short-lived, likely because the expanded polyQ region confers great conformational flexibility but misfolded states at the same time (k1). These facilitate unspecific protein-protein interactions that compromise cell function and viability. As a first line of defense, cells may therefore capture mutant htt monomeric fragments rapidly into soluble oligomers (k2). The pool size capacity of soluble oligomers may be limited by the availability of stabilization-factors (SF) of the protein quality control (chaperone, autophagy, proteosome, etc.). Chronic saturation of the soluble oligomer pool would likely increase the flux of mutant htt fragments into and out of the soluble oligomer pool into insoluble aggregates, perhaps the last resort and coping strategy cells can count on to prevent mutant htt fragments from impairing cell function (k3 and k4).

Supporting Information

Figure S1 (A) SEC elution profiles of marker proteins lead to linear correlation. The superdex 200 10/30 column was calibrated with Gel Filtration Marker Kit for Protein Molecular Weights 29,000–700,000 Da (Sigma # MWGF1000). Proteins were diluted in PBS and injected into the column. The volume of elution for each protein marker Ve was normalized to the elution volume obtained with Blue dextran (Dead volume = V0). Ratio Ve/V0 were plotted with their respective molecular weight logarithm to obtain a linear regression. **(B)** Total supernatant western blot analysis to detect mutant htt fragments with 2B7 antibody before injection onto SEC column. Western Blot analysis of wild type, Hdh Q150/− and Q150/Q150 mice forebrain supernatant extracts after ultracentrifugation at 100.000 g for 30 min (30 µg/well). 2 bands are detected: the upper band is specific for mutant htt fragment at around 80 kDa; the lower band is unspecific.

Figure S2 Quantitative analysis of aggregate size. Sizes of aggregates were calculated with the CellF software (Soft Imaging Systems/Olympus). About 100 IBs in 3 images/timepoint were analyzed. Significance was determined by Mann Whitney test, p value <0.0001 (one-tailed).

Figure S3 (A) Quantification of the area under the curve (AUC) for the peaks 1, 2a and 2b for the different ages analyzed.(B) SEC-FRET profile of HdhQ150 mice brains with TR-FRET antibody combination 2B7-Tb/MW8-D2 at 3, 4, 6 and 8 months.

Acknowledgments

We thank the CHDI foundation for support and Taconic Artemis for providing the Rosa26 ES cell lines.

Author Contributions

Conceived and designed the experiments: DM PS RRK GPL. Performed the experiments: DM DA DY JR AM JM MK GPL. Analyzed the data: DM AW MB DRS RRK HvdP PS GPL. Contributed reagents/materials/analysis tools: DA DRS RLMF GPB HvdP. Wrote the paper: GPL. Proof read the paper: DM DA RLMF GPB RRK HvdP PS.

References

1. DiFiglia M, Sapp E, Chase KO, Davies SW, Bates GP, et al. (1997) Aggregation of huntingtin in neuronal intranuclear inclusions and dystrophic neurites in brain. Science 277: 1990–1993.
2. Scherzinger E, Lurz R, Turmaine M, Mangiarini L, Hollenbach B, et al. (1997) Huntingtin-encoded polyglutamine expansions form amyloid-like protein aggregates in vitro and in vivo. Cell 90: 549–558.
3. Martindale D, Hackam A, Wieczorek A, Ellerby L, Wellington C, et al. (1998) Length of huntingtin and its polyglutamine tract influences localization and frequency of intracellular aggregates. Nat. Genet. 18: 150–154.
4. Goldberg YP, Nicholson DW, Rasper DM, Kalchman MA, Koide HB, et al.(1996) Cleavage of huntingtin by apopain, a proapoptotic cysteine protease, is modulated by the polyglutamine tract. Nat. Genet. 13: 442–449.
5. Ratovitski T, Gucek M, Jiang H, Chighladze E, Waldron E, et al.(2009) Mutant huntingtin N-terminal fragments of specific size mediate aggregation and toxicity in neuronal cells. J Biol Chem 284: 10855–10867.
6. Graham RK, Deng Y, Slow EJ, Haigh B, Bissada N, et al. (2006) Cleavage at the caspase-6 site is required for neuronal dysfunction and degeneration due to mutant huntingtin. Cell 125: 1179–11.
7. Pouladi MA, Graham RK, Karasinska JM, Xie Y, Santos RD, et al. (2009) Prevention of depressive behaviour in the YAC128 mouse model of Huntington disease by mutation at residue 586 of huntingtin Brain 132: 919–932.
8. Baldo B, Paganetti P, Grueninger S, Marcellin D, Kaltenbach LS, et al. (2012) TR-FRET-based duplex immunoassay reveals an inverse correlation of soluble and aggregated mutant huntingtin in huntington's disease. Chem.Biol. 24: 264–75.
9. Olshina MA, Angley LM, Ramdzan YM, Tang J, Bailey MF, et al.(2010) Tracking mutant huntingtin aggregation kinetics in cells reveals three major populations that include an invariant oligomer pool. J. Biol Chem 285, 21807–21816.
10. Lin CH, Tallaksen-Greene S, Chien WM, Cearley JA, Jackson WS, et al. (2001) Neurological abnormalities in a knock-in mouse model of Huntington's disease. Hum. Mol. Genet. 10: 137–144.
11. Ying QL, Wray J, Nichols J, Batlle-Morera L, Doble B, et al. (2008) The ground state of embryonic stem cell self-renewal. Nature 453: 519–523.
12. Baldo B, Weiss A, Parker CN, Bibel M, Paganetti P, Kaupmann K (2012) A screen for enhancers of clearance identifies huntingtin as a heat shock protein 90 (Hsp90) client protein. J Biol Chem 6: 1406–14.
13. Bibel M, Richter J, Lacroix E, Barde YA (2007) Generation of a defined and uniform population of CNS progenitors and neurons from mouse embryonic stem cells. Nat. Protoc. 2: 1034–1043.
14. Ko J, Ou S, Patterson PH (2001) New anti-huntingtin monoclonal antibodies: implications for huntingtin conformation and its binding proteins. Brain Res Bull 56: 319–329.
15. Weiss A, Roscic A, Paganetti P (2009) Inducible mutant huntingtin expression in HN10 cells reproduces Huntington's disease-like neuronal dysfunction. Mol. Neurodegener. Feb 09, 4: 11.
16. Paganetti P, Weiss A, Trapp M, Hammerl I, Bleckmann D, et al. (2009) Development of a method for the high-throughput quantification of cellular proteins. Chem. biochem. 10: 1678–1688.
17. Weiss A, Abramowski D, Bibel M, Bodner R, Chopra V, et al. (2009) Single-step detection of mutant huntingtin in animal and human tissues: a bioassay for Huntington's disease. Anal Biochem, 395, 8–15.
18. Weiss A, Grueninger S, Abramowski D, Giorgio FP, Lopatin MM, et al. (2011) Microtiter plate quantification of mutant and wild-type huntingtin normalized to cell count. Anal Biochem. 410: 304–306.
19. Landles C, Sathasivam K, Weiss A, Woodman B, Moffitt H, et al. (2010) Proteolysis of mutant huntingtin produces an exon 1 fragment that accumulates as an aggregated protein in neuronal nuclei in Huntington disease. J Biol Chem 285: 8808–8823.
20. Squitieri F, Gellera C, Cannella M, Mariotti C, Cislaghi G, et al. (2003) Homozygosity for CAG mutation in Huntington disease is associated with a more severe clinical course. Brain 126: 946–955.
21. Mangiarini L, Sathasivam K, Seller M, Cozens B, Harper A, et al. (1996) Exon 1 of the HD gene with an expanded CAG repeat is sufficient to cause a progressive neurological phenotype in transgenic mice. Cell 87: 493–506.
22. Benn CL, Landles C, Li H, Strand AD, Woodman B, et al. (2005) Contribution of nuclear and extranuclear polyQ to neurological phenotypes in mouse models of Huntington's disease. Hum Mol Genet 15: 3065–78.
23. Schilling G, Becher MW, Sharp AH, Jinnah HA, Duan K, et al. (1999) Intranuclear inclusions and neuritic aggregates in transgenic mice expressing a mutant N-terminal fragment of huntingtin. Hum Mol Genet 8: 397–407.
24. Graveland GA, Williams RS, DiFiglia M (1985) Evidence for degenerative and regenerative changes in neostriatal spiny neurons in Huntington's disease. Science 227: 770.
25. Myers RH, Vonsattel JP, Stevens TJ, Cupples LA, Richardson EP, et al. (1988) Clinical and neuropathologic assessment of severity in Huntington's disease. Neurology 38: 341–7.
26. Sathasivam K, Hobbs C, Turmaine M, Mangiarini L, Mahal A, et al. (1999) Formation of polyglutamine inclusions in non-CNS tissue. Hum Mol Genet 8: 813–822.
27. Scherzinger E, Sittler A, Schweiger K, Heiser V, Lurz R, et al. (1999) Self-assembly of polyglutamine-containing huntingtin fragments into amyloid-like fibrils: implications for Huntington's disease pathology. Proc Natl Acad Sci U S A 96: 4604–4609.
28. Hands SL, Wyttenbach A (2010) Neurotoxic protein oligomerisation associated with polyglutamine diseases. Acta Neuropathol.120: 419–37.
29. Legleiter J, Mitchell E, Lotz GP, Sapp E, Ng C, et al. (2010) Mutant huntingtin fragments form oligomers in a polyglutamine length-dependent manner in vitro and in vivo.J Biol Chem 285, 14777–14790.
30. Herrera F, Tenreiro S, Miller-Fleming L, Outeiro TF (2011) Visualization of cell-to-cell transmission of mutant huntingtin oligomers. PLoS Curr. 11: 3.
31. Burke KA, Godbey J, Legleiter J (2011) Assessing mutant huntingtin fragment and polyglutamine aggregation by atomic force microscopy. J. Methods. 53: 275–84.
32. Kim MW, Chelliah Y, Kim SW, Otwinowski Z, Bezprozvanny I (2009) Secondary structure of Huntingtin amino-terminal region. Structure 17: 1205–1212.
33. Bennett MJ, Huey-Tubman KE, Herr AB, West AP Jr, Ross SA, et al. (2002) A linear lattice model for polyglutamine in CAG-expansion diseases. Proc Natl Acad Sci USA 99: 11634–11639.
34. Wacker JL, Zareie MH, Fong H, Sarikaya M, Muchowski PJ (2004) Hsp70 and Hsp40 attenuate formation of spherical and annular polyglutamine oligomers by partitioning monomer. Nat Struct Mol Biol, 11: 1215–22.
35. Sathasivam K, Lane A, Legleiter J, Warley A, Woodman B, et al. (2010) Identical oligomeric and fibrillar structures captured from the brains of R6/2

and knock-in mouse models of Huntington's disease. Hum Mol Genet 19: 65–78.

36. Lotz GP, Legleiter J, Aron R, Mitchell EJ, Huang SY, et al. (2010) Hsp70 and Hsp40 functionally interact with soluble mutant huntingtin oligomers in a classic ATP-dependent reaction cycle. J Biol Chem 285: 38183–38193.
37. Behrends C, Langer CA, Boteva R, Bottcher UM, Stemp MJ, et al. (2006) Chaperonin TRiC promotes the assembly of polyQ expansion proteins into nontoxic oligomers. Mol. Cell 23: 887–897.
38. Woodman B, Butler R, Landles C, Lupton MK, Tse J, et al. (2007) The Hdh(Q150/Q150) knock-in mouse model of HD and the R6/2 exon 1 model develop comparable and widespread molecular phenotypes. Brain Res Bull 72: 83–97.
39. Labbadia J, Cunliffe H, Weiss A, Katsyuba E, Sathasivam K, et al.(2011) Altered chromatin architecture underlies progressive impairment of the heat shock response in mouse models of Huntington disease. J. Clin. Invest 121, 3306–3319.
40. Bennett EJ, Shaler TA, Woodman B, Ryu KY, Zaitseva TS, et al. (2007) Global changes to the ubiquitin system in Huntington's disease. Nature 448: 704–708.
41. Martinez-Vicente M, Talloczy Z, Wong E, Tang G, Koga H, et al. (2010) Cargo recognition failure is responsible for inefficient autophagy in Huntington's disease. Nat Neurosci. 13: 567–76.
42. Mitsui K, Doi H, Nukina N (2006) Proteomics of polyglutamine aggregates. Methods Enzymol 412, 63–76.
43. Ross CA, Poirier MA (2005) Opinion: What is the role of protein aggregation in neurodegeneration? Nat. Rev. Mol. Cell Biol. 6: 891–898.

6

Muscleblind-Like 1 Knockout Mice Reveal Novel Splicing Defects in the Myotonic Dystrophy Brain

Koichi Suenaga[1]❡, Kuang-Yung Lee[2,3]❡, Masayuki Nakamori[4¤a], Yoshiki Tatsumi[1], Masanori P. Takahashi[4], Harutoshi Fujimura[5], Kenji Jinnai[6], Hiroo Yoshikawa[1], Hongqing Du[7¤b], Manuel Ares Jr.[7], Maurice S. Swanson[2], Takashi Kimura[1]*

1 Division of Neurology, Department of Internal Medicine, Hyogo College of Medicine, Nishinomiya, Hyogo, Japan, **2** Department of Molecular Genetics and Microbiology, College of Medicine, University of Florida, Gainesville, Florida, United States of America, **3** Department of Neurology, Chang Gung Memorial Hospital, Keelung, Taiwan, **4** Department of Neurology, Osaka University Graduate School of Medicine, Suita, Osaka, Japan, **5** Department of Neurology, National Hospital Organization Toneyama Hospital, Toyonaka, Osaka, Japan, **6** Department of Neurology, National Hospital Organization Hyogo-Chuo Hospital, Ohara, Hyogo, Japan, **7** Department of Molecular, Cell and Developmental Biology, RNA Center, Sinsheimer Labs, University of California Santa Cruz, Santa Cruz, California, United States of America

Abstract

Myotonic dystrophy type 1 (DM1) is a multi-systemic disorder caused by a CTG trinucleotide repeat expansion (CTG^{exp}) in the *DMPK* gene. In skeletal muscle, nuclear sequestration of the alternative splicing factor muscleblind-like 1 (MBNL1) explains the majority of the alternative splicing defects observed in the HSA^{LR} transgenic mouse model which expresses a pathogenic range CTG^{exp}. In the present study, we addressed the possibility that MBNL1 sequestration by CUG^{exp} RNA also contributes to splicing defects in the mammalian brain. We examined RNA from the brains of homozygous $Mbnl1^{\Delta E3/\Delta E3}$ knockout mice using splicing-sensitive microarrays. We used RT-PCR to validate a subset of alternative cassette exons identified by microarray analysis with brain tissues from $Mbnl1^{\Delta E3/\Delta E3}$ knockout mice and post-mortem DM1 patients. Surprisingly, splicing-sensitive microarray analysis of $Mbnl1^{\Delta E3/\Delta E3}$ brains yielded only 14 candidates for mis-spliced exons. While we confirmed that several of these splicing events are perturbed in both *Mbnl1* knockout and DM1 brains, the extent of splicing mis-regulation in the mouse model was significantly less than observed in DM1. Additionally, several alternative exons, including *Grin1* exon 4, *App* exon 7 and *Mapt* exons 3 and 9, which have previously been reported to be aberrantly spliced in human DM1 brain, were spliced normally in the *Mbnl1* knockout brain. The sequestration of MBNL1 by CUG^{exp} RNA results in some of the aberrant splicing events in the DM1 brain. However, we conclude that other factors, possibly other MBNL proteins, likely contribute to splicing mis-regulation in the DM1 brain.

Editor: Thomas H. Gillingwater, University of Edinburgh, United Kingdom

Funding: TK was supported by Research Grant for Intractable Disease from the Ministry of Health Labour and Welfare 22-118 and Grants-in-aid for Scientific Research from JSPS 23591258. MSS was supported by the National Institutes of Health (NIH) grant NS058901. MA was supported by the NIH grant GM084317. KJ was supported by the Intramural Research Grant for Neurological and Psychiatric Disorders of NCNP 22-7. The funders had no role in study design, data collection and analysis, decision to publish, or preparation of the manuscript.

Competing Interests: The authors have declared that no competing interests exist.

* E-mail: kimura@hyo-med.ac.jp

❡ These authors contributed equally to this work.

¤a Current address: Department of Neurology, University of Rochester Medical Center, Rochester, New York, United States of America
¤b Current address: Department of Pediatrics, Stanford School of Medicine, Stanford, California, United States of America

Introduction

Myotonic dystrophy type1 (DM1) is a multi-systemic disorder affecting skeletal muscle, heart, ocular lens, testis, and the central nervous system (CNS). CNS involvement in adult-onset DM1 includes visual spatial and attention deficits, dysexecutive syndrome, apathy, avoidant behavior and excessive daytime sleepiness (review [1]). Although neuropathological studies have revealed several morphological changes [2,3,4], whether these changes contribute to the clinical symptoms observed in DM1 remains to be determined.

DM1 is caused by the unstable expansion of CTG trinucleotide repeats in the 3′ untranslated region of the DM protein kinase (*DMPK*) gene [5]. Recent evidence suggests that transcripts containing expanded CUG repeats (CUG^{exp}) accumulate in nuclear RNA foci and exert toxic effects on a variety of cellular regulatory pathways including splicing and transcription [6]. One disease model that is supported by considerable experimental evidence proposes that CUG^{exp} RNAs cause sequestration and inhibition of the RNA-binding protein MBNL1 [7]. In support of this model, *Mbnl1* knockout mice develop the muscle, eye, and RNA splicing abnormalities that are characteristic of DM1 disease [8]. In addition, we have reported a strong correlation in skeletal muscle splicing changes between two mouse models of DM1, the HSA^{LR} transgenic and the *Mbnl1* knockout [9].

In the CNS of DM1 patients, mutant *DMPK* transcripts accumulate in neuronal nuclei and sequester MBNL1 and MBNL2 [10]. Although abnormal regulation of several alternatively spliced exons has also been documented in the DM1 brain [10,11,12,13], it is not clear if MBNL1 sequestration contributes to aberrant splicing. Here we used splicing-sensitive microarrays to detect mis-splicing in the $Mbnl1^{\Delta E3/\Delta E3}$ knockout brain.

Results

Splicing perturbations in the *Mbnl1*$^{\Delta E3/\Delta E3}$ knockout brain

To test directly whether loss of MBNL1 expression contributes to aberrant splicing in the CNS, RNA was extracted from the brains of age-matched males carrying homozygous *Mbnl1*$^{\Delta E3/\Delta E3}$ knockout or wild-type alleles in the same (C57BL/6J) background and analyzed on splicing-sensitive microarrays [9]. Experience with this method indicates that differences in the $\log_2$ of the ratio of exon skipping to inclusion (the skip/include ratio) between two samples (sepscore) with an absolute value >0.3 can be validated by RT-PCR. We observed 14 events in *Mbnl1*$^{\Delta E3/\Delta E3}$ knockout mice that exceeded this score (Table S1). We used RT-PCR to validate a subset of alternative cassette exons identified by microarray analysis and found four events (*Sorbs1* exons 6 and 25, *Spag9* exon 31, *Dclk1* exon 19) that showed significant differences in splicing between wild-type and knockout mice in both the hippocampus and cerebellum (Figure 1A,B). *Sorbs1* is particularly interesting because it is expressed in multiple tissues and exon 25 is regulated during postnatal development [9,14]. In heart, MBNL1 is a major factor which regulates exon 25 splicing with nearly complete inclusion in wild-type adult heart but only ~60% inclusion in the *Mbnl1* knockout heart. While this exon is also mis-spliced in the *Mbnl1* knockout brain, the effect of MBNL1 loss on this exon is considerably less in both the hippocampus and cerebellum. This modest effect of MBNL1 loss on other mis-regulated exons was also apparent for *Spag9* exon 31, *Sorbs1* exon 6 and *Dclk1* exon 19 (Figure 1B). Nevertheless, these exons are regulated during developmental transition from neonatal (P6) to adult (P42) forebrain (Figure 1A), which indicates other factor may play a role in splicing regulation during this period.

Splicing microarrays also revealed mis-splicing of *Camk2d*, so we further investigated splicing of this gene. Importantly, *Camk2d* splicing is regulated during postnatal development with the major isoforms all containing exons 14a and 17 with alternative splicing of the exon 14b, 15 and 16 cassettes to generate several major isoforms, including δ1, δ2, δ3, δ3.1, δ4 and δ9 (Figure 2). Previous reports have indicated that the δ1 isoform is the major splice variant in the adult rat forebrain, while δ4 isoform is expressed in the neonatal rat forebrain [15]. We observed that in P1 whole brain, P6 fore- and hindbrain, δ1 and δ9 are the major isoforms while in adults (P42), exon 15 is preferentially spliced, so that in addition to δ1, δ4 is also the major form in forebrain and both δ4 and δ3 are expressed in hindbrain. In accordance with other splicing changes where immature splicing isoforms are expressed in the adult tissues, splicing of the fetal δ9 isoform significantly increased in the hippocampus of *Mbnl1* knockouts compared to controls although the increase was modest and was not observed in the cerebellum. While the δ9 isoform increased, the δ3 (+14b −15 −16) isoform decreased in *Mbnl1* knockout mouse hippocampus compared with wild-type.

Aberrant splicing in human brain samples and comparison with *Mbnl1* knockout brain

To determine whether these mis-splicing events predicted from the *Mbnl1* knockout brain microarray data were also observed in the human DM1 brain, we aligned affected mouse exons to the human genome and found 12 exons that are conserved and orthologous to MBNL1-dependent mouse exons (Table S2). We examined all of these events in post-mortem human temporal cortex and cerebellum. The most striking result in human DM1 brain was mis-splicing of *SORBS1* exon 26 (orthologous to mouse exon 25). In the temporal cortex, the average percentage of exon 26 inclusion in DM1 was ~40% while those observed in the normal controls and in the disease controls were ~85% and ~90%, respectively (Figure 3A and B, upper). In the cerebellum, exon 26 inclusion was also significantly decreased in DM1 compared with in disease controls, although this difference is subtler than that in the temporal cortex. Both *DCLK1* exon 19 inclusion and *MPRIP* exon 9 inclusion were significantly decreased in DM1 temporal cortex (Figure 3A and B, middle and bottom), whereas there is no difference in these splicing events between DM1 and disease cerebellums.

In humans, the splicing of *CAMK2D* is also regulated in a tissue-specific and developmental manner. We found that δ9 was expressed almost exclusively in human fetal whole brain (unlike rodent brain), while δ1 was predominantly expressed in adult human temporal cortex samples (Figure 3C to E). In contrast, the percentage of the δ9 isoform was significantly increased in adult DM1 temporal cortex compared to both disease and normal controls. This increase was ~30% in DM1 temporal cortex (Figure 3E), or apparently larger than that observed in the hippocampus of *Mbnl1* knockout mice (Figure 2), although we could not conclude which of the following changes will have a stronger impact: (a) an increase from 0 to ~2.5% in *Mbnl1* knockout mice (Figure 2C), or (b) an increase from ~10% to ~30% in DM1 temporal cortex (Figure 3E). As a result of the increase of δ9, the percentage of δ1 was significantly decreased in the DM1 temporal cortex. In DM1 and disease control cerebellums, δ9 was a major isoform and there is no difference between these two. Unlike mouse cerebellum, δ3 isoform was not observed in any groups of human brains.

Initially we did temporal lobe autopsy on human since a former report showed splicing defects of several exons in this region [10]. We did hippocampus analysis on mouse because it is a key region of the brain involved in learning and memory. We thought a concern of regional difference between hippocampus and temporal lobe may not be an issue since a report showed similar tau pathology in hippocampus and temporal cortex [4] and we have compared the splicing pattern of each exon in these regions of mouse brain and found similar splicing defects of *Sorbs1* exon 25 and *Camk2d* exon 14–16 (increased expression of δ9) in *Mbnl1* knockout mice (Figure S1). We also used cerebellum samples as a reference region since no apparent cerebellar symptoms in DM1 patients and the lack of RNA foci in DM1 cerebellar cortex have been reported [10]. Although we did not show a direct binding of MBNL1 on these RNA by CLIP (cross linked immuno precipitation), we identified several YGCY motifs in the upstream and downstream introns of these alternative spliced cassettes (Table S3).

We determined by Southern blot analysis the CTG repeat number of the same brain tissues from which we took RNA for RT-PCR (Table 1). Cerebral cortex showed greater CTG repeat number and larger intra-tissue CTG length heterogeneities than cerebellum, consistent with a previous observation [16]. The comparison between the degree of aberrant splicing of each exon and each shortest, median and longest CTG repeat number showed no correlation (Figure S2). Several splicing defects have been reported in DM1 brain and we confirmed some of them (exon 4 of *GRIN1*, exons 3 and 12 of *MAPT* and exon 9 of *APP*) in our human DM1 temporal cortex samples (Figure S3A). However, our splicing microarray analysis did not detect any mis-splicing of these exons in the *Mbnl1* knockout model. RT-PCR using each set of specific primer for these exons (*Grin1* exon 4, *Mapt* exons 3 and 9, and *App* exon 7) also revealed no defects of splicing (Figure S3B).

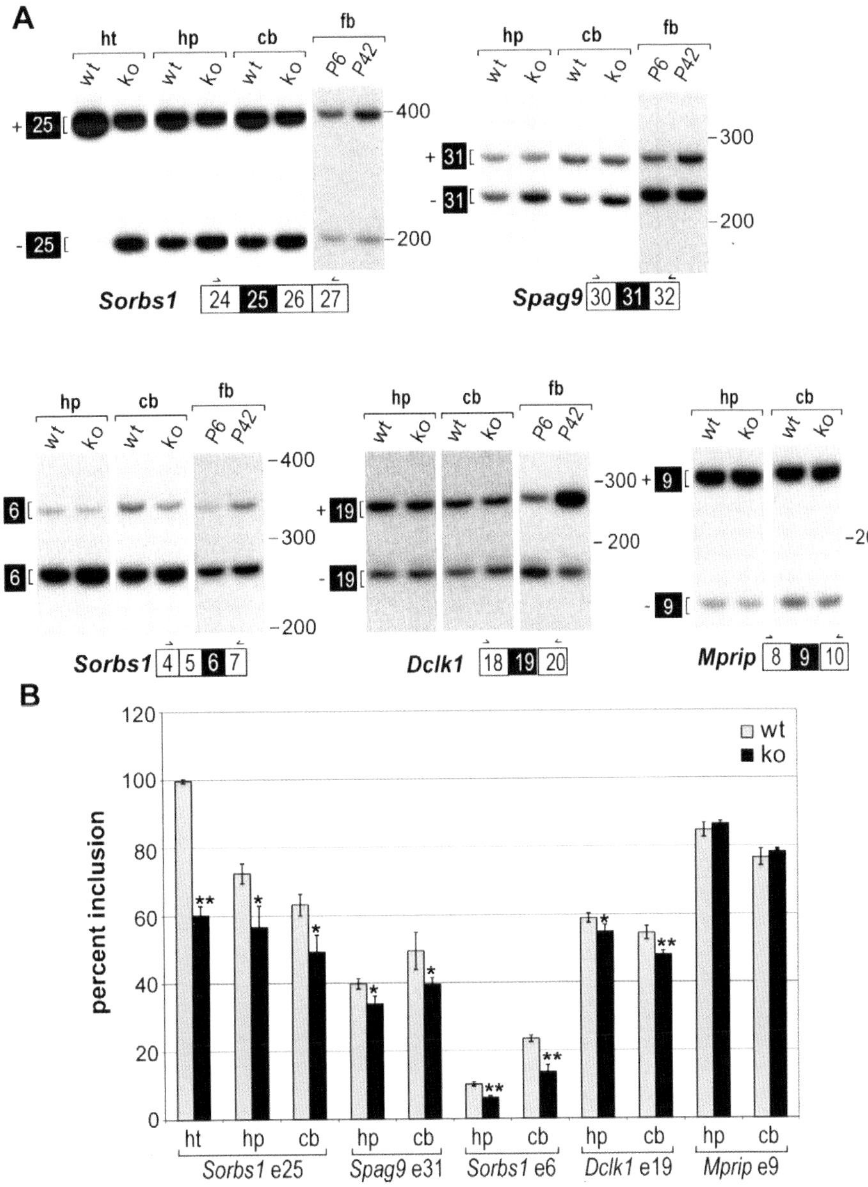

Figure 1. MBNL1 splicing targets in the mouse brain. RT-PCR analysis of wild-type (wt, n = 3, 3–6 months of age) versus *Mbnl1*$^{\Delta E3/\Delta E3}$ (ko, n = 3, 3–6months of age) brain splicing. (*A*) Representative PCR products. (*B*) Percent exon inclusion measured by phosphoimager analysis. Loss of MBNL1 expression results in reduced exon inclusion for *Sorbs1* exon 25, *Spag9* exon 31, *Sorbs1* exon 6 and *Dclk1* exon 19 in both the hippocampus (hp) and cerebellum (cb). The inclusion of these exons is enhanced in the adult (P42) forebrain (fb) compared to the neonatal (P6) forebrain. *Sorbs1* exon 25 splicing in the heart (ht) and *Mprip* splicing in the brain are included as positive and negative splicing controls. Both unpaired *t*-test and permutation test were used for calculating *p* value (**p* value$<$0.05, ***p* value$<$0.01). Averages and standard deviations were generated by unpaired *t*-test.

Discussion

In the present study, we found three novel splicing events, *Sorbs1* exon 25 (exon 26 in human), *Dclk1* exon 19, and *Camk2d* exon 14–16 (exon 14–15 in human), altered both in DM1 and in *Mbnl1* knockout brains. This is the first report of mis-splicing of orthologous exons in brain tissues from human DM1 and *Mbnl1* knockout mice, although mis-splicing of exons 3 and 12 (9 in mice) of *MAPT* has been shown in human DM1 brain [10,13] and in the CTG transgenic mouse brain [17]. In general, the *Mbnl1* knockout hippocampus and DM1 temporal cortex shared similar splicing defects. We also confirmed similar splicing defects of some genes in the hippocampus and temporal cortex of *Mbnl1* knockout mice (Figure S1). The expression of the fetal splicing isoforms in our samples is consistent with other splicing abnormalities in which fetal splice isoforms are expressed in adult DM1 patients and model mice. Interestingly, only the increase in *GRIN1* exon 4 inclusion in DM1 brain does not represent a return to a fetal splicing profile (Figure S3), which may suggest that distinct splicing factors regulate this splicing event. Our data did not demonstrate directly that MBNL1 regulates the splicing of these exons. However, we found many YGCY motifs that could potentially serve as MBNL1 binding motifs (Table S3) [9].

In human cerebellum, aberrant splicing was less apparent and only splicing of *SORBS1* exon 26 was altered significantly, while similar splicing defects were shown in the hippocampus and

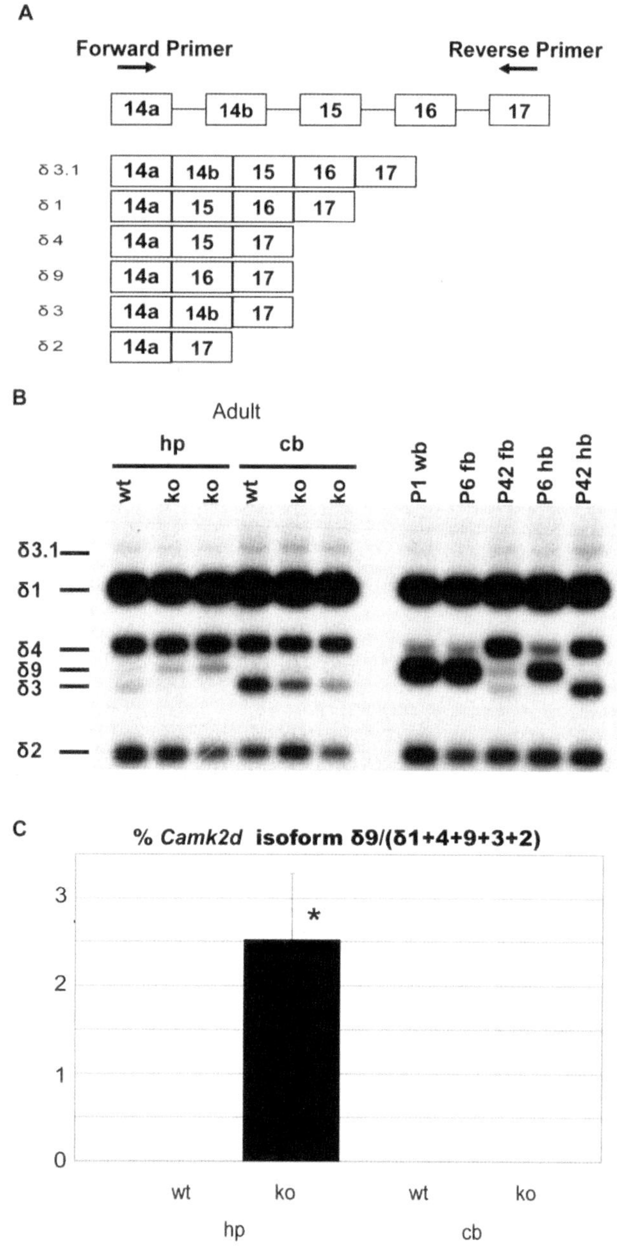

Figure 2. Spatial and temporal differences in the expression of *Camk2d*. (A) Transcripts of Camk2d. (B) Representative PCR products. Six spliced isoforms were detected by using primer pairs located in exons 14a and 17. Right panel shows isoform switching from δ9 to δ4 during the fetal (P1, P6) to adult (P42) transition in whole brain (wb), forebrain (fb) and hindbrain (hb) whereas the δ9 isoform was undetectable in adult hindbrain. Left panel shows a detectable increase in the δ9 isoform in *Mbnl1*$^{\Delta E3/\Delta E3}$ hippocampus (hp) compared with wild-type sibs. However, no δ9 isoform could be detected in the cerebellum of either wild-type or *Mbnl1* knockout mice. (C) The percentage of *Camk2d* isoform δ9 to δ1+4+9+3+2. Both unpaired *t*-test and permutation test were used for calculating *p* value (n = 3, **p* value<0.05). Averages and standard deviations were generated by unpaired *t*-test.

cerebellum of the *Mbnl1* mouse knockout model. One possible reason for this modest splicing alteration in the cerebellum of human DM1 is that fetal splicing isoforms of some genes are already dominantly expressed in human adult cerebellum and thus there is no room for any detectable difference of fetal isoforms between DM1 and control samples (e.g. *CAMK2D* in which fetal δ9 isoform is almost exclusively expressed in both disease control and DM1 cerebellums relative to fetal brain (Figure 3E)). Another possibility is that MBNL1 may not be as efficiently sequestered in RNA foci in the DM1 cerebellar nucleus because the CTG repeat expansion is much smaller in the cerebellum than in the temporal cortex (Table 1). One alternative possibility is that MBNL1 contributes less significantly to the regulation of splicing in human cerebellum. This possibility is unlikely, however, for the following reasons. First, both the immunohistochemistry and western blotting displayed similar expression of MBNL1 in different regions of the brain (Figure S4, Material and Methods S1). Second, since our RT-PCR demonstrated similar splicing defects in Mbnl1 targeted exons in both the hippocampus and cerebellum of Mbnl1 knockout mice (Figure 1), it seems that the contributions of Mbnl1 to these regions are similar.

Compared with *Mbnl1* knockout skeletal muscle, where 246 events achieved sepscore values of >0.3 [9], we observed far fewer splicing events that exceeded this score. Some exons previously reported to be mis-spliced in the DM1 brain were not observed in the *Mbnl1* knockout brain. In addition, the extent of splicing mis-regulation in the mouse model was significantly less than observed for DM1 (Figures 1, 2, 3). A possible explanation for these smaller splicing changes in *Mbnl1* knockout mouse brain is that there are species differences of splicing regulation between mouse and human. However, transgenic mouse brains carrying over 700 CTG repeat have been reported to display splicing abnormalities of *Mapt*, *Grin1*, *Mbnl1*, and *Mbnl2* [17]. These results suggest that the contribution of MBNL1 to developmental splicing transitions in the brain is less significant than in skeletal muscle or that the cellular complexity of the brain masks a larger effect of MBNL1 loss on particular cell populations. Three genes encode *MBNL* paralogs in mammals, *MBNL1*, *MBNL2* and *MBNL3*, and all of the encoded proteins have been demonstrated to colocalize with nuclear foci in DM1 cells [18]. In reconstruction experiments using transfected cells, each MBNL protein can regulate alternative splicing of pre-mRNAs that are misregulated in DM1 [19]. As MBNL3 is expressed predominantly in the placenta [18], the likely candidate which may play a more significant role in alternative splicing in the brain is MBNL2. While human MBNL1 is expressed primarily in skeletal muscle and heart, MBNL2 is expressed at a similar level in the majority of tissues [18]. Thus, the contribution of MBNL2 to splicing changes may be relatively high in brain in contrast to skeletal muscle. It has been reported that *Mbnl1* knockout mice demonstrate cognitive and behavioral abnormalities and normal spatial learning and memory [20]. This relatively mild phenotype may correlate with the modest splicing alteration. Regarding exon 31 of *Spag9* and exon 6 of *Sorbs1*, we found the significant difference between wild-type and *Mbnl1* knockout, but not in human brains. This discrepancy may contradict our hypothesis that the recruitment of MBNL1 contributes to the splicing defects in DM1 brains, but may be explained by a difference of splicing regulation between mice and human.

In vitro experiments suggested that a loss of MBNL1 or a gain of CELF1 function could repress exon 3 inclusion but not exon 9 inclusion of *Mapt*, whereas CELF2 is a repressor of both exons [21]. However, *Mbnl1* knockout mice did not show any splicing differences for these exons. This discrepancy about MBNL1 dependent regulation of the splicing of *Mapt* exon3 between in vitro and mice experiments may also indicate that some redundant factors function in this splicing regulation and loss of MBNL1

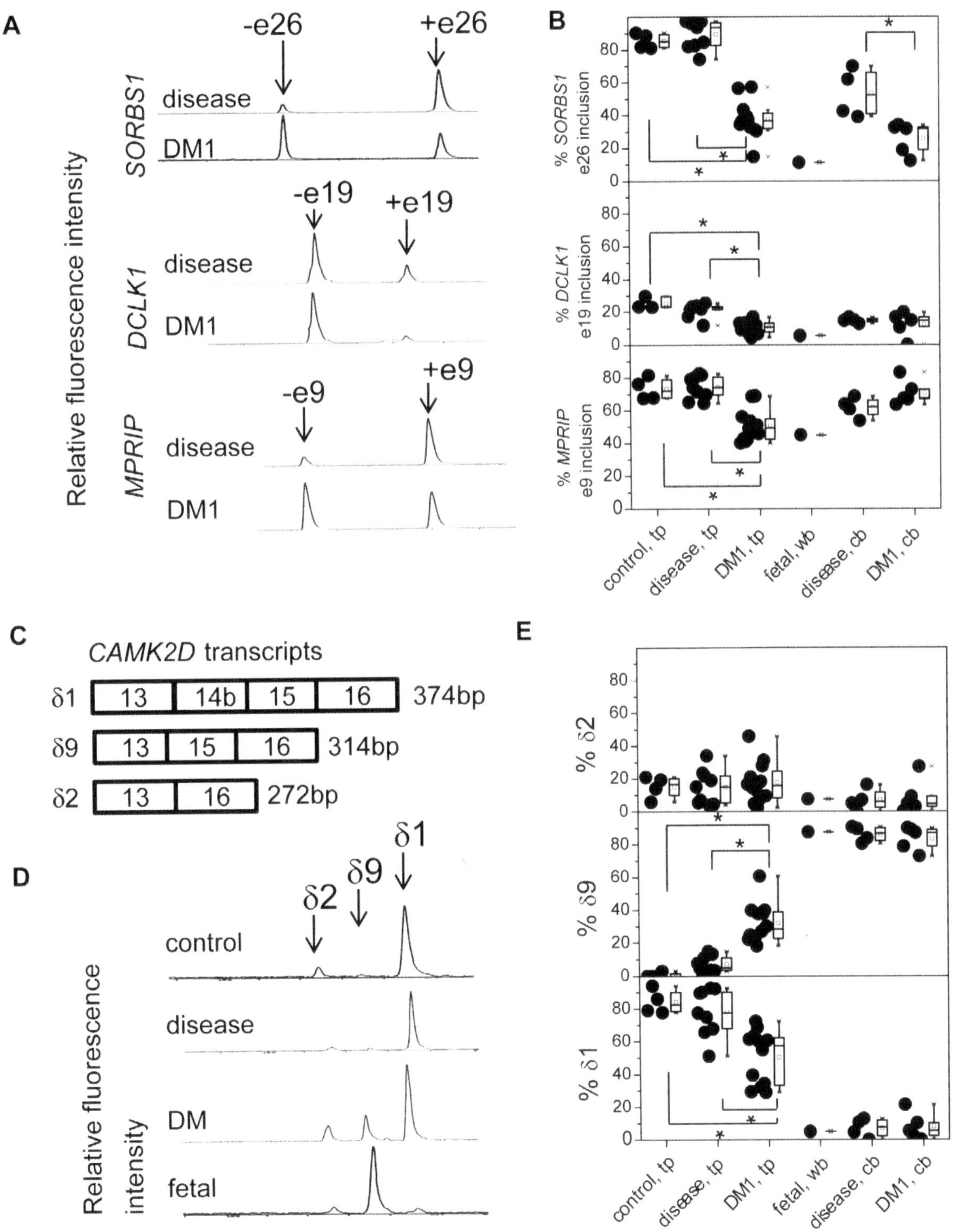

Figure 3. Aberrant splicing events in *Mbnl1*$^{\Delta E3/\Delta E3}$ brain are also observed in the human DM1 brain. We compared brain RNA from normal control temporal cortex (control, tp, n = 4), disease control temporal cortex (disease, tp, n = 9), myotonic dystrophy type 1 temporal cortex (DM1, tp, n = 12), fetal control whole brain (fetal, wb, n = 1), disease control cerebellum (disease, cb, n = 4), and DM1 cerebellum (DM1, cb, n = 5). (A) Representative RT-PCR products detected with microchip electrophoretic separation using SV1210 software on the Hitachi SV1210 from exclusion and inclusion of exon 26 of *SORBS1* (upper), exon 19 of *DCLK1* (middle), and exon 9 of *MPRIP* (bottom). (B) Graphical representation of RT-PCR analysis depicting percentages of exon 26 inclusion of *SORBS1* (upper), exon 19 inclusion of *DCLK1* (middle), and exon 9 inclusion of *MPRIP* (bottom). (C) Transcripts of *CAMK2D*. (D) Representative RT-PCR products from *CAMK2D* isoforms: δ2(−exon14b−exon15), δ9(−exon14b+exon15), and δ1(+exon14b+exon15) indicated by each arrow. (E) Graphical representation of RT-PCR analysis depicting percentages of δ2 (upper), δ9 (middle) and δ1 (bottom). Mann-Whitney U test was used for calculating the *p* value. Statistically significant differences ($p<0.05$) are indicated by an asterisk.

Table 1. Human samples analysed.

Patient no/sex	Age	disaese	Sources	CTG repeats in brain samples
C1/M	23	[a]normal	temporal cortex	
C2/M	22	[a]normal	temporal cortex	
C3/M	26	[a]normal	temporal cortex	
C4/F	78	[b]normal	temporal cortex	
D1/F	69	PD	temporal cortex	
D2/F	84	MSA-C	temporal cortex	
D3/F	80	ALS	temporal cortex	
D4/M	53	ALS	temporal cortex	
			cerebellum	
D5/F	81	ALS	temporal cortex	
			cerebellum	
D6/M	70	ALS	temporal cortex	
D7/F	75	ALS	temporal cortex	
D8/F	61	ALS	temporal cortex	
			cerebellum	
D9/M	70	ALS	temporal cortex	
			cerebellum	
DM1/M	58	DM1	temporal cortex	3000–6000
DM2/M	69	DM1	temporal cortex	3000–6000
DM3/M	50	DM1	temporal cortex	2000–6000
DM4/F	56	DM1	temporal cortex	3000–5000
			cerebellum	400
DM5/M	63	DM1	temporal cortex	1200–3000
DM6/M	59	DM1	temporal cortex	3000–9000
DM7/F	58	DM1	temporal cortex	3000–6000
			cerebellum	2200–3000
DM8/F	58	DM1	temporal cortex	2000–8000
DM9/F	58	DM1	temporal cortex	2200–6500
			cerebellum	300
DM10/F	66	DM1	temporal cortex	1900–3300
			cerebellum	150
DM11/M	64	DM1	temporal cortex	2400–5200
DM12/F	73	DM1	temporal cortex	1900–4800
			cerebellum	200
F1/F	21w	[c]fetal	whole brain	

[a]from Biochain,
[b]from Ambion,
[c]from Stratagene, PD; Parkinson's disease; MSA-C; multiple system atrophy with predominant cerebellar ataxia; ALS: amyotrophic lateral sclerosis.

alone is insufficient to change the splicing pattern of this exon in the brain.

SORBS1 was identified as a Cbl-associated protein likely to participate in insulin signaling [22]. The targeted exon encodes the nuclear localization sequence (NLS) [23], suggesting that the protein without an NLS is increased in the DM1 brain and might not be able to function as a nuclear protein. Among the four types of CAMK2 isoforms, the CAMK2D is expressed predominantly in the suprachiasmatic nucleus, substantia nigra, and striatum in the brain. Since each spliced isoform of CAMK2D has been reported to show a distinct distribution pattern [24,25], the increase in δ9 might cause abnormal localization. Interestingly, CAMK2D has been reported to play an essential role in PER1 expression, which is possibly involved in light-induced phase shifts [26]. Although excessive daytime sleepiness and dysregulation of REM sleep occur frequently in patients with DM1, it was reported that the pathophysiologic basis is distinct from narcolepsy, as patients with DM1 do not have a consistent defect of hypocretin release or receptor splicing [27]. Possibly, aberrant splicing of *CAMK2D* might be associated with excessive daytime sleepiness in DM1. DCLK1 is a microtubule-associated kinase that can undergo autophosphorylation and regulate microtubule polymerization [28]. The fetus specific C-terminal splicing variant (exon 19 exclusion), which is expressed more in DM1 adult temporal cortex, showed enhanced autophosphorylation activity and has been suggested a possible role in migrating neurons [29]. Therefore, the increase in the fetal variant of DCLK1 in DM1 brain may cause an abnormal neuronal migration. MPRIP was initially identified as an 116 kDa protein that interacts with RhoA [30]. In neuronal cells, MPRIP is essential for neurite outgrowth and may act as a scaffold to target the myosin phosphatase complex to the actin cytoskeleton [31]. Although the difference between splicing isoforms has not been reported, aberrant splicing of this gene could give rise to abnormal neurite outgrowth in DM1 brain.

In this study, we detected three novel splicing targets which were mis-regulated in both *Mbnl1* knockout mice and human DM1, two only in *Mbnl1* knockout mice, and one only in human DM1 brains. Since the brain is a heterogeneous organ consisting of many different cell types, splicing events may be regulated in a region-specific manner. Our studies support this interpretation with distinct variations in the splicing of developmentally-regulated exons observed in the hippocampus and cerebellum. Our results suggest that at least some of the aberrant splicing events in the DM1 brain result from the sequestration of MBNL1 by CUG^{exp} RNAs. Additionally, it is also likely that other RNA-associated proteins contribute to the aberrant splicing in DM1. Thus, it will be important to investigate the splicing targets in brain samples derived from other DM1 model mice, including *Celf1* transgenic, *Celf2* transgenic and *Mbnl2* knockout mice.

Materials and Methods

Ethics Statement

All experiments using mice were performed in accordance with the guidelines of the University of Florida. The protocol was approved by the University of Florida Institutional Animal Care and Use Committee (Permit Number: #200903677). All experiments using human samples were approved by the Ethics Committee of Hyogo College of Medicine (Permit number: 93) and written informed consent for specimen use for research was obtained from all patients.

Splicing Microarray Detection

RNA samples from the brain of individual 12–14-week-old male mice from the wild-type and $Mbnl1^{\Delta E3/\Delta E3}$ lines (n = 4 for each group) were compared. To identify MBNL1-dependent splicing events, RNA from $Mbnl1^{\Delta E3/\Delta E3}$ mice was compared to wild-type mice in the C57BL/6J (N10) background. RNA samples were processed for cDNA synthesis and hybridization to Affymetrix "A-chip" oligonucleotide microarrays as follows. Total RNA was primed with random hexamers and reverse transcribed. After the reaction was completed, RNA was removed from the reaction by alkaline hydrolysis and the cDNA was purified using Qiagen PCR Quick Purification Kit. A typical reaction started with 5 µg of total RNA usually yielded ~3 µg of cDNA. The cDNA was then fragmented using DNase I in an empirically controlled reaction that yields DNA fragments of 50–200 bases. This fragmented cDNA was then end labeled using terminal deoxynucleotidyl transferase and "DNA-Labeling-Reagent-1a (DLR-1a)", which is a biotinylated dideoxynucleoside triphosphate. Labeled cDNA was hybridized to arrays in standard Affymetrix hybridization buffer for 16 hrs at 50°C. Arrays were washed, processed with anti-biotin antibodies and streptavidin-phycoerythrin according to the standard Affymetrix protocol.

Microarray Data Analysis

Analysis was done according to Sugnet et al. [32], who calculate a "separation score" that measures the relative change in ratio of alternative splicing events. The equation for sepscore is:

$$\text{Separation score (sepscore)} = \text{Log}_2[\text{mut(skip/include)}/\text{wt(skip/include)}]$$

For each replicate set (each tissue from $Mbnl1^{\Delta E3/\Delta E3}$ and wild type), we estimated the $\log_2$ ratio of skipping to inclusion using robust least squares analysis. We evaluated sepscore significance by permuting the assignments of data points to replicate sets, calculating the separation score for the permuted data, and estimating the likelihood that the observed data came from the permuted distribution. The microarray data have been deposited in NCBI's Gene Expression Omnibus and are accessible through GEO series accession number GSE28640 (http://www.ncbi.nlm.nih.gov/geo/query/acc.cgi?acc=GSE28640). All data is MIAME compliant and the raw data has been deposited in a MIAME compliant database (GEO), as detailed on the MGED Society website (http://www.mged.org/Workgroups/MIAME/miame.html).

Target validation by RT-PCR for model mice

The sequences of primers used for RT–PCR assays of splicing in mouse and human brain RNA are listed in (Tables S1 and S2). To test mouse MBNL1 potential splicing targets identified by splicing microarrays, we harvested hippocampal, temporal cortex and cerebellar tissues from $Mbnl1^{+/+}$ (n = 3) and $Mbnl1^{\Delta E3/\Delta E3}$ (n = 3) mice (C57BL/6J background) ranging from 3–6 months of age. RNA was isolated using TRI Reagent (Sigma) and cDNA generated using 5 µg of RNA, oligo $(dT)_{20}$ (Invitrogen) and SuperScript III (Invitrogen) followed by digestion with 0.2 units/µl RNase H (Invitrogen) at 37°C for 20 min. Splicing targets with predicted alternately spliced cassettes were selected from microarray list and 5 ng of cDNA was PCR-amplified for 28 cycles (95°C for 30 sec, 55°C for 30 sec, 72°C for 30 sec) by using forward and reverse primers located in the flanking exons. Each PCR reaction was spiked with 2.5 µCi of $[\alpha^{32}P]$-dCTP (PerkinElmer Life Sciences). PCR products were resolved on 10% non-denaturing polyacrylamide gels followed by autoradiography using Kodak BioMax MS film (PerkinElmer Life Sciences). Exon inclusion was measured using a Typhoon 9200 imager and ImageQuant TL software (GE Healthcare).

RT-PCR and Southern blot analysis for human brain samples

Human temporal cortex and cerebellar tissues (n = 21) at autopsy were analyzed (Table 1). RNA was extracted from each sample by the ISOGEN procedure (Nippon Gene). The RNAs used as normal controls were purchased commercially as follows: human adult temporal cortex (3 male, 1female, 3 samples from Biochain, 1 sample from Ambion) and 1 sample of human fetal whole brain (Stratagene) (Table 1). The quality of RNA and the PCR product were analyzed by capillary electrophoresis using a Hitachi SV 1210 on a microchip (Hitachi Electronics Co., Tokyo, Japan) [33]. We used the samples which meet the criteria that the ratio of 28S/18S rRNA peaks was >0.8. The CTG trinucleotide repeat expansion sizes of human brain samples were determined by Southern blot analysis of genomic DNAs from each brain region tissue of DM1 as described previously [34]. cDNA was synthesized using the same method as for mouse samples except 1–3 µg of RNA and random hexamers were used. cDNA equivalent to 20 ng RNA was PCR-amplified for initial denaturation at 94°C for 10 min and 35 cycles (94°C for 30 sec, 55°C for 30 sec, 72°C for 30 sec) by using forward and reverse primers located in the exons adjacent to the human exons orthologous to mouse exons predicted by the microarray data (Table S2). We determined the percentage of each peak by dividing each signal by the total signal.

Statistical analysis

Differences for the levels of exon inclusion for age-matched genetically homogeneous mice were analyzed by unpaired t- and permutation tests. The data for human samples were analyzed using the nonparametric Mann-Whitney U test because the backgrounds such as age and CTG repeat number of each sample are regarded inhomogeneous and the data for these samples were not always normally distributed.

Supporting Information

Figure S1 *Sorbs1* exon 25 inclusion is decreased and *Camk2d* δ9 is increased to similar extent in the hippocampus (hp) and temporal cortex (tp) of $Mbnl1^{\Delta E3/\Delta E3}$ (ko) mice compared with wild type (wt) mice.

Figure S2 Comparison between the degree of aberrant splicing and CTG repeat number in DM1 brain. There was no significant correlation between each shortest, median and longest CTG repeat number, and percent inclusion of each of the exons which are mis-regulated. (A) Temporal tissues. (B) Cerebellar tissues. Spearman rank correlation coefficient was used for the analysis of correlation.

Figure S3 Some splicing defects which have been reported in DM1 brain were not reproduced in *Mbnl1* knockout brain. (A) Four splicing exons are mis-regulated in our human DM1 temporal cortex (exon4 of *GRIN1*, exons 3 and 12 of *MAPT*, and exon9 of *APP*). Mann-Whitney U test was used for calculating the *p* value. Statistically significant differences ($p<0.05$) are indicated by an asterisk. (B) These exons are normally spliced in the hippocampus (hp) of *Mbnl1* knockout mice.

Figure S4 MBNL1 distribution and expression in regions of mouse brain. (A) Immunohistochemistry with anti-MBNL1 antibody shows that MBNL1 is ubiquitously expressed in the frontal cortex (top), hippocampus (middle), and cerebellum (bottom) sections from wild-type (wt, right) but not in those from *Mbnl1* knockout (ko, left). (B) Western blot analysis shows a similar expression of MBNL1 in the cerebellum, temporal cortex, and hippocampus of a wild-type mouse. (Materials and Methods S1).

Materials and Methods S1 Supplementary Materials and Methods for Muscleblind-Like 1 Knockout Mice

Reveal Novel Splicing Defects in the Myotonic Dystrophy Brain.

Table S1 Separation score and primers for RT-PCR of mouse brain.

Table S2 Primers for RT-PCR of human brain.

Table S3 YGCY motif searching list with sequences exons aberrantly regulated in brains of *Mbnl1* knockout mice and DM1 patients. YGCY motifs are indicated by capitals.

Acknowledgments

The authors would like to acknowledge the Research Resource Network Japan for supplying human brain tissue samples.

Author Contributions

Conceived and designed the experiments: KS K-YL HF KJ MA MSS TK. Performed the experiments: KS K-YL MN YT HF KJ HD MSS. Analyzed the data: KS MN YT MPT KJ HY HD MA MSS TK. Contributed reagents/materials/analysis tools: HF KJ. Wrote the paper: KS K-YL MN YT MPT HY MA MSS TK.

References

1. Meola G, Sansone V (2007) Cerebral involvement in myotonic dystrophies. Muscle Nerve 36: 294–306.
2. Ono S, Kanda F, Takahashi K, Fukuoka Y, Jinnai K, et al. (1996) Neuronal loss in the medullary reticular formation in myotonic dystrophy: a clinicopathological study. Neurology 46: 228–231.
3. Ono S, Inoue K, Mannen T, Mitake S, Shirai T, et al. (1989) Intracytoplasmic inclusion bodies of the thalamus and the substantia nigra, and Marinesco bodies in myotonic dystrophy: a quantitative morphological study. Acta neuropathol 77: 350–356.
4. Vermersch P, Sergeant N, Ruchoux MM, Hofmann-Radvanyi H, Wattez A, et al. (1996) Specific tau variants in the brains of patients with myotonic dystrophy. Neurology 47: 711–717.
5. Harper PS (2001) Myotonic Dystrophy 3rd ed. W. B. Saunders.
6. Sicot G, Gourdon G, Gomes-Pereira M (2011) Myotonic dystrophy, when simple repeats reveal complex pathogenic entities: new findings and future challenges. Hum Mol Genet 20: R116–123.
7. Mankodi A, Logigian E, Callahan L, McClain C, White R, et al. (2000) Myotonic dystrophy in transgenic mice expressing an expanded CUG repeat. Science 289: 1769–1773.
8. Kanadia RN, Johnstone KA, Mankodi A, Lungu C, Thornton CA, et al. (2003) A muscleblind knockout model for myotonic dystrophy. Science 302: 1978–1980.
9. Du H, Cline MS, Osborne RJ, Tuttle DL, Clark TA, et al. (2010) Aberrant alternative splicing and extracellular matrix gene expression in mouse models of myotonic dystrophy. Nat Struct Mol Biol 17: 187–193.
10. Jiang H, Mankodi A, Swanson MS, Moxley RT, Thornton CA (2004) Myotonic dystrophy type 1 is associated with nuclear foci of mutant RNA, sequestration of muscleblind proteins and deregulated alternative splicing in neurons. Hum Mol Genet 13: 3079–3088.
11. Dhaenens CM, Schraen-Maschke S, Tran H, Vingtdeux V, Ghanem D, et al. (2008) Overexpression of MBNL1 fetal isoforms and modified splicing of Tau in the DM1 brain: Two individual consequences of CUG trinucleotide repeats. Exp Neurol 210: 467–478.
12. Leroy O, Wang J, Maurage CA, Parent M, Cooper T, et al. (2006) Brain-specific change in alternative splicing of Tau exon 6 in myotonic dystrophy type 1. Biochim Biophys Acta 1762: 460–467.
13. Sergeant N, Sablonniere B, Schraen-Maschke S, Ghestem A, Maurage CA, et al. (2001) Dysregulation of human brain microtubule-associated tau mRNA maturation in myotonic dystrophy type 1. Hum Mol Genet 10: 2143–2155.
14. Kalsotra A, Xiao X, Ward AJ, Castle JC, Johnson JM, et al. (2008) A postnatal switch of CELF and MBNL proteins reprograms alternative splicing in the developing heart. Proc Natl Acad Sci U S A 105: 20333–20338.
15. Donai H, Murakami T, Amano T, Sogawa Y, Yamauchi T (2000) Induction and alternative splicing of delta isoform of Ca(2+)/calmodulin-dependent protein kinase II during neural differentiation of P19 embryonal carcinoma cells and during brain development. Brain Res Mol Brain Res 85: 189–199.
16. Lopez Castel A, Nakamori M, Tome S, Chitayat D, Gourdon G, et al. (2011) Expanded CTG repeat demarcates a boundary for abnormal CpG methylation in myotonic dystrophy patient tissues. Hum Mol Genet 20: 1–15.
17. Gomes-Pereira M, Foiry L, Nicole A, Huguet A, Junien C, et al. (2007) CTG trinucleotide repeat "big jumps": large expansions, small mice. PLoS Genet 3: e52.
18. Fardaei M, Rogers MT, Thorpe HM, Larkin K, Hamshere MG, et al. (2002) Three proteins, MBNL, MBLL and MBXL, co-localize in vivo with nuclear foci of expanded-repeat transcripts in DM1 and DM2 cells. Hum Mol Genet 11: 805–814.
19. Ho TH, Charlet BN, Poulos MG, Singh G, Swanson MS, et al. (2004) Muscleblind proteins regulate alternative splicing. EMBO J 23: 3103–3112.
20. Matynia A, Ng CH, Dansithong W, Chiang A, Silva AJ, et al. (2010) Muscleblind1, but not Dmpk or Six5, contributes to a complex phenotype of muscular and motivational deficits in mouse models of myotonic dystrophy. PLoS One 5: e9857.
21. Dhaenens CM, Tran H, Frandemiche ML, Carpentier C, Schraen-Maschke S, et al. (2011) Mis-splicing of Tau exon 10 in myotonic dystrophy type 1 is reproduced by overexpression of CELF2 but not by MBNL1 silencing. Biochim Biophys Acta 1812: 732–742.
22. Ribon V, Printen JA, Hoffman NG, Kay BK, Saltiel AR (1998) A novel, multifuntional c-Cbl binding protein in insulin receptor signaling in 3T3-L1 adipocytes. Mol Cell Biol 18: 872–879.
23. Lebre AS, Jamot L, Takahashi J, Spassky N, Leprince C, et al. (2001) Ataxin-7 interacts with a Cbl-associated protein that it recruits into neuronal intranuclear inclusions. Hum Mol Genet 10: 1201–1213.
24. Xu X, Yang D, Ding JH, Wang W, Chu PH, et al. (2005) ASF/SF2-regulated CaMKIIdelta alternative splicing temporally reprograms excitation-contraction coupling in cardiac muscle. Cell 120: 59–72.
25. Takeuchi Y, Nomura K, Fukunaga K (2004) Differential subcellular distribution of Ca2+/calmodulin-dependent protein kinase II isoforms in the striatum and NG108-15 cells. J Neurosci Res 75: 480–490.
26. Nomura K, Takeuchi Y, Yamaguchi S, Okamura H, Fukunaga K (2003) Involvement of calcium/calmodulin-dependent protein kinase II in the induction of mPer1. J Neurosci Res 72: 384–392.
27. Ciafaloni E, Mignot E, Sansone V, Hilbert JE, Lin L, et al. (2008) The hypocretin neurotransmission system in myotonic dystrophy type 1. Neurology 70: 226–230.
28. Lin PT, Gleeson JG, Corbo JC, Flanagan L, Walsh CA (2000) DCAMKL1 encodes a protein kinase with homology to doublecortin that regulates microtubule polymerization. J Neurosci 20: 9152–9161.
29. Burgess HA, Reiner O (2002) Alternative splice variants of doublecortin-like kinase are differentially expressed and have different kinase activities. J Biol Chem 277: 17696–17705.
30. Gebbink MF, Kranenburg O, Poland M, van Horck FP, Houssa B, et al. (1997) Identification of a novel, putative Rho-specific GDP/GTP exchange factor and a RhoA-binding protein: control of neuronal morphology. J Cell Biol 137: 1603–1613.
31. Mulder J, Ariaens A, van den Boomen D, Moolenaar WH (2004) p116Rip targets myosin phosphatase to the actin cytoskeleton and is essential for RhoA/ROCK-regulated neuritogenesis. Mol Biol Cell 15: 5516–5527.
32. Sugnet CW, Srinivasan K, Clark TA, O'Brien G, Cline MS, et al. (2006) Unusual intron conservation near tissue-regulated exons found by splicing microarrays. PLoS Comput Biol 2: e4.
33. Kataoka M, Inoue S, Kajimoto K, Sinohara Y, Baba Y (2004) Usefulness of microchip electrophoresis for reliable analyses of nonstandard DNA samples and subsequent on-chip enzymatic digestion. Eur J Biochem 271: 2241–2247.
34. The International Myotonic Dystrophy Consortium (IDMC). (2000) New nomenclature and DNA testing guidelines for myotonic dystrophy type 1 (DM1). Neurology 54: 1218–1221.

7

Neurofibromin 1 Is a miRNA Target in Neurons

Maria Paschou, Epaminondas Doxakis*

Molecular and Cellular Neurobiology Lab, Center of Neurosciences and Social Psychiatry, Biomedical Research Foundation, Academy of Athens, Athens, Greece

Abstract

Mutations of the neurofibromin 1 gene cause neurofibromatosis type 1, a disease in which learning and behavioral abnormalities are common. The disease is completely penetrant but shows variable phenotypic expression in patients. The repertoire of regulatory interactions utilized by neurons to control neurofibromin 1 expression is poorly understood. Here, we examined the contribution of microRNAs into this regulatory network. Using reporter assays, we provided evidence that miR-128 and to a lesser extent miR-137 and miR-103 reduced neurofibromin 1 reporter levels through specific binding to *Nf1* 3′-UTR. Mutations in all three predicted binding sites eliminated the reporter response. MiR-128 and miR-137, unlike miR-103 that showed a more ubiquitous expression, were predominantly expressed in brain with a distribution that resembled neurofibromin 1 expression in different tissues as well as during the course of neuronal development. In the nervous system, all three microRNAs showed highest expression in neurons and least in Schwann cells and astrocytes. Overexpression of miR-128 alone or with miR-103 and miR-137 significantly reduced endogenous neurofibromin 1 protein levels, while antisense inhibition of these microRNAs enhanced translation of endogenous neurofibromin 1 and reporter in primary cultures of hippocampal neurons. These findings revealed a significant additional mechanism by which neurofibromin 1 is regulated in neurons and implicated new candidates for the treatment of multifarious neurofibromatosis type 1 cognitive symptoms.

Editor: Justin L. Mott, University of Nebraska Medical Center, United States of America

Funding: This work was funded by grants from General Secretariat for Research and Technology to ED. The funders had no role in study design, data collection and analysis, decision to publish, or preparation of the manuscript.

Competing Interests: The authors have declared that no competing interests exist.

* E-mail: edoxakis@bioacademy.gr

Introduction

Neurofibromatosis type 1 (NF-1) is a common autosomal dominant genetic disorder that affects 1 in 3500 individuals worldwide. The disease is characterised by a spectrum of somatic and cognitive symptoms that include café au lait macules, Lisch nodules, neurofibromas and learning disabilities [1]. Individuals affected by NF-1 are heterozygous for the *Nf1* gene mutation, as homozygous mutations appear to be lethal [2]. Neurofibromin 1 (NF1), the *Nf1* gene product, is a large protein that contains a central Ras-GTPase-activating (RasGAP) domain thought to function as a negative regulator of proto-oncogene RAS and downstream effectors [3,4,5].

Despite the fact that NF-1 is a single-gene disease, it is presented by a variable expressivity of symptoms even within families, indicating that other modifier genes are involved in the disease process. Towards this, studies have thus far recognized ubiquitination through ETEA [6] and alternative splicing mediated by RNA binding proteins HuR and CELF as possible contributing factors [6,7].

MicroRNAs (miRNAs) are short 17–24 nucleotides, non-coding RNAs that act to inhibit protein expression by hybridizing to complementary sequences in the 3′-UTR of closely related target transcripts. These recognition sequences demonstrate near perfect complementarity of a 7–8 nucleotides stretch at 5′end of the miRNA, termed the seed sequence, while interaction with the 3′end of miRNA requires less stringency [8]. MiRNAs confer robustness to developmental genetic programs by presumably two opposing ways. In the first case, the miRNA and target mRNAs are highly expressed in mutually exclusive tissues where the miRNA functions to block translation of the unwanted mRNAs expressed from leaky promoters. And in the second case, both the miRNA and target mRNAs are co-expressed in the same tissues where the miRNA acts as rheostat to dampen protein translation to optimal levels enabling customized expression [9,10]. MiRNAs display a wide variety of expression patterns and many are differentially expressed during development or disease [11]. With respect to NF-1, miR-10b and miR-34a have been shown to be up- and down- regulated in Malignant Peripheral Nerve Sheath Tumors, respectively while miR-10a also participates in the regulation of NF1 levels in these tumors [12,13].

With this in mind, we sought to further characterize the physiological regulation of NF1 expression by miRNAs. We have tested a number of predicted conserved miRNAs for NF1 regulation and identified miR-128, miR-137 and miR-103 as new regulators. These miRNAs have overlapping expression with NF1 in different tissues and are predominantly neuronal indicating they refine fluctuations of endogenous NF1 levels in the nervous system.

Materials and Methods

Ethics Statement

All rodent tissue was obtained in accordance with European Union (2003/65/CE) guidelines on the use of laboratory animals. Experimental protocols were approved by the Institutional Animal Care and Use Committee of BRFAA and the Veterinary Services of Attica prefecture (K/2134).

Generation of DNA Constructs

The murine *Nf1* 3′-UTR (NM_010897, bases 8635 to 11844) was amplified by proofreading Phusion PCR (Finnzymes, Vaanta, Finland) from mouse brain DNA by using the primers 5′-CATTAGCTCGAGAGCGTTCTTTGTTTCAC -3′ and 5′-GTAATCGCGGCCGCGAGCAGATTGAATTTACATTTT -3′. The ~3,2 kb PCR product was, then, cloned into psiCHECK-2 vector (Promega, Madison, USA) downstream from the Renilla luciferase coding sequence. Expression vectors directing the synthesis of mmu-miR-103-1 (miRBase accession no. MI0000587), mmu-miR-128-2 (miRBase accession no. MI0000726), and mmu-miR-137 (miRBase accession no. MI0000163) were prepared by introducing annealed oligonucleotides corresponding to the precursor miRNA sequences (pri-miRNA) into the pcDNA6.2-GW/EmGFP vector (Invitrogen, Carlsbad, USA). The oligonucleotide sequences were as follows:

Mmu-pri-mir-103-1 sense, 5′-TGCTGTTCTTACTGCCCTCGGCTTCTTTA-CAGTGCTGCCTTGTTGCATATGGATCAAGCAG-CATTGTACAGGGCTATGAAGGCATTGAGAC -3′ and

Mmu-pri-mir-103-1 antisense, 5′-CCTGGTCTCAATGCCTTCATAGCCCTGTA-CAATGCTGCTTGATCCATATGCAACAAGGCAGCACTG-TAAAGAAGCCGAGGGCAGTAAGAAC -3′.

Mmu-pri-mir-128-2 sense, 5′-TGCTGCAGTGGGAAGGGGGGCCGATGCACTGTAA-GAGAGTGAGTAGCAGGTCTCACAGT-GAACCGGTCTCTTTCCCTACTG-3′ and

Mmu-pri-mir-128-2 antisense, 5′-CCTGCAGTAGGGAAAGAGACCGGTTCACTGTGA-GACCTGCTACTCACTCTCTTACAGTG-CATCGGCCCCCCTTCCCACTGC-3′.

Mmu-pri-mir-137 sense, 5′-TGCTGCTTCGGTGACGGGTATTCTTGGGTGGATAA-TACGGATTACGTTGTTATTGCTTAAGAATACGCG-TAGTCGAGG -3′ and

Mmu-pri-mir-137 antisense, 5′-CCTGCCTCGACTACGCGTATTCTTAAGCAATAA-CAACGTAATCCGTATTATCCACCCAAGAATACCCGT-CACCGAAGC -3′.

The mmu-pri-mir-128/103 and mmu-pri-mir-128/137 dual miRNA expression plasmids were prepared by inserting mmu-pri-mir-103-1 or mmu-pri-mir-137 sequence after mmu-pri-mir-128-2 sequence in the pcDNA6.2-GW/EmGFP vector by restriction cloning. Scramble 1, supplied by Invitrogen is presumably predicted not to target any vertebrate gene. Scramble 2 was prepared by scrambling the mature sequence of mmu-miR-128-2 in the mmu-pri-mir-128-2 sequence (miRBase accession no. MI0000726) before inserting it in the pcDNA6.2-GW/EmGFP vector as previously described [14]. All vectors were checked by sequencing before use.

Site-directed Mutagenesis

Three point mutations, one for each miRNA binding site were inserted in *Nf1* 3′-UTR as previously described [15]. Briefly, a set of four proofreading PCR reactions with mutagenized primers was carried out using the psiCHECK2-*Nf1* 3′-UTR vector as a template. The reactions were as follows (mutations are underlined):

PCR1: External wt-*Nf1* F (5′- CATTAGCTCGA-GAGCGTTCTTTGTTTCAC -3′) + Mut-mir-103 R (5′-ATCAAAGAAAAGCACGATTAAACTTAGGCA -3′),

PCR2: Internal mut-mir-103 F (5′-CGTGCTTTTCTTTGATGTTTTTC -3′) + Internal mut-mir-137 R 5′- TTTTCCTGTACTTAAAGCTAAGACTCAAATG -3′),

PCR3: Internal mut-mir-137 F (5′- TTTAAGTACAG-GAAAATAAGC -3′) + Internal mut-mir-128 R (5′- CGGCCA-GACTTCAGTGTGACTAAATGCAA -3′),

PCR4: Internal mut-mir-128 F (5′- ACT-GAAGTCTGGCCGGCCTGTG -3′) + External wt-*Nf1* R (5′-GTAATCGCGGCCGCGAGCAGATTGAATTTACATTTT -3′).

The PCR products were purified with a gel extraction kit (Qiagen, Hilden, Germany) and equal amounts were PCR-assembled, two fragments at a time, using corresponding flanking primers. The cycling conditions were as follows: five cycles with twice as long extension times and no primers -to allow assembly of full fragment-, followed by 15 cycles of proofreading PCR to amplify the assembled fragment. The mutagenized final PCR product was then cloned into the psiCHECK-2 plasmid and sequenced.

Lentivirus Production

The vectors PLL3.7/EmGFP-pri-mir-128 and PLL3.7/EmGFP-pri-mir-128/103, and PLL3.7/EmGFP-pri-mir-128/137 were constructed by replacing the U6 promoter and GFP sequences between WRE and FLAP of the PLL3.7 vector (kindly provided by Ford E, BRFAA) with the EmGFP-pri-mir cassettes from the pcDNA6.2-GW/EmGFP-pri-mir-128, pcDNA6.2-GW/EmGFP-pri-mir-128/103 and pcDNA6.2-GW/EmGFP-pri-mir-128/137 plasmids, respectively. Viral particles were prepared by co-transfection of HEK293T cells with PLL3.7/EmGFP-pri-mirs, helper pCMV-dR8.91 and pMD2.G plasmids at 16:7: 7 μg DNA ratios per 10 cm plate by using the calcium phosphate method. After 48 hours, the supernatants were spun at 2,000 rpm for 6 minutes, filtered at 0.45 μm pore size, and spun at 26,000 rpm (Sorvall TH-641 rotor) for 1 hour 30 minutes before pellets were resuspended in 100 μl of 1% bovine serum albumin. Lentiviral titers were determined by infecting HEK293 cells with serial dilutions of the viral stock for 48 hours and followed by fluorescent-activated cytometric sorting (BD FACSAria sorter, Franklin Lakes, USA). Titers were approximately 5×10^7 infectious units per ml.

Cell-line Culture and Transfection

HEK293 cells were maintained in low-glucose DMEM (GIBCO-Invitrogen) supplemented with 10% fetal bovine serum (FBS) (Biowest, Nuaillé, France). For luciferase reporter assay, HEK293 cells were transfected a day after plating by using Lipofectamine 2000 according to the manufacturer's instructions (Invitrogen). To ensure that transfection efficiencies and NF1 reporter load onto cells were uniform across conditions both luciferase psiCHECK-2 construct and Lipofectamine 2000 reagent were prepared as master mix before aliquoting into tubes containing the different miRNA plasmids. Transfection efficiencies were at 60–80% at 48 hours as indicated by GFP. For western blotting assay, HEK293 cells were transfected at plating by using Lipofectamine 2000 according to the manufacturer's instructions. Six hours later, cells were infected with lentiviral vectors to boost transfection efficiency to near 90% by 48 hours.

Neuron Culture and Transfection

Dissociated, embryonic day 16–17 murine hippocampal or cortical neurons (>95% pure), were grown in Neurobasal medium with B-27 supplement (GIBCO, Invitrogen) and Glutamax (GIBCO, Invitrogen) in poly-L-lysine (SIGMA, St-Louis, USA) coated borosilicate glass coverslips (VWR, Radnor, USA) in the

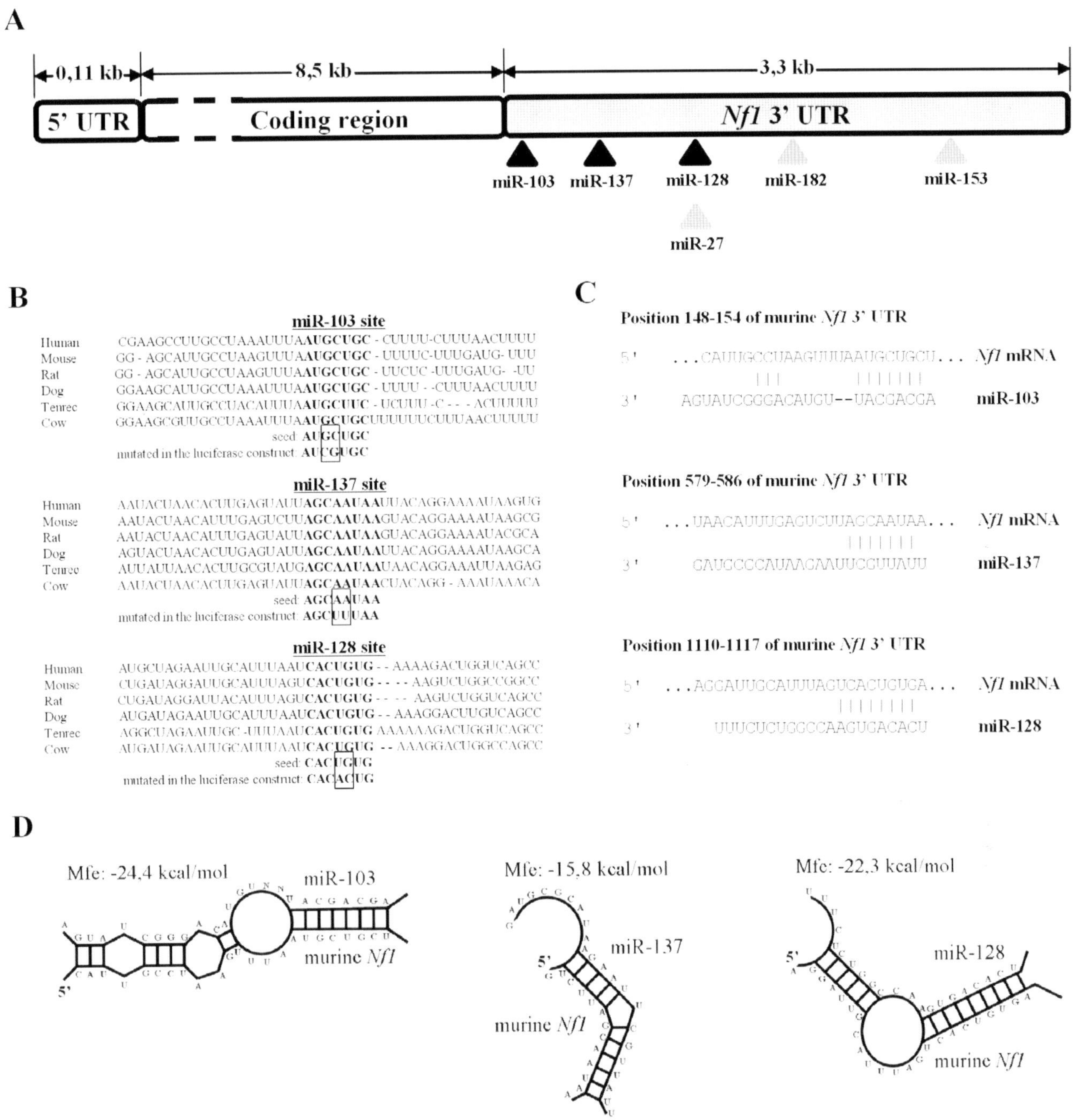

Figure 1. MiRNA binding sites in Nf1 3′-UTR. (**A**) Relative position of conserved miR-103, miR-137, miR-27, miR-128, miR-182 and miR-153 sites in *Nf1* 3′-UTR. (**B**) Sequence conservation of miR-103, miR-137 and miR-128 binding sites. (**C**) Alignment of mature miR-103, miR-137 and miR-128 sequences with *Nf1* transcript. (**D**) Predicted hybridization of miRNAs and *Nf1* transcript using the RNAhybrid algorithm [36]. The minimum free energy required for the hybridization is indicated.

absence of trophic factors [16]. For *Nf1* mRNA analysis, ~20 hours after plating, neurons were infected with miR-128 lentiviral vectors and assayed 48 hours later by RT-PCR. For NF1 protein or reporter analysis, neurons were transfected using Lipofectamine 2000 reagent straight after dissociation with the a) miRNA expression plasmids or b) the inhibitor 2′-O-methyl oligonucleotides plus luciferase psiCHECK-2 or pmaxGFP constructs (Lonza, Basel, Switzerland) according to the manufacturer's instructions (Invitrogen) and assayed ~40 hours later by immunocytochemistry or Dual-Luciferase reporter assay. The antisense (as) 2′-O-methyl RNA inhibitor sequences were: for scramble, CAGUACUUUUGUGUAGUACAA; for as-mmu-miR-103, UCAUAGCCCUGUACAAUGCUGCU; for as-mmu-miR-137, CUACGCGUAUUCUUAAGCAAUAA, and for as-mmu-miR-128, AAAGAGACCGGUUCACUGUGA (GenePharma, Shanghai, China). For co-transfection conditions, neurons received half the amount of 2′-O-methyl oligonucleotides per miRNA in order to have comparable levels of transfected oligonucleotides to control and mmu-miR-128 conditions.

Astrocyte Culture

Embryonic day 17 murine cortical tissues, free of meninges, were treated with 0.05% trypsin solution (Worthington, Lakewood, USA) for 5 min at 37°C, then dissociated using a fire-polished Pasteur glass pipette and plated in tissue culture dishes (Greiner, Kremsmünster, Austria) containing RPMI (Biosera, East Sussex, UK) and 10% FBS (Biowest). After approximately one week of culture, astrocytes were trypsinized, dispersed in RPMI plus 10% FBS and re-plated at 1:3 the original density. They were harvested for mirVana RNA isolation after becoming confluent again.

Schwann Cell Culture

Schwann cells were cultured from bilaterally excised sciatic nerves of postnatal day 0 mice. The cells were dissociated with 0.125% trypsin and 0.2% collagenase (Worthington) solutions for 40 min at 37°C, then triturated through a fire-polished Pasteur pipette and plated in poly-L-lysine coated (SIGMA) tissue culture dishes. Cells were grown in low-glucose DMEM supplemented with 10% FBS. They were harvested for mirVana RNA isolation after becoming confluent.

Measurement of miR-103, miR-137, miR-128, Nf1 and U6 RNAs

A semi-quantitative RT/PCR assay was used to compare the levels of miR-103, miR-137, miR-128, *Nf1* and *U6* mRNAs in the various cell types and tissues. Total RNA was isolated using the mirVana miRNA isolation kit (Ambion, Austin, USA) and recovered in DEPC-treated H_2O. 0.5 µg RNA was reverse transcribed for 1 hour at 42°C with superscript II enzyme (Invitrogen) in reaction containing the manufacturer's buffer and DTT supplemented with 0.5 mM dNTPs (Promega), 10 µM random hexanucleotides (Amersham/GE Healthcare, Buckinghamshire, UK) and 2.5 pmoles of gene-specific primers for mature hs/mmu-miR-103 (5′-CATGATCAGCTGGGCCAAGATCATAGCC-3′), hs/mmu-miR-137 (5′- CATGATCAGCTGGGCCAAGACTACGCGT-3′), and hs/mmu-miR-128 (5′- CATGATCAGCTGGGCCAAGAAAAGAGAC-3′). These primers included an extension sequence (underlined) to facilitate subsequent amplification and monitoring by PCR {modified from [17,18]}.

Following reverse transcription, duplicate measurements of 2 µl of 2.5 times diluted in H_2O cDNA were made in 10 µl PCR reactions containing 1 ×buffer, 0.5–1.5 mM $MgCl_2$, 0.2 mM dNTPs, 4 pmoles primers, and 1.25 units DreamTaq (Fermentas, Burlington, Canada). The forward primers were as follows: hs/mmu-miR-103 F, 5′-TGTGTGAGCAGCATTGTACAGG-3′; hs/mmu-miR-137 F, 5′-GCCGGGTTATTGCTTAAGAATAC-3′; hs/mmu-miR-128 F, 5′-TCTGGGTCACAGTGAACCGGT-3′; mmu-*Nf1* F, 5′-GTGGCCCCTACAAATCATTCTC-3′; hs-*Nf1* F, 5′-GCTTTCGTATAAGCCCTCACAA-3′; and hs/mmu-*U6* F, 5′-CGCTTCGGCAGCACATATAC-3′. The reverse primers were as follows: Universal reverse for miR-103, miR-137 and miR-128, 5′-CATGATCAGCTGGGCCAAGA-3′; mmu-*Nf1* R, 5′-TGCTTTCCGTAAACTGTCCAG-3′; hs-*Nf1* R, 5′-

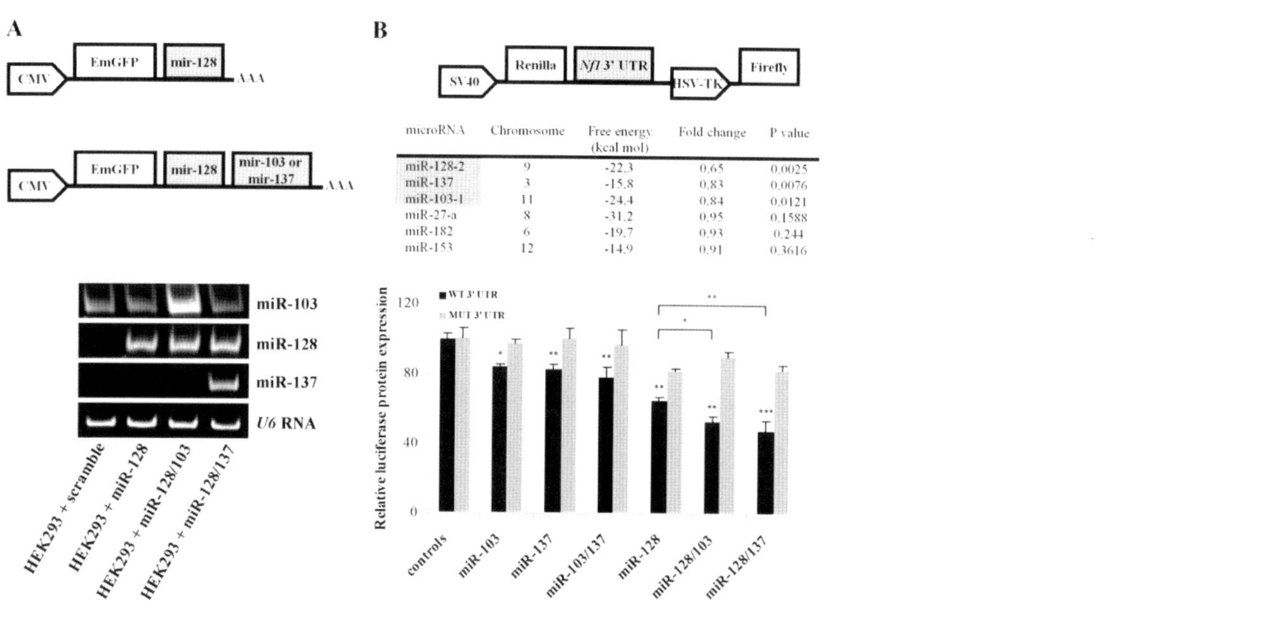

microRNA	Chromosome	Free energy (kcal/mol)	Fold change	P value
miR-128-2	9	-22.3	0.65	0.0025
miR-137	3	-15.8	0.83	0.0076
miR-103-1	11	-24.4	0.84	0.0121
miR-27-a	8	-31.2	0.95	0.1588
miR-182	6	-19.7	0.93	0.244
miR-153	12	-14.9	0.91	0.3616

Figure 2. MiR-103, miR-128 and miR-137 directly reduce NF1 reporter protein expression. (**A**) Schematic of miRNA plasmids and their expression levels in HEK293 cells. Representative gel showing the products of RT-PCR reactions amplified with primers specific for mature miR-103, miR-128, and miR-137 in HEK293 cells transfected with scramble or miR-128 vectors. The amount of starting template for each condition was equilibrated relative to *U6* RNA. Cycles were falling within the linear range of amplification for each primer pair. (**B**) Schematic of *Nf1* 3′-UTR reporter construct and miRNAs tested for *Nf1* 3′-UTR regulation of expression. HEK293 cells were co-transfected with both the reporter gene (0.2 µg/reaction) and miRNA expression vectors (pri-mir-103, pri-mir-128, pri-mir-137, pri-mir-27, pri-mir-182 and pri-mir-153) (0.8 µg/reaction) and luciferase activity was measured 48 hours later. The fold change from control values as well as the *P*-value for each miRNA condition is presented in the table. These assays demonstrated that only miR-103, miR-128 and miR-137 significantly reduce NF1 reporter protein levels. Subsequently, mutagenesis of the predicted miR-103, miR-128 and miR-137 binding sites alleviated this inhibitory effect indicating that miR-103, miR-128 and miR-137 directly suppress *Nf1* expression by targeting the identified seed regions in the *Nf1* 3′-UTR. The average value of three single (scramble 1, scramble 2, miR-218) and two double (miR-101/181, miR-218/377) miRNA constructs expressing miRNA predicted not to bind *Nf1* 3′-UTR were used as controls for the single or double expression constructs, respectively. Data show the mean ± s.e.m from 6 independent transfections (*, $P<0.05$; **, $P<0.01$).

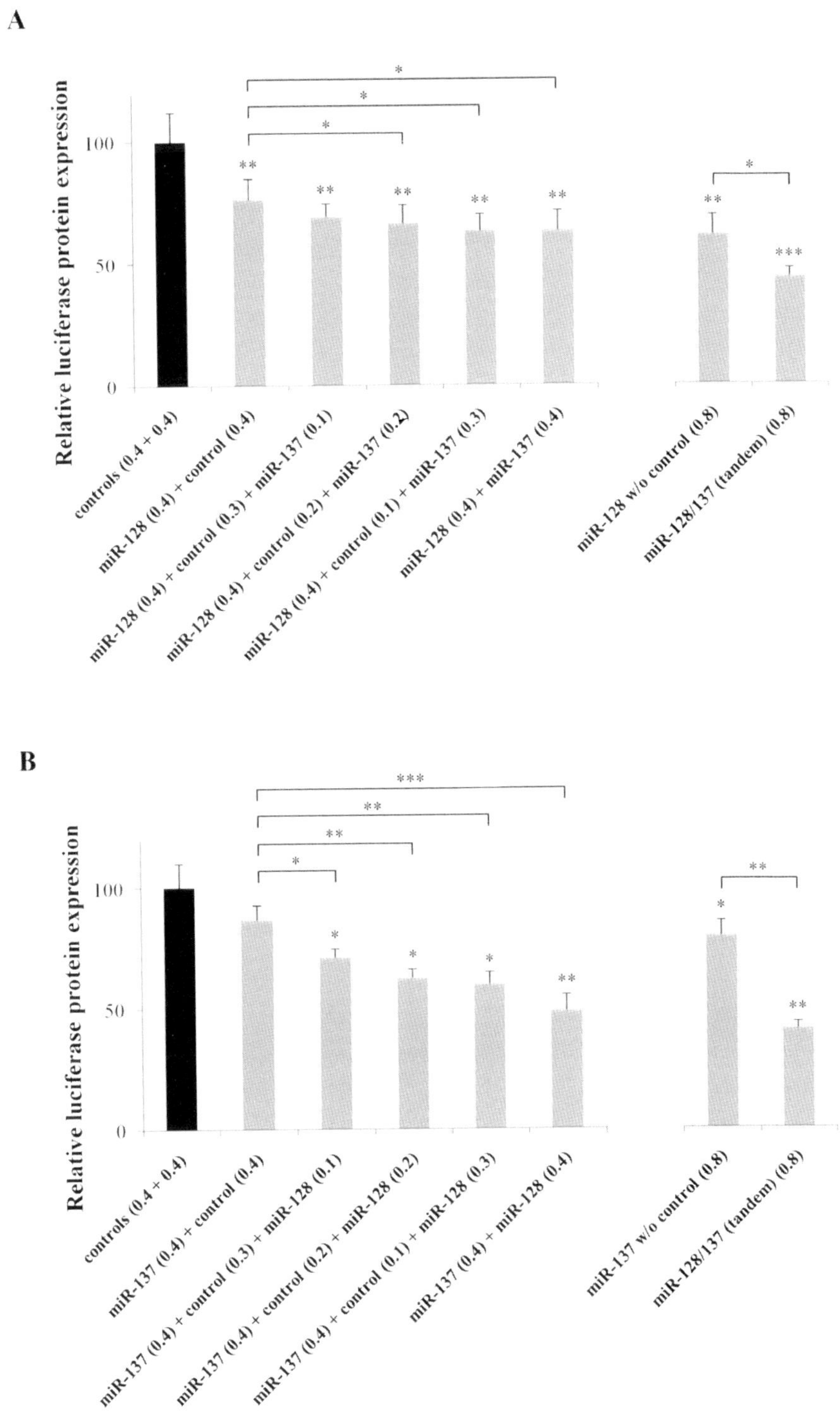

Figure 3. MiR-128 and miR-137 synergize to reduce NF1 reporter protein expression. HEK293 cells were co-transfected with both the reporter gene (0.2 µg/reaction) and variable concentrations of pri-mir-128 and pri-mir-137 expression vectors. Luciferase activity was measured 48 hours later. (**A**) pri-mir-128 plasmid concentration was kept at 0.4 µg/reaction while pri-mir-137 concentration varied from 0.1–0.4 µg/reaction. (**B**) pri-mir-137 plasmid concentration was kept at 0.4 µg/reaction while pri-mir-128 concentration varied from 0.1–0.4 µg/reaction. Scramble 2 plasmid was supplemented in some of the reactions to achieve final miRNA plasmid concentration of 0.8 µg/reaction. These assays demonstrated that miR-128 and miR-137 synergistically reduce NF1 reporter expression when levels of the less abundant miRNA in the reaction are 50% or higher of the more abundant miRNA. The average value of two single miRNA expression plasmids (combination of scramble 2 plus pri-mir-9 or pri-mir-181 or pri-mir-218) predicted not to bind *Nf1* 3′-UTR were used as controls. Data show the mean ± s.e.m from 4 independent transfections (*, P<0.05; **, P<0.01, ***, P<0.001).

GCGGAATTGGTGATGATTCGATG-3′and hs/mmu-*U6* R, 5′-TTCACGAATTTGCGTGTCAT-3′. cDNAs were amplified by cycling at 95°C for 20 sec, followed by 20 sec at 55°C, followed by 20 sec at 72°C. The reaction was then completed with a 10 min extension at 72°C. Cycles were falling within the linear range of amplification for each primer pair. These were 24–26 cycles for *U6* RNA and 27–30 cycles for miR-103, miR-128, miR-137 and *Nf1* mRNAs. The PCR products were, next, separated on 8% non-denaturing polyacrylamide gels. The gels were, subsequently, stained with SyberGold (Invitrogen) and images were captured with the Dolphin gel documentation system (Wealtech, Sparks, USA).

Luciferase Reporter Assay

Luciferase assays were performed 40–48 hours after transfection with the Dual-Luciferase reporter kit (Promega) and measured with the Lumat LB9507 luminometer (Berthold Technologies, Bad Wildbad, Germany). Changes in expression of Renilla luciferase (target) were calculated relative to firefly luciferase (internal control).

Western Blotting

Western blotting was used to assay NF1 protein levels in HEK293 cells transduced with the appropriate miRNA expression vectors. Two days later, whole-cell protein extracts were harvested with Urea lysis buffer (8 M urea, 0.5% SDS, 1 mM Na_3VO_4), sonicated and boiled for 5 min. For Western blotting, 10–30 µg of each protein extract was loaded onto denatured 7.5% polyacrylamide gel and transferred to Protran® nitrocellulose membrane (Whatman, Kent, UK). The membrane was incubated in 5% bovine serum albumin (BSA) for 1 hour followed by overnight incubation with polyclonal NF1 (sc-67, Santa Cruz Biotechnology, Santa Cruz, California, USA) and monoclonal β-tubulin (clone D66, SIGMA) antibodies. Next day, the membrane was incubated for 1 hour with anti-rabbit (sc-2054, Santa Cruz Biotechnology) for NF1 and anti-mouse (sc-2055, Santa Cruz Biotechnology) for β-tubulin secondary antibodies conjugated with horse radish peroxidase (HRP). HRP signals were, then, detected using the Western Lighting Plus ECL reagents (PerkinElmer, Waltham, USA) according to the manufacturer's instructions.

Immunocytochemistry and Densitometry

Neurons were fixed 48 hours after transfection with freshly-made 4% (w/v) paraformaldehyde solution (SIGMA) and briefly permeabilised with 0.4% Triton X-100 (SIGMA). Cells were subsequently blocked with 5% of secondary serum (normal goat serum, Santa Cruz Biotechnology) and BSA in 1:1 ratio and incubated overnight at 4°C with primary NF1 antibody. Next day, cells were incubated for 1 hour with goat anti-rabbit Alexa Fluor 546 secondary antibody (Molecular Probes/Invitrogen) and mounted with Vectashield (Molecular Probes/Invitrogen) media. Images were taken with a Leica DMRA2 upright microscope using a 60×objective. NF1 levels in scrambles, miR-128, miR-128/103 or miR-128/137 transfected cells were estimated by comparing the average intensity of five neurons with brightest Alexa Fluor 546 signal in each field with the miRNA transfected, GFP-positive, neuron in the same field (80 fields in total per miRNA condition per experiment) using ImageJ [19]. Duplicate transfections were set up for the each condition, and the data were compiled from six separate experiments. Statistical significance was assessed using the student's paired *t*-test (two-tailed distribution).

Results

Multiple miRNA Target Sites are Predicted in Nf1 3′-UTR

To identify putative miRNA target sites located within the 3.5 kb 3′-UTR of *Nf1* transcript, predictions from four different algorithms were compiled and compared. These were TargetScan [20], miRanda [21] Pictar [22] and Diana microT [23]. Several putative target sites, which were conserved at orthologous positions across multiple vertebrate species, were identified by all four software (Fig. 1*A*). They included sites for miR-27, miR-103, miR-128, miR-137, miR-153, and miR-182. Sequence conservation and bioinformatics prediction for three of these sites is shown in Fig.1*B and C*. The miR-103 predicted site (seed sequence position 148–154) has a minimum free energy of −24.4 kcal/mol, the miR-137 site (seed sequence position 579–586) has a minimum free energy of −15.8 kcal/mol and the miR-128 site (seed sequence position 1110–1117) has a minimum free energy of −22.3 kcal/mol. The predicted sites were all flanked by a large number of AU residues indicating that *Nf1* mRNA sequence may facilitate miRNA binding at these sites (Fig. 1*B*) [20].

MiR-103, miR-128 and miR-137 Functionally Interact with Nf1 3′-UTR to Reduce Protein Levels

To test whether any of the six miRNAs mediate regulatory effects on NF1 translation via *Nf1* 3′-UTR, expression plasmids, with the pri-miRNA sequences of the miRNAs inserted in the 3′UTR of Emerald GFP, were constructed (Fig. 2*A*). In addition, a reporter plasmid containing the complete *Nf1* 3′-UTR, inserted downstream of Renilla luciferase gene, was generated. This reporter plasmid, also, contained a downstream firefly luciferase gene that was used as an internal control to normalize for differences in handling and transfection efficiencies (Fig. 2*B*). For the assay, the reporter was co-transfected with the miRNA expression plasmids into HEK293 cells and luciferase reporter expression was assessed 48 hours post-transfection. HEK293 cells were used for these experiments because they express low levels of these miRNAs and are transfected with high efficiency (Fig. 2*A* and data not shown). MiR-103, miR-128, miR-137, miR-103/137, miR-128/103, and miR-128/137 (the latter three are plasmids that express two miRNAs in tandem) produced a 15.7% ($P<0.05$), 34.9% ($P<0.01$), 17% ($P<0.01$), 21.3% ($P<0.01$), 46.6% ($P<0.01$), and 51.7% ($P<0.001$) decrease in luciferase activity compared to control vectors, respectively. In contrast, miR-27, miR-182 and miR-153 did not, significantly, reduce reporter expression (Fig. 2*B*).

To confirm that this effect was mediated via the predicted sites in *Nf1* 3′-UTR, mutations in the seed sequences of miR-103, miR-137, and miR-128 were introduced in the luciferase reporter construct (Fig. 1*B*). The mutagenized reporter was then co-transfected with the miRNA expression plasmids in HEK293 cells and Renilla expression was compared to wild-type reporter. Mutations on these sites abolished the inhibitory effect of miR-103, miR-137, and miR-128 (Fig. 2*B*). These findings indicated that miR-103, miR-137, and miR-128 interact, directly, with the specified regions in *Nf1* 3′-UTR to inhibit translation from the chimaeric transcript and their effect is additive.

To determine the stoichiometric ratio at which the miRNAs were having an additive effect on reducing NF1 levels, the two most effective miRNAs, miR-128 and miR-137, were combined in different ratios (4:1, 4:2, 4:3, 4:4) and their influence on luciferase reporter expression was assessed 48 hours post-transfection. For both miRNAs, a significant additive effect was only observed when levels of the less abundant miRNA were 50% or higher of the more abundant miRNA (Figs. 3*A and B*). These findings indicated that adequate levels of both miRNAs are a prerequisite for efficient co-regulation of expression.

To examine whether miR-128, the most potent of all miRNAs, alone or together with miR-103 or miR-137, reduce endogenous NF1 levels, HEK293 cells were transfected with the miR-128 expression plasmids and *Nf1* mRNA and protein levels were

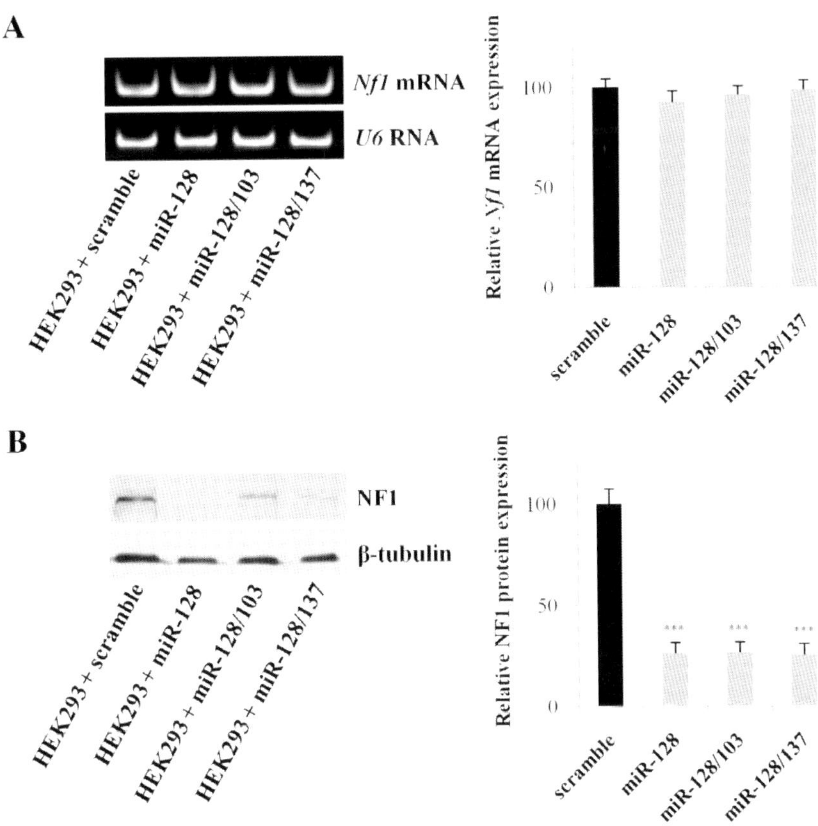

Figure 4. MiR-103, miR-128 and miR-137 reduce endogenous NF1 protein but not mRNA expression. (**A**) Representative gel of the RT-PCR amplification of *Nf1* mRNA in HEK293 cells transfected with scramble or miR-128 vectors for 48 hours. The amount of starting template for each condition was equilibrated relative to *U6* RNA. Cycles were falling within the linear range of amplification for each primer pair. (**B**) Representative Western Blot analysis demonstrating that miR-128, miR-128/103, and miR-128/137 reduce endogenous NF1 protein levels in human cells. HEK293 cells were transfected with miR-128 constructs for 48 hours. 15 µg of whole-cell lysate was then loaded in each lane. B-tubulin was used as an internal control for loading. Data show the mean ± s.e.m from 4 (for RT-PCR) and 8 (for Western Blot) independent experiments (***, $P<0.001$). B

assessed 48 hours later. RT-PCR from RNA extracts using *Nf1* specific primers revealed that *Nf1* mRNA expression was not, significantly, regulated by miR-128 or miR-128 double constructs (Fig. 4*A*). On the other hand, Western blots from whole protein extracts revealed a significant reduction in NF1 levels with all three constructs; miR-128, miR-128/103 and miR-137/128 produced a 74% ($P<0.001$), 74%, ($P<0.001$), and 75% ($P<0.001$) reduction in endogenous NF1 protein levels, respectively (Fig. 4*B*). The data indicated that these miRNAs induced translation inhibition of endogenous NF1 expression without affecting mRNA levels. Further, they showed no synergy in regulating NF1 protein levels at this cell population.

MiR-103, miR-128, miR-137 and Nf1 mRNA are Co-expressed in Neurons

To begin characterizing the physiological interaction between miR-103, miR-137, miR-128 and *Nf1*, the levels of mature miR-103, miR-137, and miR-128 as well as *Nf1* mRNA were compared in different tissues of embryonic day 18 mice. To equate the RNA levels of these tissues, the RNA levels for the ubiquitously expressed *U6* RNA were also measured. Fig. 5*A* shows that miR-103 was ubiquitously expressed in E18 tissues with highest levels in spinal cord, liver, superior cervical (SCG) and trigeminal (TG) ganglion. MiR-128 was, predominantly, expressed in neural tissues with highest levels in cortex, nodose, trigeminal and SCG ganglia, and least in spinal cord, substantia nigra and hippocampus. MiR-137 was, exclusively, expressed in the nervous system with comparable levels in all neural tissues while *Nf1* mRNA was expressed ubiquitously in all E18 tissues tested, with highest levels in the nervous system. These patterns of expression indicated that NF1 is most likely regulated by miR-103, miR-137, and miR-128 in the nervous system where levels were highest for these interactors.

Further, to determine if miR-103, miR-137, and miR-128 expression correlates with *Nf1* mRNA expression throughout development, the levels of mature miR-103, miR-137, miR-128 and *Nf1* mRNA were also profiled in cortex and hippocampus at different ages. Figs. 5*B and C* show that the levels of miR-103, miR-137, and miR-128 corresponded overall to the expression of *Nf1* mRNA, with lower levels early in embryonic development that peak in the first two weeks of postnatal development.

Since, neural tissues are a mixed population of neurons and glial cells that include astrocytes in central nervous system and Schwann cells in peripheral nervous system, the levels of mature miR-103, miR-137, miR-128 and *Nf1* mRNA were also quantified in these different cell types. Fig. 5*D* shows that the levels of miR-103, miR-137, miR-128 and *Nf1* mRNA were significantly higher in cultures of cortical neurons than astrocytes. With respect to Schwann cell cultures, miR-103, miR-137, and miR-128 showed little or no expression while *Nf1* mRNA had highest levels. Taking all together, these results indicated that miR-103, miR-137, and miR-128 are likely regulating NF1 levels in neurons only.

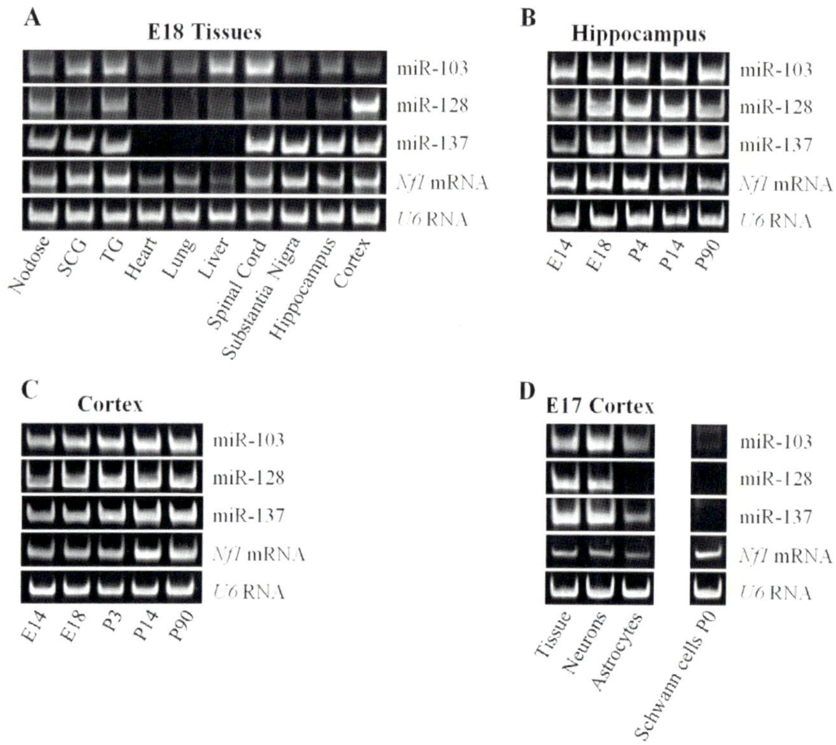

Figure 5. MiR-103, miR-128, miR-137 and Nf1 mRNA are co-expressed in the nervous system. Representative gels of the RT-PCR amplification products of miR-103, miR-128, miR-137, and *NF1* mRNA levels in: (**A**) Different murine tissues of embryonic day 18 animals; (**B**) Hippocampus of different ages; (**C**) Cortex of different ages; and (**D**) Different neural cell types. The amount of starting template for each condition was normalized to *U6* RNA. The number of PCR cycles for each miRNA RT-PCR assay is different between gels. Cycles were falling within the linear range of amplification for each primer pair. SCG, superior cervical ganglion; TG, trigeminal ganglion; E, embryonic day; P, postnatal day.

Moreover, since the three miRNAs and *Nf1* mRNA had similar rather than complementary distribution, it suggests that miR-103, miR-137, and miR-128 fine-tune, rather than block, NF1 protein levels in the nervous system.

MiR-103, miR-128 and miR-137 Modulate Endogenous NF1 Levels in Neurons

Based on the initial cell-line findings and the expression data, it was hypothesized that changes in miR-103, miR-137, and miR-128 levels would, also, impact endogenous NF1 protein but not mRNA levels in primary neurons. To test this, hippocampal neurons were transfected with miR-128 alone or in combination with miR-103 and miR-137 vectors and *Nf1* mRNA and protein levels were assessed ~48 hours later. Hippocampal neurons were selected for this experiment because they are a rather homogeneous cell population that provides enough large-size neurons for manipulation and is directly implicated in neurofibromatosis type I [24]. *Nf1* mRNA levels were assessed by RT-PCR after infecting hippocampal neurons with the pri-mir-128 lentiviral vectors. Similar to the results obtained with HEK293 cell manipulations, *Nf1* mRNA levels remained unaltered (data not shown). NF1 protein levels were assayed in GFP-positive neurons, transfected with pri-mir-128 plasmids, by immunofluorescence and quantitated by ImageJ densitometry. An average decrease of 16.1% ($P<0.01$), 33.1% ($P<0.05$), and 30% ($P<0.05$) in endogenous NF1 protein levels was measured with miR-128, miR-128/103, and miR-128/137 plasmid overexpression, respectively (Figs. *6A and B*). These findings indicated that a) miR-103, miR-137, and miR-128 function synergistically to regulate endogenous NF1 protein but not mRNA levels in neurons, and b) endogenous miR-103, miR-137, and miR-128 expression levels are not saturated for NF1 regulation of expression in neurons, thus, allowing a controlled amount of *Nf1* mRNA to be translated in accordance with the tuning hypothesis.

Next, the ability of endogenously expressed miR-103, miR-137, and miR-128 to regulate the levels of the reporter vector bearing the *Nf1* 3′-UTR was evaluated in the same cultures of hippocampal neurons. Antisense 2′-O-methyl as-miR-128, as-miR-128 plus as-miR-103 or as-miR-128 plus as-miR-137 inhibitors were transfected together with the *Nf1* reporter plasmid in freshly dissociated hippocampal neurons and luciferase activity was assayed 48 hours later. A 64% ($P<0.01$), 54% ($P<0.05$), and 68% ($P<0.05$) increase in luciferase levels were measured with antisense as-miR-128, as-miR-128/103 and as-miR-128/137 2′-O-methyl inhibitors, respectively (Fig. 6*C*) indicating that endogenous miR-128, miR-103 or miR-137 bind to mRNAs bearing *Nf1* 3′-UTR and block translation. Similar results were obtained when the inhibitors were transfected together with a GFP construct to mark transfected hippocampal neurons and NF1 protein levels were assayed by immunofluorescence and quantitated by ImageJ densitometry. An average increase of 13.4% ($P<0.05$, $n=3$), 13.5% ($P<0.05$, $n=3$), and 12.2% ($P<0.05$, $n=3$) in endogenous NF1 protein levels was measured in these neurons with miR-128, miR-128/103, and miR-128/137 inhibition, respectively (data not shown). The later effects were less pronounced than those obtained using the *Nf1* reporter maybe due to detection of NF1 protein produced before transfection, the differential distribution of NF1 inside cells (nucleocytoplasmic shuttling), and/or other factors. An additive effect for the double antisense miRNA transfections was also not observed, maybe as a result of reduced as-miR-128

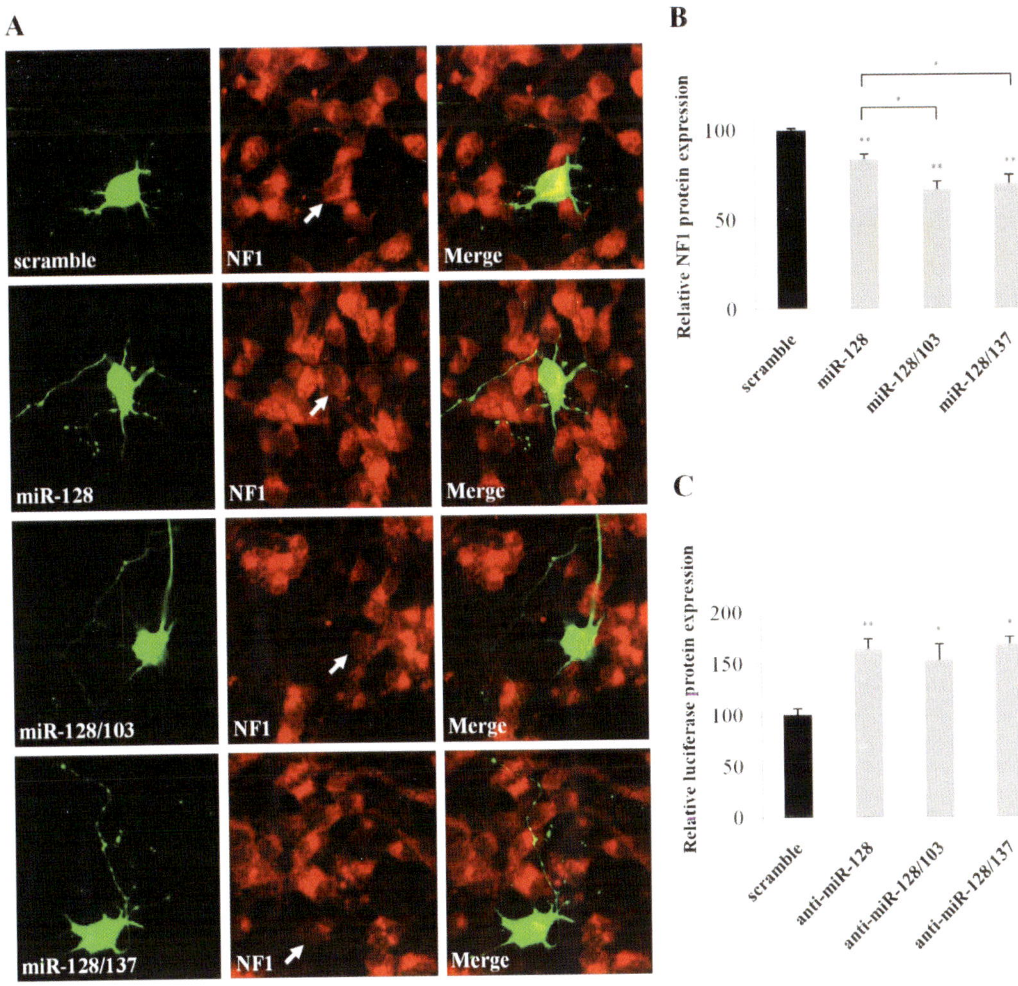

Figure 6. MiR-128 alone or together with miR-103 or miR-137 reduces endogenous NF1 protein levels in neurons. (**A**) Representative images of transfected hippocampal neurons (green) stained with NF1 antibody (red). Merged images are shown in the third column of the panel. E16 murine hippocampal neurons were transfected with scramble or pri-mir-128 plasmids immediately after plating by using Lipofectamine 2000. Immunocytochemistry was carried out 40 hours after transfection. (**B**) Average decrease in NF1 protein levels. 80 neurons were analyzed per experiment. Data show the mean ± s.e.m from 6 independent experiments (*, $P<0.05$; **, $P<0.01$). (**C**) Freshly dissociated hippocampal neurons were transfected with *Nf1* reporter vector plus antisense 2′-O-methyl inhibitors (miR-128 alone or together with miR-103 or miR-137) and assayed 48 hours later. Data show the mean ± s.e.m from 4 independent experiments (*, $P<0.05$).

delivered in neurons since for the double transfections as-miR-128 amount was halved in order to have comparable amount of 2′-O-methyl oligonucleotides loaded in all conditions.

Discussion

This study has revealed a previously unknown mechanism by which NF1 levels are regulated in the nervous system. Specifically, three miRNAs, miR-128, miR-103 and miR-137 have been shown to bind directly to the 3′-UTR of *Nf1* mRNA and significantly reduce its protein levels. This discovery has been based on: 1) conservation analysis of the recognition elements in the 3′-UTR of NF1 that show they are conserved throughout vertebrate species; 2) *in vitro* experiments in which the 'seed' regions have been mutagenized that resulted in the abrogation of protein degradation of a chimaeric luciferase reporter bearing the *Nf1* 3′-UTR; 3) gain-of-function experiments in which overexpression of miR-128, miR-128/103 or miR-128/137 resulted in down-regulation of endogenous NF1 protein levels in both cell-lines and hippocampal neurons; and 4) loss-of-function experiments in which inhibition of endogenous miR-128, miR-103 and miR-137 by antisense oligonucleotides promoted the expression of NF1 reporter and native protein in hippocampal neurons.

We have, also, presented data on miR-103, miR-128, miR-137 and *Nf1* mRNA levels across different tissues as well as different neuron types and glial cells. We found that miR-137 and miR-128, like NF1, had a neural distribution while miR-103 had a more ubiquitous tissue distribution. With respect to development, all three miRNAs and *Nf1* mRNA had their levels upregulated from their lowest levels at embryonic day 14 to peak levels around two weeks into postnatal development. Further, all three miRNAs were expressed highest in neurons and least in Schwann cells. We, also, found some lower expression of miR-103 and miR-137 in astrocytes. By considering the two opposing physiological means of miRNA function, these findings suggest that miR-103, miR-128, and miR-137 play a role in modulating, rather than blocking, NF1 expression in the nervous system and, in particular, neurons.

NF1 possesses several biochemical domains of which the RasGAP domain is best characterized for its ability to negatively regulate RAS signaling. RAS, a GTPase protein, tethered to the cell membrane, plays a central role in transmitting the extracellular signals from receptor tyrosine kinases, including growth factor receptors, to the nucleus. In cells, loss of NF1, leads to the constitutive activation of RAS signaling and decoupling from extracellular messages. As a result, patients with NF-1 develop malignancies and complex cognitive symptoms that include learning disabilities, attention deficit disorder and motor co-ordination problems. Two different splice variants, type I and II, of the NF1 RasGAP domain exist. The type I variant lacks exon 23a and it is ten times more active RasGAP than type II. Further, type I is predominantly expressed in neurons while type II in glia [25,26]. Based on these data, a likely role of the neuronal miRNAs maybe to tightly control the 'more active' NF1 in neurons and, thus, facilitate a precise fine-tuning of RAS activity in these cells.

Beyond miR-103, miR-128, and miR-137 another miRNA is capable of regulating NF1 expression. MiR-10b, an oncogenic miRNA, has recently been shown to regulate NF1 expression in non-neuronal cells [13]. Interestingly, miR-10b and NF1 are expressed in mutually exclusive cells indicating that miR-10b functions to block expression of NF1. In conjunction with our data, this indicates that different cell types of the body utilize different miRNA modes of action to regulate NF1 expression.

MiR-103, miR-128, and miR-137 have all ascribed functions apart from regulating NF1 expression. MiR-103 is downregulated in neuropathic animals while intrathecal applications relieve pain [27]; it has, also, been shown to negatively regulate BDNF, a prominent neurotrophic factor involved in neuronal ERK signaling and implicated in a plethora of neuropsychiatric diseases [28,29]. MiR-128 regulates the formation of fear-extinction memory [30] and reduces AKT signaling by repressing receptor tyrosine kinases EGFR and PDGFα [31]; it is, also, deregulated in Alzheimer's disease [32]. MiR-137 is enriched in synaptic fractions [32,33] and has been shown to regulate neuronal maturation and dendritic morphogenesis [34] while mutations in the gene have been associated with cognitive impairment [35]. All, these findings indicate that miR-103, miR-128 and miR-137 control a network of proteins previously found to be associated with NF1 signaling. Noting the spatial localization of mir-137 at synapses, it is possible that NF1 is, also, spatiotemporally regulated in neurons to control synaptic transmission.

In conclusion, this study provided strong evidence that miR-128, miR-103 and miR-137 regulate NF1 levels in neurons and set the stage to further evaluate their role in the NF-1 pathophysiological process. Future studies will reveal whether human aging, polymorphisms or environmental factors alter the expression levels of these miRNA and, thus, contribute to variability in NF-1 symptoms.

Acknowledgments

We thank Paulos Alexakos for excellent veterinary assistance. ED has received funding from the Greek General Secretariat for Research and Technology (Grant ID 13894) and the Academy of Athens.

Author Contributions

Conceived and designed the experiments: ED. Performed the experiments: MP ED. Analyzed the data: MP ED. Contributed reagents/materials/analysis tools: ED. Wrote the paper: ED.

References

1. Huson S, Hughes R (1994) The Neurofibromatoses : a pathogenetic and clinical overview. London: New York : Chapman & Hall Medical.
2. Friedman JM (1999) Epidemiology of neurofibromatosis type 1. Am J Med Genet 89: 1–6.
3. Ballester R, Marchuk D, Boguski M, Saulino A, Letcher R, et al. (1990) The NF1 locus encodes a protein functionally related to mammalian GAP and yeast IRA proteins. Cell 63: 851–859.
4. Martin GA, Viskochil D, Bollag G, McCabe PC, Crosier WJ, et al. (1990) The GAP-related domain of the neurofibromatosis type 1 gene product interacts with ras p21. Cell 63: 843–849.
5. Xu GF, Lin B, Tanaka K, Dunn D, Wood D, et al. (1990) The catalytic domain of the neurofibromatosis type 1 gene product stimulates ras GTPase and complements ira mutants of S. cerevisiae. Cell 63: 835–841.
6. Zhu H, Hinman MN, Hasman RA, Mehta P, Lou H (2008) Regulation of neuron-specific alternative splicing of neurofibromatosis type 1 pre-mRNA. Mol Cell Biol 28: 1240–1251.
7. Barron VA, Zhu H, Hinman MN, Ladd AN, Lou H (2010) The neurofibromatosis type I pre-mRNA is a novel target of CELF protein-mediated splicing regulation. Nucleic Acids Res 38: 253–264.
8. Bartel DP (2009) MicroRNAs: target recognition and regulatory functions. Cell 136: 215–233.
9. Hornstein E, Shomron N (2006) Canalization of development by microRNAs. Nat Genet 38 Suppl: S20–24.
10. Peterson KJ, Dietrich MR, McPeek MA (2009) MicroRNAs and metazoan macroevolution: insights into canalization, complexity, and the Cambrian explosion. Bioessays 31: 736–747.
11. Wienholds E, Plasterk RH (2005) MicroRNA function in animal development. FEBS Lett 579: 5911–5922.
12. Subramanian S, Thayanithy V, West RB, Lee CH, Beck AH, et al. (2010) Genome-wide transcriptome analyses reveal p53 inactivation mediated loss of miR-34a expression in malignant peripheral nerve sheath tumours. J Pathol 220: 58–70.
13. Chai G, Liu N, Ma J, Li H, Oblinger JL, et al. (2010) MicroRNA-10b regulates tumorigenesis in neurofibromatosis type 1. Cancer Sci 101: 1997–2004.
14. Doxakis E (2010) Post-transcriptional regulation of alpha-synuclein expression by mir-7 and mir-153. J Biol Chem 285: 12726–12734.
15. Ge L, Rudolph P (1997) Simultaneous introduction of multiple mutations using overlap extension PCR. Biotechniques 22: 28–30.
16. Doxakis E, Huang EJ, Davies AM (2004) Homeodomain-interacting protein kinase-2 regulates apoptosis in developing sensory and sympathetic neurons. Curr Biol 14: 1761–1765.
17. Raymond CK, Roberts BS, Garrett-Engele P, Lim LP, Johnson JM (2005) Simple, quantitative primer-extension PCR assay for direct monitoring of microRNAs and short-interfering RNAs. RNA 11: 1737–1744.
18. Lao K, Xu NL, Yeung V, Chen C, Livak KJ, et al. (2006) Multiplexing RT-PCR for the detection of multiple miRNA species in small samples. Biochem Biophys Res Commun 343: 85–89.
19. Abramoff MD, Magalhaes PJ, Ram SJ (2004) Image Processing with ImageJ. Biophotonics International 11: 36–42.
20. Grimson A, Farh KK, Johnston WK, Garrett-Engele P, Lim LP, et al. (2007) MicroRNA targeting specificity in mammals: determinants beyond seed pairing. Mol Cell 27: 91–105.
21. John B, Enright AJ, Aravin A, Tuschl T, Sander C, et al. (2004) Human MicroRNA targets. PLoS Biol 2: e363.
22. Krek A, Grun D, Poy MN, Wolf R, Rosenberg L, et al. (2005) Combinatorial microRNA target predictions. Nat Genet 37: 495–500.
23. Kiriakidou M, Nelson PT, Kouranov A, Fitziev P, Bouyioukos C, et al. (2004) A combined computational-experimental approach predicts human microRNA targets. Genes & Dev 18: 1165–1178.
24. Cui Y, Costa RM, Murphy GG, Elgersma Y, Zhu Y, et al. (2008) Neurofibromin regulation of ERK signaling modulates GABA release and learning. Cell 135: 549–560.
25. Andersen LB, Ballester R, Marchuk DA, Chang E, Gutmann DH, et al. (1993) A conserved alternative splice in the von Recklinghausen neurofibromatosis (NF1) gene produces two neurofibromin isoforms, both of which have GTPase-activating protein activity. Mol Cell Biol 13: 487–495.
26. Baizer L, Ciment G, Hendrickson SK, Schafer GL (1993) Regulated expression of the neurofibromin type I transcript in the developing chicken brain. J Neurochem 61: 2054–2060.
27. Favereaux A, Thoumine O, Bouali-Benazzouz R, Roques V, Papon MA, et al. (2011) Bidirectional integrative regulation of Cav1.2 calcium channel by microRNA miR-103: role in pain. EMBO J 30: 3830–3841.
28. Angelucci F, Brene S, Mathe AA (2005) BDNF in schizophrenia, depression and corresponding animal models. Mol Psychiatry 10: 345–352.
29. Mellios N, Huang HS, Grigorenko A, Rogaev E, Akbarian S (2008) A set of differentially expressed miRNAs, including miR-30a-5p, act as post-transcriptional inhibitors of BDNF in prefrontal cortex. Hum Mol Genet 17: 3030–3042.
30. Lin Q, Wei W, Coelho CM, Li X, Baker-Andresen D, et al. (2011) The brain-specific microRNA miR-128b regulates the formation of fear-extinction memory. Nat Neurosci 14: 1115–1117.
31. Papagiannakopoulos T, Friedmann-Morvinski D, Neveu P, Dugas JC, Gill RM, et al. (2011) Pro-neural miR-128 is a glioma tumor suppressor that targets mitogenic kinases. Oncogene 31: 1884–1895.

32. Pichardo-Casas I, Goff LA, Swerdel MR, Athie A, Davila J, et al. (2012) Expression profiling of synaptic microRNAs from the adult rat brain identifies regional differences and seizure-induced dynamic modulation. Brain Res 1436: 20–33.
33. Siegel G, Obernosterer G, Fiore R, Oehmen M, Bicker S, et al. (2009) A functional screen implicates microRNA-138-dependent regulation of the depalmitoylation enzyme APT1 in dendritic spine morphogenesis. Nat Cell Biol 11: 705–716.
34. Smrt RD, Szulwach KE, Pfeiffer RL, Li X, Guo W, et al. (2010) MicroRNA miR-137 regulates neuronal maturation by targeting ubiquitin ligase mind bomb-1. Stem Cells 28: 1060–1070.
35. Willemsen MH, Valles A, Kirkels LA, Mastebroek M, Olde Loohuis N, et al. (2011) Chromosome 1p21.3 microdeletions comprising DPYD and mir-137 are associated with intellectual disability. J Med Genet 48: 810–818.
36. Kruger J, Rehmsmeier M (2006) RNAhybrid: microRNA target prediction easy, fast and flexible. Nucleic Acids Res 34: W451–454.

8

Temporal Separation of Aggregation and Ubiquitination during Early Inclusion Formation in Transgenic Mice Carrying the Huntington's Disease Mutation

Belvin Gong[1,2]**, Catherine Kielar**[1]**, A. Jennifer Morton**[1]*

1 Department of Pharmacology, University of Cambridge, Cambridge, United Kingdom, 2 UC Davis/NIH NeuroMab Facility, Department of Neurobiology, Physiology and Behavior, University of California Davis, Davis, California, United States of America

Abstract

Abnormal insoluble ubiqitinated protein aggregates are found in the brains of Huntington's disease (HD) patients and in mice transgenic for the *HTT* mutation. Here, we describe the earliest stages of visible NII formation in brains of R6/2 mice killed between 2 and 6 weeks of age. We found that huntingtin-positive aggregates formed rapidly (within 24–48 hours) in a spatiotemporal manner similar to that we described previously for ubiquitinated inclusions. However, in most neurons, aggregates are not ubiquitinated when they first form. It has always been assumed that mutant huntingtin is recognised as 'foreign' and consequently ubiquitinated and targeted for degradation by the ubiquitin-proteasome system pathway. Our data, however, suggest that aggregation and ubiquitination are separate processes, and that mutant huntingtin fragment is not recognized as 'abnormal' by the ubiquitin-proteasome system before aggregation. Rather, mutant Htt appears to aggregate before it is ubiquitinated, and then either aggregated huntingtin is ubiquitinated or ubiquitinated proteins are recruited into aggregates. Our findings have significant implications for the role of the ubiquitin-proteasome system in the formation of aggregates, as they suggest that this system is not involved until after the first aggregates form.

Editor: Zhenyu Yue, Mount Sinai School of Medicine, United States of America

Funding: This work was supported by by Merck, Sharp and Dohme, Incorporated (PhD studentship to BG), the Cambridge Overseas Trust (BG), CHDI Foundation (CK and AJM) and the Wellcome Trust (AJM). The funders had no role in study design, data collection and analysis, decision to publish, or preparation of the manuscript. The funders had no role in study design, data collection and analysis, decision to publish, or preparation of the manuscript.

Competing Interests: This study was supported by Merck, Sharp and Dohme. There are no patents, products in development or marketed products to declare. This does not alter the authors' adherence to all the PLoS ONE policies on sharing data and materials, as detailed online in the guide for authors.

* E-mail: ajm41@cam.ac.uk

These authors contributed equally to this work.

Introduction

Huntington's disease (HD) is one of a family of progressive genetic neurodegenerative disorders caused by the pathological expansion of a CAG repeat in the *HTT* disease gene that encodes the protein huntingtin (Htt) [1]. The mechanism by which the CAG repeat expansion causes HD is not known. However, the discovery of neuronal intranuclear inclusions (NIIs) in the brains of mice transgenic for a protein fragment carrying the *HTT* mutation [2] and subsequently in brains of HD patients [2,3] has triggered a great deal of interest in both the mechanisms of inclusion formation and their potentially pathogenic role. The importance of inclusion pathology is not restricted to HD, since inclusions are present in brains of patients with other polyglutamine diseases and all mouse models thus far examined (for review, see [5]). Nevertheless, the role of inclusions in HD pathology is not only unclear, but is also hotly debated (for review see [6]). There is evidence suggesting that they may be neurotoxic ([7,8,9,10,11,12,13,14], neuroprotective [15,16,17,18,19,20,21,22,23,24] or both, depending on when and where they form [25,22].

Despite the debate about their role, there is no doubt that inclusions are a clear histopathological marker of the disease [26]. Inclusions are not found in neurologically normal subjects, but are found throughout the HD brain, particularly in striatum (STR) and cortex (CTX), the brain regions most affected in HD [3,4,16,27,28]. NIIs are defined as abnormal ubiquitinated aggregates of proteins, predominantly huntingtin and/or fragments of huntingtin and ubiquitin, although a number of other proteins have been found associated with inclusions in transgenic mouse and cell models [29,30] and human brains [31]. Importantly, it has always been assumed that mutant huntingtin is recognised as 'foreign' and consequently ubiquitinated and targeted for degradation by the ubiquitin-proteasome system pathway, because (1) a mutation in the gene coding for huntingtin causes HD, (2) mutant huntingtin is found in neuronal intranuclear inclusions, (3) neuronal nuclear inclusions are ubiquitinated, (4) the ubiquitin-proteasome pathway is responsible for recognising and disposing of abnormal proteins and (5) proteasome fragments are associated with NIIs.

To understand the role of NIIs in HD pathology, it would help if we knew what relationship exists between the appearance of inclusions, their ubiquitination and the onset of neuronal dysfunction. Here, we focused on the first stage of inclusion formation. We used juvenile R6/2 mice to study *ex vivo* the processes of Htt aggregation and inclusion formation. R6/2 mice show progressive neurological impairments [32,33,34,35] and the appearance of ubiquitinated inclusions precedes the appearance of measurable behavioral (motor and cognitive) phenotypic changes

[25] and happens at around the same time as abnormalities in synaptic plasticity [36] and early changes in brain markers [37] are first seen.

We performed an extensive and comparative immunohistochemical analysis of Htt aggregation and inclusion ubiquitination to pinpoint both the order of appearance and the regional location of aggregates in R6/2 brain. For this, we used the MW8 antibody that is specific for the aggregated conformation of mutant Htt protein [38], along with anti-ubiquitin antibodies. We showed that visible Htt-immunopositive aggregates are present in R6/2 brain as early as 2 weeks of age and appear in a region specific manner throughout the brain over the next few weeks. Notably, individual Htt-positive aggregates formed very rapidly, within the interval of a single day in most brain regions. Our data suggest that mutant Htt aggregation occurs rapidly and is then either ubiquitinated or other ubiquitinated proteins (that may include Htt itself) are recruited into inclusions.

Methods

R6/2 Mice

Mice were taken from a colony of R6/2 mice established in the Department of Pharmacology, University of Cambridge, as previously described [33]. The line was maintained by back-crossing transgenic males onto female CBA×C57BL/6 F1 mice. All mice used in this study were taken from the 21st and the 23rd generations of back-crosses. The CAG repeat lengths of transgenic mice used were measured and the mean repeat length was calculated as 188 ± 1 ($N = 122$; see genotyping section for more information). All mice were housed with a 12-hour light/dark cycle in a temperature- and humidity-controlled environment. Food (mash and dry food) and water were available *ad libitum*.

Mice used for the earliest time-points (4 weeks of age and younger) were not weaned. Older mice were weaned, separated by gender and housed in groups of mixed genotype at 4 weeks.

Time-Course Tissue Collection Scheme

We wanted to ensure that for all time-points we had at least 3 animals of each genotype from three different litters, and that for each animal we had one littermate that was exactly 24 hours younger and one that was 24 hours older (except for the 14 day timepoint where we only needed an older littermate). For time-course time-points between 14 and 28 days of age, brain tissue was collected at intervals of 24 hours. This interval was chosen because *in vitro*, aggregation is observed within this timeframe. Since most of the early time-course time-points used in this study preceded the age at which we were able to take samples for genotyping (2.5–3 weeks of age), a tissue collection 'scheme' was used for mice up to 25 days as follows. We used only litters that contained 9–12 pups. We did not distinguish between the sexes. Three or four mice were randomly selected from each litter to be killed at the same time of day on each of 3 consecutive days. Thus, any given mouse, on any given day, had at least one WT and one R6/2 littermate killed 24 hours before or 24 hours after it had been killed. This allowed us to compare regional appearance of inclusions in littermates at 24 hourly intervals. Performing the time-course in this way allowed us to examine variability between animals killed at specific time-points as well as between littermates exactly 24 hours apart. R6/2 and WT mice killed at ages greater than 25 days (4, 5, 6, 9 and 12 weeks) were killed according to their genotypes ($N = 4$ R6/2 and 3 WT littermates at each age).

Animals were genotyped to ascertain the distribution of R6/2 and WT within these groups. We used 12 litters (122 mice) for tissue collection for time course points up to 25 days, and a total of 35 mice for the other time points. All brains were dissected, frozen on powdered dry ice and stored at −80°C until use as previously described (Morton *et al.*, 2000).

Genotyping

Genotyping was performed by PCR from tail snips taken at 3 weeks of age and CAG repeat lengths were measured by Laragen (USA). All CAG repeat numbers reported are those determined directly by Genemapper software (note that the CAG repeat number measured by GeneMapper differs from that measured by sequencing). To convert the CAG repeat numbers determined by GeneMapper technique to the CAG repeat number determined by sequencing technique (which more closely represents the true CAG repeat number) the following formula needs to be applied: SEQ CAG no. (true CAG no.) = 1.0427 * GM CAG no. +1.1695; personal communication, Dr J. Li, Laragen).

Immunohistochemistry

The antibody staining procedure was performed essentially as previously described [25]. Antibodies used were either a rabbit polyclonal antibody raised against poly-ubiquitin (1:2000; Dako, Denmark) or a mouse monoclonal antibody MW8 raised against Htt (1:2000; kind gift of Dr. Paul Patterson, Caltech, CA, USA). The MW panel of antibodies was raised against synthetic peptides of polyglutamine disease protein fragments with expanded repeats [38]. MW8 was raised against the first exon of mutant Htt with antigenic boosts of aggregated Htt protein [38]. MW8 recognises the aggregated conformation of mutant Htt, and epitope-mapping studies reveal that it recognises the C-terminal portion of exon 1, specifically the sequence AVAEEPLHRPK [38]. This sequence shows no known homology to any protein other than Htt (BLAST searches). MW8 has been reported to label nuclear inclusions in R6/2 brain exclusively (although in our hands it also stains neuropil aggregates, see below). It shows no staining above background in WT animals (this study; [38]). Horseradish peroxidase (HRP)-conjugated secondary antibodies were used to label bound primary antibodies (1:2000; Vector, Peterborough, UK). Importantly, the MW8 staining here was obtained with standard histological techniques and without assistance from antigen retrieval methods that are required to 'reveal' aggregates that were not seen before (e.g. formic acid treatment [39,40]).

Cryosections of fresh frozen R6/2 and WT brain tissue were cut at 30 μm thickness onto gelatin-coated glass slides and processed for immunohistochemical staining. Sections were peroxidase-inactivated for 15 min at room temperature (20% v/v methanol, 0.2% Triton X-100 and 1% v/v hydrogen peroxide in phosphate-buffered saline (PBS)) and incubated in block solution (3% deer serum, 0.2% Triton X-100 and 0.1% sodium azide in PBS) for at least 3 hours at room temperature. At least one run of staining included sections from all of the animals used in the study and all of the sections were incubated in the same solution. Parallel sections were incubated with primary antibodies diluted in block solution at 4°C for a week, extensively washed and incubated with secondary antibodies diluted into wash solution at 4°C overnight. We used parallel sections rather than double staining to be sure that there was no false positives. Parallel sections allowed us to repeat staining on negative sections. Immunoreactivity was visualised using diaminobenzidine (Sigma, Poole, UK). All of the staining was done in parallel, timed to within 5 seconds over a 10 minute incubation period, in the same solution. A confirmation series of staining was done with one slide (a series of sections) from every animal in the study developed together. A slide with parallel sections from each brain was stained with 1% cresyl violet acetate solution in water (CV), mounted in Histoclear (CellPath, New-

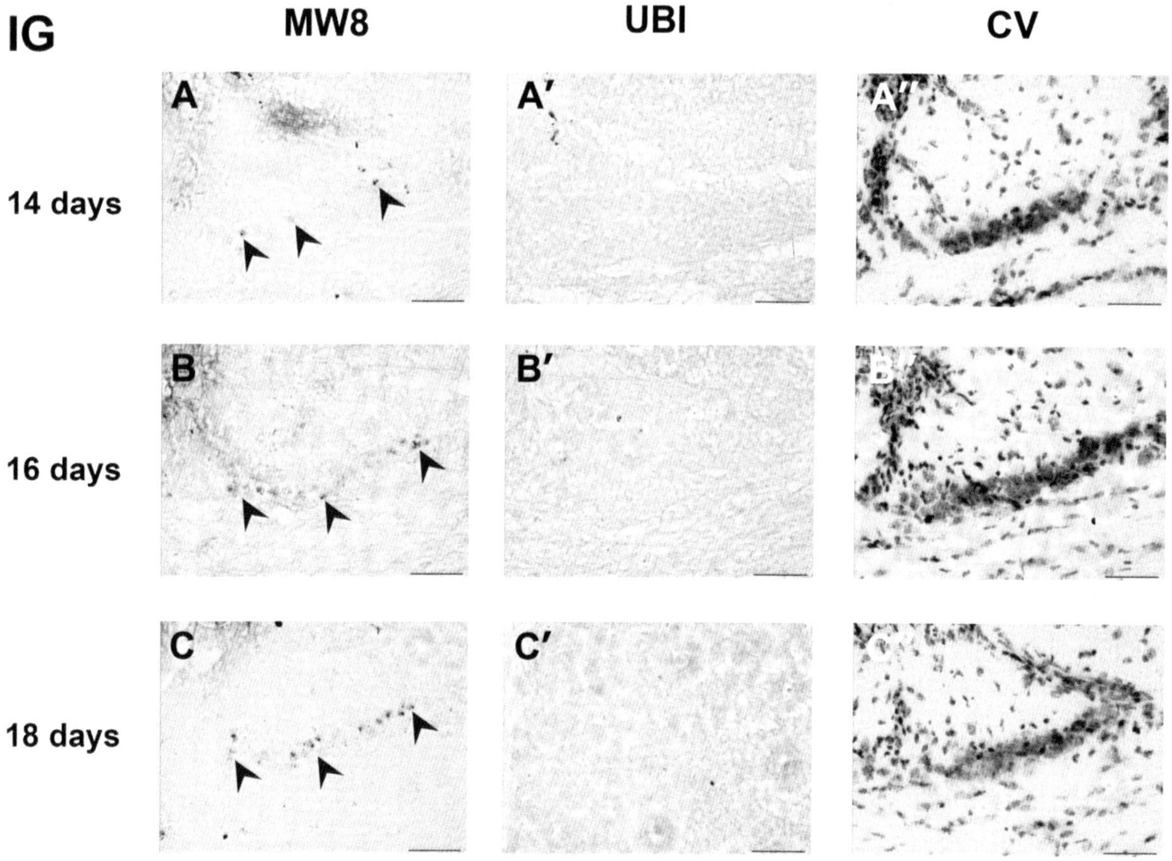

Figure 1. Aggregate appearance in indusium griseum (IG). Htt aggregates visualised by staining with the MW8 antibody were present in adjacent sections for IG of R6/2 brains as early as 14 days of age (A, black arrowheads) and increased in number with time (B, C; black arrowheads). Staining with ubiquitin antibody did not reveal the presence of inclusions in any region at these time points (A'–C'). Cell distribution in this region was visualised with a cresyl violet (CV) stain (A''–C''). Scale bar = 50 μm.

town, UK) to aid neuroanatomical identification of brain regions. All immunostained slides were counterstained with Hoechst 33258 dye (5 μg/ml in PBS for 30 min) to label nuclei, mounted in glycerol jelly, covered with a coverslip and stored in the dark at room temperature until analysis.

Light and Fluorescence Microscopy

We have shown previously that ubiquitinated NIIs appear first in juvenile R6/2 brain in the indusium griseum (IG), where they are visible by 3 weeks of age. Then, between 3 and 4.5 weeks of age NIIs appear in the CA1 region of hippocampus (Hf), layers II/III and V of frontal and parietal CTX, and STR [25]. In the current study, we again focused on these brain regions, because the different cell types in them are easily identified by their anatomical location.

Slides were analysed using an inverted fluorescence Nikon Eclipse TE-2000 microscope (Nikon, Surrey, UK). Hoechst 33342 staining of nuclei was visualised with UV light excitation and a DAPI filter. Photomicrographs were taken at X40 and X100 (under oil immersion) objective magnification with the same time exposure settings using the Nikon Still Camera DXM1200 and the Nikon Lucia software system (Nikon, Surrey, UK).

Aggregates and Inclusions

In previous studies of protein aggregation in HD brain, the terms 'aggregate' and 'inclusion' have been used interchangeably to identify ubiquitinated deposits of proteins in human and mouse HD brain. This has not caused difficulties in discussions of 'inclusions' for two main reasons. Firstly, ubiquitin antibody staining is generally accepted as the benchmark marker for identifying inclusions. Secondly, few research groups have made detailed studies of the difference between ubiquitin-positive inclusions and Htt-positive aggregates. However, the use of MW8 in the course of this study showed it was possible to clearly distinguish aggregates of Htt from aggregates with the classical morphological appearance of ubiquitinated 'inclusions'. Therefore, we have used the term 'inclusion' only[1] when referring to an aggregation of protein in the nucleus that is ubiquitinated, such as were classically described in human and mouse HD brain [2,25]. It is also important to stress that this study did not include microaggregate foci and focused solely on aggregates.

Aggregated Huntingtin

For convenience, throughout this paper, we describe the proteins that are visualised by MW8 as 'aggregated mutant huntingtin'. This is not strictly accurate, since the transgene includes only the first exon of the HD gene. Thus, the major protein species that is found in inclusions in R6/2 mice is not full length huntingtin, but rather a mutant fragment of huntingtin with a pathological length polyglutamine repeat.

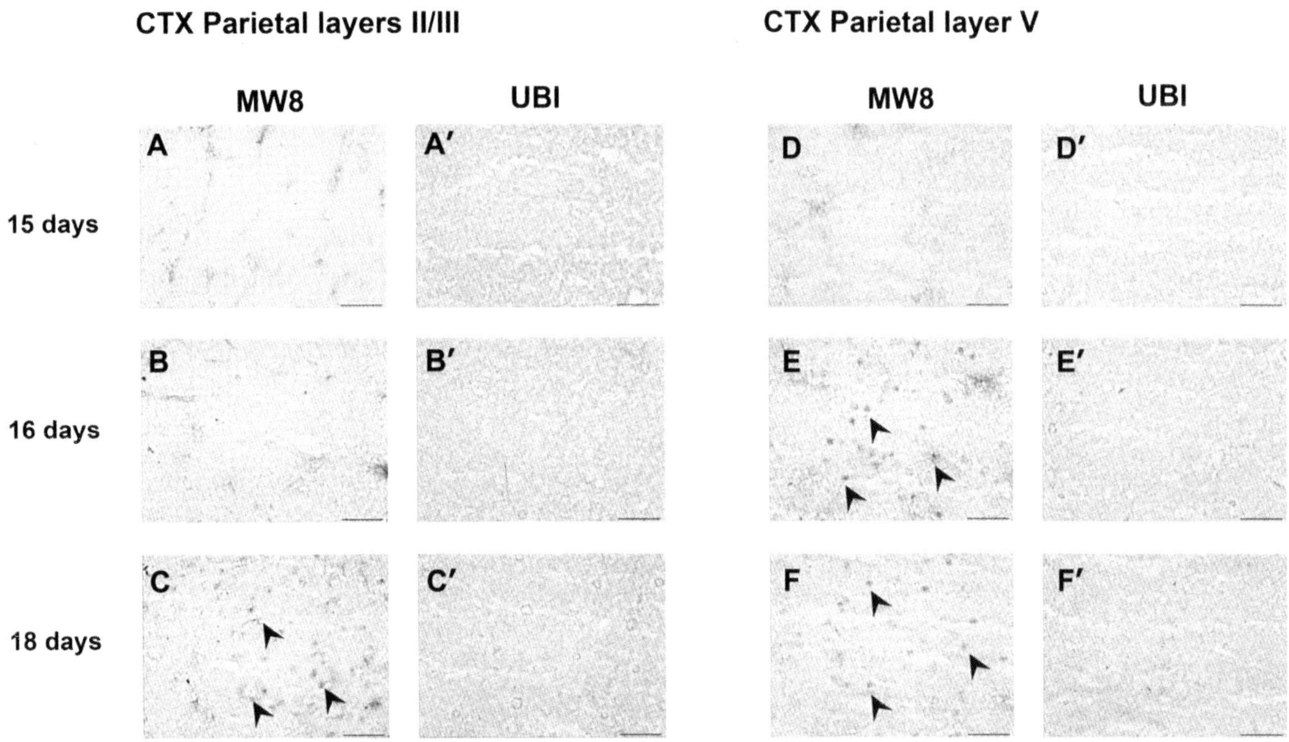

Figure 2. Aggregate appearance in parietal cortex (CTX). Htt aggregates visualised by staining with the MW8 antibody were present in the CTX of R6/2 brains at 16 days in layer V (E, F; black arrowheads) and at 18 days in layer II/III (C, black arrowheads). Staining with ubiquitin antibody did not reveal the presence of inclusions in any region at these time points (A'–F'). Scale bar = 50 μm.

Results

Htt Aggregation is a Rapid and Early Event

By comparing littermates that were killed exactly 24 hours apart, we were able to determine the age at which Htt aggregates first became visible at a light level. MW8-positive aggregates were already present in the IG of R6/2 brains by 14 days of age (Fig. 1), but were not visible in any other brain region. Thus the aggregates in IG were used as a reliable internal positive control for the MW8 antibody staining.

In many cells, Htt aggregates that could be visualised by staining with MW8 appeared almost overnight. For example, in the parietal cortex, MW8-positive aggregates were absent from all layers at 15 days (Fig. 2A, A', D and D'). Aggregates were present at 16 days in layer V (Fig. 2E and E'), but not in layer II/III (Fig. 2B and B'). By 18 days aggregates were also present in layer II/III (Fig. 2C, C'). Similarly, in CA1 cells of the hippocampus, Htt aggregates could not be seen at 18 days of age (data not shown) but were visible as diffuse aggregates in many neurons at 19 days (Fig. 3B, B' and B'') and clearly present by 22d (Fig. 3C, C' and C'').

Both the number of cells with aggregates and the levels of immunostaining intensity varied markedly in different regions of the same brain, suggesting that Htt aggregation is timed according to the identity of the cell population. However, aggregate formation appeared to follow a similar pattern in neurons of a single class. For example in pyramidal cells in the CA1 region of the hippocampus, MW8-positive aggregates first appeared with a diffuse morphology on day 19 (Fig. 3 and Fig. 4). Over the next few days, the Htt aggregates changed from being amorphous to having clear nucleation centres that became visible at 22 days (Fig. 3 and Fig. 4). This pattern was typical of all CA1 neurons. By contrast, in the dentate gyrus (DG) of the hippocampus Htt aggregates were first seen at 26 days (Fig. 3, Fig. 4), many days after they were first observed in CA1 (Fig. 3 and Fig. 4). Interestingly, it is not just the timing that varies, but also the morphology of aggregate formation. Htt aggregates in DG neurons had a more punctate morphology than those first seen in CA1 cells (Fig. 3), and they continued to grow with time (Fig. 4) until they reached the stage where MW8-stained aggregates were of similar appearance to the nucleation centres described by Chen *et al.*, [41]. By contrast, aggregates in cortical neurons were similar to those that formed in CA1 neurons, beginning as diffuse deposits in nuclei and then clustered into MW8-positive aggregates with nucleated centres.

Aggregate Formation in different Brain Regions is Differentially, but Precisely, Timed

There was a defined and consistent order to the organisation and timing of first appearance of Htt aggregates in R6/2 brains. As mentioned above, in the IG Htt aggregates were already present at 14 days of age (Fig. 1). Subsequently, Htt aggregates appeared (by 19 days of age), in the CA1 region of the Hf (Fig. 4) and the deeper layers of parietal, frontal and cingulate CTX. Aggregates also began to form in cells in layer II/III of parietal CTX (but not other parts of the CTX) at this time (Fig. 2). Between 19 and 22 days, aggregates in IG and CA1 grew larger (Fig. 3). By 22 days, almost all (>80%) cells in the deep layers of parietal CTX had visible aggregates that were MW8-positive (Fig. 2). Over the following few days marked increases in aggregate size and frequency of appearance in brain regions already containing aggregates were observed, while Htt aggregates just began to form in the DG and in STR by 26 days (Fig. 4). Finally,

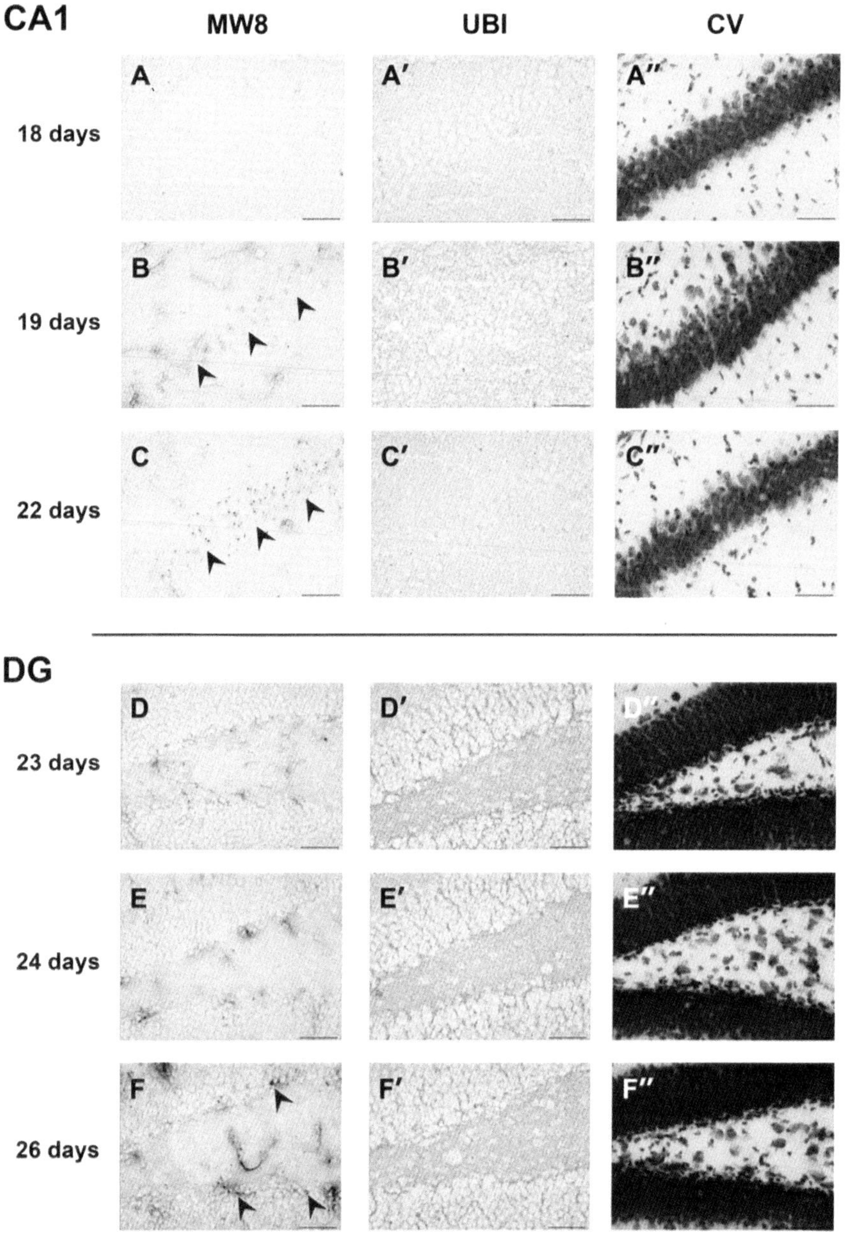

Figure 3. Aggregate appearance in CA1 and dentate gyrus (DG). In R6/2 hippocampus, Htt aggregates visualised by staining with the MW8 antibody could not be seen at 18 days of age but could be found in many neurons at 19 days in the CA1 (B, black arrowheads) and increased in number with time (C, black arrowheads). Cell distribution in this region is shown in a parallel section showed with a cresyl violet stain (A″–C″). In the DG, MW8-positive aggregates were absent up to 24 days, but were present at 26 days (F, black arrowheads). Staining with ubiquitin antibody did not reveal the presence of inclusions in any region at these time points (A′–F′). Cell distribution in both regions was visualised with a cresyl violet (CV) stain (D″–F″). Scale bar = 50 μm.

CA3 neurones began to form visible Htt-positive aggregates by 29 days (Fig. 4). By 41 days, the majority of cells contained aggregates of Htt protein in dense nuclear foci (Fig. 4). The exceptions were DG and CA3 cells, in which progression of aggregate formation was much slower.

Htt Aggregation Precedes Ubiquitination

In all R6/2 brain regions studied, the appearance of Htt-positive aggregates preceded inclusion ubiquitination. At 14 days of age, there were no ubiquitinated inclusions in any brain region, which reproduces previous observations that no NIIs could be found in any brain regions of R6/2 mice at that age [25,42]. The appearance of ubiquitinated inclusions occurred first in the IG by 19 days (Fig. 5). Ubiquitinated inclusions in other brain regions were observed at 24 days, when neurones in the CA1 region of the Hf began to show round amorphous ubiquitin-stained inclusions (Fig. 5). Over the next few days, there was a marked increase in the size and frequency of ubiquitinated inclusions in the IG as well as CA1. By 26 days, many IG and CA1 aggregates were ubiquitinated (Fig. 5). By 29 days, although Htt aggregates were present in neurons of the STR, DG and CA3 of the Hf, none of them were ubiquitinated (Fig. 5). At 41 days (nearly 6 weeks),

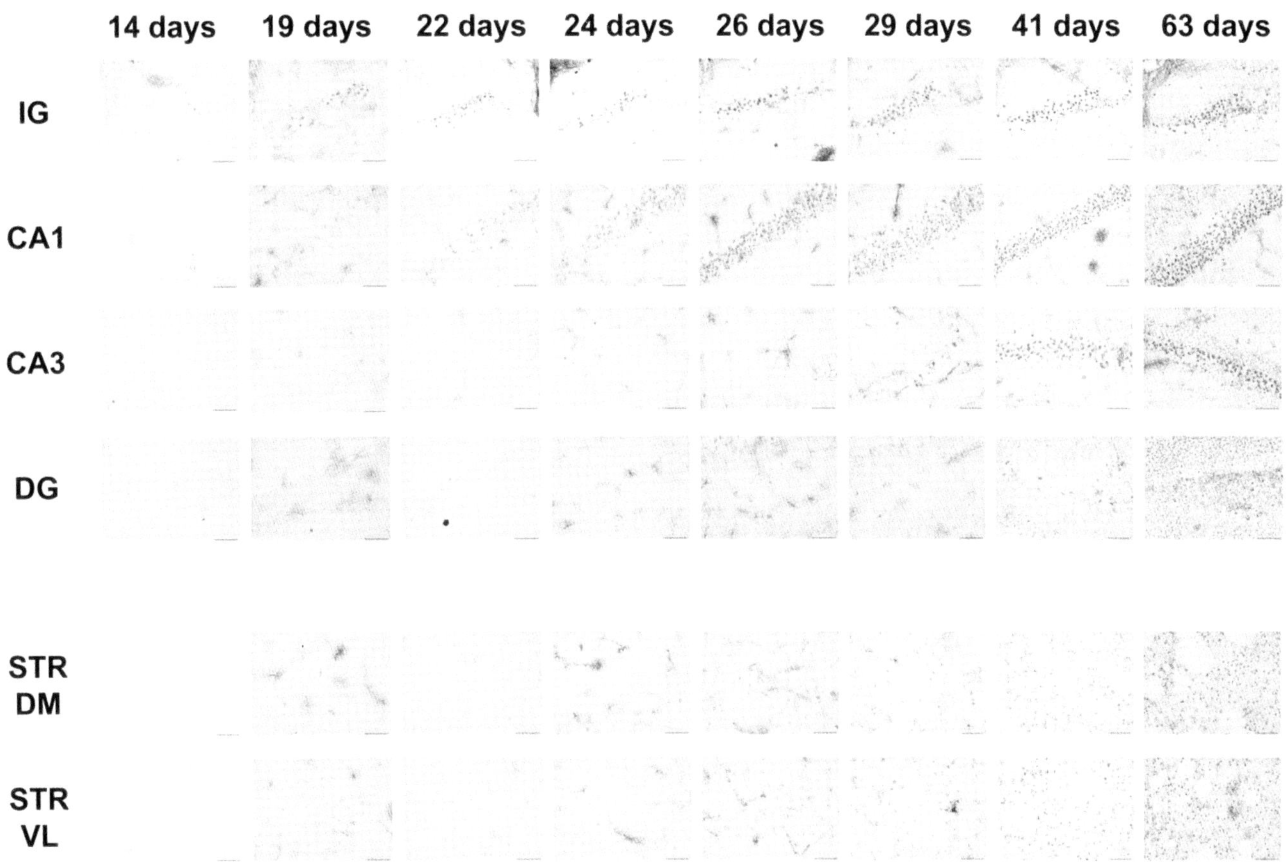

Figure 4. Aggregate appearance in different brain regions over time. Htt aggregates visualised by staining with the MW8 antibody (shown here at 14, 19, 22, 24, 26, 29, 41 and 63 days) in indisium griseum (IG), CA1, CA3, dentate gyrus (DG) and dorso-medial and ventro-lateral striatum (STR DM and STR VL) of R6/2 brains. A few aggregates were visualised in the IG as early as 14 days of age. In the hippocampus, inclusions were present at 19 days in CA1, whereas in the CA3 a few aggregates were visible at 29 days of age. In the dentate gyrus, MW8-positive aggregates were present at 26 days. In the striatum, Htt aggregates could be seen at 26 days of age in STR DM and STR VL. The number of aggregates in all the regions increased with time from the day of appearance. Scale bar =50 μm.

aggregates in many brain regions were ubiqutinated, and continued to grow bigger, as seen previously [25]. They appeared to have reached a stable density in the IG and in CA1 (Fig. 5). In addition, by that age, ubiquitinated aggregates were present in the CA3. The only brain region in which cells did not have ubiqutinated inclusions by 41 days of age was the DG (Fig. 5). These observations are generally consistent with previous studies, where ubiquitinated NIIs were seen in DG only at 7 weeks of age and beyond [25]. By 63 days (9 weeks), when all neurones studied had aggregates (see Fig. 5), most were mature, ubiquitinated inclusions.

Patterns of Ubiquitination Depend on Cell Soma Size

Previous observations have shown that increases in NII size are not due to increases in the sizes of nuclei [25], however the timing of initial aggregation formation with regard to the sizes of nuclei has not been studied until now. Here we compared cells in specific brain regions to see if a relationship existed between cell soma size, the propensity to form Htt aggregates and the time-course of ubiquitination. Neurons were classified as having small, medium or large soma. Granule cells of the DG were classified as 'small', CA1 pyramidal neurons and medium spiny striatal neurons were classified as 'medium-sized' and CA3 and cortical pyramidal neurons were classified as having 'large' soma. A direct comparison of MW8 staining patterns in cells from these brain regions showed that there was no correlation between the timing of aggregate formation and cell soma size (Fig. 6). For example, cells with medium-sized soma can form Htt aggregates as early as 22 days (CA1 neurons) or as late as 28 days of age (STR neurons). Likewise, cells with large soma can form aggregates as early as 19 days (neurons in parietal CTX) or as late as 28 days of age (CA3 neurons) (Fig. 6). However, timing of ubiquitination appeared to be related to cell soma size. Regardless of whether or not huntingtin aggregates formed early or late, aggregates that formed in cells with small and medium-sized soma were found ubiquitinated within 2–3 days of initial aggregation (Fig. 6). By contrast, there was usually lag of >3 days between initial aggregate formation and inclusion ubiquitination in cells with large soma (Fig. 6). For example, although aggregates formed early in cortical cells (19 days), ubiquitinated inclusions did not typically appear until after 22 days. In CA3 neurons, although Htt aggregates appeared by 29 days (Fig. 6), not all aggregates had been ubiquitinated before the end of the period over which we conducted 24-hour interval time-course study (that is, in CA3 neurons, some aggregates were ubiquitinated later than 41 days).

Structural Investigation of Aggregate and Inclusion Formation

In order to compare MW8 and ubiquitin staining patterns in single R6/2 neurons in the brain regions and at the time-points

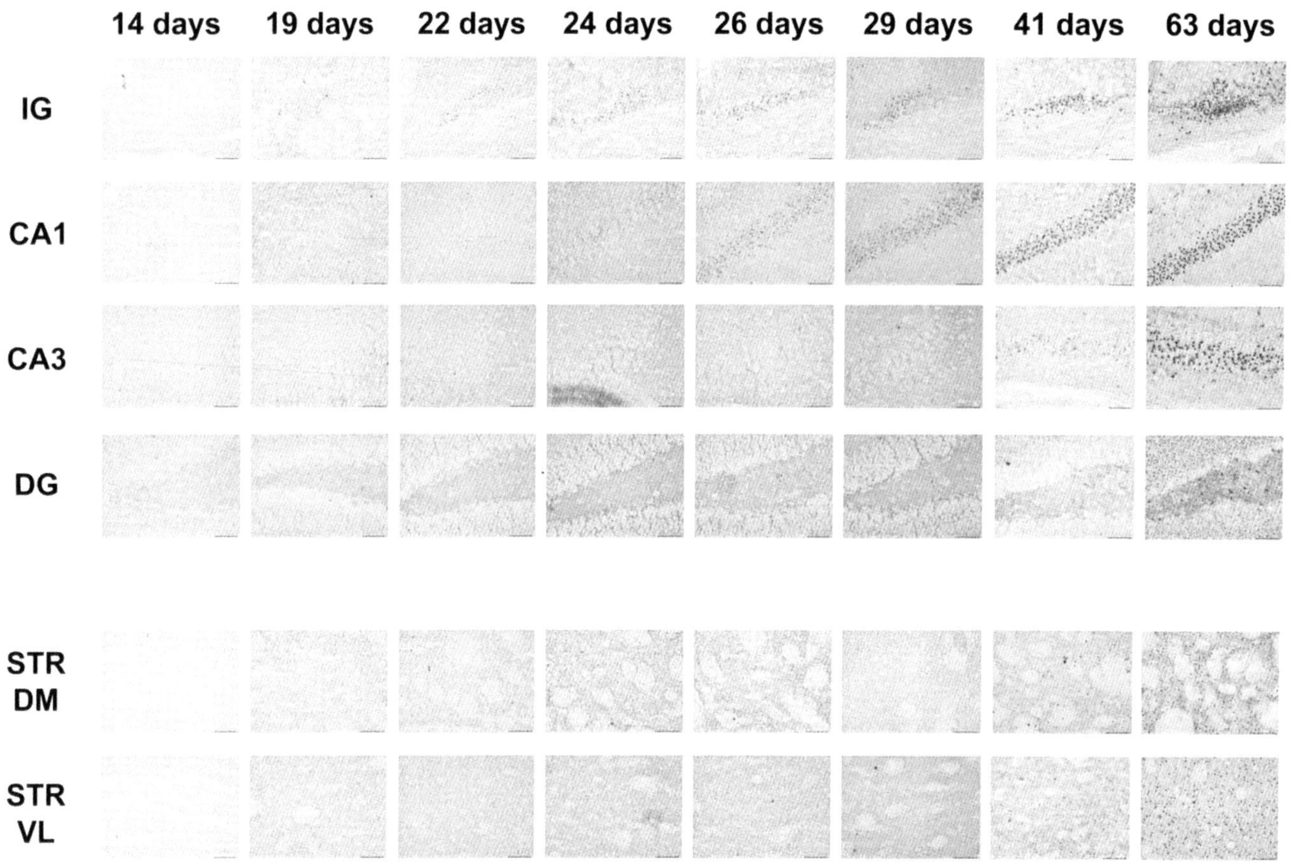

Figure 5. Inclusion appearance in different brain regions over time. Ubiquitinated Htt aggregates visualised by staining with the ubiquitin antibody (shown here at 14, 19, 22, 24, 26, 29, 41 and 63 days) in IG, CA1, CA3, DG and STR of R6/2 brains. A few inclusions are visible in the IG at 19 days of age. In the hippocampus, aggregates were present at 24 days in CA1, whereas in the CA3 a few aggregates were visible at 41 days of age. In the DG, a few ubiquitin-positive inclusions were present at 41 days. In the striatum, inclusions could be setected at 41 days of age in STR DM and STR VL. The number of aggregates in all the regions increased with time from the day of appearance. Scale bar = 50 μm.

studied in Figure 4, we used high magnification microscopy analysis. The initial morphology of MW8-positive aggregates were different from ubiquitin-positive inclusions, in that only nucleation centres of Htt aggregates were ubiquitinated (Fig. 7). Interestingly, MW8-immunolabelled Htt protein associated with the aggregate but not localised to the nucleation centre was not ubiquitinated (Fig. 7). It is possible that antigen sites on protein in parts of the aggregates may be masked by other proteins, but this seems unlikely, since the dense aggregate cores/nucleation centres were immunolabelled. It seems more likely that the MW8 antibody was labelling both aggregated and aggregating Htt, whereas ubiquitin labelled only Htt that was already aggregated. It is also notable that we could observe MW8-labelled cells before any aggregates were visible supporting the idea that there is an oligomerisation of Htt before visible aggregates form [43,44,45]. Again, this was not seen with ubiquitin staining, supporting our suggestion that the protein was not ubiquitinated before it aggregated.

By 41 days, neurons reach their developmental end-stage, there was complete overlap between MW8 and ubiquitin immonolabelling (Fig. 7), with ubiquitinated inclusion very similar to that of MW8-positive aggregates in all regions apart from CA3 neurons. Note, the precise timing of ubiquitination was not determined in the case of inclusions in CA3 neurons, because the aggregates in these cells develop later than in other regions. Htt aggregates are present in CA3 by 29 days of age, but the MW8 staining pattern in CA3 neurons was indistinguishable from the ubiquitin pattern, with regard to size and morphology, only by 63 days (Fig. 7).

The only region in which the staining pattern was different from that of Hf and CTX was the STR. In the STR, aggregates with clear nucleation centres appeared at around 25 days (Fig. 7). However, there was no lag in the appearance of ubiquitin-labelled inclusions, which were present in STR neurones at the same time (Fig. 7) and not at around 41 days (Fig. 5, 6). In contrast to what was seen in other regions, the ubiquitinated inclusions in the STR appeared to be much larger than the MW8-positive aggregates. We suggest that these aggregates formed a core or nucleation centre of Htt surrounded by ubiquitinated proteins that were not MW8-positive. While the size of the Htt-positive aggregates in the STR grew with time, the ubiquitinated inclusions did not appear to change much in size (Fig. 7), and the ubiquitinated inclusions remained larger than the Htt nucleation centres for several weeks. MW8-positive aggregate growth continued in the STR until 63 days, by which time STR inclusions appeared to have reached a stable state, and there was no longer an obvious morphological difference between the MW8-immunolabelled aggregates and the ubiquitin-labelled inclusions (Fig. 7).

Discussion

Htt aggregates have not been reported in R6/2 brains before 3 weeks of age. Here, we have been able to capture an earlier time

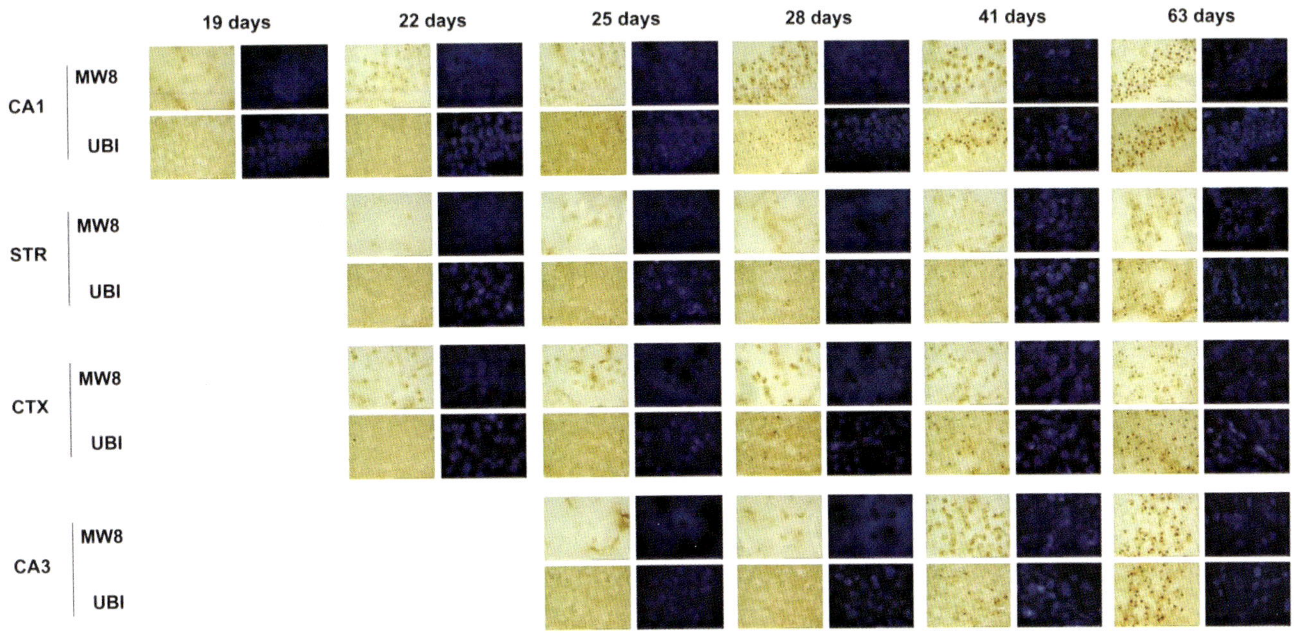

Figure 6. The timing of ubiquitination is dependent of cell soma size in R6/2 neurons. Regardless of whether or not huntingtin aggregates (visualized by staining with MW8 and ubiquitin antibodies) formed early or late, aggregates that formed in cells with small (DG neurons) and medium-sized (CA1 and STR) soma were found ubiquitinated within 2 to 3 days of initial aggregation. By contrast, there was typically a more than 3 days lag between initial aggregate formation and inclusion ubiquitination in cells with large soma (CA3). Scale bar = 50 μm.

course of aggregate formation earlier than has been shown previously. We find that aggregates are already present in R6/2 brain by 2 weeks of age. Thus, visible mutant Htt aggregation in immature R6/2 brain appears at a time much earlier than previously thought. Even though it is only a week earlier than previously reported, this is likely to be important as the first 2–3 weeks of life in a mouse is the critical time for brain and synaptic development, and cells are particularly vulnerable to excitotoxic insults in the immediate postnatal period [46]. Furthermore, and in contrast to other studies where ubiquitinated inclusions are considered to be indistinguishable from Htt-positive inclusions, we show a dissociation in the pattern of aggregate formation as shown by MW8- or ubiquitin staining. From our data we conclude that the pattern of aggregation of mutant Htt is not first recognised as foreign/abnormal, ubiquitinated, and then targeted to the proteasome where aggregation occurs, but rather that the proteins aggregate and then ubiquitination occurs (or ubiquitinated protein is recruited to the aggregates).

We showed previously that inclusions form in juvenile R6/2 brain in distinct phases that consist of (i) precipitation of aggregation centres, (ii) growth of inclusions and (iii) formation of extranuclear neuronal inclusions (ENNIs) [25]. Our previous investigations focused solely on ubiquitinated inclusions, which appear precipitously at around 3 weeks. A more recent immunostaining study of inclusion formation in R6/2 brains showed similar results, with identical overlapping patterns of inclusion labelling using EM48 and ubiquitin antibodies [42]. Our results generally agree with these of Meade *et al.*, [42] and support the present model of aggregate formation in which nucleation centres seed further aggregation of mutant proteins [41]. However, the EM48 staining done by Meade *et al.* failed to label any aggregates that were not ubiquitinated at any point in the time-course, and they describe the two immunostaining patterns as identical [42]. This discrepancy might be due to the fact that although both MW8 and EM48 bind to epitopes of the C-ter region, MW8 selectively binds aggregated Htt and is therefore more selective to the mutant form of the protein [38,47].

Aggregate Formation is a Very Rapid Event that is Differentially Timed According to Brain Region

Most prior studies, including our own, have never observed the rapidity with which the early events occur. This is because in most studies tissue is collected at weekly or even monthly intervals. Our tissue collection protocol allowed us to see changes that happened within 24 hours. We found that *in vivo*, visible aggregate formation is rapid, occurring within 24 hours. Interestingly, this parallels the situation we observed earlier with aggregation in tissue culture, where inclusions typically take 15–30 hours to form [22]. Protein aggregation has been described as a nucleation-dependent process [48]. Nucleated growth polymerization starts with the energetically unfavourable formation of a nucleus (i.e., nucleation), followed by efficient elongation of the nucleus via sequential additions of monomers [49,50]. In spite of the fact that nucleation is considered to be a slow process, and has been shown to be roughly 1,000 times slower in the cell than *in vitro* [51]. However, we show here that in most of the cells, Htt aggregates (visualised with MW8) appeared almost overnight.

Aggregates Develop Late in the Striatum

In addition to being precisely timed, aggregate formation was found to be brain region-dependent. Aggregates formed first in the IG, then in the CA1, subsequently in the CTX, followed by STR and finally in the DG and CA3. It is not clear what determines the pattern of aggregate formation, but it is unlikely to be correlated with neuronal vulnerability [52]. Nor does it relate to the putative vulnerability of neurons, since compared to the cortex and hippocampus, the appearance of aggregate formation in the STR, the region most affected by neurodegeneration in HD [52,53], lagged behind that in other regions. There are of course a number

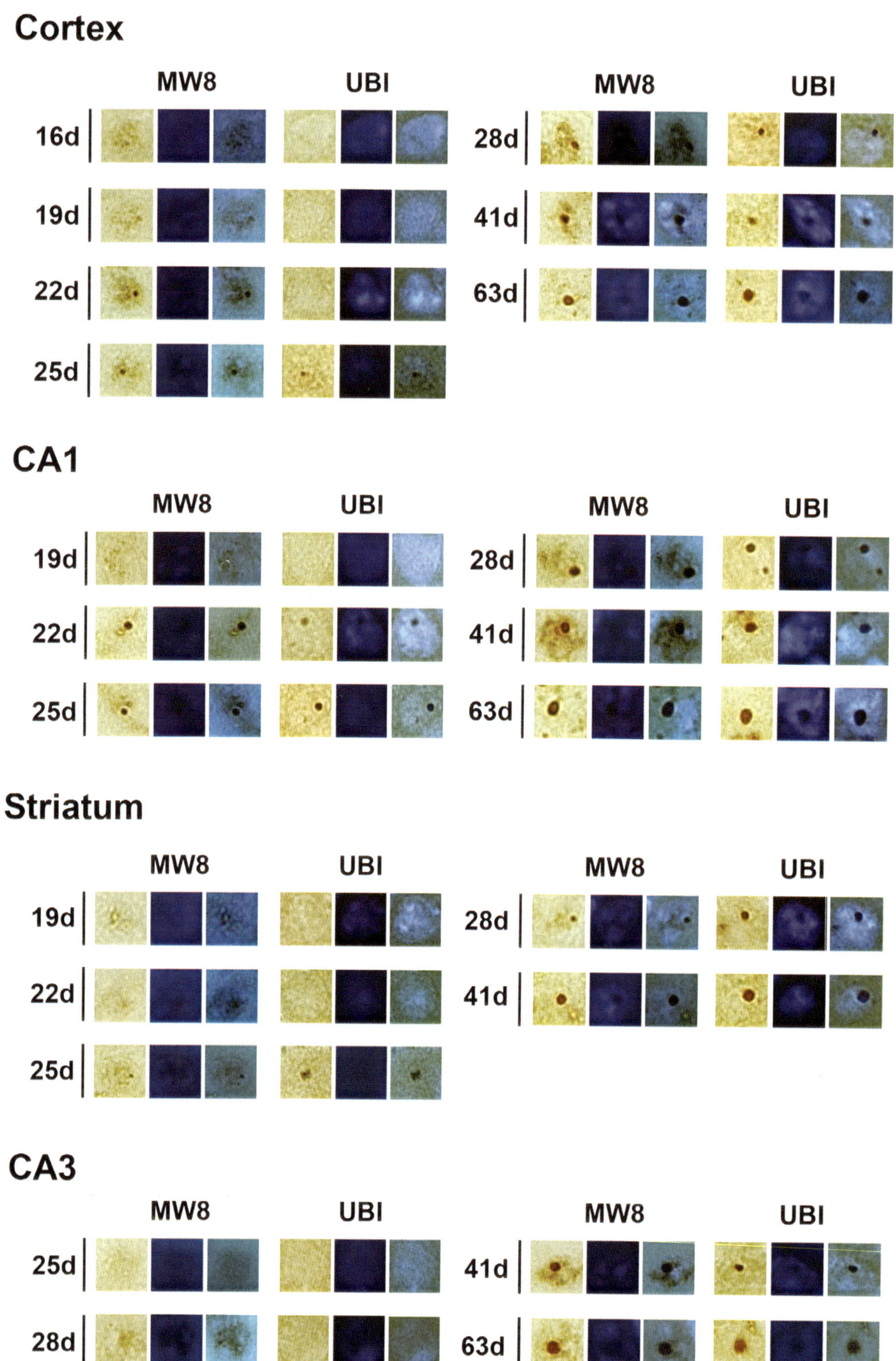
Cortex
MW8
UBI
MW8
UBI
16d
19d
22d
25d
28d
41d
63d
CA1
MW8
UBI
MW8
UBI
19d
22d
25d
28d
41d
63d
Striatum
MW8
UBI
MW8
UBI
19d
22d
25d
28d
41d
CA3
MW8
UBI
MW8
UBI
25d
28d
41d
63d

Figure 7. Comparison of MW8 and ubiquitin staining patterns. Higher magnification microscopy analysis was used in order to compare MW8 and ubiquitin staining patterns in single R6/2 neurons. In CA1, CA3 and cortex, MW8 labelling could be observed in cells before any aggregates were visible, a phenomenon that was not apparent with ubiquitin staining. The initial morphologies of MW8-positive aggregates were different from ubiquitin-positive inclusions, in that only nucleation centres of the aggregates were ubiquitinated and the MW8-immunolabelled Htt protein that was not localised to the nucleation centre did not appear to be ubiquitinated. In contrast, aggregates with clear nucleation centres were visible by 25 days in the striatum. And at the same time, larger punctate ubiquitin-labelled inclusions were already visible in STR neurones. Ubiquitinated inclusions were much bigger than MW8-positive aggregates and did not change much in size, even though Htt aggregates got bigger with time.

of different consequences of late development of aggregates in the striatum. If the aggregates are toxic, the early aggregate formation in cortical neurons could result in abnormal synaptic input to the striatum. There is ample and elegant evidence for early corticostriatal dysfunction in R6/2 mice [54,55,56,57]. On the other hand, if the aggregates are protective, the fact that aggregation of Htt in the striatal cells is delayed may make them more vulnerable to the toxicity of non-aggregated Htt [17]. Why there is such a big difference in the time-course of aggregation in the striatum compared the rest of the brain is also of particular interest, given that the striatum is most vulnerable to neurodegeneration. It is not possible to determine neuronal function or dysfunction from histopathological observations. In our opinion, it is likely that aggregate formation has complex downstream consequences that may be both beneficial and deleterious depending on the time and age of the animals [22,25].

It is important to stress that all transgenic mouse models of HD develop neuronal inclusions. In R6/2 mice NIIs develop prior to the onset of neurological symptoms [2,7]. By contrast, in N171-82Q and in YAC128 mice NIIs appear after the symptoms [58,59]. Finally in BACHHD mice inclusions are mainly (>90%) extranuclear [60]. Interestingly, the presence of aggregates is not more prevalent in neuronal subpopulations known to die earliest in HD, nor does it seem to correlate to neuronal death [16,17,59,60]. Therefore, despite studies suggesting a causal relationship, it is still not clear if aggregates play an active role in HD pathogenesis, or if they are simply markers of pathology. More studies about aggregate formation are needed.

Ubiquitination Occurs after Aggregate Formation

Our results agree with those of Meade *et al.*, where no ubiquitinated inclusions were found at all in CTX at 2 weeks (but were present in all layers by 3.5 weeks). We found that the time that elapsed between Htt aggregation and inclusion ubiquitination was dependent of the soma size, with a longer lag between initial aggregate formation and ubiquitination for large cells.

Our results support previous observations that ubiquitin associates at a relatively late stage in the maturation of aggregates into inclusions [62,63]. Although we [30] and several other groups have reported occasional aggregates [2,16,61] and microaggregates [16,61] that were not ubiquitinated, none of these have examined this in detail, and none have used tissue taken from sort interval timecourses that would allow a detailed study of this observation. In our previous study [30] we used PC12 cells to track aggregate morphology using time-lapse microscopy. We found clear evidence for aggregates that were not ubiquitinated at early stages of formation. Nevertheless, it was not clear if this phenomenon would be observed in brain tissue as well as immortalized cell lines. We have now shown that this appears to be present in the brain of R6/2 mice.

Given the early timing of the events we have reported (when aggregates are just beginning to appear), and the fact that we did not see aggregates that were partially ubiquitinated, we have interpreted our data as being due to the fact that ubiquitination of the protein in the aggregates has not yet occurred, or if it has, it is not enough to be visualised. It should be noted however that the presence of non-ubiquitinated aggregates could be due to de-ubiquitination of mutant htt. This is an interesting possibility, although testing it is beyond the scope of the current study, since the dynamics of ubiquitination/de-ubuqitination cannot be measured in post mortem tissue. Since there was little to no increase in background ubiquitin staining with the appearance of inclusions, in contrast to the increase in background expression of MW8-positive staining (data not shown), the most parsimonious explanation for our data is that monomeric mutant Htt is not recognised as 'toxic' until aggregation has started. We cannot rule out the possibility that soluble Htt might be ubiquitinated. However, in the R6/2 mice there is only normal full length Htt, so it seems unlikely that it will contribute to the pathological process at the earliest stages of aggregate formation.

We do not know the reason for the ubiquitination. It is possible that it is only after Htt has started to aggregate that it is recognised as foreign and ubiquitinated. However, importantly, to our knowledge, it has never been shown directly that mutant Htt is ubiquitinated. It has been assumed that mutant huntingtin is ubiquitinated and targeted for degradation by the ubiquitin-proteasome system pathway, because mutant huntingtin is an abnormal moiety found in neuronal intranuclear inclusions, neuronal nuclear inclusions are ubiquitinated and proteasome fragments are associated with NIIs. The possibility that mutant Htt is not recognised as foreign is consistent with the late onset of the disease in humans, where there is very little pathology for 30–40 years in the case of most adults, despite expression from both alleles [64,65,66,67,68,69]. Another possible explanation for our finding is that ubiquitin does not label mutant Htt but labels other proteins whose recruitment and inactivation trigger detrimental effects. Mutant Htt is known to recruit WT Htt via its polyglutamine tract, and normal Htt has been found to associate with an ubiquitin-conjugating enzyme (hE2-25K) in a manner that is not modulated by the length of the polyglutamine stretch [70]. Since normal Htt is larger and has more ubiquitination sites than the mutant fragments expressed in R6/2 brain [71]. It is possible that the normal Htt, rather than mutant Htt, may be the target of ubiquitination in R6/2 brain. It is also possible that proteins other than Htt containing a poly(Gln) sequence are ubiquitinated and recruited during aggregate formation [72,73,74,75,76].

Conclusion

Our results show for the first time that Htt aggregation in mouse brain is not only an early event, but that it occurs rapidly. Furthermore, ubiquitination is temporally dissociated from Htt aggregation. Both the timing of inclusion formation and the cellular recognition of the mutant protein as toxic are likely to be important events in HD pathology. The aggregation events we describe appear very early in R6/2 brain, well before any obvious detectable neurological phenotype. The onset of symptoms may signal a change in the role of aggregates from cytoprotective, to neurotoxic.

There are many controversial theories about pathological mechanisms in HD and their link with inclusion formation. However, Htt aggregation precedes symptoms in patients and mouse models. Therefore, characterizing the early stages of aggregate formation in mouse models are important steps that may help us understand the relationship between inclusion formation and mechanisms underlying cell death in HD.

Acknowledgments

We would like to thank Mrs Wendy Leavens for excellent technical assistance, and Dr. Paul Patterson and Jan Ko from the California Institute of Technology, Palo Alto, CA, USA for the kind gift of the MW8 monoclonal antibody.

Author Contributions

Conceived and designed the experiments: AJM BG. Performed the experiments: BG. Analyzed the data: BG CK AJM. Contributed reagents/materials/analysis tools: AJM. Wrote the paper: BG CK AJM. Re-designed and re-did the figures for the manuscript: CK.

References

1. The Huntington's Disease Collaborative Research Group (1993) A novel gene containing a trinucleotide repeat that is expanded and unstable on Huntington's disease chromosomes. Cell 72: 971–983.
2. Davies SW, Turmaine M, Cozens BA, DiFiglia M, Sharp AH, et al. (1997) Formation of neuronal intranuclear inclusions underlies the neurological dysfunction in mice transgenic for the HD mutation. Cell 90: 537–548.
3. Roizin L, Stellar S, Liu JC (1979) Neuronal nuclear-cytoplasmic changes in Huntington's chorea: electron microscope investigations. In Chase TN, Wexler NS and Barbeau A, eds. *Advances in Neurology, Huntington's Disease.* New York, NY: Raven Press 95–122.
4. DiFiglia M, Sapp E, Chase KO, Davies SW, Bates GP, et al. (1997) Aggregation of huntingtin in neuronal intranuclear inclusions and dystrophic neurites in brain. Science 277: 1990–1993.
5. Yamada M, Sato T, Tsuji S, Takahashi H (2008) CAG repeat disorder models and human neuropathology: similarities and differences. Acta Neuropathol 115: 71–86.
6. Gil JM, Rego AC (2009) The R6 lines of transgenic mice: a model for screening new therapies for Huntington's disease. Brain Res Rev 59: 410–431.
7. Ordway JM, Tallaksen-Greene S, Gutekunst CA, Bernstein EM, Cearley JA, et al. (1997) Ectopically expressed CAG repeats cause intranuclear inclusions and a progressive late onset neurological phenotype in the mouse. Cell 91: 753–763.
8. Cooper JK, Schilling G, Peters MF, Herring WJ, Sharp AH, et al. (1998) Truncated N-terminal fragments of huntingtin with expanded glutamine repeats form nuclear and cytoplasmic aggregates in cell culture. Hum Mol Genet 7: 783–790.
9. Rubinsztein DC, Wyttenbach A, Rankin J (1999) Intracellular inclusions, pathological markers in diseases caused by expanded polyglutamine tracts? J Med Genet 36: 265–270.
10. Rankin J, Wyttenbach A, Rubinsztein DC (2003) Intracellular green fluorescent protein-polyalanine aggregates are associated with cell death. Biochem J 15: 15–19.
11. Sánchez I, Mahlke C, Yuan J (2003) Pivotal role of oligomerization in expanded polyglutamine neurodegenerative disorders. Nature 421: 373–379.
12. Tanaka M, Machida Y, Niu S, Ikeda T, Jana NR, et al. (2004) Trehalose alleviates polyglutamine-mediated pathology in a mouse model of Huntington disease. Nat Med 10: 148–154.
13. Chopra V, Fox JH, Lieberman G, Dorsey K, Matson W, et al. ()2007 A small-molecule therapeutic lead for Huntington's disease: preclinical pharmacology and efficacy of C2–8 in the R6/2 transgenic mouse. Proc Natl Acad Sci USA 104: 16685–16689.
14. Masuda N, Peng Q, Li Q, Jiang M, Liang Y, et al. (2008) Tiagabine is neuroprotective in the N171–82Q and R6/2 mouse models of Huntington's disease. Neurobiol Dis 30: 293–302.
15. Saudou F, Finkbeiner S, Devys D, Greenberg ME (1998) Huntingtin acts in the nucleus to induce apoptosis but death does not correlate with the formation of intranuclear inclusions. Cell 95: 55–66.
16. Gutekunst CA, Li SH, Yi H, Mulroy JS, Kuemmerle S, et al. (1999) Nuclear and neuropil aggregates in Huntington's disease: relationship to neuropathology. J Neurosci 19: 2522–2534.
17. Kuemmerle S, Gutekunst CA, Klein AM, Li XJ, Li SH, et al. (1999) Huntington aggregates may not predict neuronal death in Huntington's disease. Ann Neurol 46: 842–849.
18. Hansson O, Guatteo E, Mercuri NB, Bernardi G, Li XJ, et al. (2001) Resistance to NMDA toxicity correlates with appearance of nuclear inclusions, behavioural deficits and changes in calcium homeostasis in mice transgenic for exon 1 of the huntington gene. Eur J Neurosci 14: 1492–1504.
19. Arrasate M, Mitra S, Schweitzer ES, Segal MR, Finkbeiner S (2004) Inclusion body formation reduces levels of mutant huntingtin and the risk of neuronal death. Nature 431: 805–810.
20. Slow EJ, Graham RK, Osmand AP, Devon RS, Lu G, et al. (2005) Absence of behavioral abnormalities and neurodegeneration in vivo despite widespread neuronal huntingtin inclusions. Proc Natl Acad Sci USA 102: 11402–1407.
21. Bodner RA, Outeiro TF, Altmann S, Maxwell MM, Cho SH, et al. (2006) Pharmacological promotion of inclusion formation: a therapeutic approach for Huntington's and Parkinson's diseases. Proc Natl Acad Sci USA 103: 4246–4251.
22. Gong B, Lim MC, Wanderer J, Wyttenbach A, Morton AJ (2008) Time-lapse analysis of aggregate formation in an inducible PC12 cell model of Huntington's disease reveals time-dependent aggregate formation that transiently delays cell death. Brain Res Bull 75: 146–157.
23. Zuchner T, Brundin P (2008) Mutant huntingtin can paradoxically protect neurons from death. Cell Death Differ 15: 435–442.
24. Morton AJ, Glynn D, Leavens W, Zheng Z, Faull RL, et al. (2009) Paradoxical delay in the onset of disease caused by super-long CAG repeat expansions in R6/2 mice. Neurobiol Dis 33: 331–341.
25. Morton AJ, Lagan MA, Skepper JN, Dunnett SB (2000) Progressive formation of inclusions in the striatum and hippocampus of mice transgenic for the human Huntington's disease mutation. J Neurocytol 29: 679–702.
26. Maat-Schieman M, Roos R, Losekoot M, Dorsman J, Welling-Graafland C, et al. (2007) Neuronal intranuclear and neuropil inclusions for pathological assessment of Huntington's disease. Brain Pathol 17: 31–37.
27. Martindale D, Hackam A, Wieczorek A, Ellerby L, Wellington C, et al. (1998) Length of huntingtin and its polyglutamine tract influences localization and frequency of intracellular aggregates. Nat Genet 18: 150–154.
28. Herndon ES, Hladik CL, Shang P, Burns DK, Raisanen J, et al. (2009) Neuroanatomic profile of polyglutamine immunoreactivity in Huntington disease brains. J Neuropathol Exp Neurol 68: 250–261.
29. de Pril R, Fischer DF, Maat-Schieman ML, Hobo B, de Vos RA, et al. (2004) Accumulation of aberrant ubiquitin induces aggregate formation and cell death in polyglutamine diseases. Hum Mol Genet 13: 1803–1813.
30. Wanderer J, Morton AJ (2007) Differential morphology and composition of inclusions in the R6/2 mouse and PC12 cell models of Huntington's disease. Histochem Cell Biol 127: 473–484.
31. Schwab C, Arai T, Hasegawa M, Yu S, McGeer PL (2008) Colocalization of transactivation-responsive DNA-binding protein 43 and huntingtin in inclusions of Huntington disease. J Neuropathol Exp Neurol 67: 1159–1165.
32. Mangiarini L, Sathasivam K, Seller M, Cozens B, Harper A, et al. (1996) Exon 1 of the HD gene with an expanded CAG repeat is sufficient to cause a progressive neurological phenotype in transgenic mice. Cell 87: 493–506.
33. Carter RJ, Lione LA, Humby T, Mangiarini L, Mahal A, et al. (1999) Characterization of progressive motor deficits in mice transgenic for the human Huntington's disease mutation. J Neurosci 19: 3248–3257.
34. Lione LA, Carter RJ, Hunt MJ, Bates GP, Morton AJ, et al. (1999) discrimination learning impairments in mice expressing the human Huntington's disease mutation. J Neurosci 19: 10428–10437.
35. Murphy KP, Carter RJ, Lione LA, Mangiarini L, Mahal A, et al. (2000) Abnormal synaptic plasticity and impaired spatial cognition in mice transgenic for exon 1 of the human Huntington's disease mutation. J Neurosci 20: 5115–5123.
36. Gibson HE, Reim K, Brose N, Morton AJ, Jones S (2005) A similar impairment in CA3 mossy fibre LTP in the R6/2 mouse model of Huntington's disease and in the complexin II knockout mouse. Eur J Neurosci 22: 1701–1712.
37. Bibb JA, Yan Z, Svenningsson P, Snyder GL, Pieribone VA, et al. (2000) Severe deficiencies in dopamine signaling in presymptomatic Huntington's disease mice. Proc Natl Acad Sci USA 97: 6809–6814.
38. Ko J, Ou S, Patterson PH (2001) New anti-huntingtin monoclonal antibodies: implications for huntingtin conformation and its binding proteins. Brain Res Bull 56: 319–329.
39. Landles C, Sathasivam K, Weiss A, Woodman B, Moffitt H, et al. (2010) Proteolysis of mutant huntingtin produces an exon 1 fragment that accumulates as an aggregated protein in neuronal nuclei in Huntington disease. J Biol Chem 285: 8808–8823.
40. Miller J, Arrasate M, Shaby BA, Mitra S, Masliah E, et al. (2010) Quantitative relationships between huntingtin levels, polyglutamine length, inclusion body formation, and neuronal death provide novel insight into huntington's disease molecular pathogenesis. J Neurosci 30: 10541–10550.
41. Chen S, Berthelier V, Yang W, Wetzel R (2001) Polyglutamine aggregation behavior in vitro supports a recruitment mechanism of cytotoxicity. J Mol Biol 311: 173–182.

42. Meade CA, Deng YP, Fusco FR, Del Mar N, Hersch S, et al. (2002) Cellular localization and development of neuronal intranuclear inclusions in striatal and cortical neurons in R6/2 transgenic mice. J Comp Neurol 449: 241–269.
43. Cajavec B, Bernard S, Herzel H (2005) Aggregation in Huntington's disease: insights through modelling. Genome Inform 16: 262–271.
44. Poirier MA, Jiang H, Ross CA (2005) A structure-based analysis of huntingtin mutant polyglutamine aggregation and toxicity: evidence for a compact beta-sheet structure. Hum Mol Genet 14: 765–774.
45. Zhang QC, Yeh TL, Leyva A, Frank LG, Miller J, et al. (2011) A compact beta model of huntingtin toxicity. J Biol Chem 286: 8188–8196.
46. Bhide PG, Day M, Sapp E, Schwarz C, Sheth A, et al. (1996) Expression of normal and mutant huntingtin in the developing brain. J Neurosci 16: 5523–5535.
47. Southwell AL, Patterson PH (2010) Antibody therapy in neurodegenerative disease. Rev Neurosci 21: 273–287.
48. Koo EH, Lansbury PT, Kelly JW (1999) Amyloid diseases: Abnormal protein aggregation in neurodegeneration. Proc Natl Acad Sci USA 96: 9989–9990.
49. Ferrone F (1999) Analysis of protein aggregation kinetics. Methods Enzymol 309: 256–274.
50. Wetzel R (2006) Nucleation of huntingtin aggregation in cells. Nat Chem Biol 2: 297–298.
51. Colby DW, Cassady JP, Lin GC, Ingram VM, Wittrup KD (2006) Stochastic kinetics of intracellular huntingtin aggregate formation. Nat Chem Biol 2: 319–323.
52. Fusco FR, Chen Q, Lamoreaux WJ, Figueredo-Cardenas G, Jiao Y, et al. (1999) Cellular localization of huntingtin in striatal and cortical neurons in rats: lack of correlation with neuronal vulnerability in Huntington's disease. J Neurosci 19: 1189–1202.
53. Sharp AH, Loev SJ, Schilling G, Li SH, Li XJ, et al. (1995) Widespread expression of Huntington's disease gene (IT15) protein product. Neuron 14: 1065–1074.
54. Kung VW, Hassam R, Morton AJ, Jones S (2007) Dopamine dependent long term potentiation in the dorsal striatum is reduced in the R6/2 mouse model of Huntington's disease. Neuroscience 146: 1571–1580.
55. Cepeda C, Hurst RS, Calvert CR, Hernández-Echeagaray E, Nguyen OK, et al. (2003) Transient and progressive electrophysiological alterations in the corticostriatal pathway in a mouse model of Huntington's disease. J Neurosci 23: 961–969.
56. Cummings DM, André VM, Uzgil BO, Gee SM, Fisher YE, et al. (2009) Alterations in cortical excitation and inhibition in genetic mouse models of Huntington's disease. J Neurosci 29: 10371–10386.
57. André VM, Cepeda C, Fisher YE, Huynh M, Bardakjian N, et al. (2011) Differential electrophysiological changes in striatal output neurons in Huntington's disease. J Neurosci 31: 1170–1182.
58. Gardian G, Browne SE, Choi DK, Klivenyi P, Gregorio J, et al. (2005) Neuroprotective effects of phenylbutyrate in the N171-82Q transgenic mouse model of Huntington's disease. J Biol Chem 280: 556–563.
59. Slow EJ, van Raamsdonk J, Rogers D, Coleman SH, Graham RK, et al. (2003) Selective striatal neuronal loss in a YAC128 mouse model of Huntington disease. Hum Mol Genet 12: 1555–1567.
60. Gray M, Shirasaki DI, Cepeda C, André VM, Wilburn B, et al. (2008) Full-length human mutant huntingtin with a stable polyglutamine repeat can elicit progressive and selective neuropathogenesis in BACHD mice. J Neurosci. 28: 6182–6195.
61. Menalled LB, Sison JD, Wu Y, Olivieri M, Li XJ, et al. (2002) Early motor dysfunction and striosomal distribution of huntingtin microaggregates in Huntington's disease knock-in mice. J Neurosci 22: 8266–8276.
62. Senut MC, Suhr ST, Kaspar B, Gage FH (2000) Intraneuronal aggregate formation and cell death after viral expression of expanded polyglutamine tracts in the adult rat brain. J Neurosci 20: 219–229.
63. Wyttenbach A, Swartz J, Kita H, Thykjaer T, Carmichael J, et al. (2001) Polyglutamine expansions cause decreased CRE-mediated transcription and early gene expression changes prior to cell death in an inducible cell model of Huntington's disease. Hum Mol Genet 10: 1829–1845.
64. Wexler NS, Young AB, Tanzi RE, Travers H, Starosta-Rubinstein S, et al. (1987) Homozygotes for Huntington's disease. Nature 326: 194–197.
65. Myers RH, Leavitt J, Farrer LA, Jagadeesh J, McFarlane H, et al. (1989) Homozygote for Huntington disease. Am J Hum Genet 45: 615–618.
66. Kremer B, Goldberg P, Andrew SE, Theilmann J, Telenius H, et al. (1994) A worldwide study of the Huntington's disease mutation. N Engl J Med 330: 1401–1416.
67. Durr A, Hahn-Barma V, Brice A, Pêcheux C, Dodé C, et al. (1999) Homozygosity in Huntington's disease. J Med Genet 36: 172–173.
68. Laccone F, Engel U, Holinski-Feder E, Weigell-Weber M, Marczinek K, et al. (1999) DNA analysis of Huntington's disease. Five years of experience in Germany, Austria, and Switzerland. Neurology 53: 801–806.
69. Squitieri F, Gellera C, Cannella M, Mariotti C, Cislaghi G, et al. (2003) Homozygosity for CAG mutation in Huntington disease is associated with a more severe clinical course. Brain 126: 946–955.
70. Kalchman MA, Graham RK, Xia G, Koide HB, Hodgson JG, et al. (1996) Huntingtin is ubiquitinated and interacts with a specific ubiquitin-conjugating enzyme. J Biol Chem 271: 19385–19394.
71. Bennett EJ, Shaler TA, Woodman B, Ryu KY, Zaitseva TS, et al. (2007) Global changes to the ubiquitin system in Huntington's disease. Nature 448: 704–708.
72. Huang CC, Faber PW, Persichetti F, Mittal V, Vonsattel JP, et al. (1998) Amyloid formation by mutant huntingtin: threshold, progressivity and recruitment of normal polyglutamine proteins. Somat Cell Mol Genet 24: 217–233.
73. Kazantsev A, Preisinger E, Dranovsky A, Goldgaber D, Housman D (1999) Insoluble detergent-resistant aggregates form between pathological and nonpathological lengths of polyglutamine in mammalian cells. Proc Natl Acad Sci USA 96: 11404–11409.
74. Steffan JS, Bodai L, Pallos J, Poelman M, McCampbell A, et al. (2001) Histone deacetylase inhibitors arrest polyglutamine-dependent neurodegeneration in Drosophila. Nature 413: 739–743.
75. McCampbell A, Taylor JP, Taye AA, Robitschek J, Li M, et al. (2000) CREB-binding protein sequestration by expanded polyglutamine. Hum Mol Genet 9: 2197–2202.
76. Nucifora FC Jr, Sasaki M, Peters MF, Huang H, Cooper JK, et al. (2001) Interference by huntingtin and atrophin-1 with cbp-mediated transcription leading to cellular toxicity. Science 291: 2423–2428.

9

Altered Hypothalamic Protein Expression in a Rat Model of Huntington's Disease

Wei-na Cong[1], Huan Cai[1], Rui Wang[1], Caitlin M. Daimon[1], Stuart Maudsley[2], Kerstin Raber[3], Fabio Canneva[3], Stephan von Hörsten[3], Bronwen Martin[1]*

1 Metabolism Unit, National Institute on Aging, National Institutes of Health, Baltimore, Maryland, United States of America, **2** Receptor Pharmacology Unit, National Institute on Aging, National Institutes of Health, Baltimore, Maryland, United States of America, **3** Department for Experimental Therapy, Friedrich-Alexander-Universität Erlangen-Nürnberg, Erlangen, Germany

Abstract

Huntington's disease (HD) is a neurodegenerative disorder, which is characterized by progressive motor impairment and cognitive alterations. Changes in energy metabolism, neuroendocrine function, body weight, euglycemia, appetite function, and circadian rhythm can also occur. It is likely that the locus of these alterations is the hypothalamus. We used the HD transgenic (tg) rat model bearing 51 CAG repeats, which exhibits similar HD symptomology as HD patients to investigate hypothalamic function. We conducted detailed hypothalamic proteome analyses and also measured circulating levels of various metabolic hormones and lipids in pre-symptomatic and symptomatic animals. Our results demonstrate that there are significant alterations in HD rat hypothalamic protein expression such as glial fibrillary acidic protein (GFAP), heat shock protein-70, the oxidative damage protein glutathione peroxidase (Gpx4), glycogen synthase1 (Gys1) and the lipid synthesis enzyme acylglycerol-3-phosphate O-acyltransferase 1 (Agpat1). In addition, there are significant alterations in various circulating metabolic hormones and lipids in pre-symptomatic animals including, insulin, leptin, triglycerides and HDL, before any motor or cognitive alterations are apparent. These early metabolic and lipid alterations are likely prodromal signs of hypothalamic dysfunction. Gaining a greater understanding of the hypothalamic and metabolic alterations that occur in HD, could lead to the development of novel therapeutics for early interventional treatment of HD.

Editor: Sergio T. Ferreira, Federal University of Rio de Janeiro, Brazil

Funding: The authors have no support or funding to report.

Competing Interests: The authors have declared that no competing interests exist.

* E-mail: martinbro@mail.nih.gov

Introduction

Huntington's disease (HD) has a prevalence of 5–10 cases per 100,000 worldwide, which makes it the most common monogenetically inherited neurodegenerative disorder [1,2]. HD is caused by expansion of a CAG repeat in the huntingtin (htt) gene [3]. The length of the CAG repeats correlates negatively with the age of onset and positively with severity of the disorder [4]. HD runs a debilitating and progressive course with an average survival of 10–25 years after disease onset [5]. Clinical presentations of HD typically include involuntary movements (especially chorea), progressive subcortical dementia [6,7] and psychiatric disturbances [8]. Although the neurological symptoms predominate, they are not the sole pathophysiological manifestation of HD. Continuous reports, even before the discovery of the HD gene, described pathological phenotypes in peripheral tissues of HD patients, including weight loss [9–11], appetite hormone changes [12] and altered glucose homeostasis [13–15]. A growing body of evidence has also demonstrated other non-motor symptoms of HD that include impaired energy balance [16] and a disrupted circadian rhythm [17]. A recent study by Hult *et al.* [18] even established a causal link between mutant huntingtin expression in the hypothalamus and metabolic dysfunctions, and suggested that metabolic parameters are powerful readouts for assessing HD therapies.

The neuropathology of HD is characterized by intranuclear and cytoplasmic inclusions of huntingtin aggregates, and cell death primarily in the striatum and cerebral cortex. Striatal atrophy [19] is well established in clinical diagnosis of HD and has been linked to chorea, whereas changes in the cerebral cortex have been correlated with cognitive decline [20–23]. In light of non-motor symptoms and signs of perturbed functionality of the hypothalamus in HD, it has been hypothesized that this region may also be affected in HD. Supporting this hypothesis, Soneson *et al.* found distinguishable changes in the hypothalamic region of HD gene carriers by MRI [24]. Consistently, hypothalamic atrophy was also observed in transgenic HD mice using voxel-based morphometry (VBM) of MRI images [25]. Changes in neuropeptide levels can also indicate hypothalamic dysfunctions. In cross-sectional cerebrospinal fluid (CSF) samples collected from HD patients, Bjorkqvist *et al.* reported significantly increased levels of Cocaine- and amphetamine-regulated transcript (CART) peptide. This neuropeptide has strong anorectic effects [26]. In line with this, Gabery *et al.* quantified the neuropeptide-expressing hypothalamic neurons known to regulate metabolism and confirmed the increase of CART-expressing neurons in HD patients [27]. Taken together, the evidence suggests that the delicate balance of the neuroendocrine system, which mainly depends on the hypothalamus, could be altered and likely contributes to the peripheral tissue abnormalities frequently observed in HD. However, the proteomic alterations underlying HD-related hypothalamic changes are still unclear.

With the discovery of the htt mutation in 1993, it became possible to create animal models with a similar genetic background to the disease phenotype seen in humans with HD. The R6/2 mouse is the most commonly used transgenic mouse model of HD. R6/2 mice develop symptoms as early as 4 weeks, although the average age at onset of symptoms is 9 to 11 weeks. The mean lifespan for this model is 10 to 13 weeks, and animals rarely survive past 14 weeks [28]. The N171-82Q transgenic mouse is another model for HD. Beginning at week 11, these mice show a progressive decline in performance on the rotarod test as well as the onset of clasping behavior [29]. The lifespan of N171-82Q mice is no more than 20 weeks. Early onset of symptoms and short lifespan of both these animal models restrain the depth of possible HD research. In order to overcome these problems, the only transgenic rat model currently in use for HD was created by von Hörsten and colleagues [30]. These rats express 51 human-derived CAG repeats inserted in a 1962 bp rat htt fragment of complementary DNA (cDNA). This relatively small number of CAG repeats results in an adult-onset progressive phenotype. In this transgenic rat model, motor symptoms appear at 10 to 15 months of age and the average lifespan can reach 24 months [31]. Due to the late onset of symptoms and extended lifespan compared to mouse models of HD, the tgHD rat model allows for more comprehensive evaluations such as those required to investigate metabolic and neuroendocrine function in a longitudinal manner.

As a "body-wide" disorder, symptomatic progression of HD is tightly linked with peripheral metabolic health [32]. In order to better understand the pathogenesis of hypothalamic dysfunctions in HD, we carried out a comprehensive longitudinal metabolic characterization of the tgHD rat model in the current study. Furthermore, we used the tgHD rat model to delineate alterations occurring in the hypothalamus at the proteomic level.

Results

Alterations in circulating euglycemic hormone levels in pre-symptomatic and symptomatic tgHD rats

We assessed longitudinal circulating levels of glucose, insulin, adiponectin, ghrelin (total), and leptin in rats aged 3-months (pre-symptomatic), 9-months (early-symptomatic) and 12 months (symptomatic). Longitudinal analysis demonstrated that tgHD rats possessed comparable levels of circulating glucose, compared to the WT rats across all three ages (Fig. 1A). However, significantly lower insulin levels were detected in both 3-month and 12-month tgHD rats, compared to the WT controls ($p = 0.013$, 3-month tgHD vs. 3-month WT; $p = 0.028$, 12-month tgHD vs. 12-month WT, Fig. 1B). Longitudinally, both tgHDs and WTs exhibited a progressive reduction in plasma insulin levels ($p = 0.0069$, 12-month tgHD vs. 3-month tgHD; $p = 0.009$, 9-month WT vs. 3-month WT; $p = 0.008$, 12-month WT vs. 3-month WT). There was no significant difference in plasma adiponectin levels between tgHDs and WTs across all three ages. When compared to 3-month tgHD animals, the 9-month tgHD rats displayed a significant decrease in adiponectin levels (Fig. 1C). In order to better understand peripheral metabolic alterations in tgHD rats, we further evaluated levels of leptin and ghrelin, two major appetite-modulating hormones. Compared to WT animals, the 3-month old tgHD rats demonstrated a significant decrease in plasma leptin levels ($p = 0.044$, Fig. 1D). There was also a trend towards reduction in the 12-month tgHD rats ($p = 0.067$), as well. Interestingly, compared to the 3-month tgHD animals, 9-month tgHD rats revealed a significant increase in leptin levels ($p = 0.0067$, Fig. 1D). Longitudinally, both tgHD rats and WT rats displayed a progressive elevation in plasma ghrelin levels ($p = 0.028$, 9-month tgHD vs. 3-month tgHD; $p = 0.043$, 12-month tgHD vs. 3month tgHD; $p = 0.002$, 12-month WT vs. 3-month WT) (Fig. 1E). The euglycemic hormone alterations demonstrated in the tgHD rats are similar to what has been shown previously in mouse models of HD (N171-82Q, [15]). Additionally, we also performed two-way ANOVA analysis. Two-way ANOVA analysis allows us to simultaneously consider the effects from two independent factors, *i.e.* genotype and age. With 2-way ANOVA analysis, as shown in Table S1, similar results were obtained: significantly lower insulin levels were detected in 3-month tgHD rats, compared with age-matched WTs. Compared to 12-month WT animals, the 12-month tgHD rats demonstrated a significant decrease in plasma leptin levels. Longitudinally, 9 month tgHD rats demonstrated significantly higher leptin levels compared to 3-month tgHD animals. A significant age-dependent increase in ghrelin was also found in both tgHD and WT rats.

Longitudinal alterations in metabolic hormones in the tgHD rat

We measured circulating levels of numerous metabolic hormones including amylin, gastric inhibitory polypeptide (GIP), pancreatic peptide (PP), and Peptide YY (PYY). We found that amylin (Fig. 2A) and PYY (Fig. 2D) levels were significantly decreased in 3-month tgHD rats compared to WT controls ($p = 0.0001$ for amylin; $p = 0.025$ for PYY). Compared to 12-month WT rats, we observed decreasing trends in both GIP ($p = 0.072$) (Fig. 2B) and PP ($p = 0.078$) (Fig. 2C) in 12-month tgHD rats. In addition, both tgHD and WT animals displayed significant age-dependent reductions in amylin levels ($p = 0.002$, 12-month tgHD vs. 3-month tgHD; $p < 0.001$, 9-month WT vs. 3-month WT; $p < 0.001$, 12-month WT vs. 3-month WT, Fig. 2A). Compared to 3-month tgHD rats, 12-month tgHD rats exhibited significantly decreased GIP levels (Fig. 2B), whereas 9-month tgHD rats demonstrated a significant increase in PP levels (Fig. 2C). WT rats also showed profound age-related elevations in their PP levels ($p = 0.02$, 9-month WT vs. 3-month WT; $p = 0.006$, 12-month WT vs. 3-month WT, Fig. 2C). In addition to evaluating metabolic hormone levels, we also evaluated levels of corticosterone, a stress-responsive hormone. We found that only 12-month tgHD rats demonstrated a trend of reduction in systemic corticosterone ($p = 0.068$, vs. 12-month WT) (Fig. 2E). Additionally, we also used 2-way ANOVA to assess potential changes in plasma amylin, GIP, PP, PYY and corticosterone levels. Consistently, we observed a significant decease in amylin and PYY levels in 3-month tgHD rats, compared to 3-month WT rats (Table S1).

Alterations in circulating lipid levels in the tgHD rat

We next analyzed plasma lipid levels including triglycerides, total cholesterol, high density lipoprotein (HDL), and low-density lipoprotein (LDL). The triglyceride levels of 3-month tgHD rats were significantly reduced compared to WT animals ($p = 0.0025$, vs. 3-month WT). However, this difference was abolished in both 9-month and 12-month tgHD rats. In addition, WT rats, but not tgHD rats, exhibited age-related significant decreases in plasma triglycerides ($p = 0.046$, 9-month WT vs. 3-month WT; $p = 0.008$, 12-month WT vs. 3month WT, Fig. 3A). The tgHD rats and WT rats shared similar total cholesterol levels, except for the 3-month tgHD rats, which showed a trend of reduction ($p = 0.056$, vs. 3-month WT). Longitudinally, compared to 3-month tgHD rats, both 9-month and 12-month tgHD rats possessed markedly

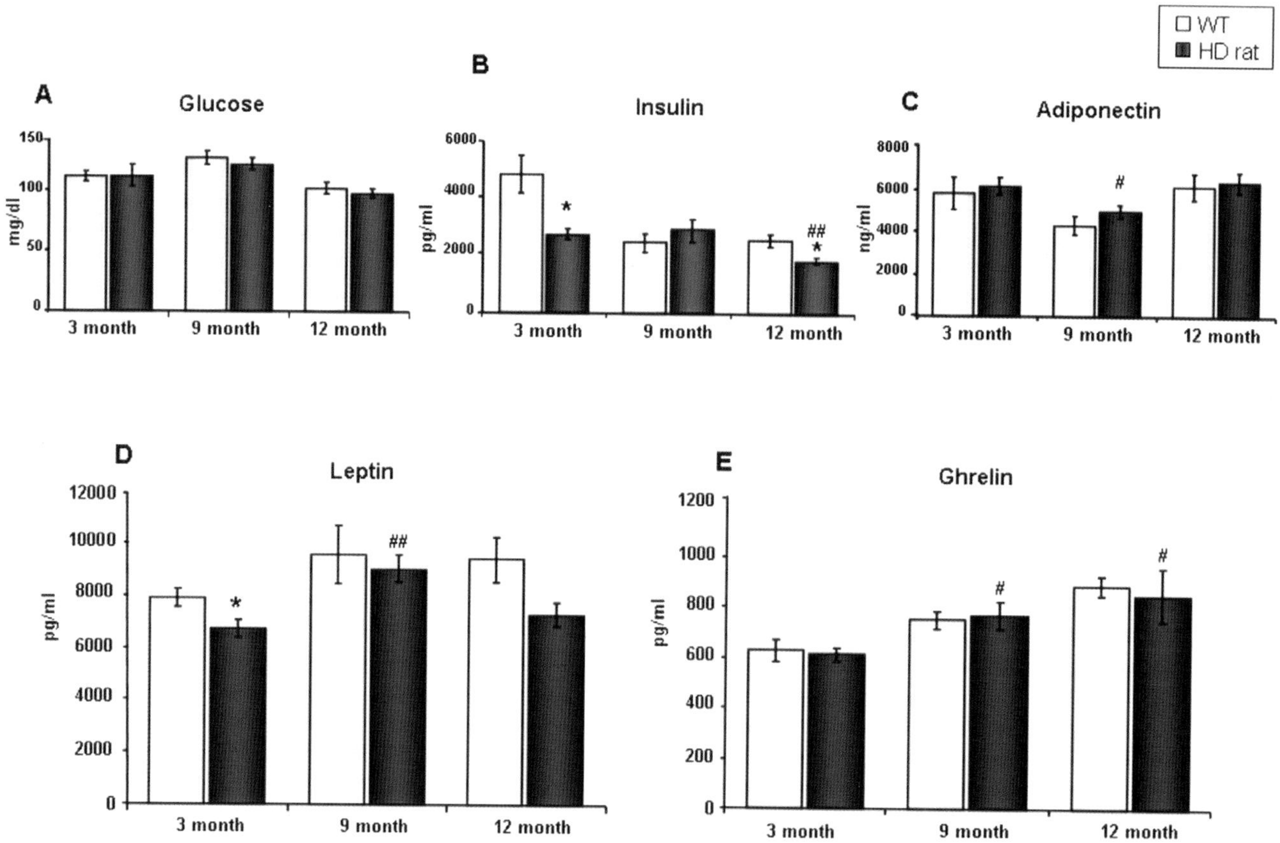

Figure 1. Altered plasma glycemic hormone and appetite hormone levels in tgHD rats. (A) Mean blood glucose concentrations for WT and tgHD rats across three ages. (B) Mean plasma insulin concentrations in WT and tgHD rats across three ages. (C) Mean plasma adiponectin concentrations in WT and tgHD rats across three ages. (D) Mean plasma leptin concentrations in WT and tgHD rats across three ages. (E) Mean plasma total ghrelin concentrations in WT and tgHD rats across three ages. Values are mean ± SEM, *: $p<0.05$; tgHD vs. WT, #: $p<0.05$; ##: $p<0.01$; 9-month or 12 month tgHD vs. 3-month tgHD, n = 5 per group.

increased levels of total cholesterol ($p = 0.0005$, 9-month tgHD vs. 3-month tgHD; $p = 0.0378$, 12-month tgHD vs. 3month tgHD, Fig. 3B). For plasma lipoproteins, a significant decrease was detected in HDL of 3-month tgHD rats compared to age-matched WTs ($p = 0.032$, Fig. 3C). No statistical difference between tgHD and WT animals was observed with respect to LDL levels (Fig. 3D). Similarly, there was no difference between tgHD and WT animals with respect to the ratio of HDL to LDL (Fig. 3E). Both 12-month tgHD and WT rats had lower HDL levels than their 3-month counterparts. Longitudinally, in terms of LDL and HDL/LDL, both tgHD rats and WT rats showed similar age-dependent changes (Fig. 3E). Using 2-way ANOVA analysis, again, we obtained similar plasma lipid results (Table S1). Triglyceride levels in 3-month old tgHD rats were significantly reduced compared to the age-matched WT animals. Longitudinally, compared to the 3-month old tgHD rats, both 9-month and 12-month tgHD rats possessed markedly increased levels of total cholesterol. Additionally, 3-month old tgHD rats also demonstrated markedly lower LDL levels, compared to 9-month or 12-month tgHD rats. In terms of the ratio of HDL/LDL, tgHD rats demonstrated an obvious age-dependent reduction.

Proteomic alterations in the hypothalamus of tgHD rats

iTRAQ mass tag ratios were calculated for proteins with reliable identifications (see Materials and Methods) based upon their collision-induced dissociation fragmentation patterns. Ratios of the tgHD mass tags (114, 115, 116) compared to the WT tags (117) that were greater than 1.2 or less than 0.8 were considered to be statistically different, *i.e.* altered expression level of the protein. Two representative iTRAQ mass spectrometry peptide identifications (glial fibrillary acidic protein (GFAP) and Lamin A) are demonstrated in Figs. 4 and 5. In total, we identified 395 significantly altered proteins in the hypothalamus of the tgHD rats (compared to the WT), which included 84 up-regulated proteins and 311 down-regulated proteins (Fig. 6, Table S2). To verify the expression changes of the identified proteins, western blots were performed by resolving tissue lysate samples onto PVDF membranes (Fig. 7). Seven proteins that were identified as significantly altered proteins by iTRAQ mass spectrometry were selected for western blot analysis. Among these proteins, G1 to S phase transition 2 (Gspt2), phosphatidylethanolamine binding protein 1 (Pebp1), muscle pyruvate kinase (Pkm2) and mTOR were up-regulated in the hypothalamus and GFAP, flotillin-2 (Flot2), and Lamin A were down-regulated in the hypothalamus of tgHD rats. Westen blotting of these proteins revealed differential protein expression, consistent with the iTRAQ results.

Phenotypic physiological signaling pathway analysis of protein alterations in tgHD rats

Both up- and down-regulated protein sets identified by iTRAQ were analyzed using the KEGG pathway algorithm. Use of the KEGG pathway algorithm allows for the potential physiological

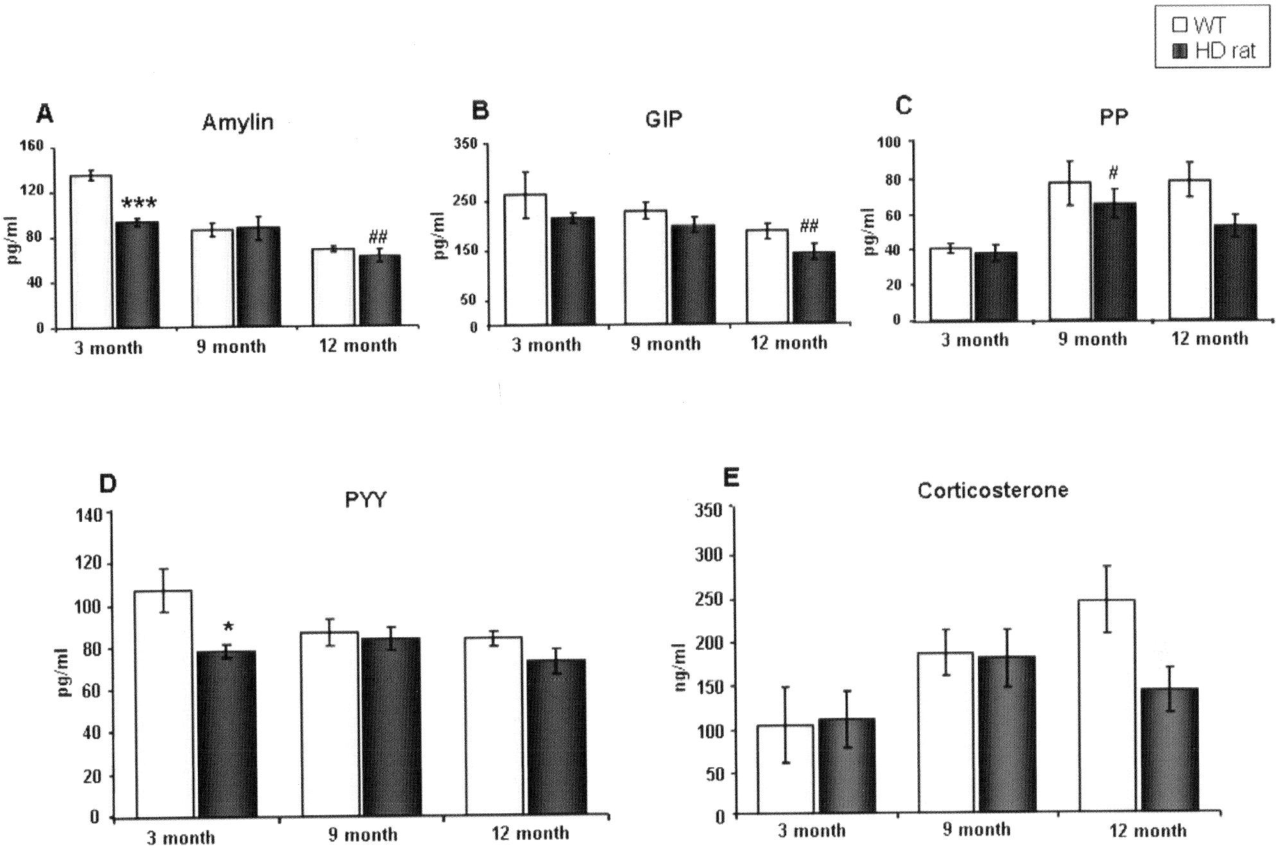

Figure 2. Alterations in metabolic hormones in tgHD rats. (A) Mean plasma amylin concentrations for WT and tgHD rats across three ages. (B) Mean plasma GIP concentrations in WT and tgHD rats across three ages. (C) Mean plasma PP concentrations in WT and tgHD rats across three ages. (D) Mean plasma PYY concentrations in WT and tgHD rats across three ages. (E) Mean plasma corticosterone concentrations in WT and tgHD rats across three ages. Values are mean ± SEM, *: $p<0.05$; ***: $p<0.001$; tgHD vs. WT, #: $p<0.05$; ##: $p<0.01$; 9-month or 12 month tgHD vs. 3-month tgHD, n = 5 per group.

role(s) of significantly altered proteins to be further delineated. We found that a major body of significantly altered proteins in tgHD rats was closely associated with energy metabolism. Calculation of subsequent hybrid scores further revealed that the significantly altered proteins were highly involved in *fatty acid metabolism*, *oxidative phosphorylation*, *glycolysis/gluconeogenesis*, *glycerolipid metabolism*, *PPAR signaling pathway* and the *insulin signaling pathway* (Fig. 8, Table 1). Other significantly altered proteins were strongly associated with cell communication (*Focal adhesion*, *Adherens junction*, *Gap junction*, *Tight junction*) and neuronal function (*Amytrophic Lateral Sclerosis*, *Long-term depression*, Fig. 8, Table 1). To further appreciate the potential hypothalamic pathophysiological ramifications of these protein alterations, we performed LSI analysis on the significantly altered proteins (Fig. 9). LSI analysis revealed that many proteins were significantly correlated to Huntingtin (arfaptin-2 (Arfip2), sacsin (Sacs), heat shock 70 kD protein 1B (Hspa1b), transglutaminase 2 (Tgm2)), chorea (Arfip2, Sacs, disco-interacting protein 2 homolog B (Dip2b)), diabetes (1-acylglycerol-3-phosphate O-acyltransferase 1 (Agpat), glycogen synthase 1 (Gys1), solute carrier family 2(Slc2a1)), and insulin (pyruvate dehydrogenase kinase isozyme 2 (Pdk2), pyruvate kinase 2 (Pkm2), branched chain aminotransferase 2 (Bcat2), carbonic anhydrase 3 (Car3)). In line with the results obtained from the KEGG analysis, upon application of LSI analysis we found that the strongest proteomic representation for tgHD rats was significantly correlated to the energy-related terms 'diabetes' and 'insulin'. A full list of LSI analysis results is provided in Table S3 (up-regulated) and Table S4 (down-regulated).

Discussion

Currently, as multiple lines of evidence have demonstrated widespread pathophysiologies in peripheral systems of both HD patients and model organisms [33], it is clear that HD is more than a purely neurological motor disorder [34]. In this study, we demonstrated significant proteomic alterations in the hypothalamus of tgHD rats, and this was accompanied by significant alterations in circulating levels of metabolic hormones and lipid factors. Unbiased bioinformatics analyses (KEGG and LSI), revealed that many pathways and proteins associated with diabetes and insulin signaling were significantly altered in the tgHD rats. Longitudinal assessments of glycemic hormones at 3-months, 9-months and 12-months of age demonstrated that even in pre-symptomatic animals (3 months) there were significant alterations in glycemic and metabolic hormones (Fig. 1, 2). In the pre-symptomatic stage, tgHD rats demonstrated significant decreases in levels of insulin, leptin, and two gut hormones (amylin and PYY). These findings are consistent with the fact that some non-motor symptoms of HD precede the onset of motor symptoms by several years in patients [35] as well as by several months in the rat model [31]. In our present study, we applied both Student's t-test analysis and 2-way ANOVA analysis for the statistical evaluation

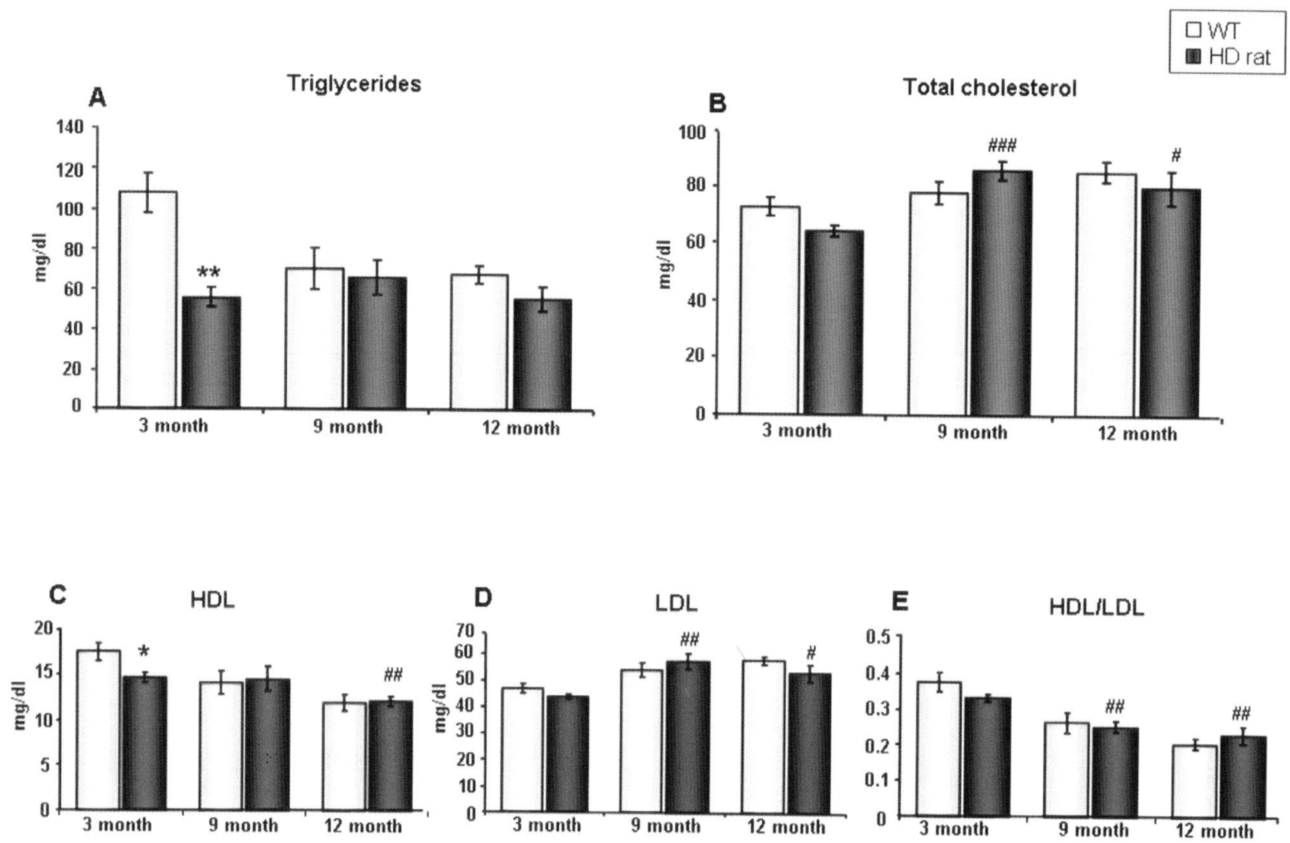

Figure 3. Changes in plasma lipid levels in tgHD rats. (A) Mean plasma triglyceride levels for WT and tgHD rats across three ages. (B) Mean plasma total cholesterol levels in WT and tgHD rats across three ages. (C) Mean plasma HDL levels in WT and tgHD rats across three ages. (D) Mean plasma LDL levels in WT and tgHD rats across three ages. (E) Mean ratio of HDL/LDL in WT and tgHD rats across three ages. Values are mean ± SEM, * : $p<0.05$; * * : $p<0.01$; tgHD vs. WT, #: $p<0.05$; ##: $p<0.01$; ###: $p<0.001$; 9-month or 12 month tgHD vs. 3-month tgHD, n = 5 per group.

of all plasma parameters. The Student's t-test allowed us to perform comparisons between tgHD rats and WT rats of each age. In the longitudinal analysis, the Student's t-test was used to compare 3-month animals with the other two ages within same genotype group. In addition to this, we also performed a 2-way ANOVA analysis which allowed us to compare two independent variables *i.e.* genotype and age at the same time.

In the clinical setting, HD patients typically develop diabetes mellitus approximately seven times more often than matched control participants [36]. Recent evidence has also demonstrated that abnormal glucose homeostasis in HD patients can be, in-part, attributed to impaired insulin secretion capacity [37]. In addition to the characteristic neurological symptoms, weight loss is also a prominent feature of HD, suggesting that considerable metabolic abnormalities are present in this disorder. Results from one clinical study [35] have subsequently shown that altered circulating leptin and ghrelin levels are strongly linked with the dysregulation of bodyweight in HD patients. In line with this clinical evidence, dysregulation of insulin and leptin in the pre-symptomatic stage tgHD rats could also be an early sign of poor glycemic control and altered appetite, which typically occurs in mid to late stages of HD [38,15]. Amylin, or Islet Amyloid Polypeptide (IAPP), is a 37-residue peptide hormone secreted by pancreatic β-cells at the same time as insulin (in a roughly 1:100 amylin:insulin ratio). Peptide YY (PYY), is found in the endocrine cells of the duodenum and exocrine pancreas, and inhibits gastric emptying and secretin-stimulated pancreatic secretion. The changes in amylin and PYY observed in the tgHD rats could further suggest impaired insulin secretion [39,40] or lack of insulin-like function, which could result in additional abnormalities in glucose homeostasis in HD. Clinically, IAPP has been shown to be co-secreted from the pancreas into the circulation with insulin in response to glucose- or amino acid-triggered insulin secretion. Hyposecretion of IAPP and insulin [41] is highly characteristic of a Type 1 diabetic state, which shares many functional and physiological aspects with the dysglycemic condition present in both HD patients [42] and rodent HD models [43].

Interestingly, in the early symptomatic animals (9-months), the difference between tgHD and WT rats in insulin, leptin, amylin and PYY were no longer apparent. It is likely that at this stage of the disease, compensatory mechanisms were activated in order to try and regain homeostatic balance [44]. However, in the symptomatic stage (12-months), alterations in metabolic hormones were apparent, including decreased GIP and PP levels. GIP is a duodenal peptide named for its ability to inhibit gastric acid secretion, but its most potent effects include its ability to mediate insulin release and its strong insulinotropic effects on adipose tissue and liver. The potent insulinotropic action of GIP, while predominantly on the pancreatic islet beta-cells, may also involve an intraislet regulation of alpha cells [45]. Pancreatic polypeptide (PP) is expressed only in the pancreatic islets. PP inhibits pancreatic secretion of enzymes, bicarbonate, and water, and may play a role in the negative feedback control of the pancreas through its inhibitory action on vagal acetylcholine release [46].

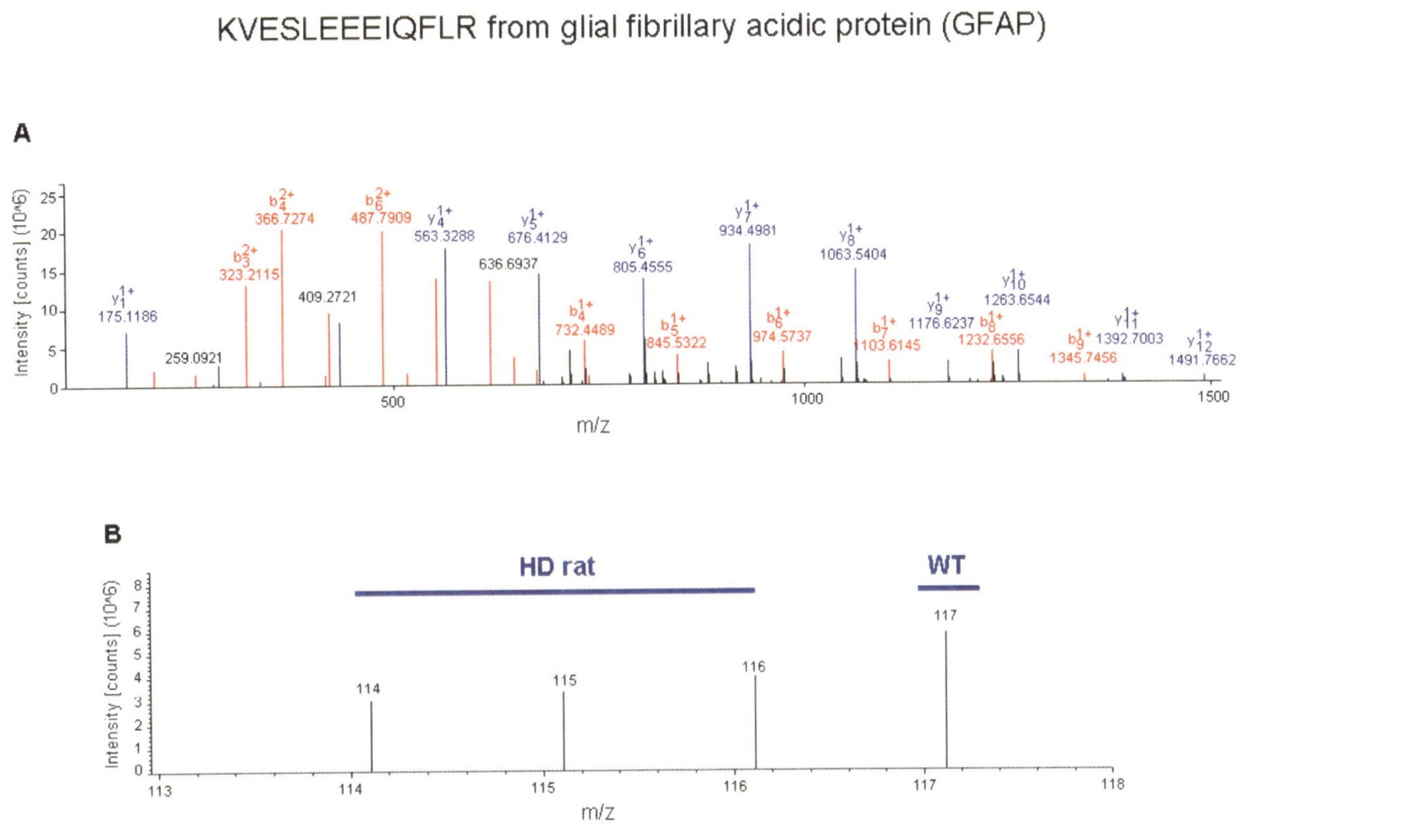

Figure 4. Sample iTRAQ analysis and iTRAQ ratio (tgHD: WT) for glial fibrillary acidic protein (GFAP) in hypothalamus. (A) Full scan MS/MS event for a single identified parent ion from GFAP with its multiple b and y series daughter ions is shown. (B) Successively expanded MS/MS spectra for identifying the low mass range end of the MS/MS scan event. The isobaric mass tag labels added were 114, 115 and 116 for tgHD rat samples and 117 for WT control samples.

The alterations in GIP and PP potentially indicate abnormalities related to pancreatic secretion, which may affect both insulin and glucagon metabolism [47,48]. In support of this, we have previously shown that there are significant alterations in pancreatic islet of Langerhans morphology and distribution of insulin and glucagon secreting cells in N171-82Q HD mice [15]. Recent evidence has also shown that GIP (glucose-dependent insulinotropic peptide) analogues can elicit beneficial effects upon synaptic plasticity and neurogenesis [49]. It is plausible therefore that a decrease of circulating GIP could be one of the hallmarks for the neurodegenerative processes that occur in HD. Even with such knowledge it is clear that further clinical HD patient studies are needed to help uncover the specific causative links between metabolic hormones such as GIP and PP and the pathophysiological etiology of HD.

Another crucial functional component of energy metabolism, plasma lipids, were also investigated in this tgHD rat model. Again, even in the pre-symptomatic stage, the tgHD rats showed a statistically significant reduction in both triglycerides and HDL. Alterations in triglycerides in tgHD rats could be due to adipose tissue dysfunction, which has been demonstrated in two HD mouse models, the R6/2 mice and CAG140K1 mice [50]. Consistently, the reduction of plasma and CSF leptin levels present in HD patients also suggests a disruption of adipose tissue function in this neurological disorder [35]. A growing body of evidence suggests that whole brain cholesterol metabolism is impaired in both HD patients [51] and HD animal models [52]. However, in our study, we did not detect any significant differences between tgHD rat and WT animals with respect to total circulating cholesterol and LDL levels. It is possible that the circulating cholesterol pool may buffer the alterations in the brain cholesterol pool. Interestingly, we also observed a profound decrease in HDL in the 3-month tgHD rats. A similar finding was reported in a recent clinical study in which HD patients demonstrated dramatically decreased HDL levels, when they displayed altered growth hormone response in the arginine test [53].

A growing body of research has established a strong association between HD and hypothalamic dysfunction such as appetite changes [16,54], circadian rhythm disturbance [55], and gut hormone alterations [15]. These hypothalamic defects can further lead to the unintended loss of bodyweight and dysfunctional energy metabolism such as diabetes and generalized insulin resistance. However, the associated underlying hypothalamic alterations are still unclear. To address this, we applied an iTRAQ proteomic approach to elucidate molecular alterations that may occur during the clinical course of HD. In the present study, we used isoflurane inhalation as an acute anesthesia method, which allows us to complete hypothalamus collection in less than 8 minutes. We specifically expedited our hypothalamic tissue collection, and minimized excessive isoflurane exposure in this as well as our previous study [56], to attenuate any potential effects our extraction procedure may have had upon protein expression or post-translational modification status. Thus, we could investigate, in a quantitative manner, proteomic changes in the hypothalamus. We identified a total of 395 significantly regulated proteins, which included 84 up-regulated proteins and

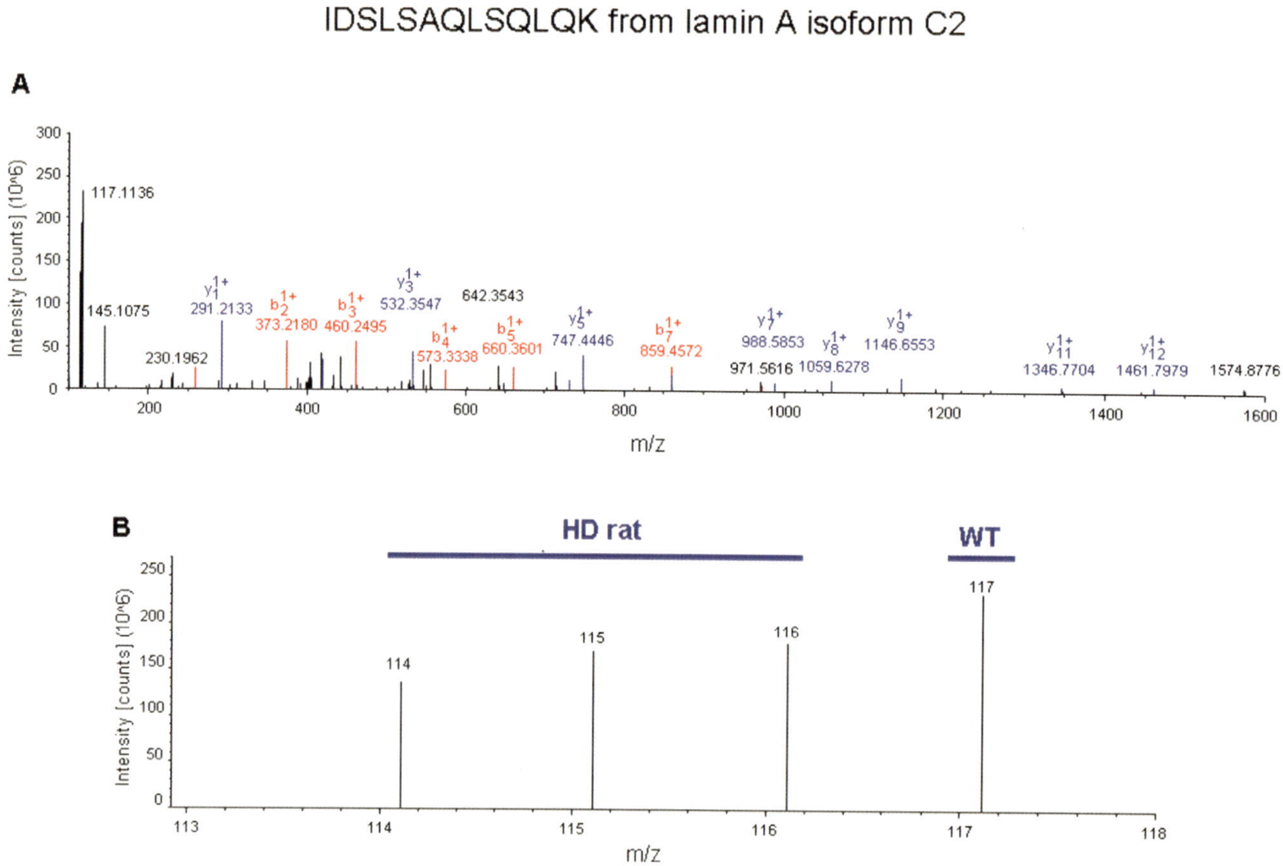

Figure 5. Sample iTRAQ analysis and iTRAQ ratio (tgHD: WT) for lamin A isoform C2 (Lamin A) in hypothalamus. (A) Full scan MS/MS event for a single identified parent ion from Lamin A with its multiple b and y series daughter ions shown. (B) Successively expanded MS/MS spectra for identifying the low mass range end of the MS/MS scan event. The isobaric mass tag labels added were 114, 115 and 116 for tgHD rats samples and 117 for WT control samples.

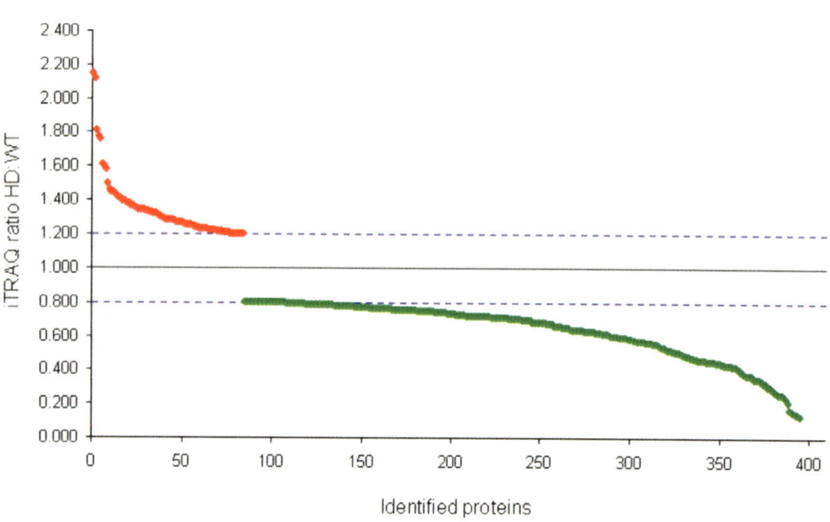

Figure 6. iTRAQ ratios of tgHD rat versus WT control for hypothalamus. Mean tgHD (114, 115,116) to the WT (117) isobaric mass tag ratios for samples resolved by MS/MS from the hypothalamus of both WT and tgHD rats. Proteins identified from peptides that displayed a ratio greater than or equal to 1.2 or less that or equal to 0.8 are considered to be statistically different according to standard protocols from unity and therefore distinctly regulated compared to WT.

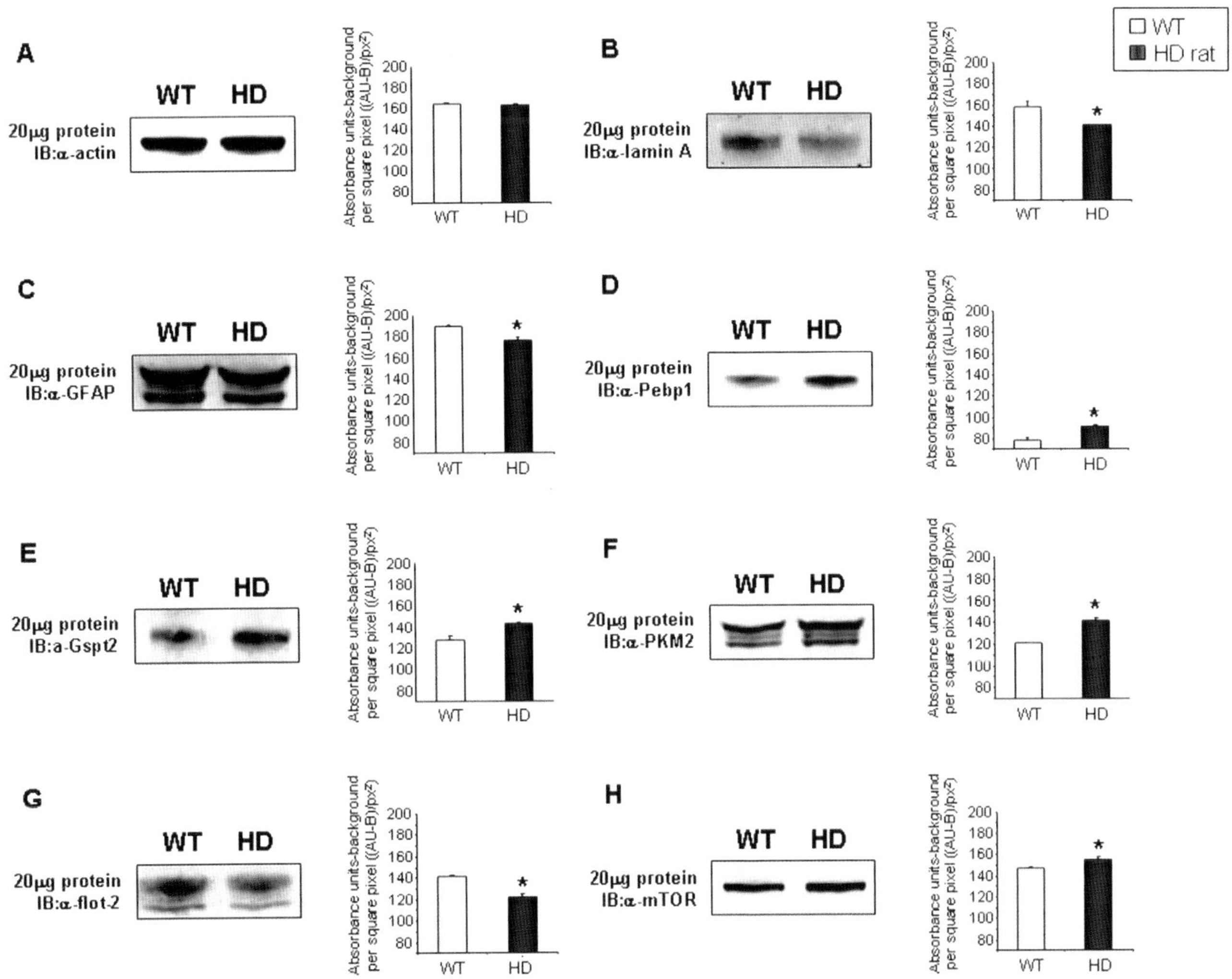

Figure 7. Western blot validation of multiple significantly regulated proteins identified by iTRAQ in tgHD hypothalami. Quantification of the representative western blots is indicated for the WT (white bars) and HD (dark bars) for the respective proteins: Lamin A (B); GFAP (C); Pebp1 (D); Gspt2 (E); PKM2 (F); Flot-2 (g); and mTOR (H). Expression variation was normalized to actin (A) expression. Assessment of statistical significance was performed with GraphPad Prism (version 5) using a Student's t-test. * : $p \leq 0.05$. Values are mean ± SEM, n = 5 per group.

311 down-regulated proteins. As expected, the majority of the top-regulated proteins are closely related to neurophysiological functions, such as glial fibrillary acidic protein (Gfap), lamin A, annexin A2 (Anxa2) and Ras-related protein Ral-A precursor (Rala). GFAP is the main intermediate filament protein in mature astrocytes, but is also an important component of the cytoskeleton in astrocytes during development. It has been shown that GFAP is involved in astrocyte functions, which are important during regeneration, synaptic plasticity and reactive gliosis [57]. The altered Lamin A/C, is associated with changes in nuclear morphology (*e.g.* increased nuclear volume). Homozygous defects in LaminA cause autosomal recessive axonal neuropathy in human (Charcot-Marie-Tooth Disorder Type 2) and mouse [58]. Anxa2 heterotetramer is involved in learning and neuronal activities [59]. RalA depletion or ectopic expression of constitutively active RalA in cultured neurons inhibits axon formation [60]. Some altered proteins are even more specifically linked to pathology of Huntington's disease, such as Heat shock protein-70 (Hspa1b), cytoplasmic dynein 1 heavy chain 1 (Dync1h1). Hsp70 is a molecular chaperone which colocalizes to inclusion bodies, which are neuroprotective in HD animal models. Recent research has also demonstrated that Hsp70 functionally interacts with soluble mutant huntingtin oligomers in a classic ATP-dependent manner [61]. Dynein dysfunction is a potential causal mechanism in neurodegenerative diseases, most notably in degenerative diseases of the striatum such as Huntington's disease [62]. In addition, we also discovered profound alterations in several oxidative stress-responsive proteins, such phospholipid hydroperoxide glutathione peroxidase (Gpx4) [63], glutathione S-transferase Mu 2 (Gstm2) and glutathione S-transferase Mu 7 (Gstm7) [64]. In order to better understand the changes of those proteins, we also used unbiased clustering of proteins into functional pathways (KEGG) as this allows for a physiological 'phenotype' of the protein set to be created that is not entirely dependent on specific protein identities in the set [65]. Using KEGG pathway analysis, the major pathways that were found to be altered in the tgHD rat hypothalami included: *fatty acid metabolism*, *oxidative phosphorylation*, *glycerolipid metabolism*, *glycolysis/gluconeogenesis*, *insulin signaling pathway*, and *PPAR signaling pathway*. In addition to KEGG analysis, LSI analysis revealed that the significantly altered proteins were highly associated with the input interrogation terms 'diabetes' and 'insulin'. Implicitly-correlating proteins of note

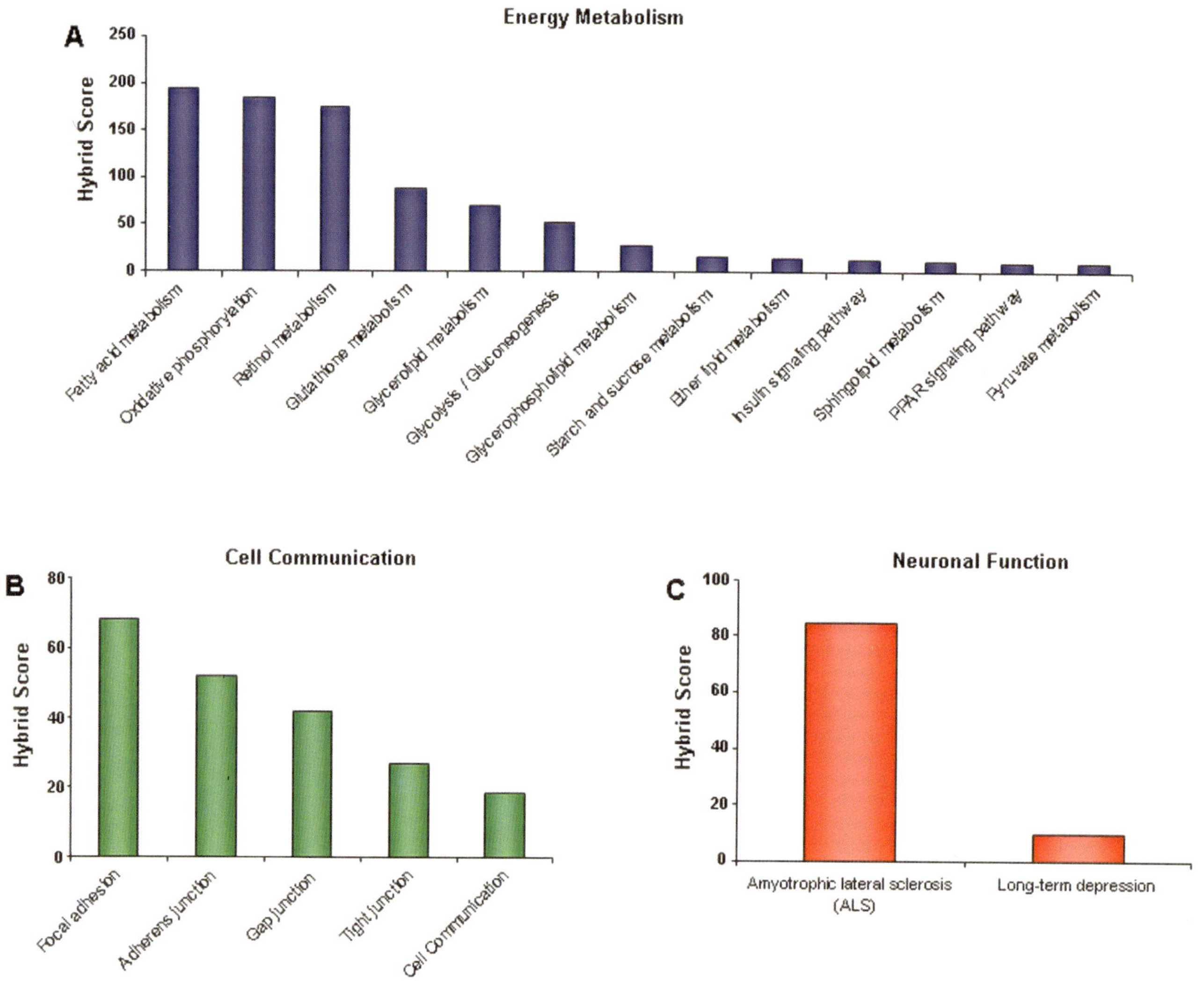

Figure 8. KEGG signaling pathway analysis of significantly regulated hypothalamic proteins. Proteins significantly regulated in tgHD rats compared to WT controls were used as input data for KEGG signaling pathway population analysis. The significantly populated pathways for tgHD rats were rationally clustered into subgroups focused upon energy metabolism (A), cell communication (B), and neuronal function (C). For each significantly-populated KEGG pathway a 'hybrid' score was generated which represents the $-\log_{10}$ of the enrichment probability multiplied with the relative enrichment factor compared to the background proteomic expression.

discovered using this informatic process included glycogen synthase1 (Gys1), pyruvate dehydrogenase kinase2 (Pdk2), pyruvate kinase M2 (Pkm2), 1-acylglycerol-3-phosphate O-acyltransferase 1 (Agpat1) and acyl-CoA synthetase family member 2 (Acsf2). Gys1, the rate-limiting enzyme in the synthesis of glycogen, is glycogen synthase encoded by two genes: Gys1 is expressed in muscle and other tissues, and Gys2, primarily expressed in liver (regulating liver glycogen synthase). Since conversion to glycogen is a major fate of ingested glucose in the body, reducing glycogen synthase activity can lead to severe glucose intolerance [66]. Pdk2 is a member of a family of pyruvate dehydrogenase kinases (Pdks 1–4). Four dedicated Pdk isoenzymes have been identified, each of which display a distinct tissue-specific expression profile, and have differential regulatory properties. Pdk plays a key role in controlling the balance between glucose and lipid oxidation according to substrate supply [67]. Increasing glucose oxidation by inhibiting Pdk may be an effective mechanism to increase glucose utilization; additionally, increasing pyruvate oxidation may further contribute to lowering glucose levels by decreasing the supply of gluconeogenic substrates [68]. The glycolytic key regulator Pkm2 (or M2-PK) can switch between a highly active tetrameric and an inactive dimeric form. In its active form, M2-Pk/Pkm2 is a metabolic sensor, which regulates cell proliferation, cell growth, and apoptotic cell death in a glucose supply-dependent manner [69]. Taken together, these three proteins play critical roles in the process of glycolysis/gluconeogenesis. The fact that we observed significant alterations in these proteins in the tgHD rat hypothalamus suggests that there is possible involvement of dysfunctional glycolysis/gluconeogenesis in HD. Most cells synthesize their glycerophospholipids and triglycerides (TG) to maintain cellular integrity and to provide energy for cellular functions. Agpat1 controls serial acylations of glycerol-3-phosphate, which is involved in *de novo* phospholipid synthesis in cells [70]. Acsf2 is one of enzymes that mediates fatty acid transportation and catalyzes the formation of acyl-CoA from fatty acids, ATP, and CoA [71]. Interestingly, these two lipid synthesis enzymes were dramatically up-regulated in the hypothalamus of the tgHD rat, which suggests increased activity of lipid

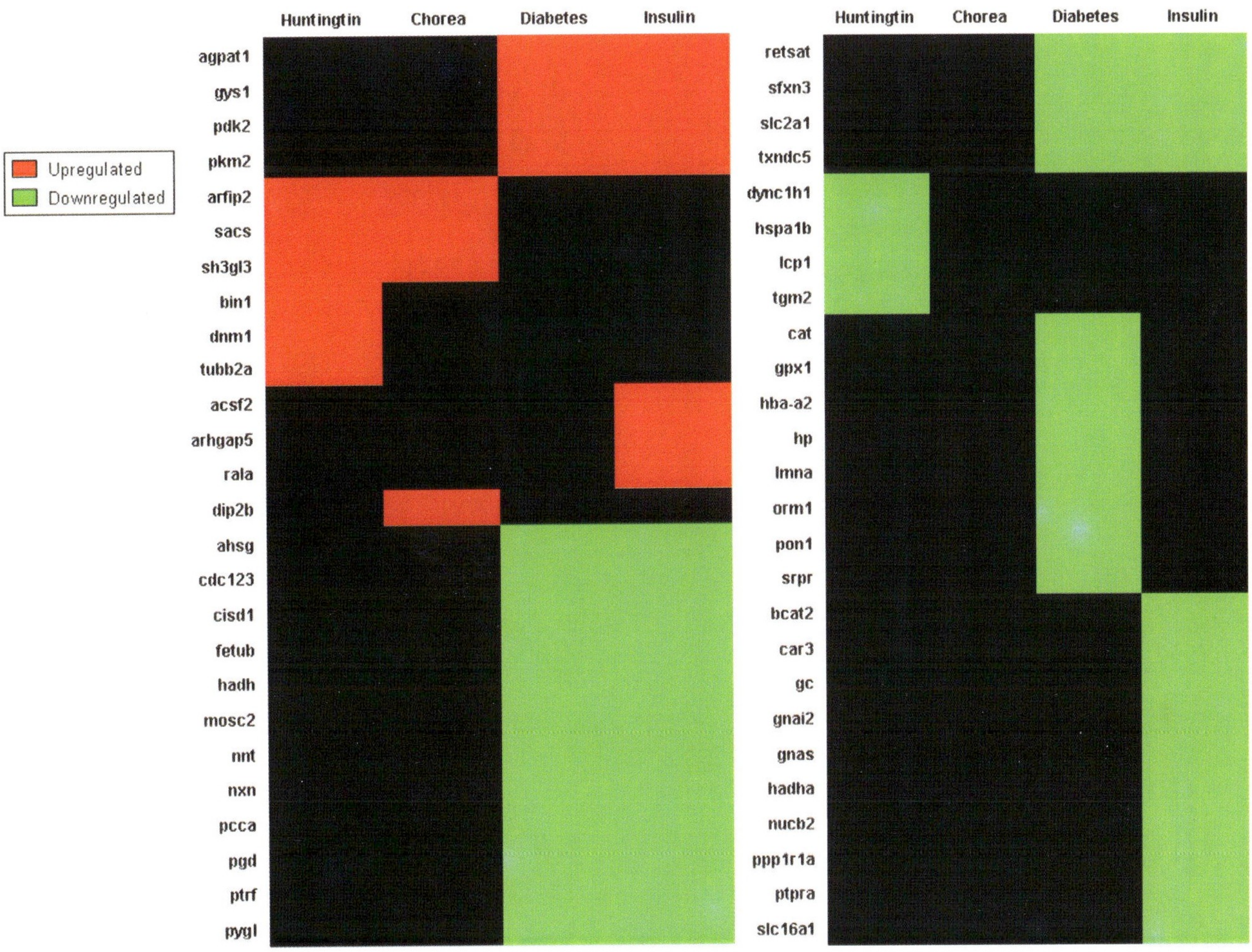

Figure 9. LSI correlation analysis of altered hypothalamic proteins in TgHD rats. LSI analysis of tgHD significantly-regulated hypothalamic proteins was performed using the following search terms: Huntingtin, Chorea, Diabetes and Insulin. Red signifies up-regulated proteins and green signifies down-regulated proteins.

synthesis in the hypothalamus. As signals of nutrient abundance, alterations of hypothalamic lipid levels might further contribute to changes in feeding behavior and other peripheral metabolic dysfunctions in HD [72]. Although it would also be interesting to investigate distinct proteomic profiles in microregions of the hypothalamus, this is not currently possible with iTRAQ technology, due to the large protein amounts that are required (150 µg).

In this study, we have gained a greater appreciation of the intricacies of alterations in the neuroendocrine system occurring throughout the Huntington's disease process. In assessing the presence of pathophysiology, one must realize that the tissue or organ that is diseased is not merely a passive entity and that its cells may react in a specific manner to the imposed insult [73]. This theory has been partly testified in our longitudinal results of tgHD rat model. Therefore, in certain important organ(s) or tissue(s) such as the hypothalamus, complicated signaling pathways and functional groups of proteins may reveal that both positive and negative regulatory mechanisms are working in concert to create the resultant diseased phenotype. By using proteomic techniques, such as iTRAQ, we gained a deeper understanding of the complex signaling pathways and functional groups of proteins that are altered in the hypothalamus of HD. With these findings, we can better understand and interpret the powerful metabolic readouts from peripheral tissues of HD and potentially open up novel therapeutic avenues for the treatment of HD.

Materials and Methods

Animals, blood collection and tissue harvesting

Male transgenic HD (tgHD) rats, containing a truncated huntingtin cDNA fragment with 51 CAG repeats under the control of the naïve rat huntingtin promoter and their male wild type (WT) littermates were used for this study. All rats were kept under a 12:12 h light-dark cycle with the light period starting at 6:00 am. All animals received *ad libitum* access to food and water. All animal procedures were approved by the Animal Care and Use Committee of the Friedrich-Alexander-Universität Erlangen-Nürnberg, Germany and conducted according the international guidelines for the use and care of laboratory animals. Longitudinal analyses were conducted on male tgHD rats and their age- and gender-mated WT littermates. Blood samples were collected from the tail vein from each animal (n = 5 per group) after an overnight fast at the following ages: 3-months (pre-symptomatic), 9-months (early symptomatic), and 12-months (symptomatic). At 12 months of age, animals were euthanized using inhalation isoflurane

Table 1. KEGG group clustering of significantly altered hypothalamic proteins in tgHD rats compared to wild-type controls.

Up-regulated proteins	Hybrid Score
Glutathione metabolism	93.9
Fatty acid metabolism	93.9
Gap junction	80.0
Starch and sucrose metabolism	62.0
Glycerophospholipid metabolism	53.6
Insulin signaling pathway	16.9
Purine metabolism	16.5
Focal adhesion	10.2
Down-regulated proteins	**Hybrid Score**
Fatty acid elongation in mitochondria	269.4
Oxidative phosphorylation	257.9
Complement and coagulation cascades	238.3
Retinol metabolism	234.0
Valine, leucine and isoleucine degradation	218.8
Benzoate degradation via hydroxylation	185.3
Fatty acid metabolism	123.0
Amyotrophic lateral sclerosis (ALS)	115.9
Propanoate metabolism	107.3
Bile acid biosynthesis	85.9
Leukocyte transendothelial migration	78.7
Adherens junction	73.8
Regulation of actin cytoskeleton	72.7
Focal adhesion	62.2
Glycerolipid metabolism	57.6
Calcium signaling pathway	53.2
Glycolysis/Gluconeogenesis	44.2
Metabolism of xenobiotics by cytochrome P450	41.8
Tight junction	39.0
Glutathione metabolism	37.8
Nitrogen metabolism	34.9
beta-Alanine metabolism	32.7
Limonene and pinene degradation	30.7
Antigen processing and presentation	28.6
Cell Communication	26.8
Arginine and proline metabolism	23.8
Cell adhesion molecules (CAMs)	19.8
Nicotinate and nicotinamide metabolism	15.5
Tryptophan metabolism	15.4
Long-term depression	13.8
ECM-receptor interaction	11.9
Butanoate metabolism	11.9
Gap junction	11.3
Lysine degradation	11.2
Fructose and mannose metabolism	10.4
Glycerophospholipid metabolism	7.8
Taste transduction	7.4
Axon guidance	5.8
Insulin signaling pathway	5.2

Table 1. Cont.

KEGG group clusters were only extracted from the differentially-regulated protein list if at least two proteins were present in each group with a compound probability of $p \geq 0.05$. To account for both KEGG enrichment (R: Observed expression frequency/Expected expression frequency) and compound probability (p) of clustered proteins, a hybrid score was used. Hybrid score = R * $-\log_{10}(p)$.

($\sim$1 ml/430 cm^3) and decapitation. Hypothalami were carefully dissected out and were stored at -80°C for proteomic analyses.

Measurement of circulating metabolic hormones and lipids

Plasma glucose levels were measured using an enzymatic assay kit (GO Assay, Sigma, St. Louis, MO), according to the manufacturer's instructions. Plasma metabolic hormones were measured using a rodent multiplex assay kit (Millipore, Billerica, MA), as described previously [74,75]. Each sample was assayed in duplicate on a 96-well plate. Analysis of quality control standards provided in the kit met expectations, validating the accuracy of panel. Additionally, this assay had an inter-assay precision of <23% and an intra-assay precision of <7%. Plasma lipid levels including triglycerides, total cholesterol, high density lipoprotein (HDL), and low density lipoprotein (LDL) were assayed using enzymatic methods with commercial kits (Wako Chemicals USA, Inc., Richmond, VA), according to the manufacturer's instructions. Plasma corticosterone levels were measured using standard radioimmunoassay (RIA) procedures as described previously [75] and according to the assay kit manufacturer's instructions.

Isobaric tag for relative and absolute quantification (iTRAQ)

Proteomic analyses of the hypothalami were conducted using iTRAQ, as described previously [44]. Briefly, iTRAQ chemistry labeling reagents were obtained from Applied Biosystems (Bedford, MA). WT and tgHD rat tissue samples were treated in parallel throughout the labeling procedure. The generic labeling protocol consisted of the following steps: protein reduction and cysteine blocking, digestion of proteins with trypsin, labeling of peptides with iTRAQ reagents, combining the samples that were to be compared, strong cation exchange chromatography, desalting with solid phase extraction, and LC/MS/MS analysis. Briefly, protein sample pellets (generated by trichloroacetic acid precipitation) were dissolved in dissolution buffer (0.5 M triethyammonium bicarbonate, TEAB), to give a 5 µg/µL concentration. Subsequently, 20 µL (100 µg) of each mixture was aliquoted and 1 µL denaturant (2% SDS) was added. Reducing reagent (2 µL, 50 mM TECP) was added and the tubes were incubated at 60°C for 1 hour. The proprietary (methyl methanethiosulphonate, Applied Biosystems, Bedford, MA) cysteine-blocking reagent (1 µL, 200 mM MMTS) was added and incubated for another 10 minutes at room temperature. Trypsin (Promega, Madison, WI) was reconstituted in water; 10 µL of the solution containing 10 µg of trypsin was added and incubated overnight at 37°C. Before labeling, the reagents were dissolved in ethanol and the contents of one vial were transferred to a sample tube. The labeling took place for 1 h at room temperature. The following labels were used for hypothalamus samples: 114-tgHD

(C1)-2 pooled Huntington's disease animals; 115-tgHD (C2)-2 pooled Huntington's disease animals; 116-tgHD (C3)-2 pooled Huntington's disease animals; 117- WT(C4)-2 pooled Wild-type animals. After labeling, sample tubes for WT and tgHD for separate tissues were combined and dried down to a volume of 50 μL to reduce the content of ethanol prior to strong cation exchange (SCX) chromatography.

Mass Spectrometry analysis

An Applied Biosystems QStar mass spectrometer was used for the isolation and collision-induced dissociation of input peptides. The electrospray voltage typically maintained was 2.5 kV. Mass spectrometer calibration was performed with a mixture of CsI (MW132.9049), synthetic peptide ALILTLVS (829.5393) and verapamil (455.2904). The general conditions for mass ion identification and isobaric mass tag resolution were: Scan Events: 1: Survey 400–1200 Da; 2–4: Data dependent MS/MS on 3 most intense ions from 1. For collision energy: rolling collision energy (automatically set according to the m/z of precursor), increased for 20% due to iTRAQ tags. The exclusion time used for analysis was 60 seconds. Mass tolerance was set to 0.15 atomic mass units for precursor and 0.1 atomic mass units for fragmented ions. Data analysis was performed using the ProQuant program suit (Applied Biosystems, Bedford, MA). Protein identification was performed using the most recently updated rodent SwissProt database. Raw peptide identification results were processed to generate a minimal set of proteins, as previously described, using the Paragon Algorithm (Applied Biosystems, Bedford, MA). Briefly, the raw peptide identification results from the Paragon Algorithm searches were further processed by the ProGroup Algorithm (Applied Biosystems, Bedford, MA) within the Protein Pilot software before final display. The ProGroup Algorithm uses the peptide identification results to determine the minimal set of proteins that can be reported for a given protein confidence threshold. For each protein, ProGroup reports two score types for each protein: unused ProtScore and total ProtScore. The total ProtScore is a measurement of all the peptide evidence for a protein (analogous to commonly reported protein scores). The unused ProtScore is a measurement of all the peptide evidence for a protein that is not better explained by a higher-ranking protein. Hence unused ProtScore is calculated by using the unique peptides that are not linked to a higher-ranking protein. The protein confidence threshold cutoff for this study was ProtScore 2.0 (unused) with at least two peptides with a 95% confidence. Proteins identified with mass tag changes (ratio = 1.2 or 0.8) that were consistent between two independent biological experiments were manually validated and quantified by two independent analysts. These arbitrary cutoffs for expression variation have been implemented by multiple researchers [44,76]. Peak areas for each of the signature ions (114, 115, 116, 117) were obtained and corrected according to the manufacturers' instructions to account for isotopic overlap. Only those signature ions with intensities less than 1500 counts were used for quantification, greater than 1500 counts results in detector saturation. To calculate the relative protein levels, proteins with a statistically significant label ratio of 114/115/116:117 greater or equal to 1.2 were considered to be proteins elevated tgHD versus WT samples. Proteins with a significant label ratio of 114/115/116:117 less than or equal to 0.8 were indicative of down-regulated proteins in tgHD versus WT. The relative expression level for 'up-regulated' proteins was calculated as follows: the mean of 114/115/116:117 label ratio. The eventual relative expression level of 'down-regulated proteins' was calculated as follows: the mean of 114/115/116:117 label ratio and then made negative to indicate the relative direction of expression compared to control.

Western blot analysis

Various proteins identified by iTRAQ were validated using western blot, as described previously [77]. 20 μg samples of the hypothalamus were mixed with a denaturing and reducing Laemmli buffer and resolved by SDS-PAGE. The proteins were then electrotransferred from the gel onto a polyvinylenedifluoride (PVDF: NEN Life Sciences) membrane. The membrane was treated with a Tris-buffered saline solution supplemented with Tween-20, NP-40 and 5% bovine serum albumin to block non-specific antibody interactions. Primary antibodies (1:500–1000) were applied to the PVDF membrane for 1 hour at room temperature and proteins were identified by the application of an alkaline-phosphatase-conjugated secondary antibody (1:10000) that recognized the species type of the primary antibody. The PVDF membrane was then exposed to an enzyme-linked chemifluorescent developing substrate (GE Heathcare, Piscataway, NJ) and was scanned using a GE Typhoon 9410 phosphorimager. Western blot images were then quantified using GE ImageQuant 5.1 software. The primary antibodies were obtained from the following sources: Lamin A antibody (sc-20680) and Gspt2 antibody (sc-135899), obtained from Santa Cruz; GFAP (#3670), Pebp1 (#4742), PKM2 (#3198), Flotillin-2 (#3436) and mTOR (#2983) antibodies were from the Cell Signaling Technology (Danvers, MA); beta-actin (A5316) antibody was purchased from Sigma (St. Louis, MO).

Bioinformatics - Protein pathway analyses and Latent Semantic Indexing

KEGG (Kyoto Encyclopedia of Genes and Genomes: http://www.genome.jp/kegg/) pathway clustering was performed using WebGestalt algorithms (http://bioinfo.vanderbilt.edu/webgestalt), as described previously [78,79]. We employed basic quantitative parameters for the significant inclusion of KEGG pathway groups, *i.e.* each group needed a minimum population of two proteins from the input experimental set and to possess a probability significance of enrichment compared to a background dataset of less than 0.05 (hypergeometric test of significance). The degree of enrichment (R: expressed as a ratio) of KEGG pathway group was calculated as follows: $R = O/E$ where O is the observed protein number in the KEGG pathway, E is the expected protein number in the KEGG pathway, and a P value is given for the pathways with $R>1$ to indicate the significance of enrichment. Based on those parameters, a hybrid score is calculated with the formula of $R*(-\log_{10}(P))$. GO analysis is an enrichment analysis for the Gene Ontology categories. The result is visualized in a directed acyclic graph (DAG) in order to maintain the relationship among the enriched GO categories. For each GO category, a hybrid score was calculated as well, based upon the same formula as KEGG analysis. The gene symbols of significantly altered hypothalamic proteins identified by iTRAQ were interrogated against a range of keywords using Latent Semantic Indexing (LSI) from GeneIndexer, as described previously [80–82]. Briefly, gene symbols of significantly altered proteins were uploaded into the Computable Genomix program (http://www.computablegenomix.com/). GeneIndexer correlates the strength of association, using LSI, between specific genes (proteins) in a dataset with user-defined interrogation terms. GeneIndexer employs a comprehensive murine database of over 2×10^6 scientific abstracts to perform this text-gene correlation analysis. LSI facilitates the specific textual interrogation of an input dataset with a specific interrogation term, *e.g.* diabetes, to ascertain which of the input dataset genes/proteins are associated with the interrogation term. The possible LSI correlation scores for a gene/protein to be associated with an input interrogation term range from 0 to 1. A score of 0 indicates neutrality of correlation, while scores ranging from 0 to −1 indicate a strengthening lack of correlation of the gene/protein to the input interrogation term. Proteins with a significant correlation (value >0.1) were extracted and labeled as either up-regulated (red) or down-regulated (green).

Statistical analyses

Both the Student's t-test and 2-way ANOVA analysis were employed in this study. A Student's t-test was used for comparison between tgHD rats and WT rats and the longitudinal alterations, in which 3-month aged animals were regarded as a control in each genotype group. Two-way ANOVA analysis was also performed to evaluate all plasma parameters, where genotype and age were regarded as 2 independent variables. $p<0.05$ was considered statistically significant throughout the study. Error bars on graphs represent the ±95% confidence interval. All data represent means ± S.E.M. (standard error of mean).

Supporting Information

Table S1 Two-way ANOVA analysis of plasma parameters. All plasma parameters were also analyzed by 2-way ANOVA, in which age and genotype were regarded as 2 independent factors. P value[a] indicates the significance for the comparison between tgHD rats and the age-matched WT rats. P value[b] indicates the significance for the comparison between 2 different ages in tgHD rats.

Table S2 Significantly regulated proteins in HD rat hypothalamic tissue compared to WT animals. The Mean ratios of significantly altered proteins between Huntington's rats (tgHD) and wild-type control animals (WT) are listed below. The mean ratios >=1.2 indicate increased expression in tgHD rats compared to WT and mean ratios <=0.8 indicate reduced expression compared to WT.

Table S3 GeneIndexer Latent Semantic Indexing (LSI) analysis of significantly up-regulated hypothalamic proteins. The search terms used were: "Huntingtin," "chorea," "diabetes," and "insulin." A score of "0" indicates no significant correlation; a score of "1" indicates a significant correlation, p≤0 .05.

Table S4 GeneIndexer Latent Semantic Indexing (LSI) analysis of significantly down-regulated hypothalamic proteins. The search terms used were: "Huntingtin," "chorea," "diabetes," and "insulin." A score of "0" indicates no significant correlation; a score of "1" indicates a significant correlation, p≤0.05.

Author Contributions

Conceived and designed the experiments: W-nC BM SM SvH. Performed the experiments: W-nC HC RW CMD SM KR FC SvH BM. Analyzed the data: W-nC BM SvH. Contributed reagents/materials/analysis tools: SVH SM . Wrote the paper: W-nC BM SM SvH.

References

1. Landles C, Bates GP (2004) Huntingtin and the molecular pathogenesis of Huntington's disease. Fourth in molecular medicine review series. EMBO Rep 5: 958–963.
2. Li SH, Li XJ (2004) Huntington and its Role in Neuronal Degeneration. Neuroscientist 10: 467–475.
3. MacDonald ME, Ambrose CM, Duyao MP, Myers RH, Lin C, et al. (1993) A novel gene containing a trinucleotide repeat that is expanded and unstable on Huntington's disease chromosomes. Cell 72: 971–983.
4. Langbehn DR, Brinkman RR, Falush D, Paulsen JS, Hayden MR, on behalf of an International Huntington's Disease Collaborative G (2004) A new model for prediction of the age of onset and penetrance for Huntington's disease based on CAG length. Clinical Genetics 65: 267–277.
5. Dewhurst K, Oliver J (1970) Huntington's disease of young people. Eur Neurol 3: 278–289.
6. Brandt J, Folstein SE, Folstein MF (1988) Differential cognitive impairment in Alzheimer's disease and Huntington's disease. Ann Neurol 23: 555–561.
7. Bamford KA, Caine ED, Kido DK, Cox C, Shoulson I (1995) A prospective evaluation of cognitive decline in early Huntington's disease: functional and radiographic correlates. Neurology 45: 1867–1873.
8. Shiwach R (1994) Psychopathology in Huntington's disease patients. Acta Psychiatr Scand 90: 241–246.
9. Sanberg PR, Fibiger HC, Mark RF (1981) Body weight and dietary factors in Huntington's disease patients compared with matched controls. Med J Aust 1: 407–409.
10. Djousse L, Knowlton B, Cupples LA, Marder K, Shoulson I, et al. (2002) Weight loss in early stage of Huntington's disease. Neurology 59: 1325–1330.
11. Hamilton JM, Wolfson T, Peavy GM, Jacobson MW, Corey-Bloom J (2004) Rate and correlates of weight change in Huntington's disease. Journal of Neurology, Neurosurgery & Psychiatry 75: 209–212.
12. Ahmad Aziz N, Pijl H, Frölich M, Maurits van der Graaf AW, Roelfsema F, et al. (2009) Leptin secretion rate increases with higher CAG repeat number in Huntington's disease patients. Clinical Endocrinology 73: 206–211.
13. Podolsky S, Leopold NA (1977) Abnormal glucose tolerance and arginine tolerance tests in Huntington's disease. Gerontology 23: 55–63.
14. Kremer HP, Roos RA, Frolich M, Radder JK, Nieuwenhuijzen Kruseman AC, et al. (1989) Endocrine functions in Huntington's disease. A two-and-a-half years follow-up study. J Neurol Sci 90: 335–344.
15. Martin B, Golden E, Carlson OD, Pistell P, Zhou J, et al. (2009) Exendin-4 Improves Glycemic Control, Ameliorates Brain and Pancreatic Pathologies, and Extends Survival in a Mouse Model of Huntington's Disease. Diabetes 58: 318–328.
16. Trejo A, Tarrats RM, Alonso ME, Boll M-C, Ochoa A, et al. (2004) Assessment of the nutrition status of patients with Huntington's disease. Nutrition 20: 192–196.
17. Morton AJ, Wood NI, Hastings MH, Hurelbrink C, Barker RA et al. (2005) Disintegration of the Sleep-Wake Cycle and Circadian Timing in Huntington's Disease. J Neurosci 25: 157–163.
18. Hult S, Soylu R, Björklund T, Belgardt BF, Mauer J, et al. (2011) Mutant huntingtin causes metabolic imbalance by disruption of hypothalamic neurocircuits. Cell Metabolism 13(4): 428–39.
19. Aylward EH, Sparks BF, Field KM, Yallapragada V, Shpritz BD, et al. (2004) Onset and rate of striatal atrophy in preclinical Huntington disease. Neurology 63: 66–72.
20. Kipps CM, Duggins AJ, Mahant N, Gomes L, Ashburner J, et al. (2005) Progression of structural neuropathology in preclinical Huntington's disease: a tensor based morphometry study. Journal of Neurology, Neurosurgery & Psychiatry 76: 650–655.
21. Paulsen JS, Magnotta VA, Mikos AE, Paulson HL, Penziner E, et al. (2006) Brain structure in preclinical Huntington's Disease. Biological Psychiatry 59: 57–63.
22. Wolf RC, Vasic N, Schönfeldt-Lecuona C, Landwehrmeyer GB, Ecker D (2007) Dorsolateral prefrontal cortex dysfunction in presymptomatic Huntington's disease: evidence from event-related fMRI. Brain 130: 2845–2857.
23. Rosas HD, Hevelone ND, Zaleta AK, Greve DN, Salat DH, et al. (2005) Regional cortical thinning in preclinical Huntington disease and its relationship to cognition. Neurology 65: 745–747.
24. Soneson C, Fontes M, Zhou Y, Denisov V, Paulsen JS, et al. (2010) Early changes in the hypothalamic region in prodromal Huntington disease revealed by MRI analysis. Neurobiology of Disease 40: 531–543.
25. Sawiak SJ, Wood NI, Williams GB, Morton AJ, Carpenter TA, et al. (2009) Voxel-based morphometry in the R6/2 transgenic mouse reveals differences between genotypes not seen with manual 2D morphometry. Neurobiology of Disease 33: 20–27.
26. Björkqvist M, Leavitt BR, Nielsen JE, Landwehrmeyer B, Ecker D, et al. (2007) Cocaine- and amphetamine-regulated transcript is increased in Huntington disease. Movement Disorders 22: 1952–1954.
27. Gabery S, Murphy K, Schultz K, Loy C, McCusker E, et al. (2010) Changes in key hypothalamic neuropeptide populations in Huntington disease revealed by neuropathological analyses. Acta Neuropathologica 120: 777–788.

28. Mangiarini L, Sathasivam K, Seller M, Cozens B, Harper A, et al. (1996) Exon 1 of the HD gene with an expanded CAG repeat is sufficient to cause a progressive neurological phenotype in transgenic mice. Cell 87: 493–506.
29. McBride JL, Ramaswamy S, Gasmi M, Bartus RT, Herzog CD, et al. (2006) Viral delivery of glial cell line-derived neurotrophic factor improves behavior and protects striatal neurons in a mouse model of Huntington's disease. Proceedings of the National Academy of Sciences 103: 9345–9350.
30. von Hörsten S, Schmitt I, Nguyen HP, Holzmann C, Schmidt T, et al. (2003) Transgenic rat model of Huntington's disease. Human Molecular Genetics 12: 617–624.
31. Nguyen HP, Kobbe P, Rahne H, Wörpel T, Jäger B, et al. (2006) Behavioral abnormalities precede neuropathological markers in rats transgenic for Huntington's disease. Human Molecular Genetics 15: 3177–3194.
32. Martin B, Golden E, Keselman A, Stone M, Mattson MP et al. (2008) Therapeutic perspectives for the treatment of Huntington's disease: treating the whole body. Histol Histopathol 23: 237–250.
33. van der Burg JMM, Björkqvist M, Brundin P (2009) Beyond the brain: widespread pathology in Huntington's disease. The Lancet Neurology 8: 765–774.
34. Cai H, Cong WN, Ji S, Rothman S, Maudsley S, et al. (2012) Metabolic dysfunction in Alzheimer's disease and related neurodegenerative disorders. Curr Alzheimer Res 9: 5–17.
35. Hult S, Schultz K, Soylu R, Petersén A (2010) Hypothalamic and neuroendocrine changes in Huntington's disease. Curr Drug Targets 11: 1237–1249.
36. Lalic NM, Maric J, Svetel M, Jotic A, Stefanova E, et al. (2008) Glucose Homeostasis in Huntington disease. Arch neurol 65: 476–480.
37. Farrer LA. (1985) Diabetes Mellitus in Huntington's disease. Clin Genet 27: 62–67.
38. Popovic V, Svetel M, Djurovic M, Petrovic S, Doknic M, et al. (2004) Circulating and cerebrospinal fluid ghrelin and leptin: potential role in altered body weight in Huntington's disease. Eur J Endocrinol 151: 451–5.
39. Scherbaum WA (1998) The role of amylin in the physiology of glycemic control. Exp Clin Endocrinol Diabetes 106: 97–102.
40. Boey D, Sainsbury A, Herzog H (2007) The role of peptide YY in regulating glucose homeostasis. Peptides 28: 390–395.
41. Tomita M. (2011) Islet amu;oid polypeptide in pancreatic islets from type 1 diabetic subjects. Islets 3: 166–174
42. Hashimoto K-I, Ito Y, Tanahashi H, Hayashi M, Yamakita N, et al. (2012) Hyperglycemic Chorea-Ballism or Acute Exacerbation of Huntington's Chorea? Huntington's DiseaseUnmasked by Diabetic Ketoacidosis in Type 1 Diabetes Mellitus. Clin Endocrinol Metab [Epub ahead of print]
43. Hurlbert MS, Zhou W, Wasmeier C, Kaddis FG, Hutton JC, et al. (1999) Mice transgenic for an expanded CAG repeat in the Huntington's disease gene develop diabetes. Diabetes 48:649–651
44. Martin B, Brenneman R, Becker KG, Gucek M, Cole RN, et al. (2008) iTRAQ Analysis of Complex Proteome Alterations in 3×TgAD Alzheimer's Mice: Understanding the Interface between Physiology and Disease. PLoS ONE 3: e2750.
45. Ding WG, Gromada J (1997) Protein kinase A-dependent stimulation of exocytosis in mouse pancreatic beta-cells by glucose-dependent insulinotropic polypeptide. Diabetes 46: 615–621.
46. Schwartz TW, Holst JJ, Fahrenkrug J, Jensen SL, Nielsen OV, et al. (1978) Vagal, cholinergic regulation of pancreatic polypeptide secretion. J Clin Invest 61: 781–789.
47. Baggio LL, Drucker DJ (2007) Biology of Incretins: GLP-1 and GIP. Gastroenterology 132: 2131–2157.
48. Field BCT, Chaudhri OB, Bloom SR (2010) Bowels control brain: gut hormones and obesity. Nat Rev Endocrinol 6: 444–453.
49. Faivre E, Hamilton A, Holscher C (2012) Effects of acute and chronic administration of GIP analogues on cognition, synaptic plasticity and neurogenesis in mice. European Journal of Pharmacology 674:294–306
50. Phan J, Hickey MA, Zhang P, Chesselet MF, Reue K (2009) Adipose tissue dysfunction tracks disease progression in two Huntington's disease mouse models. Hum Mol Genet 18: 1006–1016
51. Leoni V, Mariotti C, Nanetti L, Salvatore E, Squitieri F, et al. (2011) Whole body cholesterol metabolism is impaired in Huntington's disease. Neurosci Lett 494: 245–9.
52. Valenza M, Leoni V, Karasinska JM, Petricca L, Fan J, et al. (2010) Cholesterol defect is marked across multiple rodent models of Huntington's disease and is manifest in astrocytes. J Neurosci 30: 10844–10850.
53. Salvatore E, Rinaldi C, Tucci T, Di Maio L, Di Somma C, et al. (2011) Growth hormone response to arginine test differentiates between two subgroups of Huntington's disease patients. J Neurol Neurosurg Psychiatry 82: 543–7.
54. Whittier JR (1976) Letter: Asphyxiation, bulimia, and insulin levels in Huntington disease (chorea). JAMA 235: 1423–1424.
55. Peterson A, Hult S, Kirik D (2009) Huntington's Disease :New Perspectives Based on Neuroendocrine Changes in Rodent Models. Neurodegenerative Diseases 6: 154–164.
56. Chadwick W, Martin B, Chapter MC, Park SS, Wang L, et al. (2012). GIT2 acts as a potential keystone protein in functional hypothalamic networks associated with age-related phenotypic changes in rats. PLoS One 7(5):e36975.
57. Middeldorp J, Hol EM (2011) GFAP in health and disease. Prog Neurobiol 93: 421–43.
58. De Sandre-Giovannoli A, Chaouch M, Kozlov S, Vallat JM, Tazir M, et al. (2002) Homozygous defects in LMNA, encoding lamin A/C nuclear-envelope proteins, cause autosomal recessive axonal neuropathy in human (Charcot-Marie-Tooth disorder type 2) and mouse. Am J Hum Genet 70: 726–36.
59. Zhao WQ, Lu B (2007) Expression of annexin A2 in GABAergic interneurons in the normal rat brain. J Neurochem 100: 1211–23.
60. Lalli G (2009) RalA and the exocyst complex influence neuronal polarity through PAR-3 and aPKC. J Cell Sci 122: 1499–506.
61. Lotz GP, Legleiter J, Aron R, Mitchell EJ, Huang SY, et al. (2010) Hsp70 and Hsp40 functionally interact with soluble mutant huntingtin oligomers in a classic ATP-dependent reaction cycle. J Biol Chem 285: 38183–93.
62. Braunstein KE, Eschbach J, Rona-Vörös K, Soylu R, Mikrouli E, et al. (2010) A point mutation in the dynein heavy chain gene leads to striatal atrophy and compromises neurite outgrowth of striatal neurons. Hum Mol Genet 19: 4385–98.
63. Bellinger FP, Bellinger MT, Seale LA, Takemoto AS, Raman AV, et al. (2011) Glutathione peroxidase 4 is associated with neuromelanin in Substantia Nigra and dystrophic axons in putamen of Parkinson's brain. Mol Neurodegener 6: 8.
64. Raza H (2011) Dual localization of glutathione S-transferase in the cytosol and mitochondria: implications in oxidative stress, toxicity and disease. FEBS J 278: 4243–51.
65. Stranahan AM, Lee K, Becker KG, Zhang Y, Maudsley S, et al. (2010) Hippocampal gene expression patterns underlying the enhancement of memory by running in aged mice. Neurobiology of Aging 31: 1937–1949.
66. Irimia JM, Meyer CM, Peper CL, Zhai L, Bock CB, et al. (2010) Impaired Glucose Tolerance and Predisposition to the Fasted State in Liver Glycogen Synthase Knock-out Mice. Journal of Biological Chemistry 285: 12851–12861.
67. Holness MJ, Bulmer K, Smith ND, Sugden MC (2003) Investigation of potential mechanisms regulating protein expression of hepatic pyruvate dehydrogenase kinase isoforms 2 and 4 by fatty acids and thyroid hormone. Biochem J 369: 687–695.
68. Mayers RM, Leighton B, Kilgour E (2005) PDH kinase inhibitors: a novel therapy for Type II diabetes? Biochem Soc Trans 33: 367–370.
69. Spoden GA, Rostek U, Lechner S, Mitterberger M, Mazurek S, et al. (2009) Pyruvate kinase isoenzyme M2 is a glycolytic sensor differentially regulating cell proliferation, cell size and apoptotic cell death dependent on glucose supply. Experimental Cell Research 315. 2765–2774.
70. Takeuchi K, Reue K (2009) Biochemistry, physiology, and genetics of GPAT, AGPAT, and lipin enzymes in triglyceride synthesis. American Journal of Physiology - Endocrinology And Metabolism 296: E1195–E1209.
71. Pohl J, Ring A, Herrmann T, Stremmel W (2004) New concepts of cellular fatty acid uptake: role of fatty acid transport proteins and of caveolae. Proceedings of the Nutrition Society 63: 259–262.
72. López M, Vidal-Puig A (2008) Brain lipogenesis and regulation of energy metabolism. Curr Opin Clin Nutr Metab Care 11: 483–490.
73. Martin B, Shin YK, White CM, Ji S, Kim W, et al. (2010) Vasoactive intestinal peptide-null mice demonstrate enhanced sweet taste preference, dysglycemia, and reduced taste bud leptin receptor expression. Diabetes 59: 1143–52.
74. Martin B, Pearson M, Kebejian L, Golden E, Keselman A, et al. (2007) Sex-dependent metabolic, neuroendocrine, and cognitive responses to dietary energy restriction and excess. Endocrinology 148: 4318–33.
75. Rothman SM, Herdener N, Camandola S, Texel SJ, Mughal MR, et al. (2012) 3×TgAD mice exhibit altered behavior and elevated Aβ after chronic mild social stress. Neurobiol Aging 33: 830.e1–12.
76. Griffiths SD, Burthem J, Unwin RD, Holyoake TL, Melo JV, et al. (2007) The use of isobaric tag peptide labeling (iTRAQ) and mass spectrometry to examine rare, primitive hematopoietic cells from patients with chronic myeloid leukemia. Mol Biotechnol 36: 81–89.
77. Martin B, Brenneman R, Golden E, Walent T, Becker KG (2009) et al. Growth factor signals in neural cells: coherent patterns of interaction control multiple levels of molecular and phenotypic responses. J Biol Chem 284: 2493–511.
78. Chadwick W, Boyle JP, Zhou Y, Wang L, Park SS, et al. (2011) Multiple oxygen tension environments reveal diverse patterns of transcriptional regulation in primary astrocytes. PLoS One 6: e21638.
79. Martin B, Pearson M, Brenneman R, Golden E, Wood W, et al. (2009) Gonadal transcriptome alterations in response to dietary energy intake: sensing the reproductive environment. PLoS One 4: e4146.
80. Chadwick W, Zhou Y, Park SS, Wang L, Mitchell N, et al. (2010) Minimal peroxide exposure of neuronal cells induces multifaceted adaptive responses. PLoS One 5: e14352.
81. Chadwick W, Brenneman R, Martin B, Maudsley S (2010) Complex and multidimensional lipid raft alterations in a murine model of Alzheimer's disease. Int J Alzheimers Dis 604792.
82. Chadwick W, Park SS, Zhou Y, Wang L, Brenneman R, et al. (2011) Repetitive peroxide exposure reveals pleiotropic mitogen-activated protein kinase signaling mechanisms. J Signal Transduct pii: 636951.

10

Investigation of the *In Vitro* Therapeutic Efficacy of Nilotinib in Immortalized Human *NF2*-Null Vestibular Schwannoma Cells

Nesrin Sabha[1], Karolyn Au[1], Sameer Agnihotri[1], Sanjay Singh[1], Rupinder Mangat[1], Abhijit Guha[1,2], Gelareh Zadeh[1,2]*

1 Arthur and Sonia Labatt Brain Tumour Research Centre, Hospital for Sick Children Research Institute, University of Toronto, Toronto, Canada, **2** Department of Surgery (Neurosurgery), Western Hospital, University of Toronto, Toronto, Canada

Abstract

Vestibular schwannomas (VS) are a common posterior fossa brain tumor, and though benign can cause significant morbidity, particularly loss of hearing, tinnitus, vertigo and facial paralysis. The current treatment options for VS include microsurgical resection, stereotactic radiosurgery or close surveillance monitoring, with each treatment option carrying associated complications and morbidities. Most importantly, none of these options can definitively reverse hearing loss or tinnitus. Identification of a novel medical therapy, through the use of targeted molecular inhibition, is therefore a highly desirable treatment strategy that may minimize complications arising from both tumor and treatment and more importantly be suitable for patients whose options are limited with respect to surgical or radiosurgical interventions. In this study we chose to examine the effect of Nilotinib on VS. Nilotinib (Tasigna®) is a second-generation receptor tyrosine kinase (RTK) inhibitor with a target profile similar to that of imatinib (Gleevec®), but increased potency, decreased toxicity and greater cellular and tissue penetration. Nilotinib targets not only the BCR-ABL oncoprotein, but also platelet-derived growth factor (PDGF) receptor signalling. In this preclinical study, the human *NF2*-null schwannoma cell line HEI-193 subjected to nilotinib inhibition demonstrated decreased viability, proliferation and anchorage-independent growth, and increased apoptosis. A daily dose of nilotinib for 5 days inhibited HEI-I93 proliferation at a clinically-relevant concentration in a dose-dependent manner (IC_{50} 3–5 μmol/L) in PDGF-stimulated cells. These anti-tumorigenic effects of nilotinib were correlated to inhibited activation of PDGFR-α and PDGFR-β and major downstream signalling pathways. These experiments support a therapeutic potential for Nilotinib in VS.

Editor: Nikos K. Karamanos, University of Patras, Greece

Funding: Novartis provided Nilotinib and partial funding for this study; grant agreement for academic research - MTA #MTD 33832. Operating funds for AG were provided by the Cancer Research Society (CRS) of Canada. The funders had no role in study design, data collection and analysis, decision to publish, or preparation of the manuscript. No additional external funding received for this study.

Competing Interests: The authors have the following interests to declare: Novartis provided Nilotinib and partial funding for this study. There are no patents, products in development or marked products to declare. This does not alter the authors' adherence to all the PLoS ONE policies on sharing data and materials, as detailed online in the guide for authors.

* E-mail: Gelareh.Zadeh@uhn.on.ca

Introduction

Vestibular schwannomas (VS) are typically slow-growing tumors that arise from the Schwann cell sheath of the vestibulocochlear nerve. Though benign, they can cause significant morbidity through compression of neurologic structures and obstruction of cerebrospinal fluid flow. Effects on the vestibulocochlear nerve result in permanent hearing loss, tinnitus and disequilibrium, and facial nerve compression can cause facial weakness or paralysis and disfiguration. Symptoms leading to diagnosis occur in 0.7–1 per 100 000 and are generally unilateral, although in 5–10% of cases tumors are bilateral and associated with the cancer predisposition syndrome neurofibromatosis type 2 (NF2). Management options include observation, surgical excision and radiosurgery, all of which have significant short- and long-term adverse effects [1–3]. However, for a distinct population of NF2 patients, surgery and radiosurgery are not feasible and no additional therapy is currently available.

The tumor suppressor gene *NF2*, located on chromosome 22 at 22 q12.2, encodes the protein merlin [4], also called schwannomin [5], an ezrin, moesin and radixin (ERM) family protein that associates the actin cytoskeleton with the cell membrane [6]. Schwann cell-specific knockout of merlin in mice leads to initiation of schwannomas [7], likely through loss of inhibition of the AKT [8] and ERK1/2 [9] signalling pathways. These mediators of survival and proliferation are activated by cell surface receptors such as stem cell factor receptor (c-KIT) and platelet-derived growth factor (PDGF) receptor-α and -β, which are over-expressed and over-activated in sporadic and NF2-associated peripheral and vestibular schwannomas [10].

These *in vitro* studies using the immortalized *NF2*-null VS cell line HEI-193 [10] demonstrated that the receptor tyrosine kinase (RTK) inhibitor imatinib mesylate (Gleevec, STI571) decreased the activation of c-KIT, PDGFR-α and PDGFR-β, as well as ERK-1/2, AKT and FAK. Furthermore, imatinib treatment increased apoptosis and cell cycle arrest, while inhibiting cell growth and proliferation and decreasing anchorage-independent growth. While developed as an inhibitor of the kinase activity of the BCR-ABL oncoprotein in chronic myelogenous leukemia (CML) [11,12], the efficacy of imatinib against other RTKs has led to its application as a therapy for several human cancers, including myeloid malignancies [13] and gastrointestinal stromal tumors [14]. The emergence of imatinib-resistant kinase mutants, however, warranted the development of new RTK inhibitors. The compound nilotinib (Tasigna, AMN107) was rationally designed to improve potency and selectivity over imatinib towards the BCR-ABL kinase [15]. Nilotinib is also effective against c-KIT, PDGFR-α, PDGFR-β, and discoidin domain receptor (DDR) −1 and −2 [16], but has a better toxicity profile [17] and greater cellular and tissue penetration [18] than imatinib, this latter consideration of particular significance for chemotherapeutic agents that must penetrate the blood-brain barrier. Nilotinib is currently in clinical use for treatment of imatinib-resistant CML and Philadelphia chromosome-positive acute lymphoblastic leukemia.

In the current study, we chose to investigate the in vitro therapeutic efficacy of nilotinib in the immortalized human NF2-null VS cell line HEI-193 in two different growth conditions: in Schwann cell growth medium (GM) or in media supplemented with PDGF-BB. We demonstrate that activation of PDGFR-α and PDGFR-β was inhibited, as well as their downstream mediators AKT and mTOR. Functional assays demonstrated decreased viability, proliferation and anchorage-independent growth, and increased apoptosis, in a dose-dependent manner. Taken together these results suggest that nilotinib may be a viable option for treatment of patients with vestibular schwannoma.

Materials and Methods

Nilotinib Treatment

HEI-193 is an HPV E6-E7 immortalized human vestibular schwannoma cell line (gift from Marco Giovannini and David Lim: Department of Cell and Molecular Biology, House Ear Institute, Los Angeles, CA), established after they obtained informed patient consent [19]. For cell viability, proliferation and apoptosis experiments, HEI-193 cells were plated at a density of 1×10^3 cells/well in 96-well plates and grown for 24 hours in DMEM supplemented with 10% FBS. Cultures were then incubated with vehicle or nilotinib (Novartis, Switzerland) at concentration 0, 1, 3, 5, 10 or 20 μM for four days in the presence of one of two growth media: 100 ng/mL PDGF-BB (Cell Signaling) in DMEM, or Schwann cell growth medium (GM; [9]) consisting of DMEM, 10% FCS, 0.5 μM forskolin (Sigma), 10 nM β-heregulin, 0.5 mM 3-isobutyl-1-methylxanthine (IBMX; Sigma), and 2.5 μg/mL insulin (Sigma). Media containing nilotinib was refreshed daily, extrapolating from the 18-hour half-life of nilotinib in human serum. Functional assays were carried out on the fifth day as described below.

Viability Assays

HEI-193 cells were plated, grown and incubated with nilotinib as described above. Trypan blue based viable cell counting was done every day for 5 days, or on the fifth day of nilotinib treatment, by using the Vi-CELL Coulter Analyzer (Beckman). The percentage of viable cells is plotted against each dose level and normalized to HEI-193 cells in PDGF-BB or GM with vehicle only. Cell viability was also evaluated by the 3-(4,5-dimethylthiazol-2yl)-5-(3-carboxymethoxyphenyl)-2-(4-sulfophenyl)-2H-tetrazolium (MTS) assay (CellTiter 96 AQueous Assay System; Promega) as well as CellTiter-Fluor™ CelViability Assay (Promega) according to the manufacturer's instructions. MTS labelling reagent was added on the fifth day of nilotinib inhibition, and the absorbance at 490 nm determined following four hours of incubation using plate reader (Versa max, Molecular Devices). CellTiter-Fluor reagent was added for 3 hours on the fifth day of nilotinib inhibition, and the fluorescence was measured according to the manufacturing instructions. The mean of six experimental replicates from three independent experiments was determined for each nilotinib concentration. Statistical analysis was carried out using Student's t-test.

Proliferation Assay

HEI-193 cells were grown and incubated with nilotinib as described above. On the fourth day of nilotinib inhibition, bromodeoxyuridine (BrdU) was added to cell cultures and incubated for the final 18 hours of growth. Cells were fixed and the ELISA carried out according to the manufacturer's instructions (Roche, Switzerland). Sample absorbance was measured at 450 nm. The mean of six experimental replicates from three independent experiments was determined for each nilotinib concentration. Statistical analysis was carried out using Student's t-test.

Apoptosis Assay

HEI-193 cells were plated, grown and incubated with nilotinib as described above. Apoptosis was evaluated using the Apo-One Homogeneous Caspase-3/7 Assay (Promega), with addition of Apo-One reagent at 5 days following the final dose of nilotinib. The reagent was incubated for 6 hours and fluorescence measured according to the manufacturer's instructions (485 nm excitation/527 nm emission). The mean of six experimental replicates from three independent experiments was determined for each nilotinib concentration. Statistical analysis was carried out using Student's t-test.

Cell Cycle Analysis

HEI-193 cells were grown in DMEM supplemented with 10% FBS for 2 days, serum-starved for 24 hours and then inhibited with nilotinib (0, 3, 5, 10, or 20 μM) in PDGF-BB or GM for 2 days. Cell cycle analysis was carried out using propidium iodide (PI; BD Pharmingen) staining and fluorescence-activated cell sorting (FACScan; Becton Dickinson). Cells were fixed with 80% ethanol for 18 hours at 4°C, centrifuged at 1500 rpm, resuspended in solution containing PI (0.1 mg/mL) and RNaseA (2 mg/mL), and incubated for 40 minutes at room temperature. Following repeat centrifugation, cells were resuspended in 500 μL PBS for FACS analysis. Samples were analyzed using CellQuest Pro (Becton Dickinson) software. Sub G_1, G_1, S, G2/M-phase fractions were calculated as the mean of duplicate experiments.

Soft Agar Clonogenic Assay

Growth media containing 0.5% agar was added to the bottom of each 60 mm well. HEI-193 cells (1.0×10^4) were suspended in a mixture of 0.35% low-melting point agar (Cambrex), RPMI 1640 and 10% FBS, and plated over solidified base agar. Either PDGF-BB medium or GM containing vehicle or nilotinib (5, 10 or 20 μM) was added to the agar surface, and changed 5 times per week. Plates were incubated at 37°C for 3 weeks. Colonies growing in the agar were stained with 0.005% crystal violet (Sigma) and visualised using AxioVision (Carl Zeiss, Canada) on an inverted microscope. Clusters larger than 500 μm were counted as discrete colonies, and the maximal diameter of colonies was recorded. The soft agar assay was performed in triplicate, with two independent experiments analyzed by Student's t-test.

Western Blot Analysis

HEI-193 cells grown in DMEM with 10% FBS to 50% confluence, then serum-starved for 24 hours. Cells were treated with vehicle or nilotinib (3, 5, 10 or 20 μM) for 30 minutes or 24 hours, followed by a 10-minute incubation in PDGF-BB medium or GM in the presence or absence of nilotinib.

Ras-GTP was extracted by applying 600 μg of protein to glutathione S-transferase-Ras-binding domain of Raf1 (GST-RBD; Ras Activation Assay Kit, Upstate Biotech). In brief, cells were lysed in Mg^{2+} buffer containing protease (Roche) and phosphatase (Calbiochem) inhibitors and then incubated for 1 hour at 4°C with glutathione-sepharose beads bound to 6.0 μg of GST-RBD. The beads were then washed in lysis buffer, followed by immunoblotting of the supernatant with the anti-Ras antibody (1:2000; Upstate Biotech).

Immunoblotting of activated receptor and other downstream mediators was carried out on whole-cell lysate. In brief, cells inhibited and stimulated as described above were lysed on ice in modified PLC lysis buffer supplemented with protease (Roche) and phosphatase (Calbiochem) inhibitors, and protein concentration determined using BCA assay. Equal quantities of whole-cell lysate were separated on 7% SDS-PAGE gel and transferred to PVDF membrane (NEN) using a semi-dry transfer apparatus (Bio-Rad). Membranes were probed overnight with activation-specific phosphotyrosine antibodies to PDGFR-α (Tyr754, Abcam; 1:500), PDGFR-β (Tyr771, Cell Signaling; 1:250), AKT (Ser473, Cell Signaling; 1:1000), ERK1/2 (Thr202/Tyr204, Cell Signaling; 1:1000), S6 ribosomal protein (Ser240/244, Cell Signaling; 1:1000), and mTOR (Ser2448, Cell Signaling; 1:1000). Total protein expression was determined using non–activation-specific antibodies: PDGFR-α (Cell Signaling; 1:400), PDGFR-β (Cell Signaling; 1:400), AKT (Cell Signaling; 1:1000), ERK1/2 (Cell Signaling; 1:1000), S6 ribosomal protein (Cell Signaling; 1:1000), mTOR (Cell Signaling; 1:1000) and β-actin (Sigma; 1:20,000). Horseradish peroxidase–conjugated secondary antibody (Bio-Rad) was used, with visualization carried out using Chemiluminescence Reagent Plus (Perkin-Elmer). Densitometric analysis was undertaken to determine the ratio of phosphorylated-to-total protein levels. The mean ratio of phosphorylated/total protein as a function of nilotinib dose was analyzed by Student's t-test. All densitometric analyses were undertaken within the linear range with the AlphaEaseFC software. Fold changes were calculated using the vehicle-containing PDGF- or GM-stimulated treatment as a standard value of 1.

Results

Optimal Inhibition Conditions

Initial experiments were carried out to establish concentration of nilotinib which is most tolerated by cells when exposed for longer duration (Fig. 1). Our results show that 3 μM concentration of nilotinib was tolerated by cells for at least 5 days before a significant reduction in viability was observed (1b), and 5 μM for cells grown in GM. This concentration of nilotinib also happens to be clinically relevant, below the mean peak inhibitor concentration (4.27 μM) found in the serum of patients treated for CML [18].

Reduction in Cell Viability and Proliferation

HEI-193 cells grown either in media supplemented with PDGF-BB or in GM were administered daily doses of nilotinib. The lowest concentration of nilotinib which resulted in significant reduction in viable cells for PDGF-BB condition after 5 days treatment, was determined to be 3 μM, by two separate assays, MTS (Fig. 2A) and fluorescent based viability assay (Fig. 2B). Higher concentrations did not provide additional advantage in terms of decreased cell viability except very high (20 μM) concentration of nilotinib.

Decrease in cell viability is also reflected by significant and concomitant decrease in proliferating cells upon treatment with 3 μM nilotinib for 5 days (Fig. 2C). For the cell cultured in GM conditions, a higher nilotinib concentration (5 μM) is effective for significant decrease in cell viability (as shown by two separate assays; Fig. 2A and B) and proliferation (Fig. 2C). A further decrease in viability and proliferation was observed at higher concentrations of nilotinib.

As shown in Fig. 1A and B, cells cultured in PDGF-BB conditions and exposed to 3 μM concentrations of nilotinib was well tolerated for longer time as compared to 20 μM, as well as 5 μM for cells grown in GM (data not shown and Fig. 1c). Nilotinib thus decreased cell viability and proliferation in a manner that is dependent upon drug concentration as well as growth conditions.

Increase in Caspase-dependent Apoptosis

As determined by caspase-3/7 activity assay normalized ratio to cell number, nilotinib induced apoptosis in HEI-193 in a dose-dependent manner. In cultures grown in media containing PDGF-BB, in the presence of ≥3 μM nilotinib, caspase-3/7 activity was significantly increased ($p<0.005$) at 5 days following the final inhibitor dose (Fig. *3a*). When cells grown in GM were assayed for caspase-3/7 activity at 5 days following the final nilotinib dose, an increase in apoptosis ($p<0.005$) was observed at ≥5 μM nilotinib compared to vehicle (Fig. *3a)*.

Induction of Cell Cycle Arrest

To explore the cell cycle status of cells treated with nilotinib, concentration and duration of exposure was selected where control and treated cells were phenotypically comparable (3 μM for 2 days in PDGF and 5 μM for 2 days in GM conditions). Measurement of propidium iodide (PI) staining demonstrated a significant increase ($p<0.05$) in the number of cells in G1 phase following 2 days of nilotinib treatment (Fig. 3*b*). For cells grown in PDGF-BB, this increase was observed in the presence of ≥3 μM nilotinib with no further increase at higher concentrations. This increase in G1 was accompanied by a reduction in the number of cells in S-phase, as well as reduction in the G2/M cycle. An increase in the number of cells in G1 phase, with a corresponding reduction in G2/M-phase cells, was observed in the presence of ≥5 μM nilotinib for cells grown in GM (Fig. 3c), with not statistically changes in the S-phase.

Reduction in Anchorage-independent Growth

HEI-193 cells treated with nilotinib showed a dose-dependent decrease in the number and size of colonies formed in soft agar (Fig. 4*a*). Cells grown in PDGF-BB formed fewer (Fig. 4*b*) and smaller (Fig. 4*c*) colonies in ≥3 μM nilotinib, compared to vehicle. In GM, the presence of ≥5 μM nilotinib reduced the total number (Fig. 4*b*) of colonies formed, as well as their diameter (Fig. 4*c*).

Reduced Activation of Targeted Receptors

HEI-193 cells were pre-treated for 30 minutes with nilotinib of different concentrations prior to stimulation with PDGF-BB or GM. Quantification of phosphorylation-specific immunoblot

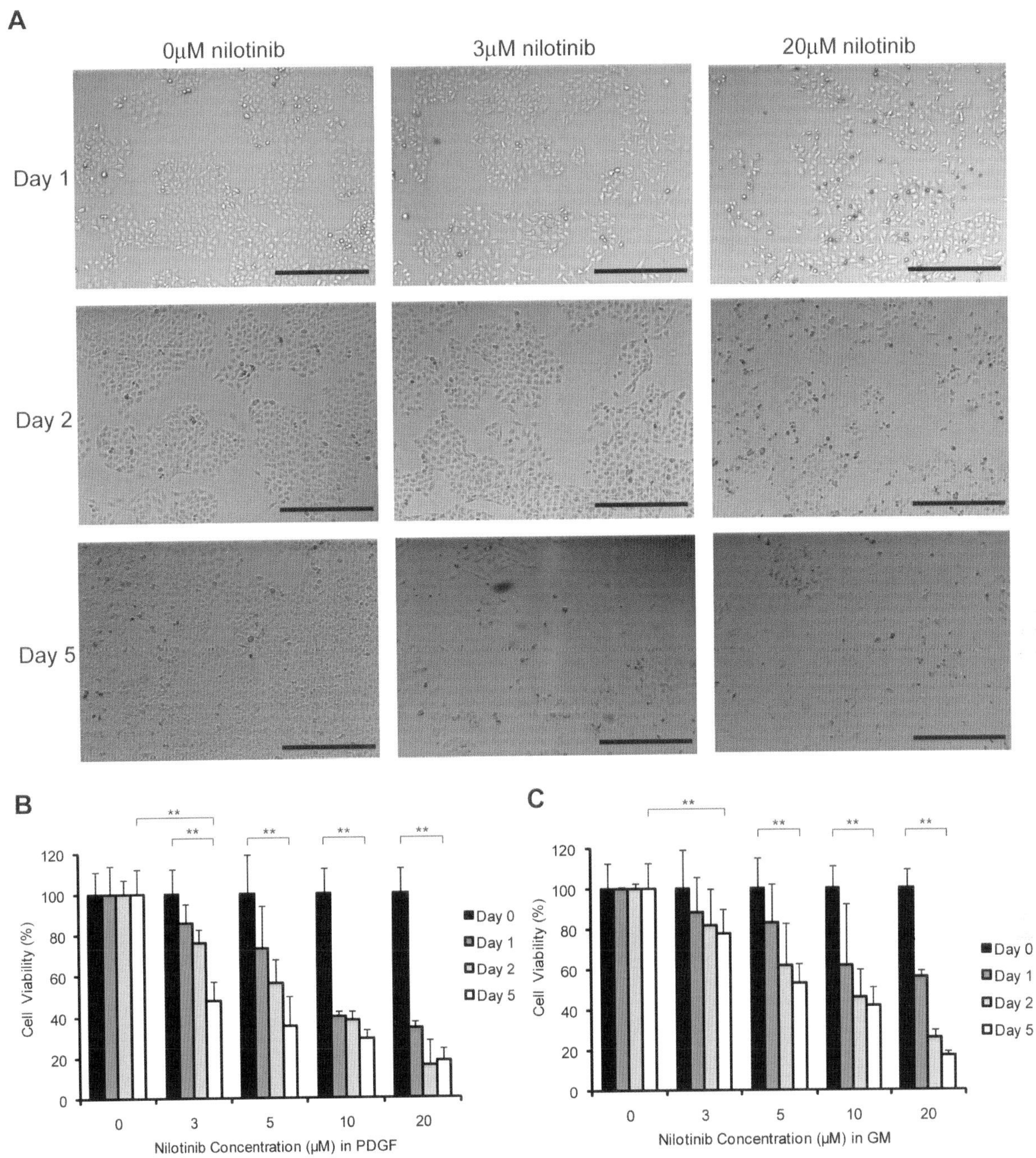

Figure 1. Nilotinib decreases HEI-193 cell viability in a time-, dose-, and growth condition- dependent manner. (A) HEI-193 grown in (PDGF or GM) were treated with 0, 3 or 20 μM nilotinib. Phase contrast microscopy images obtained at 1, 2 and 5 days show fewer cells with increasing nilotinib concentration. Scale bar = 500 μm. (B) HEI-193 grown in PDGF media were treated with 0, 3, 5, 10 or 20 μM nilotinib up to 5 days. Trypan blue viability assay shows decreased number of viable cells at 5 days in 3 μM nilotinib, compared to vehicle shown, mean and SD of six technical replicates. **denotes significant ($p<0.005$) difference between treated and untreated samples. (C) HEI-193 grown in GM were treated with 0, 3, 5 or 20 μM nilotinib up to 5 days. Trypan blue viability assay shows decreased number of viable cells at 5 days in 5 μM nilotinib. Shown, mean and SD of six technical replicates. **denotes significant ($p<0.005$) difference between treated and untreated samples.

assays, normalized to total receptor expression, showed that PDGF-BB stimulation for 10 minutes resulted in high activation of the PDGFR-α and PDGFR-β receptors (Fig. 5a). Stimulation with GM activated PDGFR-β (Fig. 5b); however, phosphorylation of PDGFR-α did not increase above baseline (data not shown). A significant decrease in receptor activation was seen with both PDGF-BB and GM stimulation at nilotinib concentration as low as 3 μM. The expression for total PDGFR-α and PDGFR-β receptors decreased upon stimulation with PDGF-BB, likely due to rapid receptor endocytosis kinetics upon ligand binding.

Inhibition of Downstream Mediators

HEI-193 cells were pre-incubated with nilotinib for 24 hours then stimulated with PDGF-BB or GM for 10 minutes. The

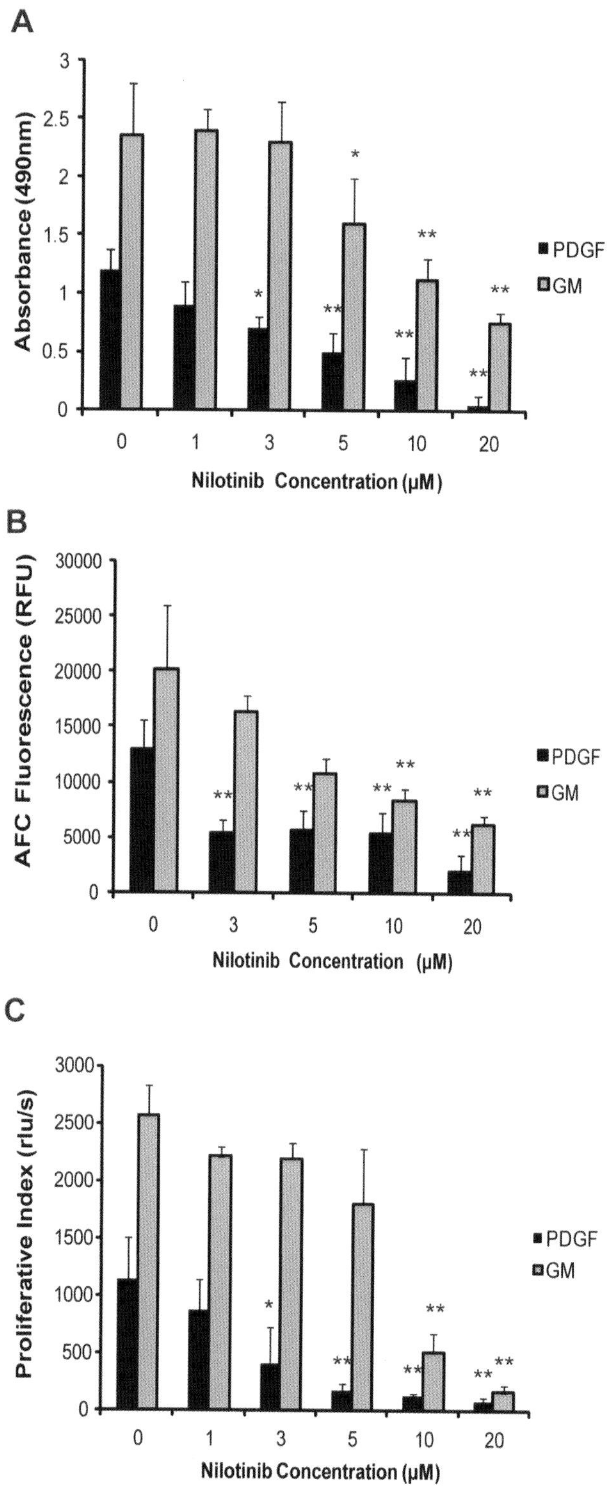

Figure 2. Nilotinib decreases viability and proliferation of HEI-193 cells in a dose-dependent manner. HEI-193 cells grown in PDGF-BB or GM were evaluated after 5 days of treatment with 0, 3, 5, 10 or 20 µM nilotinib. Shown, mean value of six technical replicates. *denotes significant value ($p<0.05$), **denotes significant value ($p<0.005$) (A) Nilotinib decreased absorbance on MTS viability assay in both growth conditions. (B) Compared to cells grown in vehicle control, nilotinib reduced the absorbance on fluorescence viability assay in both growth conditions. (*c*) Proliferation measured by BrdU incorporation was decreased by nilotinib in both growth conditions.

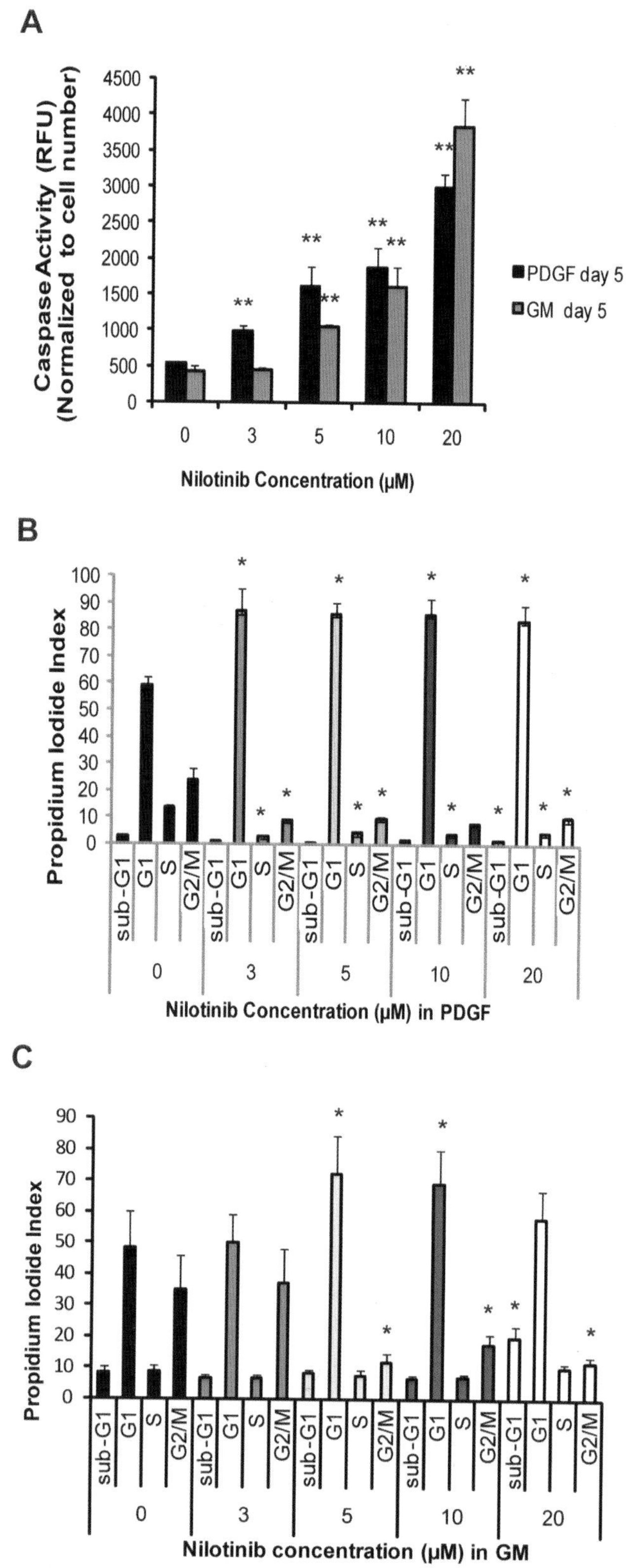

Figure 3. Nilotinib induces apoptosis and cell cycle arrest in HEI-193 cells at clinically-relevant concentrations. (A) HEI-193 cells were treated with 0, 3, 5, 10 or 20 µM nilotinib for 5 days. In PDGF-BB, an increase in caspase-3/7 activity is seen at ≥3 µM; in GM, caspase-3/7 activity is increased at ≥5 µM. Fluorescence signal normalized to number of viable cells. Shown, mean value of six technical replicates. (B) HEI-193 cells were treated with 0, 3, 5, 10 or 20 µM nilotinib for 2 days.

In PDGF-BB-supplemented media, the proportion of cells in G1-phase is increased, and the proportion in S- and G2/M-phase decreased, at all concentrations tested. Shown, mean of two replicate experiments. (C) In GM, the proportion of cells in G1-phase is increased and the proportion in G2/M decreased at ≥5 μM nilotinib. Shown, mean of two replicate experiments.

addition of either PDGF-BB or GM resulted in activation of effectors involved in multiple pro-tumorigenic pathways, including Ras, AKT, mTOR, and S6 ribosomal protein (Fig. *6a, b*). In PDGF-BB media, Nilotinib was effective, in inhibiting activation of AKT at 3 μM, of Ras and mTOR at 5 μM nilotinib. With the addition of GM, activation of Ras was inhibited at 3 μM nilotinib, and of mTOR at 5 μM nilotinib. Decrease of phosphorylation of AKT was seen at 20 μM nilotinib in GM. For both conditions, decrease in phosphorylation of S6 ribomsomal protein was seen at 20 uM of nilotinib and levels of mTOR activity fluctuates as nilotinib concentrations increases (*Fig. 6a*, b), (see discussion). Activation of ERK1/2 was not inhibited by nilotinib to any significant extent (data not shown).

Discussion

Vestibular schwannomas are benign tumors that grow slowly and can often be managed with close observation. In instances of large or growing and symptomatic tumors, surgery or radiosurgery may be indicated, with potential complications and adverse effects. In addition, for a distinct population of NF2 patients, surgery and RT are not feasible and no additional therapy is currently

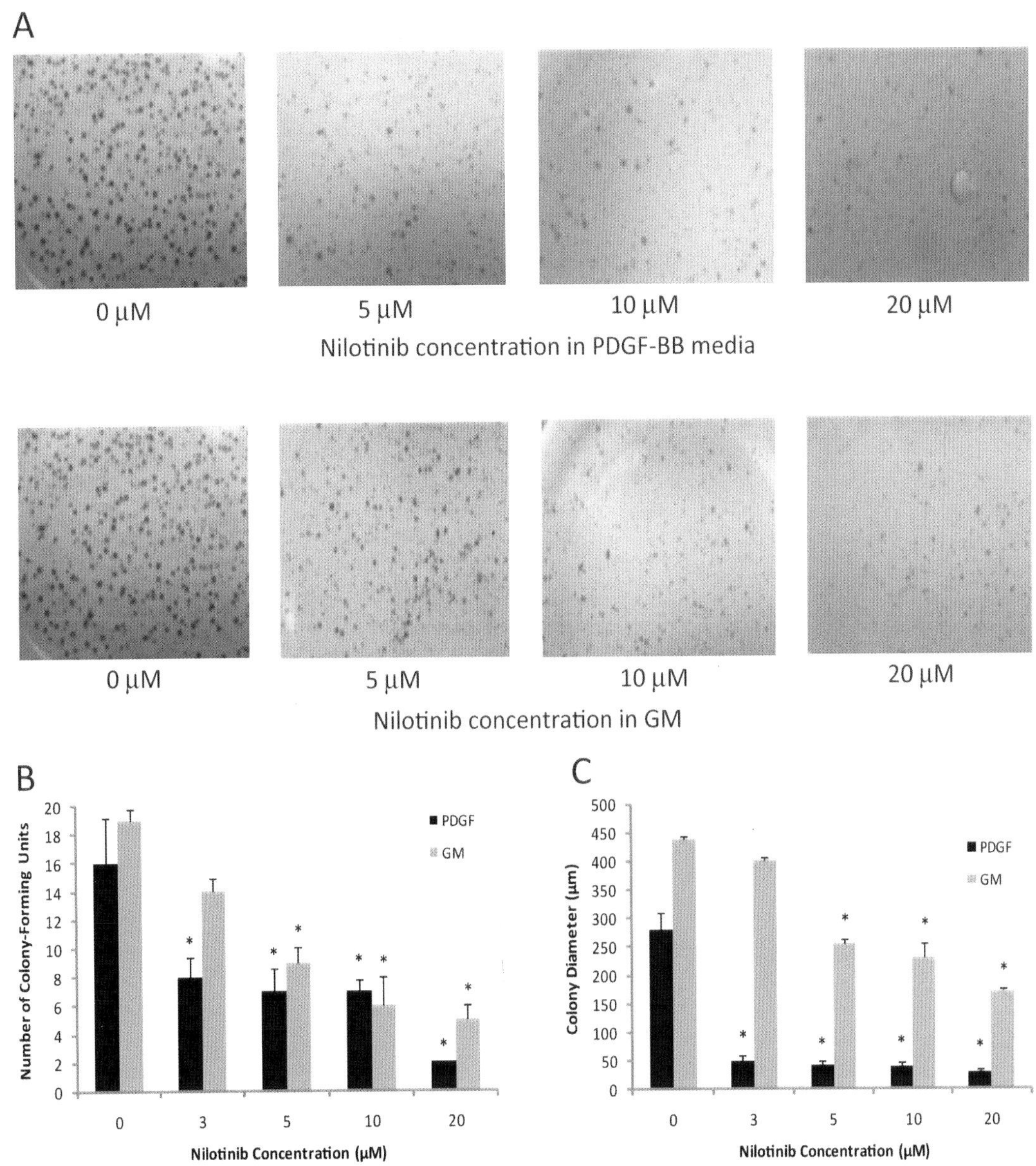

Figure 4. Nilotinib decreases the *in vitro* tumorigenicity of HEI-193 cells. Anchorage-independent growth in soft agar was inhibited in the presence of nilotinib. (A) Visual assessment of agar plates shows qualitative decrease of colony formation by nilotinib. (B) The number of colonies was reduced at ≥3 μM nilotinib in media containing PDGF-BB, and at ≥5 μM in GM. *denotes significant value ($p<0.05$). (C) The mean maximal colony diameter was decreased by nilotinib at ≥3 μM in PDGF-BB media, and at ≥5 μM in GM. *denotes significant value ($p<0.05$).

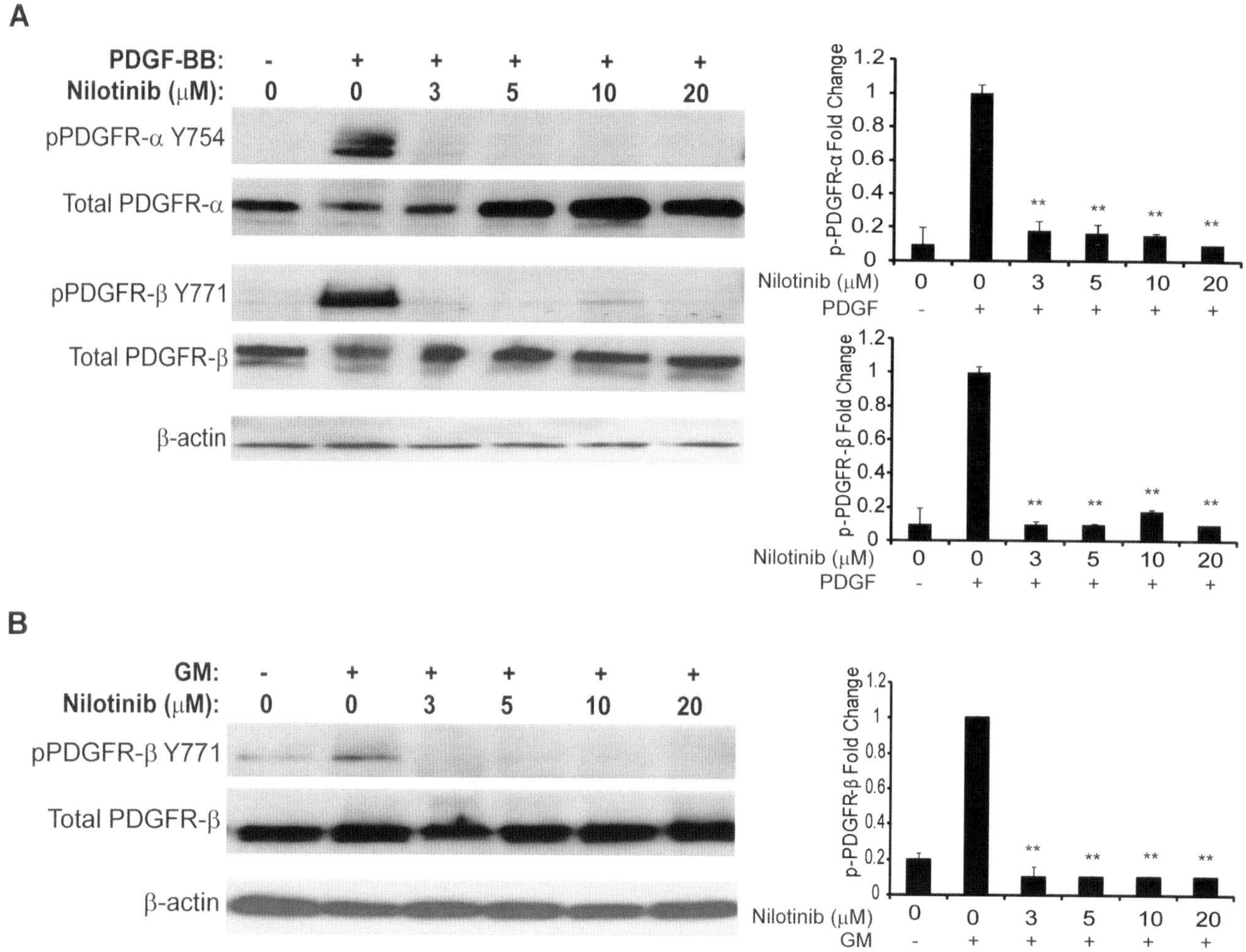

Figure 5. Nilotinib inhibition of HEI-193 cells decreases activation of PDGFR-α and PDGFR-β. HEI-193 cells inhibited with nilotinib and stimulated with PDGF-BB or GM were lysed and analyzed by Western immunoblot using phophorylation-specific antibodies. Comparison was made to total protein expression, as determined by immunoblotting using non-activation specific antibodies. Densitometry was used to evaluate fold-change in phosphorylation, with values normalized to activation in the presence of vehicle control. **denotes significant ($p<0.05$) difference compared to phosphorylation in vehicle control. (A) PDGF-BB activation of both PDGFR-α and PDGFR-β is abrogated in the presence of ≥3 μM nilotinib. (B) GM-stimulated activation of PDGFR-β is inhibited by ≥3 μM nilotinib.

available. Hence, there is a compelling need to identify efficacious and well-tolerated systemic therapy. Such therapy must have minimal adverse effects over the long term, and can ideally be administered at a low dose. The efficacy and utility of targeted tyrosine kinase inhibition was demonstrated by imatinib in the chronic treatment of CML driven by the BCR-ABL oncogene [11,12]. Its sister compound nilotinib also targets BCR-ABL, as well as c-KIT and PDGFRs, and is an appealing candidate for management of VS due to its improved side-effect profile and greater cell and tissue penetration.

Previous studies have demonstrated increased expression and activation of RTKs, particularly PDGFR-β, in human schwannoma specimens and primary schwannoma cells [9,20]. Nilotinib has been shown to reduce proliferation in primary schwannoma cell cultures at concentrations significantly lower than imatinib [20]. These are promising results, but examine PDGFR-β in isolation; as patient-derived schwannomas express and activate both PDGFR isoforms, the paradoxical decreased effect observed at higher nilotinib concentration could be due to increased activation of alternative receptors, such as PDGFR-α. Furthermore, the cell viability maintained at the very low nilotinib concentration (0.5 μM) examined in this study may lead to emergence of resistant mutants over time in a disease that requires life-long treatment.

In contrast, in our study, we aimed to assess the role of PDGFR-α in addition to PDGFR-β. We show that nilotinib administered continuously at 3 μM for five days reduces viability of HEI-193 cells, which results from reduction of proliferation and increase of cell cycle arrest and apoptosis. This prolonged treatment is critical to achieve continuous inhibition of the receptors and to determine whether resistant mutants will arise over time. In addition, nilotinib reduces the number and size of colonies formed in anchorage-independent growth assay. The observed reduction in cell viability and clonogenicity results from nilotinib inhibiting the PDGF-BB-mediated activation of PDGFR- α, PDGFR- β, AKT, and mTOR, which it effects at a concentration below the mean peak inhibitor concentration (4.27 μM) found in the serum of patients treated for CML [18]. Thus, by increasing apoptosis and reducing viability among cells of an established tumor, nilotinib may be able to reduce tumor mass with tolerable systemic toxicity.

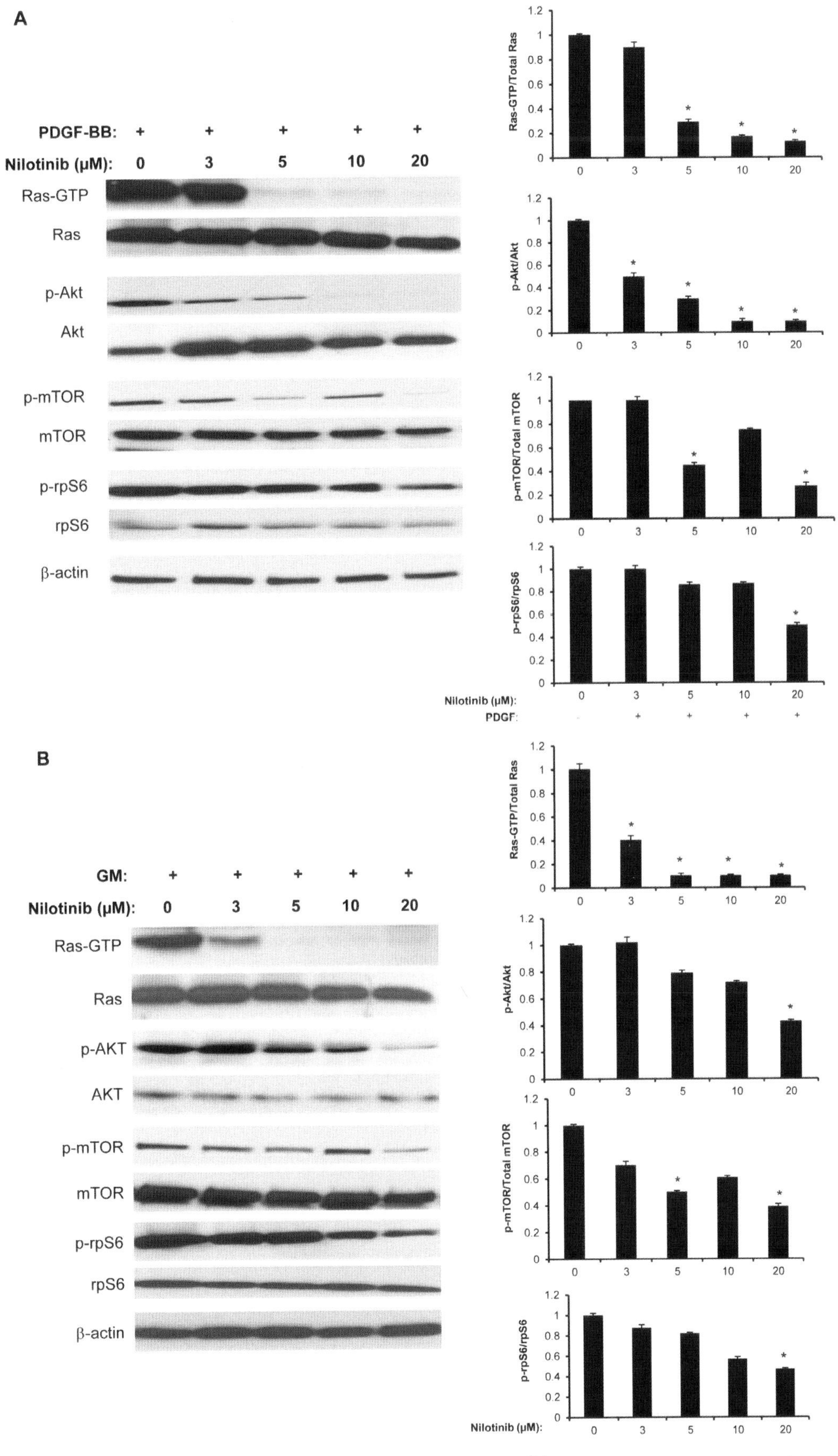
A
PDGF-BB: + + + + +
Nilotinib (μM): 0 3 5 10 20
Ras-GTP
Ras
p-Akt
Akt
p-mTOR
mTOR
p-rpS6
rpS6
β-actin
Ras-GTP/Total Ras
p-Akt/Akt
p-mTOR/Total mTOR
p-rpS6/rpS6
Nilotinib (μM): 0 3 5 10 20
PDGF: - + + + +
B
GM: + + + + +
Nilotinib (μM): 0 3 5 10 20
Ras-GTP
Ras
p-AKT
AKT
p-mTOR
mTOR
p-rpS6
rpS6
β-actin
Ras-GTP/Total Ras
p-Akt/Akt
p-mTOR/Total mTOR
p-rpS6/rpS6
Nilotinib (μM): 0 3 5 10 20
GM: + + + + +

Figure 6. Nilotinib inhibition of HEI-193 decreases signaling downstream of PDGFR. HEI-193 cells inhibited with nilotinib and stimulated with PDGF-BB or GM were lysed and analyzed by Western immunoblot using phophorylation-specific antibodies. Comparison was made to total protein expression, as determined by immunoblotting using non-activation specific antibodies. Densitometry was used to evaluate fold-change in phosphorylation, with values normalized to activation in the presence of vehicle control. *denotes significant ($p<0.05$) difference compared to phosphorylation in vehicle control. (A) PDGF-BB-mediated activation of Ras and AKT are inhibited at low nilotinib concentration. Inhibition of S6 ribosomal protein phosphorylation is seen at high nilotinib concentration, and mTOR phosphorylation is variable with nilotinib concentration. (B) GM-mediated activation of Ras is inhibited at low nilotinib concentration. Inhibition of AKT and S6 ribosomal protein phosphorylation is seen at high nilotinib concentration, and mTOR phosphorylation is variable.

When cells are grown in GM, similar anti-tumorigenic effects are observed, but at slightly higher inhibitor concentration. This difference in sensitivity to nilotinib is likely due to activation of other receptors by factors released from the cells. As strong activation of PDGFR-α is observed only when cells are grown in PDGF-BB, and not in GM, the former better recapitulates the growth environment of schwannomas, which exhibit increased PDGFR-α expression and activation compared to Schwann cells [10].

While the prolonged treatment used in the viability assays demonstrated a sustained inhibition of PDGFR, a trend toward decreased cell viability was observed as early as 24 hours into treatment of cells cultured in PDGF-BB with 3 μM nilotinib, and a significant decrease at 5 days. This correlated with a significant increase in cell cycle arrest, as evidenced by accumulation of cells in G1 phase, observed two days after start of treatment with 3 μM nilotinib, as well as an increase in caspase-3/7 activity at 5 days of treatment. A similar pattern was observed for cells cultured in GM conditions (Fig. 1*c*).

The effect of nilotinib on receptor activation and tumorigenic behavior correlate with its inhibition of PDGF-BB- and GM-stimulated activation of downstream signaling mediators AKT and mTOR. These findings are in keeping with established evidence of the PI3K and mTOR pathways as critical regulators of schwannoma growth [21]. Inhibition of PDGFR-α and -β occurs at a low concentration of 3 μM which leads to inactivation of downstream signaling but at different nilotinib concentrations. While Ras activation is decreased at low nilotinib concentrations, there is no significant effect on ERK1/2 phosphorylation, which is in part explained by the presence of non-PDGFR-mediated means of activating ERK1/2, as previously described in schwannomas [9]. This supports the concept proposed by Ammoun *et al.* [20] that nilotinib may be beneficial as one component in combinatorial therapy. Phosphorylation of AKT is inhibited by 3 μM niltonib in PDGF-BB-stimulated cells, but mTOR activity fluctuates between 3 and 10 μM in both PDGF-BB and GM. This might be due to the regulation of mTOR activity not only at the PDGFR level but also by positive feedback mechanisms downstream of the receptor, such as saturation of PI3K activity [22]. Similarly, Ammoun *et al.* [20] showed that nilotinib at high concentration (10 μM) completely loses effect in down-regulating AKT and ERK1/2. Furthermore, decreased phosphorylation of S6 ribosomal protein is seen only at high nilotinib concentration, indicating the presence of alternative activation pathways further downstream.

One limitation of this study is the use of a single cell line for the investigations. The HEI-193 cell line was derived from a vestibular schwannoma in a NF2 patient, and immortalized with human papilloma E6–E7. A point mutation in NF2 results in a merlin mutant that has attenuated, but not absent, tumor suppressor activity [23]. Nevertheless, as HEI-193 cells have an expression and activation profile for RTK targets of nilotinib similar to human surgical VS specimens [10], it remains a valid model for the functional experiments carried out here and elsewhere. Similar to our work, Fraenzer *et al.* [24] stimulated HEI-193 cells with PDGF to study the effects of NF2 restoration on PDGFR degradation. Using the PDGF and GM stimulation strategy previously shown [9,20,24], we established the *in vivo* PDGFR receptor status in order to understand the mechanisms of nilotinib-mediated effect.

In summary, these *in vitro* results support the anti-tumorigenic activity of nilotinib in human vestibular schwannoma cells. These preclinical results provide the basis to support testing Nilotinib as potential biological therapy for growing VS. Given that there is demonstrated safety and tolerability of Nilotinib through extensive clinical experience with this compound in other tumor types, it would be safe to proceed with clinical studies testing the efficacy of Nilotinib in growing VS.

Acknowledgments

This work is dedicated in memory of Dr Abhijit Guha, who passed away on November 8, 2011. We thank Dr David Lim and Dr Marco Giovannini (Department of Cell and Molecular Biology, House Ear Institute, Los Angeles, CA) for providing the HEI-193 cells.

Author Contributions

Conceived and designed the experiments: NS AG GZ. Performed the experiments: NS. Analyzed the data: NS. Contributed reagents/materials/analysis tools: KA SA SS RM. Wrote the paper: NS KA AG GZ.

References

1. Balasubramaniam A, Shannon P, Hodaie M, Laperriere N, Michaels H, et al. (2007) Glioblastoma multiforme after stereotactic radiotherapy for acoustic neuroma: case report and review of the literature. Neuro-Oncology 9: 447–53.
2. Johnson WD, Loredo LN, Slater JD (2008) Surgery and radiotherapy: complementary tools in the management of benign intracranial tumors. Neurosurg Focus 24: E2.
3. Martin TPC, Tzifa K, Kowalski C, Holder RL, Walsh R, et al. (2008) Conservative versus primary surgical treatment of acoustic neuromas: a comparison of rates of facial nerve and hearing preservation. Clin Otolaryngology 33: 228–235.
4. Trofatter JA, MacCollin MM, Rutter JL, Murrell JR, Duyao MP, et al. (1993) A novel moesin-, ezrin-, radixin-like gene is a candidate neurofibromatosis 2 tumor suppressor. Cell 72: 791–800.
5. Rouleau GA, Merel P, Lutchman M, Sanson M, Zucman J, et al. (1993) Alteration in a new gene encoding a putative membrane-organizing protein causes neuro-fibromatosis type 2. Nature 363: 515–521.
6. Bretscher A, Edwards K, Fehon RG (2002) ERM proteins and merlin: integrators at the cell cortex. Nat Rev Mol Cell Biol 3: 586–99.
7. Giovannini M, Robanus-Maandag E, van der Valk M, Niwa-Kawakita M, Abramowski V, et al. (2000) Conditional biallelic *Nf2* mutation in the mouse promotes manifestations of human neurofibromatosis type 2. Genes Dev 14: 1617–1630.
8. Rong R, Tang X, Gutmann DH, Ye K (2004) Neurofibromatosis 2 (NF2) tumor suppressor merlin inhibits phosphatidylinositol 3-kinase through binding to PIKE-L. Proc Natl Acad Sci USA 101: 18200–5.
9. Ammoun S, Flaiz C, Ristic N, Schuldt J, Hanemann CO (2008) Dissecting and targeting the growth factor-dependent and growth factor-independent extracellular signal-regulated kinase pathway in human schwannoma. Cancer Res 68: 5236–5245.
10. Mukherjee J, Kamnasaran D, Balasubramaniam A, Radovanovic I, Zadeh G, et al. (2009) Human schwannomas express activated platelet-derived growth factor

receptors and c-KIT and are growth inhibited by Gleevec (imatinib mesylate). Cancer Res 69: 5099–5107.

11. Druker BJ, Talpaz M, Resta D, Peng B, Buchdunger E, et al. (2001) Efficacy and safety of a specific inhibitor of the BCR-ABL tyrosine kinase in chronic myeloid leukemia. NEJM 344: 1031–7.
12. Druker BJ, Sawyers CL, Kantarjian H, Resta DJ, Fernandes Reese S, et al. (2001) Activity of a specific inhibitor of the BCR-ABL tyrosine kinase in the blast crisis of chronic myeloid leukemia and acute lymphoblastic leukemia with the Philadelphia chromosome. NEJM 344: 1038–42.
13. Apperley JF, Gardembas M, Melo JV, Russell-Jones R, Bain BJ, et al. (2002) Response to imatinib mesylate in patients with chronic myeloproliferative diseases with rearrangements of the platelet-derived growth factor receptor beta. NEJM 347: 481–7.
14. Demetri GD, von Mehren M, Blanke CD, Van den Abbeele AD, Eisenberg B, et al. (2002) Efficacy and safety of imatinib mesylate in advanced gastrointestinal stromal tumors. NEJM 347: 472–80.
15. Weisberg E, Manley PW, Breitenstein W, Bruggen J, Cowan-Jacob SW, et al. (2005) Characterization of AMN107, a selective inhibitor of native and mutant BCR-ABL. Cancer Cell 7: 129–141.
16. Manley PW, Drueckes P, Fendrich G, Furet P, Liebetanz J, et al. (2010) Extended kinase profile and properties of the protein kinase inhibitor Nilotinib. Biochim Biophys Acta 1804: 445–453.
17. Kantarjian H, Giles F, Wunderle L, Bhalla K, O'Brien S, et al. (2006) Nilotinib in imatinib-resistant CML and Philadelphia chromosome-positive ALL. NEJM 354: 2542–51.
18. Tanaka C, Yin OQP, Sethuraman V, Smith T, Wang X, et al. (2010) Clinical pharmacokinetics of the BCR-ABL tyrosine kinase inhibitor nilotinib. Clinical Pharmacol Ther 87: 197–203.
19. Hung G, Li X, Faudoa R, Xeu Z, Kluwe L, et al. (2002) Establishment and characterization of a schwannoma cell line from a patient with neurofibromatosis 2. Int J Oncol. Mar; 20(3): 475–82.
20. Ammoun S, Schmid M, Triner J, Manley P, Clemens Oliver Hanemann (2011) Nilotinib alone or in combination with selumetinib is a drug candidate for neurofibromatosis type 2. Neuro-Oncology 13(7): 759–766.
21. James MF, Han S, Polizzano C, Plotkin SR, Manning BD, et al. (2009) NF2/Merlin is a novel negative regulator of mTOR Complex 1, and activation of mTORC1 is associated with meningioma and schwannoma growth. Mol Cell Bio 29: 4250–61.
22. Park CS, Schneider IC, Haugh JM (2003) Kinetic analysis of platelet-derived growth factor receptor/phosphoinositide 3-kinase/Akt signaling in fibroblasts. J Biol Chem 278: 37064–72.
23. Lepont P, Stickney JT, Foster LA, Meng JJ, Hennigan RF, et al. (2008) Point mutation in the NF2 gene of HEI-193 human schwannoma cells results in the expression of a merlin isoform with attenuated growth suppressive activity. Mutat Res. 1; 637(1–2): 142–51.
24. Fraenzer JT, Pan H, Minimo L, Jr, Smith GM, Knauer D, et al. (2003) Overexpression of the NF2 gene inhibits schwannoma cell proliferation through promoting PDGFR degradation. Int J Oncol. 23(6): 1493–500.

Regional Brain Differences in Cortical Thickness, Surface Area and Subcortical Volume in Individuals with Williams Syndrome

Shashwath A. Meda[1], Jennifer R. Pryweller[2], Tricia A. Thornton-Wells[1]*

1 Department of Molecular Physiology and Biophysics, Center for Human Genetics and Research, Vanderbilt University, Nashville, Tennessee, United States of America, 2 Interdisciplinary Studies in Neuroimaging of Neurodevelopmental Disorders, The Graduate School, Vanderbilt University, Nashville, Tennessee, United States of America

Abstract

Williams syndrome (WS) is a rare genetic neurodevelopmental disorder characterized by increased non-social anxiety, sensitivity to sounds and hypersociability. Previous studies have reported contradictory findings with regard to regional brain variation in WS, relying on only one type of morphological measure (usually volume) in each study. The present study aims to contribute to this body of literature and perhaps elucidate some of these discrepancies by examining concurrent measures of cortical thickness, surface area and subcortical volume between WS subjects and typically-developing (TD) controls. High resolution MRI scans were obtained on 31 WS subjects and 50 typically developing control subjects. We derived quantitative regional estimates of cortical thickness, cortical surface area, and subcortical volume using FreeSurfer software. We evaluated between-group ROI differences while controlling for total intracranial volume. In post-hoc exploratory analyses within the WS group, we tested for correlations between regional brain variation and Beck Anxiety Inventory scores. Consistent with our hypothesis, we detected complex patterns of between-group cortical variation, which included lower surface area in combination with greater thickness in the following cortical regions: post central gyrus, cuneus, lateral orbitofrontal cortex and lingual gyrus. Additional cortical regions showed between-group differences in one (but not both) morphological measures. Subcortical volume was lower in the basal ganglia and the hippocampus in WS versus TD controls. Exploratory correlations revealed that anxiety scores were negatively correlated with gray matter surface area in insula, OFC, rostral middle frontal, superior temporal and lingual gyrus. Our results were consistent with previous reports showing structural alterations in regions supporting the socio-affective and visuospatial impairments in WS. However, we also were able to effectively capture novel and complex patterns of cortical differences using both surface area and thickness. In addition, correlation results implicate specific brain regions in levels of anxiety in WS, consistent with previous reports investigating general anxiety disorders in the general population.

Editor: Yong He, Beijing Normal University, Beijing, China

Funding: This research was supported by the following grants: National Institute of Health Roadmap for Medical Research, Grant T32 MH075883; National Institutes of Health/National Institute of Child Health and Development P30-HD15052 to the Vanderbilt Kennedy Center, National Center for Research Resources (Vanderbilt Clinical and Translational Science Award grant 1-UL1-RR024975); National Institute of Mental Health K01-MH083052; a Vanderbilt University Discovery Grant, and National Institute of Aging P30AG036445-01. The funders had no role in study design, data collection and analysis, decision to publish, or preparation of the manuscript.

Competing Interests: The authors have declared that no competing interests exist.

* E-mail: t.thornton-wells@vanderbilt.edu

Introduction

Williams syndrome (WS) is a rare genetic neurodevelopmental disorder caused by a microdeletion of approximately 25 genes on chromosome 7q11.23. WS is associated with a unique behavioral and cognitive profile, which involves mild to moderate intellectual disability. Individuals with WS often demonstrate increased non-social anxiety and phobias, paired with hypersociability and heightened empathy. In social interactions, persons with WS are often impulsive, lack social inhibition and have a lack of fear of strangers [1,2,3]. The WS cognitive profile is characterized by deficits in visuospatial, motor and visuomotor abilities and relative strengths in face and object recognition, expressive language and music processing skills [3,4,5,6,7].

Over the past 10–15 years, several structural and functional neuroimaging studies have characterized brain anatomical differences in WS and have identified putative neural correlates for specific aspects of the WS phenotype. Post-mortem and *in vivo* structural studies have shown a global reduction in brain volume [8,9,10,11]. The literature also describes a higher ratio of frontal to posterior cerebral volume in WS compared to typically developing (TD) controls [8]. Previous magnetic resonance imaging (MRI) studies that employed automated methods, such as voxel-, tensor- or deformation-based morphometry, consistently showed reduced grey matter volume in the intraparietal sulcus, occipitoparietal sulcus, brain stem and occipital lobe regions in WS versus TD controls [12,13,14,15]. Other regional differences, such as in the orbitofrontal cortex (OFC), superior temporal gyrus, insula and the anterior cingulate cortex are often reported inconsistently across studies, with some studies reporting greater grey matter volume and others reporting less or no differences [9,10,12,13,14,15]. More recent studies have used surface- and mesh-based analyses to measure sulcal and gyral pattern differences in WS. Gaser et al. [16] used an automated measure of gyrification and found greater gyrification in the cuneus, occipital and medial frontal lobes in the WS group versus TD controls. A surface-based analysis by Van Essen et al. [17] reported reductions in sulcal depth in the cingulate, frontal operculum, and anterior and posterior intraparietal regions, along with increases in sulcal depth in the hippocampus, cuneus, angular gyrus, superior temporal gyrus, medial frontal gyri, and parieto-occipital regions.

Several studies have now reported using diffusion tensor imaging (DTI) to detect differences in white matter (WM) structure and connectivity. Marenco and colleagues [18] analyzed a unique subset of high functioning WS individuals and found significant differences in fiber orientation underlying the posterior regions of the brain. Hoeft et al. [19] investigated the integrity of the superior and inferior longitudinal fasciculi that connect the fronto-parietal and the temporo-parietal brain systems respectively and found increased fractional anisotropy in WS relative to normal individuals. Furthermore, this increase in anisotropy was associated with visuo-spatial deficits in WS [19]. Arlinghaus and colleagues [20] used tract-based DTI in WS and found decreased structural connectivity between regions previously reported to have morphometric differences in the WS brain, primarily in posterior regions. Most recently, Avery et al. [21] reported alterations in the structural integrity of the prefrontal-amydala white matter pathway might underlie the altered emotional reactivity and the heightened non-social fear and anxiety observed in WS.

Although a substantial body of literature exists to characterize anatomical brain differences in WS, few studies have made simultaneous, within-subject measurement of distinct morphological traits. Discrepant or lack of significant findings may be due to the likelihood that the brain volume phenotype is a combination of at least two genetically and developmentally independent traits: cortical surface area and cortical thickness [22,23]. In order to disentangle this potential confound, we made concurrent regional cortical measurements of surface area and thickness. However, for subcortical regions, we instead used brain volume as the most appropriate measure. We hypothesized that concurrent measures of surface area and thickness would increase the sensitivity and specificity of cortical morphometric measurement and better characterize complex patterns of structural brain differences in WS, informing how those findings relate to particular aspects of the WS cognitive and behavioral phenotype [22].

Individuals with WS have preserved face and object recognition but impaired visuospatial processing, implicating a specific impairment in the dorsal (versus ventral) stream of processing. Reports from high resolution structural imaging studies, as well as from functional MRI (fMRI) studies have confirmed the anatomical specificity of these findings [14,24]. Moreover, structural studies have also found regional alterations in brain regions governing visuospatial functioning in WS. Reiss et al. [15] used an automated voxel based morphometry method to identify decreases in gray matter volume in several areas including the superior parietal, cuneus and the middle occipital gyrus in individuals with WS. Also, the prior mentioned DTI study by Arlinghaus and colleagues [20] provides support for poor white matter integrity in tracts connecting visuo-spatial regions in WS. Thus, we expected to find cortical differences in areas related to visuospatial processing and visuomotor abilities, such as the cuneus, superior parietal, inferior parietal, premotor and other occipital regions.

Many individuals with WS have increased auditory sensitivities, heightened empathy, and with an increased emotional response and interest in music [25,26,27,28]). MRI studies have implicated functional differences in the auditory cortex as well as emotional brain regions, such as the amygdala, insula and posterior cingulate [29,30]. One study also found evidence for altered auditory processing that might involve cross-modal sensory connections between auditory (temporal) and visual (occipital) cortices [30]. Morphometric studies have also implicated increased GM volume in the superior temporal gyrus and left planum temporale with the WS musical phenotype [10,31]. Given the above evidence, we hypothesized that we would observe morphological differences in temporal and limbic lobe regions related to the unique behavioral phenotype of WS.

Several fMRI studies have looked at WS from a social cognition perspective [32,33,34]. One study found that WS subjects had increased activation in the amygdala in response to threatening scenes but a blunted response to threatening faces and concluded that abnormal interactions between the OFC and amygdala are a possible neural basis for dysregulated social behavior in WS [32]. Supporting this particular functional finding, a recent DTI study found reduced integrity of WM tracts between the OFC and amygdala in WS versus TD controls [21]. In the current study, we further explored this putative neural correlate of anxiety and tested for correlations between morphometric measures and scores on the Beck Anxiety Inventory. Based on prior research, we predicted that anxiety scores would be significantly correlated with structural morphological measures in the frontal-amygdala circuit, anterior cingulate, OFC and insula [33,35,36]. We expected to detect specific structural alterations in additional regions governing emotional regulation and social cognition, such as the amygdala, OFC and medial frontal gyrus.

Many individuals with WS are impulsive and qualify as having attention deficit disorder. In a recent study by Mobbs et al. [5], subjects with WS demonstrated poor response inhibition in a Go/NoGo task and showed gross hypofunction of the basal ganglia system relative to TD subjects. Other behavioral studies have documented visuomotor deficits that support anecdotal reports of difficulty with balance, coordination and gait [6,7]. Given these findings, we further hypothesized there would be differences in the basal ganglia circuit.

Materials and Methods

The current study included 31 WS subjects (20 males; mean age 26.3) and 50 TD control subjects (27 males; mean age 28). WS participants were recruited through the annual Academy of Country Music Lifting Lives Music Camp, which is organized by the Vanderbilt Kennedy Center. All WS participants exhibited the physical, cognitive and behavioral profile of WS and previously had received a clinical diagnosis of WS and confirmatory genetic testing. TD controls were recruited using flyers and website postings with IRB-approved language targeting healthy individuals from the general population. Although many WS subjects are literate, to allow for consistent administration, regardless of reading level, the Beck Anxiety Inventory was administered to each WS participant by reading the items out loud and asking for a verbal response, which was then recorded by the trained interviewer. The two groups were tested for differences in age and sex, using an independent samples t-test and a chi-square test, respectively. Demographic characteristics along with their corresponding statistical values are detailed in Table 1.

High resolution 3D T1-weighted MRI scans were obtained on a 3T Philips Achieva scanner housed at the Vanderbilt University Institute of Imaging Science (Nashville, TN) with the following parameters: field of view = 256×256 mm^2; in plane voxel

Table 1. Sample summary statistics.

	TD (N = 50)	WS (N = 31)	Group Contrasts	
	Mean (SD)	**Mean (SD)**	**t**	**p-value**
Age (years)	28.0 (9.0)	26.3 (7.7)	0.41	0.74
Intracranial Volume (Z norm)	0.46 (0.84)	−0.75 (0.74)	6.6	4.20E-09
Beck Anxiety Inventory	-	6.5 (6.2)	-	-
	N (%)	**N (%)**	**Chi-square**	**p-value**
Male Sex	27 (54)	20 (64)	0.35	0.24

Group means and standard deviations for age, total intracranial brain volume estimates, and Beck Anxiety Inventory scores (in WS only), along with test statistics for between-group analyses are provided. Proportion of males is also reported by group.

resolution = 1×1 mm^2; TR = 8.9 ms; TE = 4.6 ms; flip angle = 8°; slice thickness = 1 mm and 170 slices with no slice gap. TD control subjects and caregivers of individuals with WS gave informed consent, while participants with WS gave assent. The study was approved by the Vanderbilt University Institutional Review Board. We used an automated, non-biased atlas-based Bayesian segmentation procedure, applied in Freesurfer v.5.0 (http://surfer.nmr.mgh.harvard.edu/), to derive quantitative estimates of brain structure and to label cortical and subcortical tissue classes [37,38,39]. Freesurfer processing for volumetric T1-weighted images included: motion correction, brain extraction and removal of non-brain tissue using a hybrid watershed/surface deformation procedure [40]; automated spatial transformation and WM segmentation of subcortical volumetric structures [41]; intensity normalization, tessellation of GM/WM boundary and automated topology correction [42]; and surface deformation following intensity gradients to optimally place GM/WM and GM/CSF borders at the location where the greatest shift in intensity defines the transition to the other tissue class [37]. Image outputs from each stage of Freesurfer processing were visually inspected and edited by an experienced imaging analyst (S.M.).

Quantitative estimates were derived in a large set of spatially distinct region of interests (ROIs) that covered the whole brain [38]. Surface area and cortical thickness were estimated for cortical areas, and GM volume was estimated for subcortical ROIs. We also measured total intracranial volume (ICV). All ROI measures were normalized to a Z-score before evaluating between-group differences using a general linear model (MANCOVA) with ICV as a covariate and group status (WS versus TD) as the independent factor. The significance threshold was adjusted using the Benjamin-Hochberg false discovery rate (FDR; $q<0.05$) correction for multiple comparisons. Exploratory analyses were conducted to test for correlations between regional brain variations and Beck Anxiety Inventory scores using Pearson correlation statistics. Anxiety scores were not available for TD controls; therefore, correlation tests were only conducted within the WS group. Analyses were limited to brain regions that showed significant between-group differences. Due to the exploratory nature of the correlation analysis, results are reported at an unadjusted p-value<0.05.

Results

There were no significant group differences in age or sex (see Table 1). For all cortical regions showing significant group differences in morphology, we observed a consistent pattern of lower surface area (SA) and greater cortical thickness (CT), although in some cases, only one measure reached significance for a given ROI. The cortical regions with significantly lower SA and significantly greater CT in the WS group compared to the TD control group included the left cuneus, left lateral OFC, right lingual gyrus, and bilateral postcentral gyrus. Only one region—the left temporal pole—showed significantly higher SA and significantly lower CT in WS versus TD controls. Additional regions were significantly different only for SA (21 ROIs lower in WS) or only for CT (4 ROIs greater in WS). Table 2 presents the test statistics and p-values for all regions showing a significant group difference in morphology at either SA or CT, along with annotations of morphological results from prior studies for these same ROIs. Figures 1 and 2 depict significant between group differences in cortical surface area and cortical thickness ROI measurements, respectively, overlaid on a standard reference brain. Figure 3 shows subcortical volume differences in the form of scatter plots.

Exploratory correlation analyses identified several brain ROIs correlated with anxiety scores, such that higher anxiety scores were associated with lower regional surface area or thickness. In the WS group, surface area was negatively correlated with Beck Anxiety Inventory scores in the left and right insula, left precentral gyrus, left rostral middle frontal gyrus, left superior temporal lobe, left superior frontal lobe, right lateral OFC and right lingual gyrus, such that higher anxiety scores were related to lower surface area. In contrast, cortical thickness was positively correlated with anxiety scores in the postcentral gyrus, such that higher anxiety scores were associated with greater cortical thickness. It is important to note that while these correlation trends are interesting and have good face validity, none would have survived correction for multiple comparisons and, thus, should be interpreted with caution. Table 3 details all nominally significant correlations.

Discussion

Using simultaneous ROI measures of cortical surface area, cortical thickness and subcortical volume, we were able to investigate complex patterns in brain morphological differences in WS relative to TD control subjects. Further, we explored brain-behavior relationships to identify possible neural correlates of anxiety in this genetically-driven disorder.

One of the most striking phenotypic features of WS is the characteristic hypersociability, paired with heightened empathy and a lack of fear of strangers. However, this pattern of over-friendliness is also accompanied by increased non-social anxiety [3]. An fMRI study by Meyer-Lindenberg et al. [32] examined the

Table 2. Complete list of cortical ROIs with significant group differences in surface area and/or thickness.

		Current Study						Prior Studies		
		Surface Area			Thickness			[11,12,14,15]	[16]	[17]
Cortical ROI	Hemi-sphere	F	FDR q value	Higher(+) or Lower(−) in WS	F	FDR q value	Higher(+) or Lower(−) in WS	Volume/ Concen-tration	Gyrifi-cation	Sulcal Depth
Caudal Anterior Cingulate	R	6.38	**4.05E-02**	**−**	0.21	NS	+		+	+
Caudal Middle Frontal Gyrus	R	14.49	**1.70E-03**	**−**	0.98	NS	+			
Cuneus	L	15.08	**1.41E-03**	**−**	7.84	**2.07E-02**	**+**	−[15]	+	−
	R	0.21	NS	−	9.14	**1.16E-02**	**+**		+	−
Inferior Parietal Cortex	R	22.41	**9.34E-05**	**−**	1.98	NS	+			+
Insular Cortex	L	9.95	**8.14E-03**	**−**	0.27	NS	+	+[11,15], −[15]		−
	R	20.17	**2.21E-04**	**−**	1.65	NS	+			−
Lateral Orbital Frontal Cortex	L	18.02	**4.46E-04**	**−**	2.34	NS	+	+[11],−[14,15]		
	R	11.1	**5.16E-03**	**−**	10.64	**6.25E-03**	**+**	+[11], −[14]		
Lingual Gyrus	L	31.85	**3.84E-06**	**−**	2.66	NS	+			
	R	31.6	**3.86E-06**	**−**	6.97	**3.03E-02**	**+**			
Medial Orbital Frontal Cortex	R	0.48	NS	−	11.9	**4.15E-03**	**+**			−
	L	0.43	NS	−	12.29	**3.78E-03**	**+**			−
Parahippocampal gyrus	R	11.82	**4.17E-03**	**−**	0.2	NS	+	−[15]		−
	L	7.33	**2.62E-02**	**−**	3.66	NS	+	−[15]		−
Pars Opercularis	R	13.19	**2.75E-03**	**−**	0.69	NS	+			+
	L	18.84	**3.64E-04**	**−**	2.44	NS	+			+
Pars Triangularis	R	32.92	**3.19E-06**	**−**	0.01	NS	+			
	L	18.65	**3.76E-04**	**−**	0.73	NS	+			
Pericalcarine Cortex	R	18.23	**4.26E-04**	**−**	0.17	NS	+			+
Postcentral Gyrus	L	10.09	**7.77E-03**	**−**	13.61	**2.34E-03**	**+**	−[11], +[15]	+	−
	R	15.07	**1.00E-03**	**−**	9.43	**1.02E-02**	**+**	−[11,15], +[15]	+	
Posterior Cingulate Cortex	R	11.45	**4.84E-03**	**−**	0.73	NS	+		+	+
Precentral Gyrus	L	30.59	**5.17E-06**	**−**	0.1	NS	+		+	
	R	12.1	**3.87E-03**	**−**	0.44	NS	+		+	
Rostral Middle Frontal Gyrus	L	10.52	**6.49E-03**	**−**	1.05	NS	+			
Superior Frontal Gyrus	L	11.12	**5.38E-03**	**−**	0.27	NS	+	−[15]		
Superior Parietal Cortex	L	40.33	**1.08E-06**	**−**	1.67	NS	+	−[11,12,14,15]		−
	R	39.53	**7.08E-07**	**−**	1.07	NS	+	−[11,15]		−
Temporal Pole	L	7.21	**2.74E-02**	**+**	6.16	**4.37E-02**	**−**			
Transverse Temporal Gyrus	L	0.01	NS	−	12.76	**3.23E-03**	**+**			−

neural correlates of social cognition abnormalities in WS and found a deficient negative feedback circuit between OFC and amygdala that might underlie non-social anxiety and social disinhibition in WS. Avery et al. [21] found structural connectivity differences between amygdala and OFC that support the anxiety-related phenotype of WS. Morphometric findings in the OFC for WS have been inconsistent, with some reports of increases [14] and other reports of decreases in OFC volume in WS versus controls [15]. We found increased cortical thickness in the right lateral OFC and bilateral medial OFC, paired with reduced surface area bilaterally in the lateral (but not medial) OFC, in WS versus TD. These data may lend support to a previously published meta-analysis of fMRI and lesion studies suggesting a medio-lateral OFC distinction, wherein the medial OFC was related to monitoring reward value of reinforcers and lateral OFC function was related to evaluating negative reinforcers of ongoing behavior [43]. We found relative preservation of amygdala volume in WS. Our finding is consistent with a previous report in WS that used a tensor-based morphometric technique [9]; but conflicts with another that used voxel-based morphometry to detect a significant increase in GM density and volume in the amygdala [15]. The above discrepancy could be due to a couple reasons: 1) the nature of the analytic method that we employed uses a surface based registration algorithm to do inter-subject registration that yields a superior matching of homologous cortical regions compared to volumetric techniques such as voxel-based morphometry and 2) the VBM study had a small sample size and very different demographic characteristics compared to ours. Consistent with the report by Cohen et al. (2010) [44] of decreased volume in insular cortex, our study found bilaterally decreased insular surface area

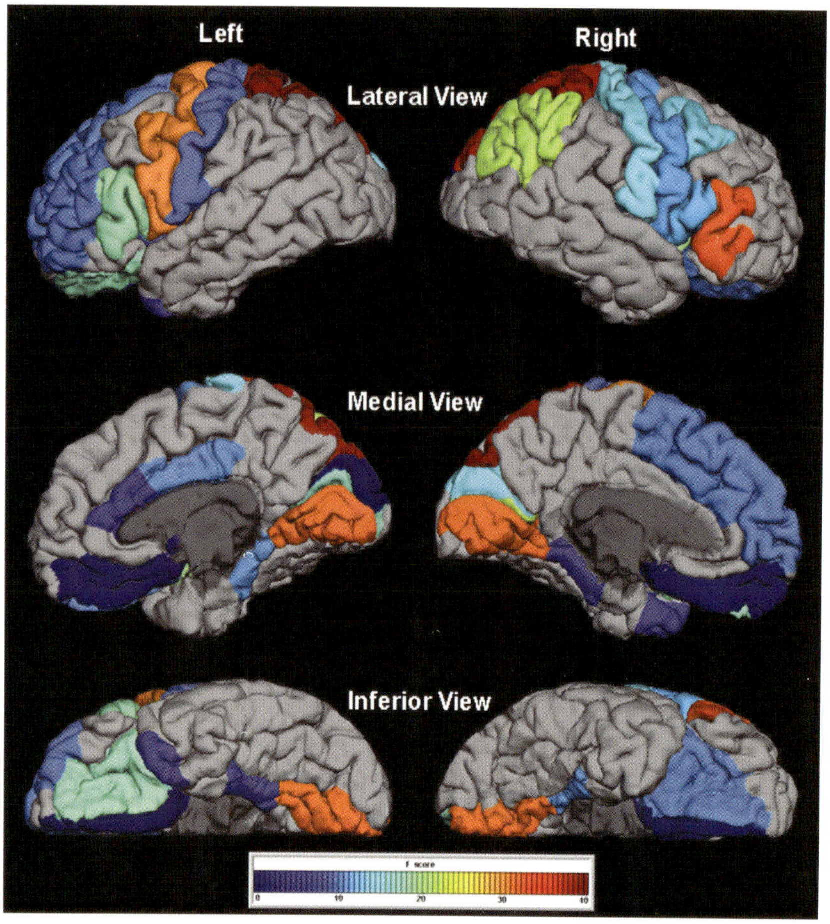

Figure 1. Significant reductions in gray matter surface area measures in WS versus TD controls. Figure 1 shows an overlay of F-test statistics (with values indicated by the color bar) on each Freesurfer-labeled ROI that was significantly different between groups. Surface area measures in gray regions were not significantly different between WS and TD.

(with no significant differences in thickness). Insular function is thought to be critical to processing introceptive awareness, motor control and social and emotional processing, all of which are affected in WS [3,45,46,47,48,49,50]. Taken together, our findings indicate that a pattern of complex structural variations in the OFC, amygdala and insula may underlie impaired social and emotional processing in WS.

Persons with WS often demonstrate an impaired ability to suppress inappropriate social behavior, coupled with hypersociability. Recently, Mobbs et al. [5] conducted a functional MRI experiment using the Go/NoGo task, concluding that individuals with WS failed to activate a frontal network of regions, including both cortical and sub-cortical regions such as the basal ganglia that are critical to successful behavioral inhibition. Reductions in basal ganglia and brain stem volume in WS have been consistently reported in previous studies using voxel- and tensor-based morphometry [9,10]. Similarly, in the WS group from our study, we found a marked volumetric reduction in the brainstem and several subcortical regions within the basal ganglia. We also found evidence for decreased surface area (with no alterations in thickness) in other frontal regions such as the rostral middle frontal gyrus, caudal middle frontal gyrus, superior frontal gyrus and precentral gyrus. These findings lend further support for significant structural alterations in the fronto-basal circuit that might underlie impaired social restraint, inhibitory control of action and social cognition in WS [51,52,53].

Individuals with WS have difficulty performing tasks that require visual-spatial information to be analyzed and transmitted to motor and executive control processes primarily performed in the frontal lobes, such as drawing and block construction tasks, suggesting an overall deficiency in the visuospatial cognitive system governed by fronto-parietal circuits [54]. Reductions in surface area in the cuneus, inferior parietal, superior parietal, inferior frontal, medial frontal, superior frontal, premotor and lingual gyri seen in our study all lend further support to the widely accepted dorsal-visual stream impairment that likely underlies poor visuospatial abilities in WS [16,54].

Even though short-term verbal working memory is a relative strength in WS [55], our study found reduced volume of the hippocampus and reduced surface area of the parahippocampal gyrus in WS. This might be consistent with the study results from Meyer-Lindenberg et al. [32] that used multi-modal imaging (positron emission tomography and fMRI) to show a profound reduction in blood flow to the hippocampal formation in WS.

We also found increased thickness and relatively preserved surface area of the transverse temporal gyrus in WS that might underpin an increased affinity to music, ability to remember lyrics and auditory sensitivity [4]. This is consistent with a report from

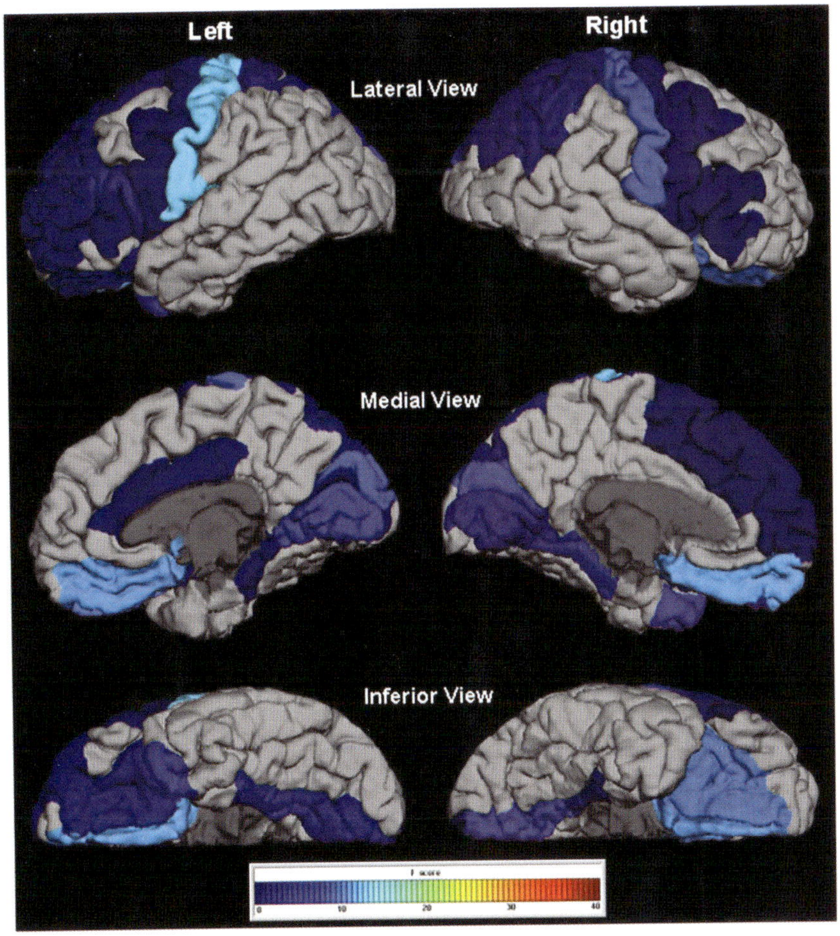

Figure 2. Significant increases in gray matter thickness measures in WS versus TD controls. Figure 2 shows an overlay of F-test statistics (with values indicated by the color bar) on each Freesurfer-labeled ROI that was significantly different between groups. Thickness measures in gray regions were not significantly different between WS and TD.

Thompson et al. [56] that employed a different 3D cortical reconstruction method (using cortical pattern matching and fractal dimension analysis) to capture only thickness profiles in WS. They also found a pattern of increased gyrification and cortical thickness in WS in the perisylvian region that encompassed the superior temporal and transverse temporal gyri.

Although preliminary, our supplementary analyses aimed to shed more light on the influential role of observed structural alterations on levels of anxiety in WS. Individuals with WS show high rates of symptoms of generalized and anticipatory anxiety, and more than 50% of the population meets DSM-IV criteria for specific (non-social) phobias [1,50]. In our study, participants with WS demonstrated mild-to-moderate levels of anxiety as measured by the Beck Anxiety Inventory questionnaire. Functional neuro-imaging studies have attributed regional impairments in the amygdala and OFC to heightened anxiety in WS [33,34,57]. Killgore et al. [58] recently demonstrated that functional activation in the middle rostral insula was associated with anxiety sensitivity, or the tendency to fear the thoughts, symptoms and social consequences associated with the experience of anxiety, in controls and in individuals with social phobia. Insula has also been implicated in specific animal phobia [59].

In addition to the aforementioned regions, individuals with generalized anxiety disorder exhibit reduced regional cerebral blood flow in the frontal and temporal lobes [60,61]. Our study consistently implicates these regions in anxiety that is characteristic of WS by showing significant negative correlations between anxiety scores and surface area in the insula, lateral OFC, superior temporal gyrus, and superior and rostral middle frontal gyri. However, none of the thickness measures were correlated with anxiety scores.

A novel aspect of our study was the concurrent investigation of cortical surface area and thickness as opposed to volume or thickness measurements alone. This enabled us to capture specific patterns of morphological differences in critical regions such as the lateral and medial OFC, postcentral gyrus, temporal pole, lingual gyrus and cuneus that are often inconsistently reported in WS studies that examine only volumetric differences [8]. It is possible that increased surface area of a particular region might be associated with decreased thickness or vice-versa, negating between-group volumetric differences. Thus, studies limited to volume- or tensor-based measurement might not capture these complex structural variations or their associations with neuropsychological scores.

Despite its novel aspects and strengths, our study was limited by the fact that we did not investigate differences in white matter (WM) pathologies. Future studies incorporating concurrent WM measurements using tensor-based techniques, such as DTI, could further inform structural pathology in WS. We also did not directly test for laterality differences, which might provide

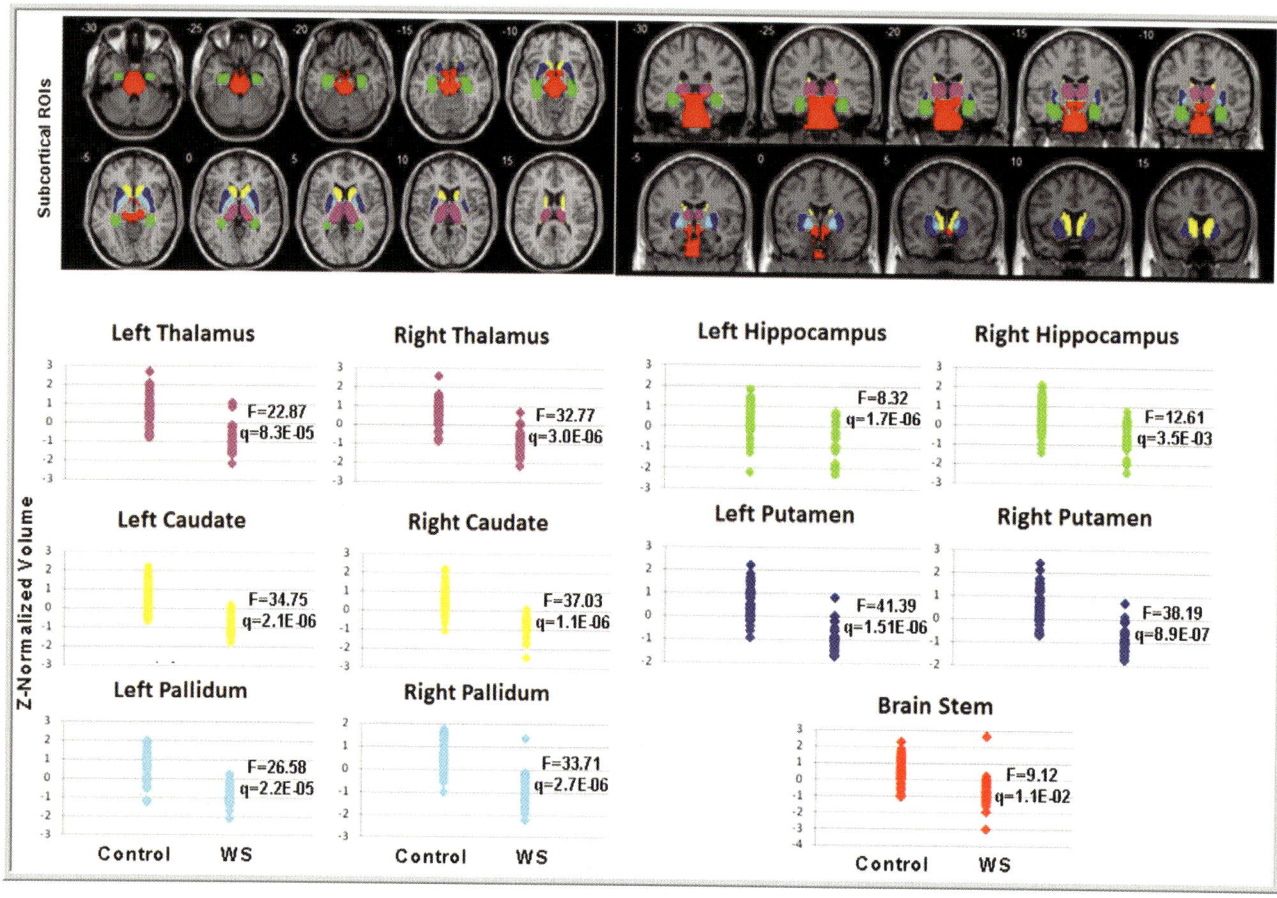

Figure 3. (Top) Color coded anatomical ROI masks of subcortical regions, which showed significant group differences in volume. (Bottom) Scatter plots of volume estimates (Z-normalized) in corresponding subcortical regions demonstrating overall decreases in volume in the areas in the WS brain versus TD controls. Presented statistical values correspond to F scores and FDR corrected q values derived from the MANCOVA. Colors in scatter plots correspond to in the color-coded anatomical ROIs in the Top portion of Figure 3.

Table 3. Results from exploratory correlation analyses of brain morphological measures and Beck Anxiety Inventory scores in WS subjects.

				Beck Anxiety Index	
ROI	**Hemi-sphere**	**Measure**	**N**	**Pearson Correlation Coefficient (r)**	**Unadjusted p-value**
Insular Cortex	L	SA	30	−0.39	**0.03**
Parahippocampal Gyrus	L	SA	30	−0.21	NS
Pars Opercularis	L	SA	30	−0.45	**0.01**
Postcentral Gyrus	L	T	30	0.46	**0.01**
Precentral Gyrus	L	SA	30	−0.56	**0.001**
Rostral Middle Frontal Gyrus	L	SA	30	−0.36	**0.05**
Superior Frontal Gyrus	L	SA	30	−0.39	**0.04**
Superior Temporal Gyrus	L	SA	30	−0.39	**0.04**
Lingual Gyrus	R	SA	30	−0.38	**0.04**
Insula Cortex	R	SA	30	−0.37	**0.04**
Lateral Orbital Frontal Cortex	R	SA	30	−0.42	**0.02**
Posterior-cingulate Cortex	R	SA	30	−0.09	NS

additional insight to help describe unique morphological differences. Future studies could use an analytic approach similar to ours but also include other clinical populations, such as Down syndrome or autism, to evaluate comprehensive WS brain-behavior differences in the context of other neurodevelopmental disorders. Also, it would be necessary and interesting to explore and replicate our brain-behavior correlations in larger samples and in control subjects to validate and elucidate behavioral relationships with structural brain variations. Alternative neuropsychological measures, which might better capture aspects of non-social anxiety most relevant to WS should be considered as well.

In conclusion, this is the first study to examine a comprehensive set of surface- and volume-based ROIs in WS using Freesurfer methods. Our results were consistent with previous reports and also identified novel structural differences in regions related to impaired visuospatial construction, impulsivity, and altered social and emotional processing in WS. Furthermore, we were able to elucidate the complexity of structural gray matter differences in our WS cohort by measuring regional increases and decreases in the cortical surface area and thickness. Additionally, the study tested for associations of specific structural variations with levels of anxiety in WS, in an effort to elucidate their roles in the disorder. Overall, the study demonstrates the utility of concurrently measuring independent structural phenotypes to investigate the complex brain-behavior relationships in a neurodevelopmental disorder such as WS.

Author Contributions

Conceived and designed the experiments: SAM TATW. Performed the experiments: JRP TATW. Analyzed the data: SAM. Contributed reagents/materials/analysis tools: SAM JRP TATW. Wrote the paper: SAM JRP TATW.

References

1. Dykens EM (2003) Anxiety, fears, and phobias in persons with Williams syndrome. Dev Neuropsychol 23: 291–316.
2. Mervis CB, John AE (2010) Cognitive and behavioral characteristics of children with Williams syndrome: implications for intervention approaches. Am J Med Genet C Semin Med Genet 154C: 229–248.
3. Morris CA (2010) The behavioral phenotype of Williams syndrome: A recognizable pattern of neurodevelopment. Am J Med Genet C Semin Med Genet 154C: 427–431.
4. Dykens EM, Rosner BA, Ly T, Sagun J (2005) Music and anxiety in Williams syndrome: a harmonious or discordant relationship? Am J Ment Retard 110: 346–358.
5. Mobbs D, Eckert MA, Mills D, Korenberg J, Bellugi U, et al. (2007) Frontostriatal dysfunction during response inhibition in Williams syndrome. Biol Psychiatry 62: 256–261.
6. Tsai SW, Wu SK, Liou YM, Shu SG (2008) Early development in Williams syndrome. Pediatr Int 50: 221–224.
7. Hocking DR, Rinehart NJ, McGinley JL, Moss SA, Bradshaw JL (2011) A kinematic analysis of visually-guided movement in Williams syndrome. J Neurol Sci 301: 51–58.
8. Jackowski AP, Rando K, Maria de Araujo C, Del Cole CG, Silva I, et al. (2009) Brain abnormalities in Williams syndrome: a review of structural and functional magnetic resonance imaging findings. Eur J Paediatr Neurol 13: 305–316.
9. Chiang MC, Reiss AL, Lee AD, Bellugi U, Galaburda AM, et al. (2007) 3D pattern of brain abnormalities in Williams syndrome visualized using tensor-based morphometry. Neuroimage 36: 1096–1109.
10. Reiss AL, Eliez S, Schmitt JE, Straus E, Lai Z, et al. (2000) IV. Neuroanatomy of Williams syndrome: a high-resolution MRI study. J Cogn Neurosci 12 Suppl 1: 65–73.
11. Eckert MA, Tenforde A, Galaburda AM, Bellugi U, Korenberg JR, et al. (2006) To modulate or not to modulate: differing results in uniquely shaped Williams syndrome brains. Neuroimage 32: 1001–1007.
12. Boddaert N, Mochel F, Meresse I, Seidenwurm D, Cachia A, et al. (2006) Parieto-occipital grey matter abnormalities in children with Williams syndrome. Neuroimage 30: 721–725.
13. Eckert MA, Galaburda AM, Mills DL, Bellugi U, Korenberg JR, et al. (2006) The neurobiology of Williams syndrome: cascading influences of visual system impairment? Cell Mol Life Sci 63: 1867–1875.
14. Meyer-Lindenberg A, Kohn P, Mervis CB, Kippenhan JS, Olsen RK, et al. (2004) Neural basis of genetically determined visuospatial construction deficit in Williams syndrome. Neuron 43: 623–631.
15. Reiss AL, Eckert MA, Rose FE, Karchemskiy A, Kesler S, et al. (2004) An experiment of nature: brain anatomy parallels cognition and behavior in Williams syndrome. J Neurosci 24: 5009–5015.
16. Gaser C, Luders E, Thompson PM, Lee AD, Dutton RA, et al. (2006) Increased local gyrification mapped in Williams syndrome. Neuroimage 33: 46–54.
17. Van Essen DC, Dierker D, Snyder AZ, Raichle ME, Reiss AL, et al. (2006) Symmetry of cortical folding abnormalities in Williams syndrome revealed by surface-based analyses. J Neurosci 26: 5470–5483.
18. Marenco S, Siuta MA, Kippenhan JS, Grodofsky S, Chang WL, et al. (2007) Genetic contributions to white matter architecture revealed by diffusion tensor imaging in Williams syndrome. Proc Natl Acad Sci U S A 104: 15117–15122.
19. Hoeft F, Barnea-Goraly N, Haas BW, Golarai G, Ng D, et al. (2007) More is not always better: increased fractional anisotropy of superior longitudinal fasciculus associated with poor visuospatial abilities in Williams syndrome. J Neurosci 27: 11960–11965.
20. Arlinghaus LR, Thornton-Wells TA, Dykens EM, Anderson AW (2011) Alterations in diffusion properties of white matter in Williams syndrome. Magn Reson Imaging 29: 1165–1174.
21. Avery SN, Thornton-Wells TA, Anderson AW, Blackford JU (2011) White matter integrity deficits in prefrontal-amygdala pathways in Williams syndrome. Neuroimage 59: 887–894.
22. Winkler AM, Kochunov P, Blangero J, Almasy L, Zilles K, et al. (2011) Cortical thickness or grey matter volume? The importance of selecting the phenotype for imaging genetics studies. Neuroimage 53: 1135–1146.
23. Panizzon MS, Fennema-Notestine C, Eyler LT, Jernigan TL, Prom-Wormley E, et al. (2009) Distinct genetic influences on cortical surface area and cortical thickness. Cereb Cortex 19: 2728–2735.
24. Paul BM, Stiles J, Passarotti A, Bavar N, Bellugi U (2002) Face and place processing in Williams syndrome: evidence for a dorsal-ventral dissociation. Neuroreport 13: 1115–1119.
25. Doyle TF, Bellugi U, Korenberg JR, Graham J (2004) "Everybody in the world is my friend" hypersociability in young children with Williams syndrome. Am J Med Genet A 124A: 263–273.
26. Dykens EM, Rosner BA (1999) Refining behavioral phenotypes: personality-motivation in Williams and Prader-Willi syndromes. Am J Ment Retard 104: 158–169.
27. Levitin DJ, Cole K, Chiles M, Lai Z, Lincoln A, et al. (2004) Characterizing the musical phenotype in individuals with Williams Syndrome. Child Neuropsychol 10: 223–247.
28. Levitin DJ, Cole K, Lincoln A, Bellugi U (2005) Aversion, awareness, and attraction: investigating claims of hyperacusis in the Williams syndrome phenotype. J Child Psychol Psychiatry 46: 514–523.
29. Levitin DJ, Menon V, Schmitt JE, Eliez S, White CD, et al. (2003) Neural correlates of auditory perception in Williams syndrome: an fMRI study. Neuroimage 18: 74–82.
30. Thornton-Wells TA, Cannistraci CJ, Anderson AW, Kim CY, Eapen M, et al. (2010) Auditory attraction: activation of visual cortex by music and sound in Williams syndrome. Am J Intellect Dev Disabil 115: 172–189.
31. Schlaug G, Jancke L, Huang Y, Steinmetz H (1995) In vivo evidence of structural brain asymmetry in musicians. Science 267: 699–701.
32. Meyer-Lindenberg A, Hariri AR, Munoz KE, Mervis CB, Mattay VS, et al. (2005) Neural correlates of genetically abnormal social cognition in Williams syndrome. Nat Neurosci 8: 991–993.
33. Munoz KE, Meyer-Lindenberg A, Hariri AR, Mervis CB, Mattay VS, et al. (2010) Abnormalities in neural processing of emotional stimuli in Williams syndrome vary according to social vs. non-social content. Neuroimage 50: 340–346.
34. Thornton-Wells TA, Avery SN, Blackford JU (2011) Using novel control groups to dissect the amygdala's role in Williams Syndrome. Dev Cogn Neurosci 1: 295–304.
35. Ding J, Chen H, Qiu C, Liao W, Warwick JM, et al. (2011) Disrupted functional connectivity in social anxiety disorder: a resting-state fMRI study. Magn Reson Imaging 29: 701–711.
36. Pietrini F, Godini L, Lazzeretti L, Benni L, Pracucci C, et al. (2010) [Neuroimaging and neurobiology of social anxiety]. Riv Psichiatr 45: 349–360.
37. Dale AM, Fischl B, Sereno MI (1999) Cortical surface-based analysis. I. Segmentation and surface reconstruction. Neuroimage 9: 179–194.
38. Desikan RS, Segonne F, Fischl B, Quinn BT, Dickerson BC, et al. (2006) An automated labeling system for subdividing the human cerebral cortex on MRI scans into gyral based regions of interest. Neuroimage 31: 968–980.
39. Fischl B, Sereno MI, Dale AM (1999) Cortical surface-based analysis. II: Inflation, flattening, and a surface-based coordinate system. Neuroimage 9: 195–207.
40. Segonne F, Dale AM, Busa E, Glessner M, Salat D, et al. (2004) A hybrid approach to the skull stripping problem in MRI. Neuroimage 22: 1060–1075.

41. Fischl B, van der Kouwe A, Destrieux C, Halgren E, Segonne F, et al. (2004) Automatically parcellating the human cerebral cortex. Cereb Cortex 14: 11–22.
42. Segonne F, Pacheco J, Fischl B (2007) Geometrically accurate topology-correction of cortical surfaces using nonseparating loops. IEEE Trans Med Imaging 26: 518–529.
43. Kringelbach ML, Rolls ET (2004) The functional neuroanatomy of the human orbitofrontal cortex: evidence from neuroimaging and neuropsychology. Prog Neurobiol 72: 341–372.
44. Cohen JD, Mock JR, Nichols T, Zadina J, Corey DM, et al. (2010) Morphometry of human insular cortex and insular volume reduction in Williams syndrome. J Psychiatr Res 44: 81–89.
45. Phan KL, Wager T, Taylor SF, Liberzon I (2002) Functional neuroanatomy of emotion: a meta-analysis of emotion activation studies in PET and fMRI. Neuroimage 16: 331–348.
46. Singer T (2006) The neuronal basis and ontogeny of empathy and mind reading: review of literature and implications for future research. Neurosci Biobehav Rev 30: 855–863.
47. Craig AD (2009) How do you feel–now? The anterior insula and human awareness. Nat Rev Neurosci 10: 59–70.
48. Fink GR, Frackowiak RS, Pietrzyk U, Passingham RE (1997) Multiple nonprimary motor areas in the human cortex. J Neurophysiol 77: 2164–2174.
49. Perez-Garcia D, Granero R, Gallastegui F, Perez-Jurado LA, Brun-Gasca C (2011) Behavioral features of Williams Beuren syndrome compared to Fragile X syndrome and subjects with intellectual disability without defined etiology. Res Dev Disabil 32: 643–652.
50. Udwin O, Yule W (1991) A cognitive and behavioural phenotype in Williams syndrome. J Clin Exp Neuropsychol 13: 232–244.
51. Aron AR, Durston S, Eagle DM, Logan GD, Stinear CM, et al. (2007) Converging evidence for a fronto-basal-ganglia network for inhibitory control of action and cognition. J Neurosci 27: 11860–11864.
52. Jahfari S, Waldorp L, van den Wildenberg WP, Scholte HS, Ridderinkhof KR, et al. (2011) Effective connectivity reveals important roles for both the hyperdirect (fronto-subthalamic) and the indirect (fronto-striatal-pallidal) fronto-basal ganglia pathways during response inhibition. J Neurosci 31: 6891–6899.
53. Masterman DL, Cummings JL (1997) Frontal-subcortical circuits: the anatomic basis of executive, social and motivated behaviors. J Psychopharmacol 11: 107–114.
54. Atkinson J, Braddick O, Anker S, Curran W, Andrew R, et al. (2003) Neurobiological models of visuospatial cognition in children with Williams syndrome: measures of dorsal-stream and frontal function. Dev Neuropsychol 23: 139–172.
55. Jarrold C, Baddeley AD, Hewes AK (1999) Genetically dissociated components of working memory: evidence from Down's and Williams syndrome. Neuropsychologia 37: 637–651.
56. Thompson PM, Lee AD, Dutton RA, Geaga JA, Hayashi KM, et al. (2005) Abnormal cortical complexity and thickness profiles mapped in Williams syndrome. J Neurosci 25: 4146–4158.
57. Meyer-Lindenberg A, Mervis CB, Berman KF (2006) Neural mechanisms in Williams syndrome: a unique window to genetic influences on cognition and behaviour. Nat Rev Neurosci 7: 380–393.
58. Killgore WD, Britton JC, Price LM, Gold AL, Deckersbach T, et al. (2011) Neural correlates of anxiety sensitivity during masked presentation of affective faces. Depress Anxiety 28: 243–249.
59. Rosso IM, Makris N, Britton JC, Price LM, Gold AL, et al. (2010) Anxiety sensitivity correlates with two indices of right anterior insula structure in specific animal phobia. Depress Anxiety 27: 1104–1110.
60. de Bellis MD, Keshavan MS, Shifflett H, Iyengar S, Dahl RE, et al. (2002) Superior temporal gyrus volumes in pediatric generalized anxiety disorder. Biol Psychiatry 51: 553–562.
61. Zhao XH, Wang PJ, Li CB, Wang JH, Yang ZY, et al. (2006) Prefrontal and superior temporal lobe hyperactivity as a biological substrate of generalized anxiety disorders. Nat Med J China 86: 955–960.

12

Alterations in White Matter Microstructure in Neurofibromatosis-1

Katherine H. Karlsgodt[1,2*], Tena Rosser[4], Evan S. Lutkenhoff[3], Tyrone D. Cannon[1,2,3], Alcino Silva[1,3,5], Carrie E. Bearden[1,2,3]

1 Semel Institute for Neuroscience and Behavior, University of California Los Angeles, Los Angeles, California, United States of America, 2 Center for Cognitive Neuroscience, University of California Los Angeles, Los Angeles, California, United States of America, 3 Department of Psychology, University of California Los Angeles, Los Angeles, California, United States of America, 4 Children's Hospital Los Angeles, Los Angeles, California, United States of America, 5 Department of Neurobiology, University of California Los Angeles, Los Angeles, California, United States of America

Abstract

Neurofibromatosis (NF1) represents the most common single gene cause of learning disabilities. NF1 patients have impairments in frontal lobe based cognitive functions such as attention, working memory, and inhibition. Due to its well–characterized genetic etiology, investigations of NF1 may shed light on neural mechanisms underlying such difficulties in the general population or other patient groups. Prior neuroimaging findings indicate global brain volume increases, consistent with neural over-proliferation. However, little is known about alterations in white matter microstructure in NF1. We performed diffusion tensor imaging (DTI) analyses using tract-based spatial statistics (TBSS) in 14 young adult NF1 patients and 12 healthy controls. We also examined brain volumetric measures in the same subjects. Consistent with prior studies, we found significantly increased overall gray and white matter volume in NF1 patients. Relative to healthy controls, NF1 patients showed widespread reductions in white matter integrity across the entire brain as reflected by decreased fractional anisotropy (FA) and significantly increased absolute diffusion (ADC). When radial and axial diffusion were examined we found pronounced differences in radial diffusion in NF1 patients, indicative of either decreased myelination or increased space between axons. Secondary analyses revealed that FA and radial diffusion effects were of greatest magnitude in the frontal lobe. Such alterations of white matter tracts connecting frontal regions could contribute to the observed cognitive deficits. Furthermore, although the cellular basis of these white matter microstructural alterations remains to be determined, our findings of disproportionately increased radial diffusion against a background of increased white matter volume suggest the novel hypothesis that one potential alteration contributing to increased cortical white matter in NF1 may be looser packing of axons, with or without myelination changes. Further, this indicates that axial and radial diffusivity can uniquely contribute as markers of NF1-associated brain pathology in conjunction with the typically investigated measures.

Editor: Emanuele Buratti, International Centre for Genetic Engineering and Biotechnology, Italy

Funding: This work was supported by the Carol Moss Spivak Foundation and National Institutes of Health grant MH084315 to AS, and the National Institute of Mental Health (R34 MH089299-01 to CEB). The funders had no role in study design, data collection and analysis, decision to publish, or preparation of the manuscript.

Competing Interests: The authors have declared that no competing interests exist.

* E-mail: kkarlsgodt@nshs.edu

Introduction

Neurofibromatosis Type 1 (NF1) is caused by a mutation in the neurofibromin gene at locus 17q11.2, and is one of the most common single-gene genetic disorders (prevalence 1:3000) affecting cognitive function in humans [1]. It is also characterized by multi-system clinical findings, including including café au lait spots, neurofibromas, scoliosis, bone dysplasias, optic pathway gliomas and Lisch nodules [2]. However, the accompanying cognitive deficits lead to significant difficulties in functioning, particularly in the school environment, and in fact are often the most significant cause of lifetime morbidity in this population [3]. The NF1 cognitive profile is characterized by severe impairments in 'cognitive control', or the ability to maintain attentional focus and resist distraction, which is generally considered to be a key function of the frontal lobe. These cognitive control deficits are particularly notable in the areas of working memory, cognitive flexibility, and inhibitory control [1,4,5,6].

About 65% of children with NF1 have sustained attentional difficulties and 38–50% meet diagnostic criteria for ADHD, with the vast majority fulfilling criteria for the inattentive subtype [7,8]. In addition, a substantial proportion of individuals with NF1 demonstrate social deficits similar to those observed in autism spectrum disorders (ASD) [9,10]. Due to its well-characterized genetic etiology, investigation of the neural mechanisms underlying these deficits in NF1 could shed light on the pathogenesis of attentional dysfunction and social deficits in the broader population.

Neurofibromin, the NF1 gene product, appears early during embryonic development, with high levels of expression in the brain, suggesting that it is important for the orderly differentiation of CNS neurons [11]. Gray and white matter volume increases relative to healthy individuals have been consistently documented,

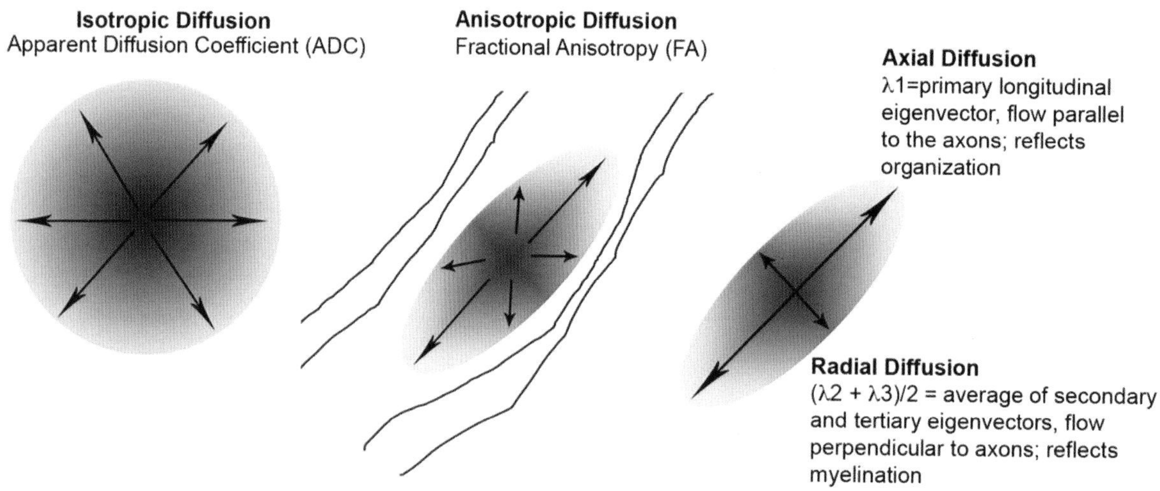

Figure 1. DTI diagram showing radial diffusion, axial diffusion and ADC as related to FA.

although the origins and significance of these brain changes is unclear [12,13,14]. Overall macrocephaly (i.e. brain circumference greater than the 95th percentile) characterizes about half of children with NF1 [15]. Corresponding to increased overall white matter volume, increased corpus callosum area and/or callosal thickening also appears to be characteristic of NF1 [16,17,18]. Also, two studies have found increased corpus callosum size to be associated with lower IQ and poorer performance on measures of academic achievement, abstract concept formation, verbal memory and visual-spatial and motor skills [13,19], indicating that this structural change has functional importance.

NF1 mutations are known to impact myelin, as the gene encoding the oligodendrocyte-myelin glycoprotein (OMgp) is embedded within an intron of the NF1 gene [20]. This protein has been the focus of much interest as a potential mechanism underlying overproliferation of oligodendrocytes, which may explain structural neuroanatomic findings of enlarged white matter. However, while increases in oligodendrocyte progenitors have been demonstrated in the spinal cords of NF1 mutant mice [21], Lee et al. [22] recently showed that NF1 deletion increases neuroglial progenitor/stem cells (NSCs) in the brainstem, but not in the cortex. Consistent with findings that tumors commonly appear in the optic nerve, hypothalamus, and brain stem but rarely in the cortex, they also found no increased proliferation or gliogenesis in cortex. Therefore, the mechanisms underlying the observed white matter changes still require further investigation. However, few studies have examined indices of brain myelination in adult patients with NF1 to determine how these changes are reflected *in vivo*. Diffusion tensor imaging (DTI) is the only currently available non-invasive method for investigating white matter microstructure and connectivity in vivo, based on patterns of water diffusion in neural tissue [23]. The fractional anisotropy (FA; or directional variability) of diffusion is higher in heavily myelinated fiber tracts, and increases with progressive myelination during development [24]. While traditional magnetic resonance imaging (MRI) allows for only a gross overview of white matter, the current study employs diffusion-based methods to examine the integrity of white matter microstructure and inter-regional axonal connectivity.

To date, only a handful of studies have employed DTI measures in NF1 patients, none of which have taken a whole-brain approach. Previous studies have noted increased apparent diffusion coefficient (ADC) values, indicating more diffuse or less organized cerebral tissue, in both children and adults with NF1 relative to control subjects [25,26,27]. More recently, studies have begun exploring the FA properties of white matter using a region of interest (ROI)-based approach. These studies have generally shown decreases in FA, the primary DTI index of white matter microstructural integrity, as well as increases in overall diffusivity [28,29,30]. However, these studies have had a limited focus on specific brain regions. A major limitation of an ROI-based approach is that it does not address the possibility that the changes observed may be widespread. In addition, it is not known to what extent the observed increases in overall diffusivity (as indexed by FA and ADC) reflect alterations in radial versus axial diffusion. Axial and radial diffusion measures of the length of the longest and shortest axes of the elliptical area of diffusion (see Figure 1), and are thought to index tract organization or axonal integrity and myelination, respectively [31,32,33] particularly in the case of confluent white matter changes [34]. However, it is known that myelination is not the only factor that contributes to radial diffusion [35]. In addition, there may be a role for axonal packing density (amount of space between axons); this measure has been shown to be positively correlated with ADC and radial diffusion, and negatively correlated with FA [36,37,38].

Here, we conducted the first study to date to investigate changes in white matter microstructure across the whole brain using voxel-wise methods in NF1. Secondly, we examined volumetric differences in grey and white matter between groups, to determine whether previously observed global volume alterations were also present in our sample. Based on findings from prior mouse and human studies we predicted that individuals with NF1 would have larger overall grey and white matter volumes, concomitant with increases in overall diffusivity and decreased FA. Moreover, since neurofibromin is expressed throughout the brain and not just in the localized regions that were the focus of prior analyses, we hypothesized that a voxel-wise approach would reveal more widespread differences than had been previously reported.

Methods

Participants

14 individuals with NF1 and 12 unaffected, demographically matched control subjects participated in the study (see Table 1 for

demographics). NF1 participants were recruited via advertisement, and had been previously diagnosed with NF1 by a physician. All NF1 participants fulfilled the diagnostic criteria specified by the National Institutes of Health Consensus Development Conference [39] as confirmed by clinical interview. Healthy controls were recruited from a community sample through advertisements for ongoing research studies at UCLA, and did not have any Axis-I psychiatric disorders, nor any medical conditions that may affect cognitive function, as assessed by the Structured Clinical Interview for DSM-IV [40]. Individuals in NF1 and control groups were excluded for significant substance use in the last six months, history of head injury, mental retardation (IQ less than 70) and/or insufficient fluency in the English language.

Ethics Statement

All participants provided written consent for participation, as approved by the institutional review board of the University of California, Los Angeles (UCLA).

Scanning Procedures

Subjects were scanned on a 1.5 T Siemens Sonata scanner (Siemens, Erlagen, Germany) at the Ahmanson-Lovelace Brain Mapping Center at UCLA. Head motion was restricted using foam padding. DTI data were acquired using a 6-direction EPI sequence with 75 contiguous 2 mm AC-PC aligned interleaved slices with no gap (TR = 9.5 s, TE = 77 ms, flip angle = 90 deg, matrix = 128×96, b-value = 1000, FOV 256 mm x 192 mm resulting in 2 mm isotropic voxels). Five repetitions of the sequence were acquired, with a total scan time of 6 minutes 20 seconds. In addition, a high resolution T1-weighted structural image was acquired (1 mm cubic voxels on 160 slices, TR = 1900 ms, TE = 4.38 ms).

Image Processing

The five image acquisitions for each direction were merged, aligned with McFlirt (FMRIB Software Library; FSL [41]), and averaged to create one file each for the 6 directions and the b0 image. Eddy current correction was done using Flirt (FSL), and images were skull stripped using the Brain Extraction Tool. FA images were calculated using DTIFit (FMRIB's Diffusion Toolbox), which fits a diffusion tensor model at each voxel, and then were registered to MNI-152 space using a 12-parameter affine registration with a mutual information cost function implemented in Flirt (FSL). A group map was created using Tract-Based Spatial Statistics (TBSS, [42]). An average FA image was created and the tracts were narrowed to generate an FA "skeleton" representing the center of all tracts common to the entire group. The area around the skeleton in each subjects' aligned FA map was searched and the highest local FA value was assigned to the skeleton. These procedures ensure that each subject's skeleton is in the group space, yet represents the center of that subject's own unique fiber tracts. Apparent diffusion coefficient (ADC) was utilized as it is implemented in the FDT toolkit. Radial diffusion was calculated using the value from the primary eigenvector (L1), and axial diffusion was calculated using the average of the secondary and tertiary eigenvectors (L2+L3/2). Each measure was projected on the skeleton and analyzed in TBSS accordingly.

Grey and white matter volumes were assessed using the FSL-VBM tools, in a voxel-based morphometry style analysis [43,44] carried out with FSL tools [41]. First, structural images were brain-extracted using BET [45]. Next, tissue-type segmentation was carried out using FAST4 [46]. The resulting grey-matter partial volume images were then aligned to MNI152 standard space using the affine registration tool FLIRT [47,48], followed optionally by nonlinear registration using FNIRT [49,50], which uses a b-spline representation of the registration warp field [51]. The resulting images were averaged to create a study-specific template, to which the native grey matter images were then non-linearly re-registered. The registered partial volume images were then modulated (to correct for local expansion or contraction) by dividing by the Jacobian of the warp field. The modulated segmented images were then smoothed with an isotropic Gaussian kernel with a sigma of 3 mm. Grey and white matter volumes were determined by counting the number of voxels in each of the segmented (grey and white matter) images. To create a count of voxels in the frontal lobe alone, a mask of the frontal lobe (i.e., brain tissue in front of the central sulcus) was created and warped from MNI space to each individual subjects' space, and then used as a mask for voxel count extractions.

Region of interest definition. White matter regions of interest (ROIs) were defined in the anterior thalamic radiation (ATR), cingulate bundle, hippocampal cingulum, inferior longitudinal fasciculus (ILF), superior longitudinal fasciculus (SLF) and uncinate fasciculus (UF), corticospinal tract, and inferior fronto-occipital fasciculus (IFO) based on the John Hopkins University DTI-based probabilistic tractography atlas [52,53,54]. To ensure the validity of the tractography-based ROIs for our TBSS skeleton, all ROIs were overlaid with the skeleton and manually edited. Each subjects' FA skeleton was masked using each of the ROIs, and the average FA was calculated for each region, as previously described in Karlsgodt et al., 2009 [55].

Statistical analysis. Statistics on the ROI data were performed in Stata (v8). Independent samples t-tests were performed on the DTI regions, as well as the structural MRI regions. Voxel-wise statistics on the DTI data were performed in FSL's randomise tool, which performs a permutation analysis. We performed 5000 permutations using the Threshold Free Cluster Environment (TFCE), a rigorous approach to cluster analysis that avoids the need to define and initial cluster-forming threshold or to perform large amounts of data smoothing. Age and sex (de-meaned) were included in the model as confound regressors, with

Table 1. Demographics.

	Patients	Controls	Statistics
Age (yrs ± stdev)	24±4.93	22.66±4.54	$t(24) = .713$, $p = .483$
Sex (M/F)	6/8	5/7	$X^2 = .0038$, $p = .951$
Estimated IQ (avg ± stdev)	96.79±8.68	109.62±9.78	$t(20) = 2.189$, $p = .0046$*
Yrs Education (avg ± stdev)	14.21±2.12	15.00±2.28	$t(24) = -.613$, $p = .5459$
Race/Ethnicity:			$X^2 = .1806$, $p = .671$**
Caucasian	7	5	
Hispanic/Latino	5	1	
Asian/Pacific Islander	2	0	
African American	0	3	
Other	0	3	

*IQ data was only available for 8/12 control subjects.
**Race and ethnicity statistics were calculated for Caucasian vs non-Caucasian subjects.

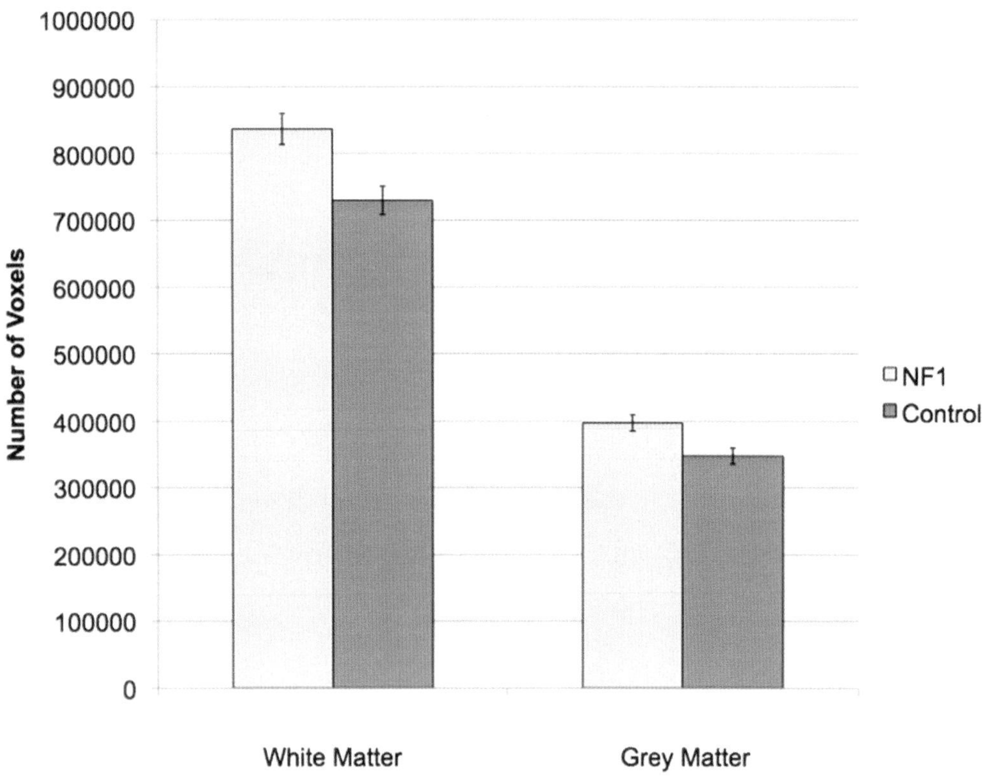

Figure 2. Gray and White Matter volumetric differences between groups.

groups modeled separately. Family-wise error rate (FWE) was used to correct for multiple comparisons.

In order to directly test whether the observed FA effects were secondary to radial or axial changes, we performed an exploratory analysis in which we re-ran two additional versions of the FA randomize analysis (again with demeaned age and sex as covariates), once with demeaned radial diffusion and once with demeaned axial diffusion as covariates. Then, the number of remaining significant voxels were compared to the number of original significant voxels in the FA analysis.

Results

Structural MRI Results

The structural volume analysis revealed significantly larger total grey matter volume [$t(24) = 2.84$, $p = .009$; effect size = .987] and white matter volume [$t(24) = 3.38$, $p = .003$; effect size = 1.12] in NF1 patients relative to controls. This finding remained significant when restricted to an ROI of the frontal lobe white matter [$t(24) = 3.62$, $p = .0014$; effect size (Cohen's d) = 1.17], however, frontal lobe grey matter was significantly larger in controls [$t(24) = 3.64$,$p = .0013$; effect size = 1.174; see Figure 2].

DTI Results

When corrected for multiple comparisons at $p < .05$, permutation analysis revealed highly significant reductions in FA in NF1 patients relative to controls, which were spread broadly across the entire brain (Figure 3). Radial diffusion showed a similar pattern of global changes (here, NF1 patients were higher than controls) (Figure 4). However, there were less widespread increases in axial diffusion in the NF1 group (Figure 5). Finally, NF1 patients showed overall increases in ADC (Figure 6) across the brain, at both high and lower thresholds.

Given the widespread nature of the findings at conventional thresholding levels, we took two approaches to ascertain whether these effects were more pronounced in any particular region. First, we performed a secondary voxel-wise analysis at an increased statistical threshold ($p = .005$) to look for areas that remained significant at suprathreshold levels, indicating more robust differences. We found that the alterations in FA (Figure 3) and radial diffusion (Figure 4) did show regional effects, with only voxels in the frontal lobe surviving the more stringent thresholding. However, increased thresholding for axial diffusion (Figure 5) and ADC maps (Figure 6) did not reveal any suprathreshold patterns: no voxels survived the higher thresholding for axial diffusion, and for ADC the affected regions remained significant throughout the brain. In the exploratory analysis of the relationship between FA and radial and axial diffusion we found that when axial diffusion was entered as a covariate, it did not impact the overall FA findings and 98.23% of the voxels remained the same as in the original FA analysis. However, when radial diffusion was used as the covariate, only 63.32% of voxels remained significant, indicating that radial diffusion may specifically contribute to the FA changes more than axial diffusion.

Our second approach to probing regional variation was to perform a ROI analysis in a set of white major matter association tracts (ROI definition described above) including those that do and do not connect to the frontal lobe. When corrected for multiple comparisons using Bonferroni correction, the significant p-value threshold was set at.005 (.05/10 = .005) (see Table 2). At this threshold the left and right anterior thalamic radiations (ATR), which connect the thalamus and frontal lobes, showed significantly lower FA in NF1 patients, as did the left cingulate bundle. There

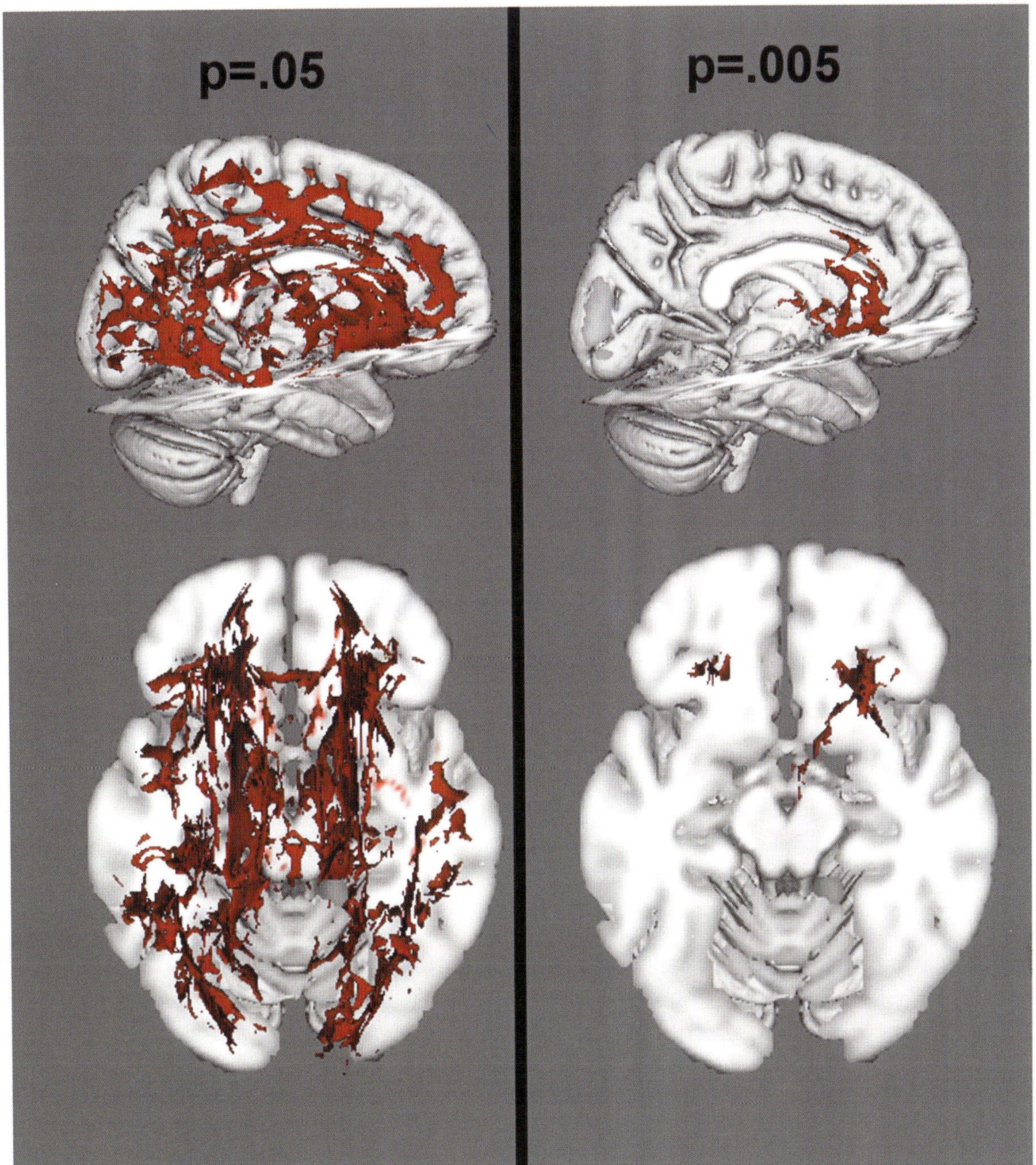

Figure 3. Voxelwise analysis of FA, at a threshold of p<.05 (left) and p<.005 (right). Red colors reflect areas of decreased FA in the NF1 group.

were trend level effects in the forceps minor, a tract that travels through the genu of the corpus callosum and connects the two hemispheres of the frontal lobe, and the inferior fronto-occipital fasciculus (which projects from the frontal lobe back through the temporal and occipital lobes) bilaterally. Finding significant results in tracts that originate in the frontal lobe confirmed the predominantly frontal nature of the FA alterations (See Figure 2). To probe the basis of these differences, a post-hoc analysis was performed within ROIs showing significant differences in FA; namely, the left and right ATR and the left cingulate bundle (see Table 3), this time assessing radial and axial diffusion as well as ADC. We found that while radial diffusion and ADC were significantly increased in these ROIs, there were no significant differences between groups in axial diffusion. Given the more robust effects in radial diffusion in both the voxelwise and ROI approaches, this convergent evidence supports the hypothesis that the observed FA changes may be driven by alterations in radial diffusion.

Discussion

This is the first paper to investigate diffusion tensor imaging measures in adults with NF1 across the entire brain using

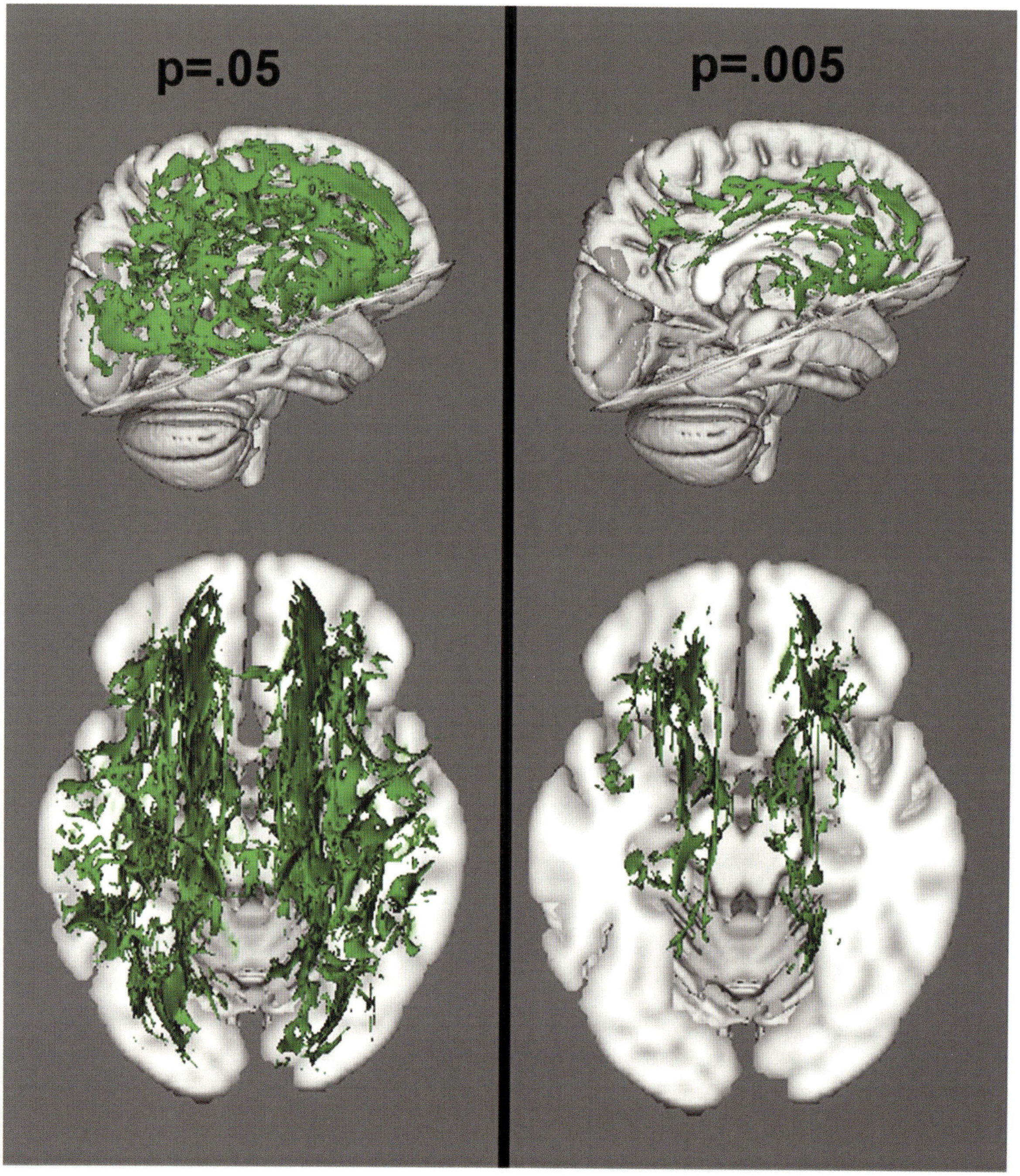

Figure 4. Voxelwise analysis of radial diffusion, at a threshold of $p < .05$ and $p < .005$. Green colors reflect increased radial diffusion in the NF1 group.

a rigorous registration approach, tract-based spatial statistics (TBSS). First, our data replicate and support previous sMRI findings indicating white matter volumetric enlargement in NF1 patients [12,13,14]. However, our study sheds new light on the widespread nature of white matter microstructural alterations in NF1, a pattern that has not been observed in previous studies that focused on a limited selection of white matter tracts. Furthermore, by using two approaches (ROI analysis and a suprathreshold voxel-wise analysis) to probe these widespread effects for regional specificity, we were able to determine that the alterations are more pronounced in the frontal lobe. The finding that alterations in white matter integrity are most pronounced in the frontal lobe in adults with NF1 is highly consistent with the nature of their cognitive deficits. We have previously demonstrated deficits in frontally-mediated working memory processes [1]. Moreover, the attentional, executive, language, and other academic deficits characteristic of NF1 may be reliant either in whole or in part on frontal lobe functions.

By using multiple DTI measures, this study uniquely contributes to our broader understanding of the previously observed white matter volume increases. Our finding of increased ADC reflects a general increase in diffusivity that can arise through a variety of

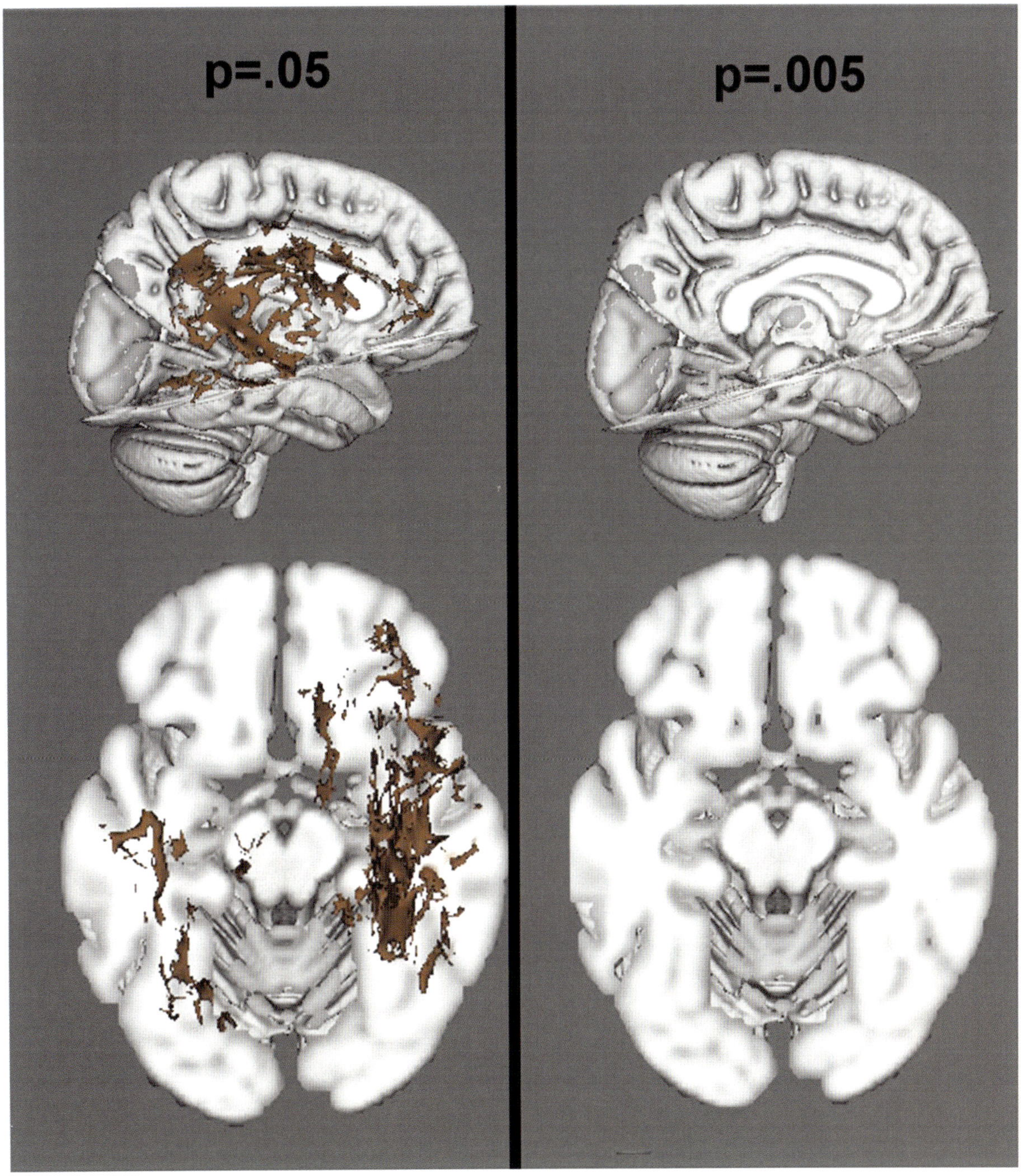

Figure 5. Voxelwise analysis of axial diffusion, at a threshold of p<.05 and p<.005. Brown colors reflect increased axial diffusion in the NF1 group.

mechanisms (see Figure 6). One post-mortem study using ADC alone has proposed that the increase in ADC commonly reported in NF1 could be result of increased vacuoles in the myelin [56]. This explanation has been used to explain subsequent findings of ADC increases [57], as has the hypothesis that the ADC difference reflects demyelination [25,27]. However, while ADC is sensitive to determining whether there is more global diffusion, it cannot inform whether diffusion in a particular direction is differentially impacted, as can be assessed using FA. Our finding of significantly decreased FA in patients with NF1 indicates that diffusion is not globally increased, but is specifically less constrained perpendicular to the tracts (the ellipse describing the diffusion is less eccentric, or narrow, than in controls). Because of the directionality of this effect, it is unlikely that an increase in diffusion within circular vacuoules, which would not be associated with diffusion changes in any particular direction, could explain the observed differences. However, the finding of decreased FA may still be driven by either decreased organization of tracts, which prevents diffusion along the long (axial) axis of the ellipse, or alternatively by decreased myelination or increased axonal spacing that allows for more room between axons for water molecules to move perpendicular to the tract (radially). Therefore, the separate investigation of radial and

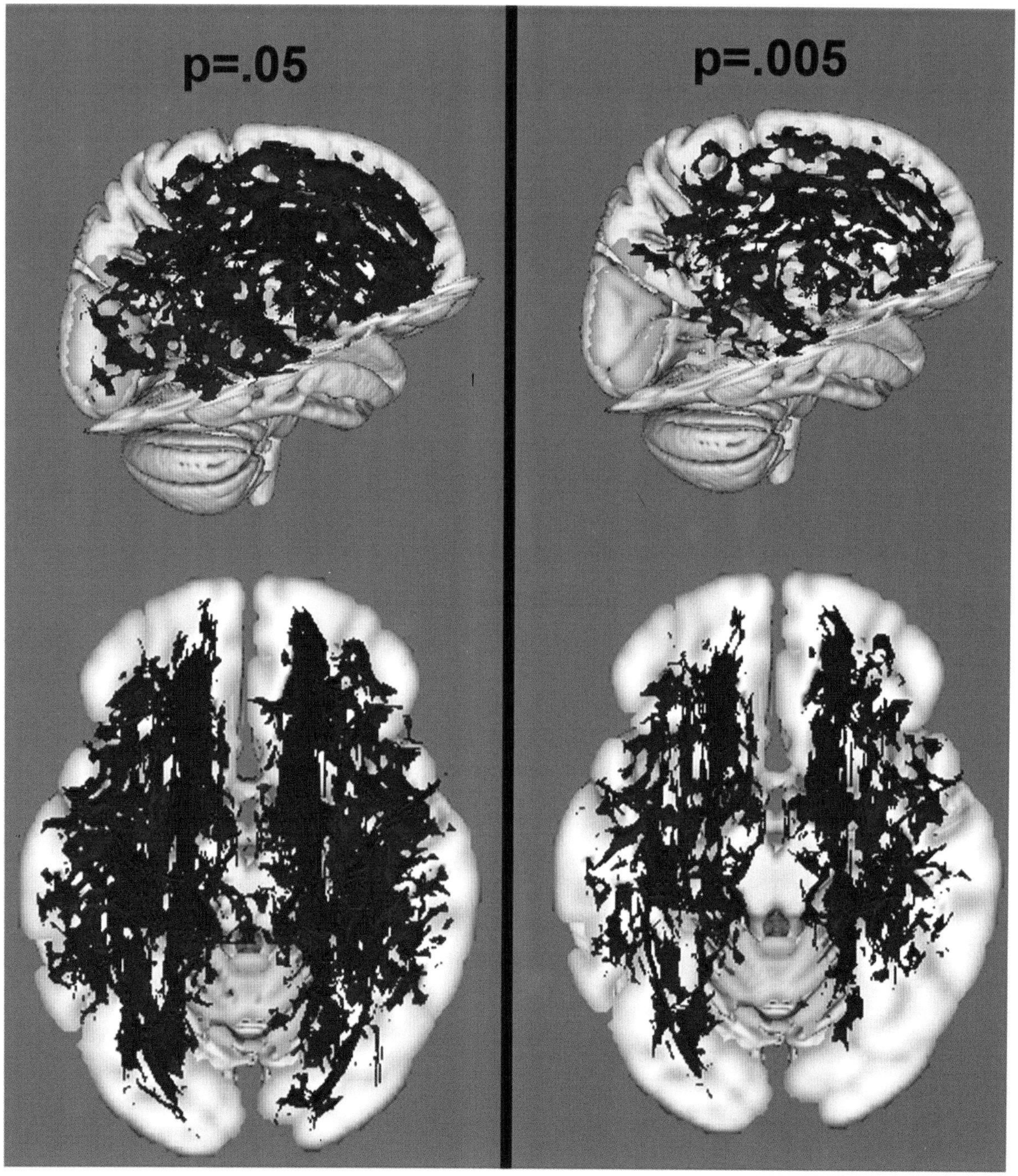

Figure 6. Voxelwise analysis of ADC, at a threshold of p<.05 and p<.005. Blue colors reflect increased ADC in the NF1 group.

axial diffusivity measures was critical to help elucidate the basis of the white matter microstructural changes. We demonstrated that within the tracts showing significant FA alteration the change is driven by radial diffusion with no significant change in axial diffusion. Thus, we have evidence indicating that the cause of the differences in FA and ADC between groups is likely based on either myelination differences, density of axonal packing, or both. Further, additional analyses using radial and axial diffusion as covariates had different effects on the significance of the FA analysis, further, indicating that radial diffusion may play a particularly important role.

A limitation of DTI methodology is that it is an indirect measure of the distance between axons, and must remain agnostic to which factor (myelin or axonal spacing) is driving the results. However, given that white matter volume is increased in this sample and in other samples in the literature, a simple finding of decreased myelination (which would typically result in a decrease in white matter volume) is not sufficient to explain the larger pattern of results. Therefore, our data support the novel hypothesis that while there may be myelination differences in NF1, there are also likely to be differences in the degree of axonal packing, with the larger distances between axons contributing to the white matter volume increase. Given our findings of increased ADC and

Table 2. Differences in Fractional Anisotropy (NF1 Patients vs. Controls).

Region	Hemisphere	Patients	Controls	Statistics
Anterior Thalamic Radiation	L	**.4153 (.0155)**	**.4424 (.0182)**	**t(24) = 4.10, p = .0004; effect size = 1.30**
Anterior Thalamic Radiation	R	**.4171 (.0140)**	**.4480 (.0233)**	**t(24) = 4.16, p = .0003; effect size = 1.6**
Corticospinal Tract	L	.5567 (.0207)	.5654 (.0228)	t(24) = 1.01, p = .321; effect size = .390
Corticospinal Tract	R	.5391 (.0182)	.5433 (.0187)	t(24) = 5.74, p = .572; effect size = .229
Cingulate Bundle	L	**.5253 (.0221)**	**.5639 (.0273)**	**t(24) = 3.99, p = .0005; effect size = 1.24**
Cingulate Bundle	R	.5315 (.0374)	.5555 (.0300)	t(24) = 1.786, p = .087; effect size = .692
Hippocampal Cingulum	L	.3305 (.0195)	.3379 (.0423)	t(24) = .591, p = .2815; effect size = .235
Hippocampal Cingulum	R	.2968 (.0231)	.3093 (.0345)	t(24) = 1.10, p = .282; effect size = .432
Forceps Major	L+R	.7215 (.0351)	.7349 (.0313)	t(24) = 1.023, p = .316; effect size = .402
Forceps Minor	L+R	.5538 (.0186)	.5561 (.0278)	t(24) = 1.838, p = .078; effect size = .691
Inferior fronto-occipital fasciculus	L	.4359 (.0184)	.4592 (.0215)	t(24) = 2.98, p = .0066; effect size = 1.02
Inferior fronto-occipital fasciculus	R	.4329 (.0203)	.4567 (.0204)	t(24) = 2.97, p = .0066; effect size = 1.02
Inferior longitudinal fasciculus	L	.4064 (.0139)	.4178 (.0257)	t(24) = 1.44, p = .164; effect size = .553
Inferior longitudinal fasciculus	R	.4154 (.0175)	.4282 (.0203)	t(24) = 1.72, p = .098; effect size = .652
Superior longitudinal fasciculus	L	.4400 (.0229)	.4550 (.0312)	t(24) = 1.41, p = .172; effect size = .543
Superior longitudinal fasciculus	R	.4538 (.0273)	.4568 (.0208)	t(24) = .312, p = .754; effect size = .125
Uncinate fasciculus	L	.4265 (.0216)	.4308 (.0259)	t(24) = 4.64, p = .647; effect size = .185
Uncinate fasciculus	R	.4072 (.0196)	.4239 (.0260)	t(24) = 1.87, p = .074; effect size = .70

Region of interest based FA analysis.

radial diffusion in the context of decreased FA, this hypothesis is consistent with histological findings that axonal packing density (amount of space between axons) is positively correlated with ADC and radial diffusion and negatively correlated with FA [36,37,38].

The possibility that the alterations in axial diffusion may be the result of increased space between axons (less dense tract packing) is supported by some of the known functions of neurofibromin and the molecules it interacts with. Developmentally, when white matter tracts are formed, cellular adhesion molecules play an

Table 3. Radial and Axial Diffusion and ADC: NF1 Patients vs. Controls.

Tract	Measure	Patients	Controls	Statistics
Left ATR	**Radial**	**.000614 (2.24 $\times 10^{-5}$)**	**.000579 (2.15 $\times 10^{-5}$)**	**t(24) = 4.097, p = .0004**
	Axial	.001190 (2.67 $\times 10^{-5}$)	.001180 (2.74 $\times 10^{-5}$)	t(24) = .9817, p = .3361
	ADC	**.000810 (2.16 $\times 10^{-5}$)**	**.000778 (1.95 $\times 10^{-5}$)**	**t(24) = 3.31, p = .003**
Right ATR	**Radial**	**.000603 (2.75 $\times 10^{-5}$)**	**.000563 (2.57 $\times 10^{-5}$)**	**t(24) = 3.79, p = .0009**
	Axial	.001175 (3.09 $\times 10^{-5}$)	.001162 (3.25 $\times 10^{-5}$)	t(24) = .996, p = .3292
	ADC	**.000794 (2.74 $\times 10^{-5}$)**	**.000763 (2.22 $\times 10^{-5}$)**	**t(24) = 3.103, p = .0049**
Left Cingulate	**Radial**	**.00052 (2.08 $\times 10^{-5}$)**	**.000470 (2.61 $\times 10^{-5}$)**	**t(24) = 5.60, p<.0001**
	Axial	.001260 (4.11 $\times 10^{-5}$)	.001249 (2.87 $\times 10^{-5}$)	t(24) = .803, p = .430
	ADC	**.000768 (2.04 $\times 10^{-5}$)**	**.000730 (1.70 $\times 10^{-5}$)**	**t(24) = 5.10, p<.0001**
Right Cingulate	**Radial**	**.000515 (3.69 $\times 10^{-5}$)**	**.000480 (3.52 $\times 10^{-5}$)**	**t(24) = .247, p = .021**
	Axial	.001267 (5.47 $\times 10^{-5}$)	.001252 (3.65 $\times 10^{-5}$)	t(24) = .808, p = .427
	ADC	**.000766 (2.18 $\times 10^{-5}$)**	**.000737 (2.78 $\times 10^{-5}$)**	**t(24) = 2.93; p = .0073**

Supplementary ROI analysis testing radial diffusion, axial diffusion, and ADC in regions with significant FA findings.

important role in axon guidance along tracts, and in holding tracts together. There is some evidence that OMgp has the potential to function as an adhesion molecule [58,59], and thus may be affected by NF1 mutation. OMgp expression across development coincides with the progression of myelination, which moves in a caudal to rostral direction [59], and it may have a particularly important effect in thalamocortical tracts (such as the ATR found to be significantly affected in the current study) [60]. Furthermore, neurofibromin itself has been shown to regulate not only Ras, but also Akt and focal adhesion kinase (FAK), which impacts cell adhesion, migration, and survival [61,62]. While the current data cannot directly address this issue, the findings are consistent with a disruption in fasciculation during early development, and future histological and molecular studies addressing the relationship of these factors to white matter alterations will be highly informative.

Certain limitations of the current study must be noted. First of all, the sample size is small, due to limitations in recruiting individuals with this rare disorder and future studies in larger populations, as well as prospective longitudinal studies in developmental samples, will be useful for further probing the etiology and developmental trajectory of structural brain changes in NF1. Secondly, our DTI acquisition sequence had a limited number of directions and thus, we were not able to do tractography analyses. Further, while an increasing number of studies are beginning to include measures of radial and axial diffusion, as they provide more specific information about the nature of white matter microstructural changes than do FA and ADC, there are limitations to these measures. One particular issue is related to the reliability of these measures in areas where there are crossing fibers. This issue may be intensified in low directional data, as we have here. While our results indicate widespread changes across large areas of white matter, regional interpretation of these measures should be considered with caution. This may be better addressed in future studies with higher directional data. Finally, particularly interesting for future studies will be explorations of the relationship of these changes to clinical symptoms, such as those associated with ADHD. Although no studies, to our knowledge, have previously examined the impact of ADHD diagnosis on DTI indices in NF1, Cutting et al. [12] noted that NF1 children with an ADHD diagnosis had smaller frontal gray matter volumes relative to NF1 patients without ADHD. Similarly, it is possible that those individuals with the greatest deficits in white matter organization are also those for whom NF1 has resulted in ADHD symptoms. Based on the literature in idiopathic ADHD showing white matter deficits in prefrontal regions [63,64,65], we would anticipate that alterations in these regions in NF1 may also be associated with attentional symptoms. However, unlike in NF1, such studies have revealed deficits in axial as well as radial diffusion, Thus, further longitudinal developmental studies aimed at elucidating the similarities and differences in frontal lobe white matter development in NF1 and ADHD are warranted.

Overall, the current study demonstrates that the finding of white matter overgrowth, as measured by sMRI, persists into adulthood in NF1 patients and that white matter microstructural changes, as measured by DTI, also persist and are more pronounced in the frontal lobe. Notably, we show a novel pattern of DTI findings that may indicate that one contributing factor to this increase in volume may be related to looser fiber packing. Further, our findings indicate that indices of axial and radial diffusivity have added utility as markers of NF1-associated brain pathology beyond the typically investigated measures of diffusion (i.e., fractional anisotropy and ADC).

Acknowledgments

We would like to thank the following individuals for their contributions: Theo van Erp, Molly Hardt, Jennifer K. Johnson.

Author Contributions

Conceived and designed the experiments: KHK TDC AS CEB. Performed the experiments: KHK TR. Analyzed the data: KHK ESL. Contributed reagents/materials/analysis tools: TDC AS CEB. Wrote the paper: KHK TR ESL TDC AS CEB.

References

1. Shilyansky C, Karlsgodt K, Cummings DM, Sidiropoulou K, Hardt M, et al. (2010) Neurofibromin regulates corticostriatal inhibitory networks during working memory performance. Proceedings of the National Academy of Sciences 107: 13141–13146.
2. Huson SM (1989) Recent developments in the diagnosis and management of neurofibromatosis. Arch Dis Child 64: 745–749.
3. Ozonoff S (1999) Cognitive impairment in neurofibromatosis type 1. Am J Med Genet 89: 45–52.
4. Rowbotham I, Pit-ten Cate IM, Sonuga-Barke EJ, Huijbregts SC (2009) Cognitive control in adolescents with neurofibromatosis type 1. Neuropsychology 23: 50–60.
5. North K, Joy P, Yuille D, Cocks N, Mobbs E, et al. (1994) Specific learning disability in children with neurofibromatosis type 1: significance of MRI abnormalities. Neurology 44: 878–883.
6. North KN, Riccardi V, Samango-Sprouse C, Ferner R, Moore B, et al. (1997) Cognitive function and academic performance in neurofibromatosis. 1: consensus statement from the NF1 Cognitive Disorders Task Force. Neurology 48: 1121–1127.
7. Hyman SL, Shores A, North KN (2005) The nature and frequency of cognitive deficits in children with neurofibromatosis type 1. Neurology 65: 1037–1044.
8. Mautner VF, Kluwe L, Thakker SD, Leark RA (2002) Treatment of ADHD in neurofibromatosis type 1. Dev Med Child Neurol 44: 164–170.
9. Huijbregts SC, de Sonneville LM (2011) Does cognitive impairment explain behavioral and social problems of children with neurofibromatosis type 1? Behav Genet 41: 430–436.
10. Gillberg C, Forsell C (1984) Childhood psychosis and neurofibromatosis–more than a coincidence? J Autism Dev Disord 14: 1–8.
11. North K (2000) Neurofibromatosis type 1. Am J Med Genet 97: 119–127.
12. Cutting LE, Cooper KL, Koth CW, Mostofsky SH, Kates WR, et al. (2002) Megalencephaly in NF1: predominantly white matter contribution and mitigation by ADHD. Neurology 59: 1388–1394.
13. Moore BD, 3rd, Slopis JM, Jackson EF, De Winter AE, Leeds NE (2000) Brain volume in children with neurofibromatosis type 1: relation to neuropsychological status. Neurology 54: 914–920.
14. Greenwood RS, Tupler LA, Whitt JK, Buu A, Dombeck CB, et al. (2005) Brain morphometry, T2-weighted hyperintensities, and IQ in children with neurofibromatosis type 1. Arch Neurol 62: 1904–1908.
15. Payne JM, Moharir MD, Webster R, North KN (2010) Brain structure and function in neurofibromatosis type 1: current concepts and future directions. J Neurol Neurosurg Psychiatry 81: 304–309.
16. Dubovsky EC, Booth TN, Vezina G, Samango-Sprouse CA, Palmer KM, et al. (2001) MR imaging of the corpus callosum in pediatric patients with neurofibromatosis type 1. AJNR Am J Neuroradiol 22: 190–195.
17. Kayl AE, Moore BD, 3rd, Slopis JM, Jackson EF, Leeds NE (2000) Quantitative morphology of the corpus callosum in children with neurofibromatosis and attention-deficit hyperactivity disorder. J Child Neurol 15: 90–96.
18. Margariti PN, Blekas K, Katzioti FG, Zikou AK, Tzoufi M, et al. (2007) Magnetization transfer ratio and volumetric analysis of the brain in macrocephalic patients with neurofibromatosis type 1. Eur Radiol 17: 433–438.
19. Pride N, Payne JM, Webster R, Shores EA, Rae C, et al. (2010) Corpus callosum morphology and its relationship to cognitive function in neurofibromatosis type 1. J Child Neurol 25: 834–841.
20. Viskochil D, Cawthon R, O'Connell P, Xu GF, Stevens J, et al. (1991) The gene encoding the oligodendrocyte-myelin glycoprotein is embedded within the neurofibromatosis type 1 gene. Mol Cell Biol 11: 906–912.
21. Bennett A O MR (2008) Dual constraints on synapse formation and regression in schizophrenia: neuregulin, neuroligin, dysbindin, DISC1, MuSK and agrin. Aust NZ J Psychiatry 42: 662–677.
22. Lee JS, Padmanabhan A, Shin J, Zhu S, Guo F, et al. (2010) Oligodendrocyte progenitor cell numbers and migration are regulated by the zebrafish orthologs of the NF1 tumor suppressor gene. Hum Mol Genet 19: 4643–4653.
23. Basser PJ, Jones DK (2002) Diffusion-tensor MRI: Theory, experimental design and data analysis - A technical review. NMR in Biomedicine 15: 456–467.

24. Karlsgodt KH, Jacobson SC, Seal M, Fusar-Poli P (2012) The relationship of developmental changes in white matter to the onset of psychosis. Curr Pharm Des 18: 422–433.
25. Eastwood JD, Fiorella DJ, MacFall JF, Delong DM, Provenzale JM, et al. (2001) Increased brain apparent diffusion coefficient in children with neurofibromatosis type 1. Radiology 219: 354–358.
26. Tognini G, Ferrozzi F, Garlaschi G, Piazza P, Patti A, et al. (2005) Brain apparent diffusion coefficient evaluation in pediatric patients with neurofibromatosis type 1. J Comput Assist Tomogr 29: 298–304.
27. Alkan A, Sigirci A, Kutlu R, Ozcan H, Erdem G, et al. (2005) Neurofibromatosis type 1: diffusion weighted imaging findings of brain. Eur J Radiol 56: 229–234.
28. Wignall EL, Griffiths PD, Papadakis NG, Wilkinson ID, Wallis LI, et al. (2010) Corpus callosum morphology and microstructure assessed using structural MR imaging and diffusion tensor imaging: initial findings in adults with neurofibromatosis type 1. AJNR Am J Neuroradiol 31: 856–861.
29. Zamboni SL, Loenneker T, Boltshauser E, Martin E, Il'yasov KA (2007) Contribution of diffusion tensor MR imaging in detecting cerebral microstructural changes in adults with neurofibromatosis type 1. AJNR Am J Neuroradiol 28: 773–776.
30. van Engelen SJ, Krab LC, Moll HA, de Goede-Bolder A, Pluijm SM, et al. (2008) Quantitative differentiation between healthy and disordered brain matter in patients with neurofibromatosis type I using diffusion tensor imaging. AJNR Am J Neuroradiol 29: 816–822.
31. Wozniak JR, Lim KO (2006) Advances in white matter imaging: a review of in vivo magnetic resonance methodologies and their applicability to the study of development and aging. Neuroscience and Biobehavioral Reviews 30: 762–774.
32. Song AW, Harshbarger T, Li T, Kim KH, Ugurbil K, et al. (2003) Functional activation using apparent diffusion coefficient-dependent contrast allows better spatial localization to the neuronal activity: Evidence using diffusion tensor imaging and fiber tracking. NeuroImage.
33. Song SK, Yoshino J, Le TQ, Lin SJ, Sun SW, et al. (2005) Demyelination increases radial diffusivity in corpus callosum of mouse brain. Neuroimage 26: 132–140.
34. Acosta-Cabronero J, Williams GB, Pengas G, Nestor PJ (2010) Absolute diffusivities define the landscape of white matter degeneration in Alzheimer's disease. Brain 133: 529–539.
35. Song SK, Sun SW, Ramsbottom MJ, Chang C, Russell J, et al. (2002) Dysmyelination revealed through MRI as increased radial (but unchanged axial) diffusion of water. Neuroimage 17: 1429–1436.
36. Ford JC, Hackney DB, Lavi E, Phillips M, Patel U (1998) Dependence of apparent diffusion coefficients on axonal spacing, membrane permeability, and diffusion time in spinal cord white matter. J Magn Reson Imaging 8: 775–782.
37. Hikida T, Jaaro-Peled H, Seshadri S, Oishi K, Hookway C, et al. (2007) Dominant-negative DISC1 transgenic mice display schizophrenia-associated phenotypes detected by measures translatable to humans. Proc Natl Acad Sci U S A 104: 14501–14506.
38. Golabchi FN, Brooks DH, Hoge WS, De Girolami U, Maier SE (2010) Pixel-based comparison of spinal cord MR diffusion anisotropy with axon packing parameters. Magn Reson Med 63: 1510–1519.
39. Conference NIoHCD (1988) Neurofibromatosis: Conference Statement. Archives of Neurology. 575–578.
40. First MB, Spitzer R, Gibbon M, Williams J (1997) Structured Clinical Interview for DSM-IV Axis I Disorders. New York: Biometrics Research Department, New York State Psychiatric Institute.
41. Smith SM, Jenkinson M, Woolrich MW, Beckmann CF, Behrens TE, et al. (2004) Advances in functional and structural MR image analysis and implementation as FSL. Neuroimage 23 Suppl 1: S208–219.
42. Smith SM, Jenkinson M, Johansen-Berg H, Rueckert D, Nichols TE, et al. (2006) Tract-based spatial statistics: Voxelwise analysis of multi-subject diffusion data. Neuroimage 31: 1487–1505.
43. Ashburner J, Friston KJ (2000) Voxel-based morphometry the methods. Neuroimage 11: 805–821.
44. Good CD, Johnsrude IS, Ashburner J, Henson RN, Friston KJ, et al. (2001) A voxel-based morphometric study of ageing in 465 normal adult human brains. Neuroimage 14: 21–36.
45. Smith S (2002) Fast robust automated brain extraction. Human Brain Mapping 17: 143–155.
46. Zhang Y, Brady M, Smith S (2001) Segmentation of brain MR images through a hidden Markov random field model and the expectation maximization algorithm. IEEE Trans Med Imaging 20: 45–57.
47. Jenkinson M, Smith S (2001) A global optimisation method for robust affine registration of brain images. Med Image Anal 5: 143–156.
48. Jenkinson M, Bannister P, Brady M, Smith S (2002) Improved optimization for the robust and accurate linear registration and motion correction of brain images. Neuroimage 17: 825–841.
49. Andersson J, Jenkinson M, Smith S (2007) Non-linear optimisation. FMRIB Technical Report TR07JA1 www.fmrib.ox.ac.uk/analysis/techrep.
50. Andersson J, Jenkinson M, Smith S (2007) Non-linear registration, aka Spatial normalisation. FMRIB Technical Report TR07JA2 www.fmrib.ox.ac.uk/analysis/techrep.
51. Rueckert D, Sonoda LI, Hayes C, Hill DL, Leach MO, et al. (1999) Nonrigid registration using free-form deformations: application to breast MR images. IEEE Trans Med Imaging 18: 712–721.
52. Mori S, Wakana S, Nagae-Poetscher LM, van Zijl PC (2005) MRI Atlas of Human White Matter. Amsterdam: Elsevier.
53. Wakana S, Caprihan A, Panzenboeck MM, Fallon JH, Perry M, et al. (2007) Reproducibility of quantitative tractography methods applied to cerebral white matter. Neuroimage 36: 630–644.
54. Hua K, Zhang J, Wakana S, Jiang H, Li X, et al. (2008) Tract probability maps in stereotaxic spaces: analyses of white matter anatomy and tract-specific quantification. Neuroimage 39: 336–347.
55. Karlsgodt K, Niendam TA, Bearden CE, Cannon TD (2009) White matter integrity and prediction of social and role functioning in subjects at ultra-high risk for psychosis. Biol Psychiatry 66: 562–569.
56. DiPaolo DP, Zimmerman RA, Rorke LB, Zackai EH, Bilaniuk LT, et al. (1995) Neurofibromatosis type 1: pathologic substrate of high-signal-intensity foci in the brain. Radiology 195: 721–724.
57. Sheikh SF, Kubal WS, Anderson AW, Mutalik P (2003) Longitudinal evaluation of apparent diffusion coefficient in children with neurofibromatosis type 1. J Comput Assist Tomogr 27: 681–686.
58. Johnson MR, Ferner RE, Bobrow M, Hughes RA (2000) Detailed analysis of the oligodendrocyte myelin glycoprotein gene in four patients with neurofibromatosis 1 and primary progressive multiple sclerosis. J Neurol Neurosurg Psychiatry 68: 643–646.
59. Mikol DD, Rongnoparut P, Allwardt BA, Marton LS, Stefansson K (1993) The oligodendrocyte-myelin glycoprotein of mouse: primary structure and gene structure. Genomics 17: 604–610.
60. Gil V, Bichler Z, Lee JK, Seira O, Llorens F, et al. (2010) Developmental expression of the oligodendrocyte myelin glycoprotein in the mouse telencephalon. Cereb Cortex 20: 1769–1779.
61. Kweh F, Zheng M, Kurenova E, Wallace M, Golubovskaya V, et al. (2009) Neurofibromin physically interacts with the N-terminal domain of focal adhesion kinase. Mol Carcinog 48: 1005–1017.
62. Boyanapalli M, Lahoud OB, Messiaen L, Kim B, Anderle de Sylor MS, et al. (2006) Neurofibromin binds to caveolin-1 and regulates ras, FAK, and Akt. Biochem Biophys Res Commun 340: 1200–1208.
63. Tamm L, Barnea-Goraly N, Reiss AL (2012) Diffusion tensor imaging reveals white matter abnormalities in Attention-Deficit/Hyperactivity Disorder. Psychiatry Res 202: 150–154.
64. de Zeeuw P, Mandl RC, Hulshoff Pol HE, van Engeland H, Durston S (2012) Decreased frontostriatal microstructural organization in attention deficit/hyperactivity disorder. Hum Brain Mapp 33: 1941–1951.
65. Nagel BJ, Bathula D, Herting M, Schmitt C, Kroenke CD, et al. (2011) Altered white matter microstructure in children with attention-deficit/hyperactivity disorder. J Am Acad Child Adolesc Psychiatry 50: 283–292.

Perceptual Learning in Williams Syndrome: Looking Beyond Averages

Patricia Gervan*, **Ferenc Gombos, Ilona Kovacs**

Department of Cognitive Science, Budapest University of Technology and Economics, Budapest, Hungary

Abstract

Williams Syndrome is a genetically determined neurodevelopmental disorder characterized by an uneven cognitive profile and surprisingly large neurobehavioral differences among individuals. Previous studies have already shown different forms of memory deficiencies and learning difficulties in WS. Here we studied the capacity of WS subjects to improve their performance in a basic visual task. We employed a contour integration paradigm that addresses occipital visual function, and analyzed the initial (i.e. baseline) and after-learning performance of WS individuals. Instead of pooling the very inhomogeneous results of WS subjects together, we evaluated individual performance by expressing it in terms of the deviation from the average performance of the group of typically developing subjects of similar age. This approach helped us to reveal information about the possible origins of poor performance of WS subjects in contour integration. Although the majority of WS individuals showed both reduced baseline and reduced learning performance, individual analysis also revealed a dissociation between baseline and learning capacity in several WS subjects. In spite of impaired initial contour integration performance, some WS individuals presented learning capacity comparable to learning in the typically developing population, and vice versa, poor learning was also observed in subjects with high initial performance levels. These data indicate a dissociation between factors determining initial performance and perceptual learning.

Editor: Tricia A. Thornton-Wells, Vanderbilt University, United States of America

Funding: This study was supported by OTKA (Hungarian Scientific Research Fund) NF60806 and TÁMOP-4.2.2.B-10/1′2010-0009 (Social Renewal Operational Programme). The funders had no role in study design, data collection and analysis, decision to publish, or preparation of the manuscript.

Competing Interests: The authors have declared that no competing interests exist.

* E-mail: pgervan@cogsci.bme.hu

Introduction

Genetically determined neurodevelopmental disorders (GNDs) involve impairment in the growth and development of the central nervous system and refer to a variety of disorders of brain functions, which can affect social behavior, emotions, learning ability and memory. Reduced learning capacity is a main feature of GNDs, e.g. Williams-, Rett-, fragile X- and Down syndrome [1].

Variations and anomalies in the structural and neurocomputational features of neurodevelopmentally disordered systems are extensive, and it is these altered features that determine the limits of plasticity and learning capacity. Pennington [2] suggests three groups of genetic effects on brain development that are possibly disrupted in neurodevelopmental disorders. Genetically driven alterations might be detected (i) in brain size, by altering the number of neurons or synapses; (ii) in the pattern of neuronal migration, occasionally in a regionally specific manner; and (iii) in the features of neurotransmission, either in terms of changed neurotransmitter levels or altered binding properties of receptor proteins.

In addition to genetically determined structural abnormalities [3–11] and altered features of neurotransmission [12–14], the characteristic difficulty to learn may occur because of disruption in terms of classic 'epigenetic factors,' such as sleep [15–21].

Our aim was to assess the ability to learn in a simple visual task in a group of subjects living with a GND, and to compare their initial and after-learning performance to that of a group of typically developing subjects. Perceptual learning is exceptionally helpful when assessing learning abilities in GNDs, since it requires relatively low cognitive load. Another advantage of employing a perceptual learning paradigm is that perceptual learning has been extensively studied and its neural background has been clarified (e.g. [22–24]). Because of the relatively small genetic deletion, and the well-defined functional and structural impairments of the visual system, we have decided to study perceptual learning in Williams syndrome (WS). WS is a genetic disorder caused by a hemizygous microdeletion of cc. 20–30 genes on chromosome 7q11.2, and it causes –among other problems - mild to moderate mental retardation and is associated with poor visuo-spatial abilities [25–26]. Earlier studies reported impaired short-term visuo-spatial memory deficits (e.g. [27–28]), relatively poor performance on tests of visual and verbal long-term memory [29] and poor episodic retrieval of both verbal and visuo-perceptual stimuli [28]. Reduced learning rate was found in procedural tasks [30–31] in groups of WS children; however, perceptual learning has not yet been studied in this population.

We employed a Contour Integration paradigm (CI) that was originally developed by Kovacs and Julesz [32] to study low-level visual integration processes. CI images are composed of collinear chains of Gabor elements forming a horizontally placed egg shape on a background of randomly positioned and oriented Gabor patches (Figure 1A). At the neuronal level, visual contour integration involves spatial integration and it is thought to be mediated by the long-range horizontal connections of orientation selective neurons in the primary visual cortex (e.g. [32–34]). Behavioral studies found an unexpectedly late development of contour integration abilities, improving until the early teen-age years [35–36].These results are in line with the neuroanatomical findings on the prolonged development of horizontal connections in layer II/III of the human primary visual cortex, which extends well into childhood [37]. Perceptual learning in CI is specific to stimulus features, such as orientation and color [35,38], indicating that the process involves use-dependent changes in connectivity within the orientation selective neuronal network in the primary visual cortex. More recently, it has been demonstrated that after an initial acquisition phase, significant performance increase in this task occurs only after a night of sleep, indicating that learning in CI is sleep dependent [39].

It is especially challenging to evaluate the different aspects of behavior, perception and cognition in GNDs, and well-controlled comparisons across subject groups are difficult. GND populations are frequently studied as groups, and individual variability is not always taken into account. Large individual differences have been shown to exist in GND populations (e.g. in Down Syndrome (DS): [40]; in WS: [41]), therefore, averaging across subjects leads to significant information loss. It has also been suggested that group matching can be misleading in GND research when only the equivalency of means across groups is monitored routinely, and the homogeneity of their variances or the shapes of their distributions are not [42]. It is extremely common to choose a control group by matching for IQ or using IQ as a covariate in group-matching studies [43]. Generally, GNDs result in significant disparity between chronological and mental age, so researchers have the options to either appoint chronologically younger typically developing (TD) persons with similar mental

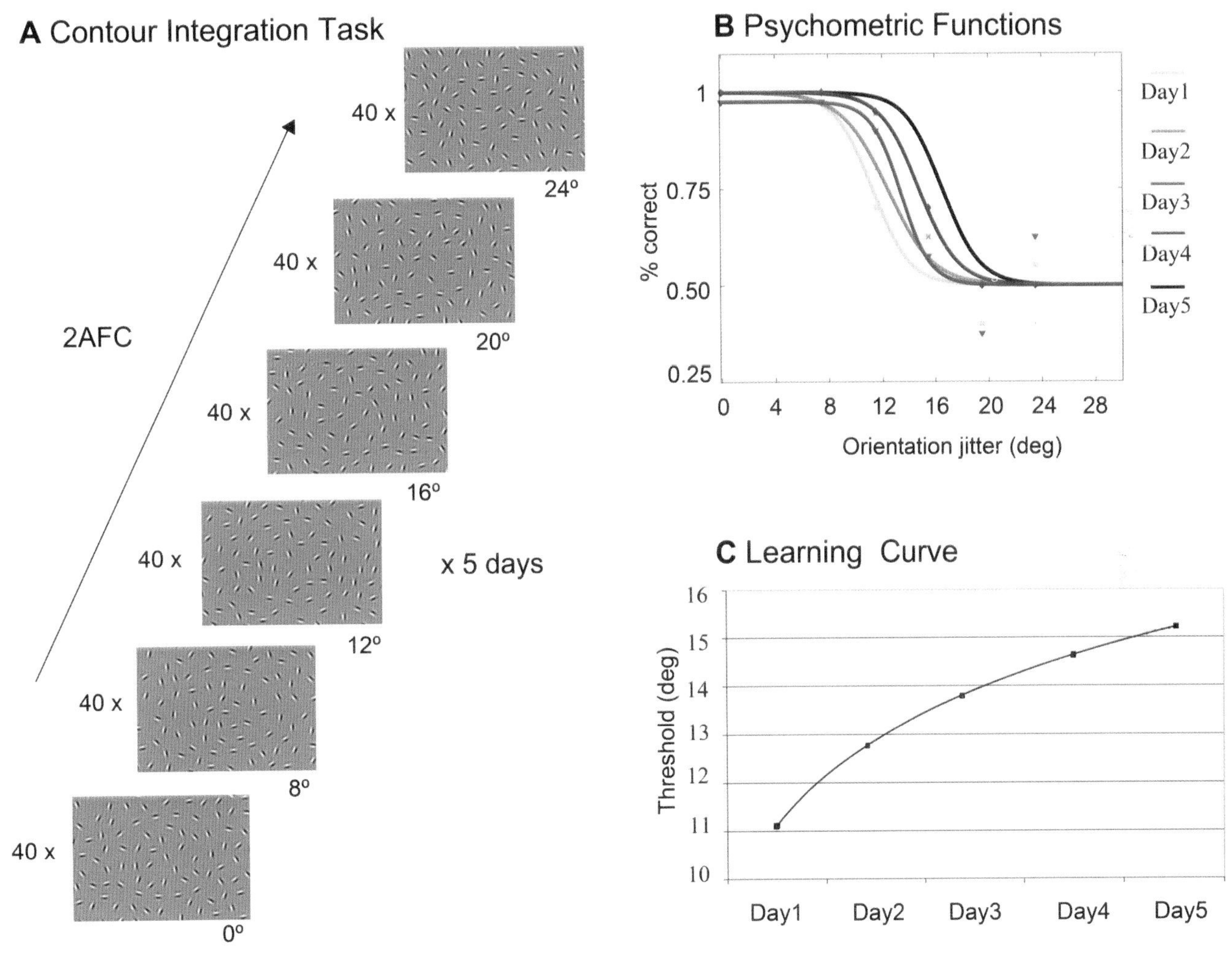

Figure 1. Procedure. (A) Contour Integration task. The visual stimulus consists of a collinear chain of Gabor elements forming a horizontally placed egg shape embedded in random noise. The contour elements were jittered from the original path of the contour in an increasing order of difficulty, between 0° to 24,° across six difficulty levels. Observers were presented with forty stimuli at each difficulty level and had to decide in a 2AFC procedure which direction the narrower part of the egg points to. Subjects practiced on five consecutive days. (B) Calculating perceptual threshold. This panel shows an example of how the perceptual threshold was calculated for every subject during the five-day training. Percentage of correct responses (on the y axis) was recorded at each of the six difficulty levels (on the x axis). Individual marks (triangles, squares etc.) are the measured data points. Perceptual threshold was calculated by fitting a logistic psychometric function on the data points. Threshold was defined by orientation jitter at 75% correct performance. Threshold increased (i.e. performance increased and this resulted in shifting of the fitted curves to the right) during the five-day-long training as a consequence of perceptual learning. (C) Example of a learning curve. The learning curve shows how the perceptual threshold increases through a five-day long training as a result of perceptual learning. These curves were drawn for each TD age-group by plotting the perceptual thresholds of the groups across the five practice days (see Figure 2B).

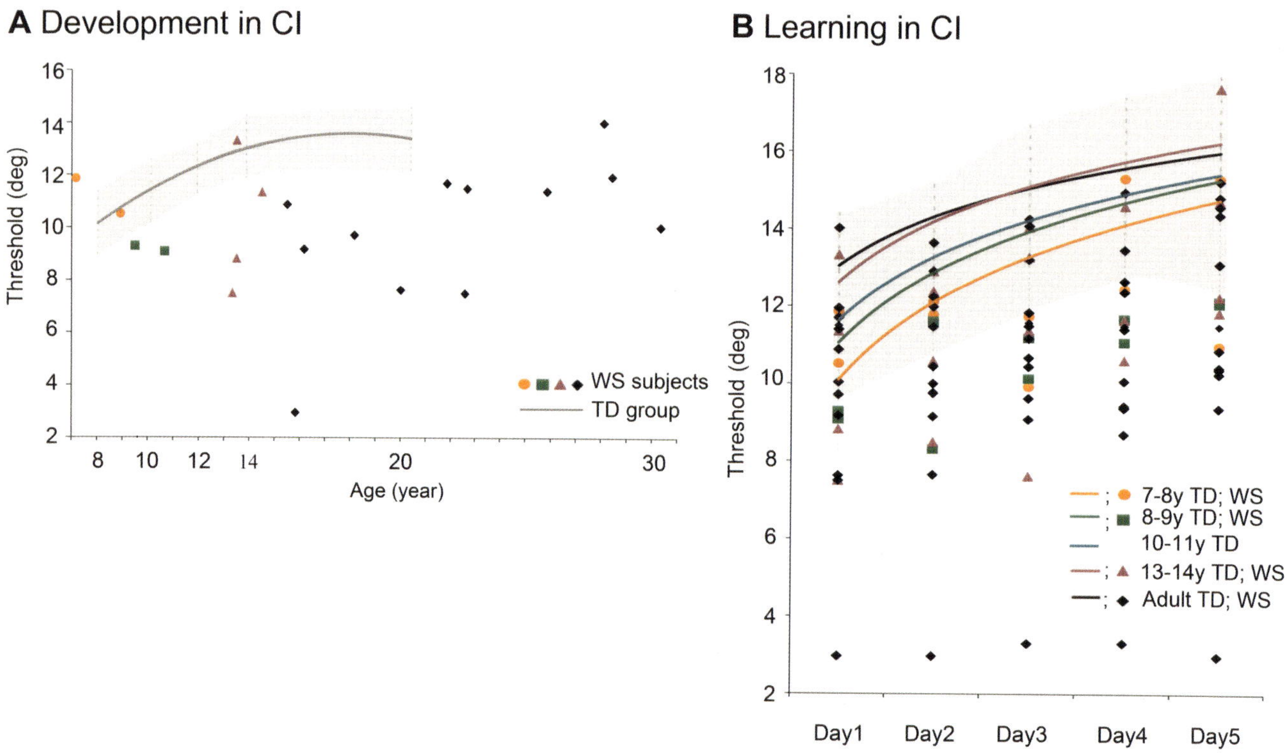

Figure 2. Development and learning in CI. (A) Development in CI. The developmental curve of the TD group was fitted on the baseline averages of the six age-groups (goodness of fit: R = 0,9162*), the shaded area designates standard deviation. Visual CI performance increases as a function of age showing a slow developmental course of contour integration, reaching the adult level by 13–14 years of age. Colored symbols stand for individual WS subjects. Colors correspond to the appropriate age-groups shown in Fig. 2B. Performance of WS subjects has an extremely high variability and only a few subjects are within the TD range. (B) Learning in CI. Colored lines represent learning curves of each TD age-group (standard deviation is shown by light-grey shading). Younger TD subjects seem to learn at a greater speed. Colored symbols stand for individual WS subjects. Colors correspond to the appropriate age-groups. WS subjects vary a great deal in terms of learning capacity, and only a few subjects are in the TD range.

age as a control group, or select a control population with a different disorder and similar mental and chronological age. In the case of selecting TD controls, maturational and experience-related concerns arise as younger controls will be at a more immature neural level, and a shorter amount of time will be available for them for perceptual, social and cognitive experiences. On the other hand, choosing atypically developing controls brings on the problem of uneven cognitive profiles, which is fairly common in GNDs (e.g. in DS: [44]; in WS: [41]). Similar overall IQ scores can arise from entirely different response profiles, i.e. from dissimilar cognitive profiles, in different GNDs [45]. Moreover, it has been suggested that IQ is not sufficient as a covariate in cognitive studies, and using IQ as a matching variable or covariate has resulted in over-corrected, inconsistent, and counterintuitive findings about neurocognitive functions [43]. Here we attempt to overcome the above mentioned difficulties arising in the classical matched-control design, and strive to obtain more informative and reliable evaluation of WS individuals. According to this effort, we analyzed individual WS data as compared to the data of typically developing subject groups of corresponding ages in a perceptual learning paradigm.

We assume typically low initial (baseline) performance, and, at the same time, relatively high individual variability both in the initial contour integration performance and in learning capacity within the WS population. We assume that initial performance and learning capacity might be dissociated: low initial performance may not be linked with reduced learning capacity, and, vice versa, reduced learning may not be coupled with low initial performance.

Materials and Methods

Participants

Williams syndrome subjects. 19 individuals (7 males, 12 females, age range: 7 to 30 years) with WS took part in the experiment. Detailed demographic data of the WS group is described in Table 1. In case of each WS subject, the genetic diagnosis was established using fluorescent in situ hybridization (FISH) probes for elastin. All participants had normal or corrected to normal vision.

Typically developing (TD) subjects. The TD control children and adults were recruited from primary schools and universities in Budapest. The TD population consisted of eighty children in four age-groups (40 females, 40 males; age range: 7–14 years) and twenty adults (10 males, 10 females; age range: 18–23 years). Further details of the TD population are summarized in Table 2. Those with a history of neurological or psychiatric illnesses were excluded. All observers had normal or corrected to normal vision. During the course of the experiment participants were asked about the amount of night sleep. Those who did not have at least seven hours of sleep were also excluded from the study.

Table 1. Demographic data of participating WS subjects.

WS code	Age (years)	Gender
WS1	7	Male
WS2	9	Female
WS3	10	Male
WS4	11	Female
WS5	13	Female
WS6	14	Male
WS7	14	Female
WS8	15	Male
WS9	16	Female
WS10	16	Male
WS11	18	Female
WS12	20	Female
WS13	22	Female
WS14	23	Male
WS15	16	Female
WS16	26	Male
WS17	28	Female
WS18	28	Female
WS19	30	Female

Ethics

Written informed consent was obtained from adult subjects and the parents of participating children. Subjects participated voluntarily and were unpaid. Ethical approval was granted by the Social Sciences Ethical Review Board of the Budapest University of Technology and Economics.

Procedure

In this altered version of the CI task, orientation jitter was introduced along the contour (see also in [46]). Orientation jitter of the contour elements was varied between 0° to 24° across six difficulty levels (0°, 8°, 12°,16°, 20°, 24°, see Figure 1A). The carrier spatial frequency of the Gabor patches was 5 c/deg and their contrast was 95%. The spacing between the contour elements was kept constant (8 λ; where λ is the wavelength of the Gabor stimulus) at the average spacing value between the background elements. The signal-to-noise ratio as defined by a D parameter (D = average background spacing/contour spacing) of each image was 0.9. The stimulus onset time was maximum 2000 milliseconds (or until the subject responded), with a fixation cross between stimuli (500 milliseconds). Observers had to determine which direction the egg shaped contour pointed to. A set of 40 images was presented at each of the six difficulty levels in four blocks of 10 trials, which means 240 trials/session. Stimuli were presented in the order of increasing difficulty levels. The experiment took a maximum of 20 minutes to complete. The percentage of correct responses was recorded at each difficulty level. Threshold was determined by a psychometric function at 75% correct performance. Observers practiced in the CI task through five consecutive days in the same design. Thresholds were calculated for each day (see example in Figure 1B), and these thresholds outlined a learning curve for the five-day-long training period (see example in Figure 1C). Day1 performance was considered as baseline and we measured perceptual improvement by Day5. No feedback was provided to the participants.

Table 2. Age-groups of TD participants.

Group	Age(months)	SD	Male (n)	Female(n)
7–8 years	95,3	7,6	10	10
9–10 years	120,5	8,2	9	11
11–12 years	142,3	7,3	9	11
13–14 years	165,5	7,4	10	10
Adults	243,9	20	10	10

Results

Typically Developing Subjects

Adults vs. children. Table 3 presents the baseline and learning data of TD age-groups. Independent t-test revealed significant differences in baseline performance between Adults and Group 7–8y, Group 9–10y, Group 11–12y (Adults vs. Group 7–8y: $t = -6.244$, $df = 38$, $p<0.01$; Adults vs. Group 9–10y: $t = -4.653$, $df = 38$, $p<0.01$; Adults vs. Group 11–12y: $t = -2.836$, $df = 38$, $p<0.01$).

In order to determine the learning capacity of the different age-groups, a learning rate was calculated by subtracting Day1 threshold from Day 5 threshold. Independent t-test showed significantly lower learning rate in Adults than in Group 7–8y, Group 9–10y, Group 11–12y (Adults vs. Group 7–8y: $t = 2.959$, $df = 38$, $p<0.01$; Adults vs. Group 9–10y: $t = 2.931$, $df = 38$, $p<0.01$; Adults vs. Group 11–12y: $t = 2.246$, $df = 38$, $p<0.05$).

No significant differences were found between Adults and Group 13–14y in baseline (independent t-test; $t = -0.808$, $df = 38$, $p = 0.424$) or in learning rate (independent t-test; $t = 1.602$, $df = 38$, $p = 0.118$).

Differences between age-groups of children. Independent t-test revealed significant differences in baseline performance between Group 7–8y and all the other child groups (Group 9–10y: $t = -2.534$, $df = 33.798$, $p<0,05$; Group 11–12y: $t = -4.395$, $df = 31.605$, $p<0.01$, Group 13–14y: $t = -5.321$, $df = 38$, $p<0.01$). Group 9–10y's baseline performance was significantly lower than that of Group 11–12y and Group 13–14y (independent t-test: Group 11–12y: $t = -2.246$, $df = 38$, $p<0.05$; Group 13–14y: $t = -3.580$, $df = 38$, $p<0,01$). Independent t-tests showed no significant differences in the learning rate of the different groups of children.

Williams Syndrome Subjects

Normalization and correction of the TD and WS data. As Figure 2 demonstrates, there are enormous individual differences among WS subjects. Some subjects are within the typically developing performance range, while some are far below the average TD performance. Since evaluating WS subjects as a group would have lead to loss of information, we analyzed the performance of WS subjects individually. In order to perform normalization on the TD population data we converted individual baseline values (Day1 perceptual threshold in jitter) and learning rate (the improvement by Day5 expressed in jitter; i.e. subtracting Day1 threshold from Day5 threshold) into z-scores. Baseline performance and learning rate of the TD individuals were normalized with respect to the age-group they belonged to. Baseline performance and learning rate of WS individuals were

Table 3. TD baseline and learning data.

Group	Baseline group means and SE (in degree)	Learning group means and SE (in degree)
7 – 8 years	10,02 (0,4)	4,46 (0,44)
9 – 10 years	11,24 (0,29)	4,15 (0,3)
11 – 12 years	12,07 (0,33)	3,87 (0,32)
13 – 14 years	12,91 (0,38)	3,57 (0,27)
Adults	13,22 (0,36)	2,81 (0,34)

The raw baseline and learning data of the TD age-groups. The table shows mean baseline data (threshold on Day1) and the average learning data (improvement from Day1 to Day5 expressed in degree) of the TD participants.

normalized with respect to their TD age-group as well, calculating z-scores for WS individuals from the mean and standard deviation of the corresponding TD age-group. Although previous studies have shown age-related performance reduction in contour integration, this was only found well beyond the age of 30 [47–48]. Therefore, it is safe to compare our older WS subjects to the younger TD adult group.

Figure 3A presents the relationship between the baseline and learning z-score values. There is a significant negative correlation ($r = -0.372$, $p < 0.0001$) between the baseline and learning z-score values of the TD population. The lower the baseline, the greater the improvement is during the five-day learning course. Regression analysis showed linear connection between learning and baseline z-score values (regression coefficient $= -0.372$; $R^2 = 0.1384$; $F = 15.7373$; $p < 0,0001$; error variance $= 0.8353$). Most WS subjects have poor baseline z-score values, thus the amount of their improvement does not represent adequately their learning abilities compared to the TD population, who start from a higher baseline value. In order to eliminate the baseline effect and to create an improvement measure that is comparable across TD and WS populations, we corrected the learning z-score values of every subject. Correction was performed by subtracting the baseline value multiplied by the regression coefficient from the learning z-score values, thereby subtracting the regression line value at the baseline z-score value from the learning z-score value (see Figure 3B).

TD subjects flock together around zero, while WS subjects are typically outside of the TD range both with respect to baseline and corrected learning z-score. However, they also show large individual differences. After the correction of the learning z-score values, mean of the baseline and the corrected learning z-score values of the TD population were 0 with a standard deviation of 0.9796 and 0.9093, respectively. The range of one and two standard deviations around the mean of the baseline z-score (shaded and colored vertical strips in Figure 3B) and the corrected learning z-score (shaded and colored horizontal strips in Figure 3B) of the TD population were calculated respectively. Table 4 shows the individual baseline and corrected learning z-score data of the WS subjects.

Discussion

According to Figure 3B and Table 4, WS subjects' performances show four major patterns: (1) subjects performing in the normal range (or even above) both in terms of baseline performance and learning rate, (2) subjects in the normal range in terms of baseline, but handicapped in learning, (3) subjects in the normal range in terms of learning, but handicapped in terms of baseline performance, (4) subjects handicapped both in terms of baseline performance and learning. We would like to draw attention to the fact that (2) and (3) are particularly interesting with respect to the potential dissociation between the factors determining initial (baseline) performance and learning. According to the current state of knowledge (see references below), these factors might be related to genetically determined structural brain damage (in the case of initial performance); and genetically determined changes in the morphology, altered features of neurotransmission or epigenetic factors (learning).

The observer is assumed to rely on the horizontal connections of the orientation selective neurons in V1 while carrying out the CI task [32,49], therefore, baseline performance in CI might be considered as an indicator of V1 function, and poor performance suggests structural and/or functional damage in V1. Brain imaging and anatomical studies found an overall smaller brain volume in WS with structural abnormalities, including abnormally increased gyrification and a relatively large loss of gray matter volume in parieto-occipital areas (e.g. [50–53]). Studies identified a well-differentiated area V1 in WS; however, the volume of this area is smaller compared to controls [50,52]. Besides the volumetric abnormalities, increased cell packing and neuronal size differences were described in this region [52–53]. The above mentioned findings imply atypical V1 functioning in WS. However, in order to directly demonstrate the connection between the behavioral scores in CI (baseline performance) and V1 structural abnormality at the level of WS individuals, further imaging and anatomical studies are needed.

There might be a number of different factors behind reduced learning capacity in WS. Functional, morphological or cell–cell interaction- and connection abnormalities are likely to be involved. Genetically determined changes in the morphology, shape and number of dendritic spines, or alterations of synaptic transmission and subsequent impairment of synaptic function will likely underlie learning and memory deficits. One of the genes commonly missing in WS is Limk1 [54]. Limk1 is thought to be involved in regulating dendritic spine size [55]. Dendritic spines are localized at the postsynaptic sites of excitatory synapses, and as sites of axonal-dendritic contacts, they are potential mediators of the connective plasticity underlying learning, memory, and cognition [56]. In addition to Limk1, Cyln2 [57] is another possible candidate gene contributing structural–functional abnormalities and impaired plasticity in WS. Cyln2 encodes proteins that regulate dynamic aspects of the cytoskeleton of the cells. Altered regulation might lead to defects during brain development and/or deficits in synaptic plasticity in adulthood [58]. Stx1a is also mentioned as a relevant gene in terms of cognitive features in WS. This gene encodes Syntaxin-1A, a protein that plays a crucial role in synaptic exocytosis of neurotransmitters from neuronal cells [59]. Growing evidence support the role of Stx1a in deficits of

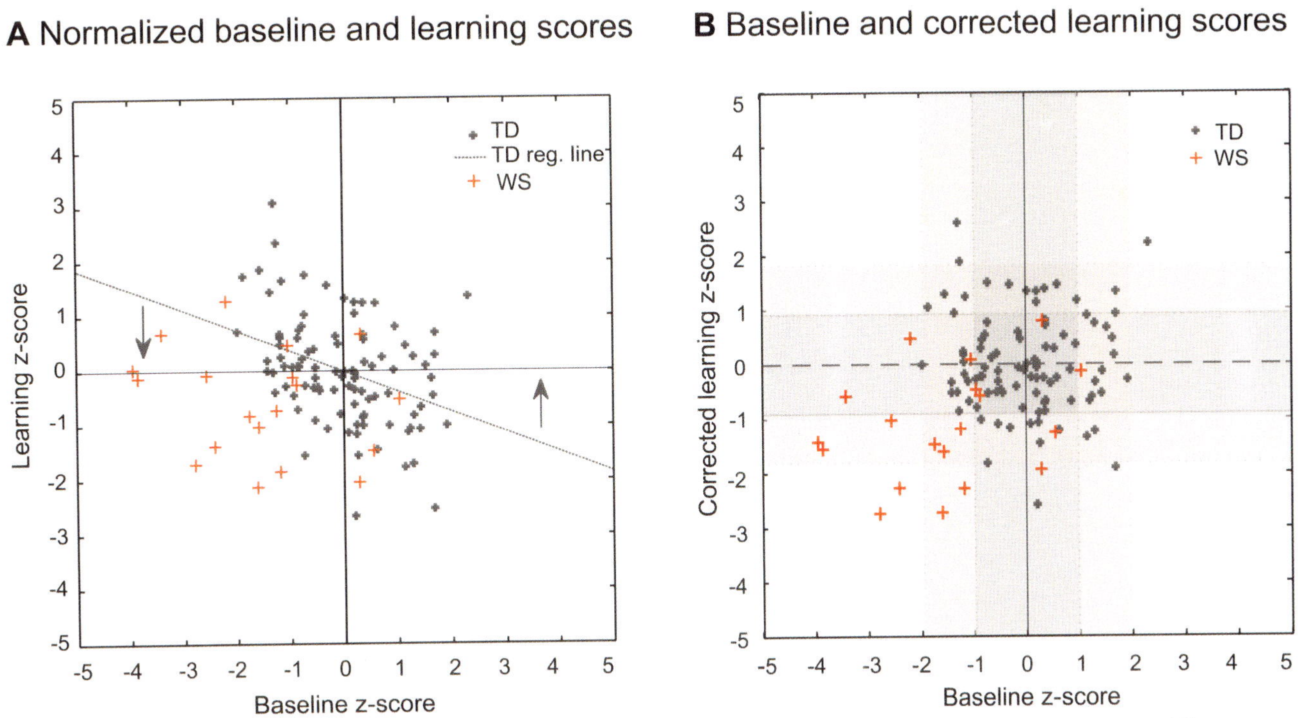

Figure 3. Normalized and corrected scores in CI. (A). Normalized baseline and learning scores. The scatter-plot shows individual baseline (threshold on Day1) and learning (Day5 threshold - Day1 threshold) z-score of individual TD (dark grey cross) and WS (red cross) subjects. Average performance on both axes is at zero. The dotted grey line represents the linear regression line fitted on the TD data set. There is a significant negative correlation between baseline performance and the amount of learning in the task ($r = -0{,}372$, $p < 0{,}0001$): the lower the baseline is the greater the improvement will be by the fifth day. (B). Baseline and corrected learning scores. In order to eliminate the effect of the baseline on improvement we corrected the learning data. Corrected learning z-scores were obtained by subtracting baseline values multiplied by the regression coefficient from the learning z-scores. The scatter plot represents individual baseline z-scores and corrected learning z-scores of the TD (dark grey cross) and WS (red cross) participants. Light grey and light pink zones show the range of one and two standard deviations around the mean of the baseline z-score (vertical strip) and the corrected learning z-score (horizontal strip) of the TD population, respectively.

learning and memory in WS [60–61]. In spite of the genetic determination of the cognitive symptoms in WS, it is important to recognize that there is also variability in the amount and type of genetic impairment. Studies reported atypical, partial deletions [62–63], providing a potential explanation for the inhomogeneous behavioral performance in the WS population.

In addition to the genetically determined morphological, functional, neurotransmission related alterations, another possible factor determining reduced learning capacity is disturbed sleep in WS. Polysomnographic studies report decreased sleep time, fragmented sleep, atypical limb movements, increased slow wave sleep, decreased REM sleep and irregular sleep cycles in WS [64–66]. In the spectral analysis of the polysomnographic recordings Gombos and colleagues [65] also showed increased frontal slow wave activity in NREM sleep as well as decreased alpha and sigma activity in both NREM and REM sleep of WS subjects. The higher frequency of NREM sleep EEG sigma activity was shown to be a characteristic feature of WS suggesting an alteration of sleep-dependent thalamocortical activity in this population [66]. Normal baseline CI performance associated with poor learning in some of our WS subjects might suggest that impaired sleep might be the culprit. However, this hypothesis needs confirmation from polysomnographic sleep studies.

In addition to gaining further insight about the learning abilities of WS subjects, we also intended to highlight variability in this atypically developing group. Individual differences are amplified even during typical development as a consequence of interactive effects of genetic and epigenetic factors. These emerging differences are greater in atypical development. Several difficulties may arise with respect to group-matching studies, involving loss of information about individual differences, missing the link between behavioral phenotypes and genes, and also between altered cognition and abnormal structural organization of the neural system. And finally, merging individual data in atypically developing groups might prevent the development of optimal treatment strategies. Effective treatment requires that exact determination of factors underlying cognitive/behavioral symptoms. Here we compared the individual results of WS subjects to that of the typically developing age-groups in order to avoid the above mentioned drawbacks.

We studied initial performance and perceptual learning capacity of Williams Syndrome and typically developing subjects in a basic visual task involving the Contour Integration paradigm. In order to avoid the usual drawbacks arising in group-matching studies, we compared WS individuals to typically developing populations in a novel way. Instead of pooling the very inhomogeneous results of WS subjects together, we evaluated individual performance by expressing it in terms of the deviation from the average performance of the group of typically developing subjects of similar age. We have chosen the contour integration task since we wanted to study an assumed dissociation between measured baseline performance and learning capacity in a given task. We assumed that the majority of the WS subjects would have difficulty and lower than TD level performance in this task. This choice allowed us to highlight and emphasize that structural/functional impairments would not necessarily lead to reduced/impaired

Table 4. Individual data of the WS individuals.

WS subject code	Raw Baseline Data (in deg)	Raw Learning data (in deg)	Baseline (B) z-score	Corrected Learning (CL) z-score	Deviation from average B	Deviation from average CL
WS1	11,86	3,46	1,0344	−0,1283	+	N
WS7	13,3292	4,3382	0,313	0,79	n	N
WS8	11,349	3,3856	−0,9527	−0,465	n	N
WS18	11,9511	2,4351	−0,8777	−0,5768	n	N
WS2	10,5258	0,4629	0,2823	−1,9329	n	- -
WS17	14,02	0,58	0,5479	−1,2563	n	-
WS13	11,7	3,55	−1,0508	0,0858	-	n
WS19	10,0418	4,7975	−2,1934	0,4743	- -	n
WS5	7,5	4,357	−3,413	−0,5806	- -	n
WS3	9,29973	2,78907	−1,587	−1,6059	-	-
WS4	9,09	3,06	−1,7578	−1,4682	-	-
WS16	11,3988	1,7173	−1,2583	−1,1865	-	-
WS15	11,5	0,0004	−1,6158	−2,7197	-	- -
WS9	10,88	−0,43	−1,6158	−2,7197	-	- -
WS12	7,63	2,638	−3,8553	−1,5521	- -	-
WS14	7,5	2,887	−3,9449	−1,4231	- -	-
WS6	8,82892	3,43368	−2,5636	−1,0246	- -	-
WS10	9,18383	0,21007	−2,7846	−2,7371	- -	- -
WS11	9,72214	0,71536	−2,4136	−2,2696	- -	- -

Note:
+: z-scores above one standard deviation.
n: z-scores within one standard deviation.
-: z-scores below one standard deviation.
- -: z-scores below two standard deviations.

learning capacity. Some of those who gave very low baseline level performance presented learning capacity within the normal range, and vice versa. The detailed analysis we offer might affect treatment strategies at the level of the individual. Exploring individual differences and looking at each subject individually with a goal-oriented and comprehensive approach shall enable substantial advancement in the field of neurorehabilitation in the future.

Acknowledgments

The authors would like to thank the Hungarian Williams Syndrome Foundation for connecting us with the families of WS subjects.

Author Contributions

Conceived and designed the experiments: PG IK. Performed the experiments: PG. Analyzed the data: PG FG. Contributed reagents/materials/analysis tools: PG IK FG. Wrote the paper: PG IK FG.

References

1. Ewen JB, Shapiro BK (2005) Disorders of Attention or Learning in Neurodevelopmental Disorders. Sem Pediat Neurol 12: 229–241.
2. Pennington BF (2001) Genetic methods. In: Nelson CA, Luciana M, editors. Handbook of developmental cognitive neuroscience. Cambridge, MA: MIT Press. 149–158.
3. Weiss S, Weber G, Neuhold A, Rett A (1991) Down syndrome: MR quantification of brain structures and comparison with normal control subjects, Am J Neuroradiol 12: 1207–1211.
4. Raz N, Torres IJ, Briggs SD, Spencer WD, Thornton AE, et al. (1995) Selective neuroanatomic abnormalities in Down's syndrome and their cognitive correlates: evidence from MRI morphometry, Neurology 45: 356–366.
5. Reiss AL, Aylward E, Freund LS, Joshi PK, Bryan RN (1991) Neuroanatomy of fragile X syndrome: the posterior fossa. Ann Neurol 29: 26–32.
6. Reiss AL, Faruque F, Naidu S, Abrams M, Beaty T, et al. (1993) Neuroanatomy of Rett syndrome: a volumetric imaging study. Ann Neurol 34: 227–234.
7. Reiss AL, Lee J, Freund L (1994) Neuroanatomy of fragile X syndrome: the temporal lobe. Neurolgy 44: 1317–24.
8. Carter JC, Lanham DC, Pham D, Bibat G, Naidu S, et al. (2008) Selective cerebral volume reduction in Rett syndrome: a multiple-approach MR imaging study. Am J Neuroradiol 29: 436–41.
9. Takashima S, Becker LE, Armstrong DL, Chan F (1981) Abnormal neuronal development in the visual cortex of the human fetus and infant with Down's syndrome. A quantitative and qualitative Golgi study. Brain Res 225: 1–21.
10. Armstrong DD, Dunn JK, Antalffy B, Trivedi R (1995) Selective dendritic alterations in the cortex of Rett syndrome. J Neuropath Exp Neur 53: 195–201.
11. Irwin SA, Patel B, Idupulapati M, Harris B, Crisostomo A, et al. (2001) Abnormal dendritic spine characteristics in the temporal and visual cortices of patients with fragile-X syndrome: a quantitative examination. Am J Med Genet 98: 161–167.
12. Temudo T, Rios M, Prior C, Carrilho I, Santos M, et al. (2009) Evaluation of CSF neurotransmitters and folate in 25 patients with Rett disorder and effects of treatment. Brain and Dev 31: 46–51.
13. Jørgensen SO, Brooksbank BWL, Balázs R (1990) Neuronal plasticity and astrocytic reaction in Down syndrome and Alzheimer disease. Neurol Sci 98: 63–79.
14. Weiler IJ, Irwin SA, Klintsova AY, Spencer CM, Brazelton AD, et al. (1997) FragileX mental retardation protein is translated near synapses in response to neurotransmitter activation. PNAS 94: 5395–540.
15. Didden R, Sigafoos J (2001) A review of the nature and treatment of sleep disorders in individuals with developmental disabilities. Res Dev Disabil 22: 255–72.
16. Dyken ME, Lin-Dyken DC, Poulton S, Zimmerman MB, Sedars E (2003) Prospective polysomnographic analysis of obstructive sleep apnea in Down syndrome. Arch Pediat Adol Med 157: 655–660.
17. Harvey M, Kennedy C (2002) Polysomnographic phenotypes in developmental disabilities. Int J Dev Neurosci 20: 443–8.

18. Marcus CL, Keens TG, Bautista DB, von Pechmann WS, Ward SL (1991) Obstructive sleep apnea in children with Down syndrome. Pediatrics 88: 132–139.
19. De Miguel-Diez J, Villa-Asensi JR, Alvarez-Sala JL (2003) Prevalence of sleep-disordered breathing in children with Down syndrome: polygraphic findings in 108 children. Sleep 26: 1006–1009.
20. Kronk R, Bishop EE, Raspa M, Bickel JO, Mandel DA, et al. (2010) Prevalence, Nature, and Correlates of Sleep Problems Among Children with Fragile X Syndrome Based on a Large Scale Parent Survey. Sleep 33: 679–687.
21. Young D, Nagarajana L, deKlerka N, Jacobya P, Ellaway C, et al. (2007) Sleep problems in Rett syndrome. Brain and Development 29: 609–616.
22. Karni A, Sagi D (1991) Where practice makes perfect in texture discrimination: evidence for primary visual cortex plasticity. Proc Natl Acad Sci USA 88: 4966–4970.
23. Karni A, Sagi D (1993) The time course of learning a visual skill. Nature 365: 250–252.
24. Schwartz S, Maquet P, Frith C (2002) Neural correlates of perceptual learning: a functional MRI study of visual texture discrimination. Proc Natl Acad Sci USA 99: 17137–17142.
25. Bellugi U, Marks S, Bihrle A, Sabo H (1988) Dissociation between language and cognitive functions in Williams syndrome. In: Bishop D, Mogford K, editors. Language development in exceptional circumstances. East Sussex: Lawrence Erlbaum Associates. 177–189.
26. Atkinson J, Braddick O, Anker S, Curran W, Andrew R, et al. (2003) Neurobiological models of visuospatial cognition in children with Williams syndrome: measures of dorsal-stream and frontal function. Dev Neuropsychol 23: 139–172.
27. Wang PP, Bellugi U (1994) Evidence from two genetic syndromes for a dissociation between verbal and visual-spatial short-term memory. J Clin Exp Neuropsychol 16: 317–322.
28. Vicari S, Brizzolara D, Carlesimo GA, Pezzini G, Volterra V (1996) Memory abilities in children with Williams syndrome. Cortex 32: 503–14.
29. Jarrold C, Baddeley AD, Phillips C (2007) Long-term memory for verbal and visual information in Down syndrome and Williams syndrome: Performance on the doors and people test. Cortex 43: 233–247.
30. Vicari S, Bellucci S, Carlesimo GA (2003) Visual and Spatial working memory dissociation: evidence from a genetic syndrome. Dev Med Child Neurol 45: 269–273.
31. Mandolesi L, Addona F, Foti F, Menghini D, Petrosini L, et al. (2009) Spatial competences in Williams syndrome: a radial arm maze study. Int J Dev Neurosci 27: 205–213.
32. Kovacs I, Julesz B (1993) A closed curve is much more than an incomplete one – effect of closure on figure ground segmentation. Proc Natl Acad Sci USA 90: 7495–7.
33. Angelucci A, Levitt JB, Walton EJS, Hupper J-M, Bullier J, et al. (2002) Circuits for local and global signal integration in primary visual cortex. J Neurosci 22: 8633–8646.
34. Chisum HJ, Fitzpatrick D (2004) The contribution of vertical and horizontal connections to the receptive field center and surround in V1. Neural Networks 17: 681–693.
35. Kovacs I, Kozma P, Feher A, Benedek G (1999) Late maturation of visual spatial integration in humans. Proc Natl Acad Sci USA 96: 12204–122.
36. Gervan P, Berencsi A, Kovacs I (2011) Vision first? The development of primary visual cortical networks is more rapid than the development of primary motor networks in humans. PloS ONE 6: e25572. doi: 10.1371/journal.pone.0025572.
37. Burkhalter A (1993) Development of Forward and Feedback Connections between Areas V1 and V2 of Human Visual Cortex. Cereb Cortex 3: 476–487.
38. Kozma P, Kovács I, Feher A (2002) Learning only after sleep in a contour integration task. Second Annual Meeting of the Vision Sciences Society, Sarasota, FL, USA.
39. Gervan P, Kovacs I (2010) Two phases of offline learning in contour integration. J Vision 10: 241–7.
40. Epstein CJ (2001) Down Syndrome (trisomy 21). In: Scriver CR, Beaudet AL, Sly WS, Valle D, editors. The metabolic and molecular bases of inherited diseases, New York: McGraw-Hill. 1223–1256.
41. Bellugi U, Lichtenberger L, Jones W, Zona Lai Z, St. George M. (2000) The Neurocognitive Profile of Williams Syndrome: A Complex Pattern of Strength sand Weaknesses. J Cognitive Neurosci 12: 7–29.
42. Facon B, Magis D, Belmont JM (2011) Beyond matching on the mean in developmental disabilities. Res Dev Disabil 32: 2134–2147.
43. Dennis M, Francisa DJ, Cirinoa PT, Schachar R, Barnes MA, et al. (2009) Why IQ is not a covariate in cognitive studies of neurodevelopmental disorders. J Int Neuropsych Soc 15: 331–343.
44. Silverman W (2007) Down syndrome: cognitive phenotype. Ment Retard Dev D R 13: 228–36.
45. Spitz HH (1982) Intellectual extremes, mental age, and the nature of human intelligence. Merrill-Palmer Q Beh 28: 167–192.
46. Kozma-Wiebe P, Silverstein S, Feher A, Kovacs I, Ulhaas P, et al. (2006) Development of a World-Wide Web based contour integration test: Reliability and validity. Comput Hum Behav 22: 971–980.
47. Roudaia E, Bennett PJ, Sekuler AB (2008) The effect of aging on contour integration. Vision Res 48: 2767–2774.
48. McKendrick MA, Weymouth AE, Battista J (2010) The effect of normal aging on closed contour shape discrimination. J Vision 10: 1–9.
49. Kovacs I. (1996) Gestalten of today: Early processing of visual contours and surfaces. Behav Brain Res 82: 1–11.
50. Thompson PM, Lee AD, Dutton RA, Geaga JA, Hayashi KM, et al. (2005) Abnormal cortical complexity and thickness profiles mapped in Williams syndrome. J Neurosci 25: 4146–4158.
51. Chiang MC, Reiss AL, Lee AD, Bellugi U, Galaburda AM, et al. (2007) 3D pattern of brain abnormalities in Williams syndrome visualized using tensor-based morphometry. Neuroimage 36: 1096–109.
52. Galaburda AM, Holinger DP, Bellugi U, Sherman GF (2002) Williams syndrome: Neuronal size and neuronal-packing density in primary visual cortex. Arch Neurol 59: 1461–1467.
53. Galaburda AM, Bellugi U (2000) Multi-level analysis of cortical neuroanatomy in Williams syndrome. J Cog Neurosci 12: 74–88.
54. Tassabehji M, Metcalfe K, Fergusson WD, Carette MJ, Dore JK, et al (1996) LIM-kinase deleted in Williams syndrome. Nat Genet 13: 272–273.
55. Schratt GM, Tuebing F, Nigh EA, Kane CG, Sabatini ME, et al. (2006) A brain-specific microRNA regulates dendritic spine development. Nature 439: 283–289.
56. Calverley RK, Jones DG (1990) Contributions of dendritic spines and perforated synapses to synaptic plasticity. Brain Res Rev 15: 215–49.
57. Hoogenraad CC, Koekkoek B, Akhmanova A, Krugers H, Dortland B, et al. (2002) Targeted mutation of Cyln2 in the Williams syndrome critical region links CLIP-115 haploinsufficiency to neurodevelopmental abnormalities in mice. Nature Genet 32: 116–127.
58. Meyer-Lindenberg A, Mervis CB, Berman KF (2006) Neural mechanisms in Williams syndrome: a unique window to genetic influences on cognition and behaviour. Nat Rev Neurosci 7: 380–93.
59. Nakayama T, Matsuoka R, Kimura M, Hirota H, Mikoshiba K, et al. (1998) Hemizygous deletion of the HPC-1/syntaxin 1A gene (STX1A) in patients with Williams syndrome. Cytogenet Cell Genet 82: 49–5.
60. Botta A, Sangiuolo F, Calza L, Giardino L, Potenza S, et al. (1999) Expression Analysis and Protein Localization of the Human HPC-1/Syntaxin 1A, a Gene Deleted in Williams Syndrome. Genomics 62: 525–528.
61. Gao MC, Bellugi U, Dai L, Mills DL, Sobel EM, et al. (2010) Intelligence in Williams Syndrome Is Related to STX1A, Which Encodes a Component of the Presynaptic SNARE Complex. PLoS ONE 5: e10292.
62. Botta A, Novelli G, Mari A, Novelli A, Sabani M, et al. (1999) Detection of an atypical 7q11.23 deletion in Williams syndrome patients which does not include the STX1A and FZD3 genes. J Med Genet 36: 478–480.
63. Ashkenas J (1996) Williams syndrome starts making sense. Am J Hum Genet 59: 756–761.
64. Arens R, Wright B, Elliott J, Zhao H, Wang PP, et al. (1998) Periodic limb movement in sleep in children with Williams syndrome. J Pediatr 133: 670–4.
65. Gombos F, Bódizs R, Kovács I (2011) Atypical sleep architecture and altered EEG spectra in Williams syndrome. J Intell Disabil Res 55: 255–262.
66. Bodizs R, Gombos F, Kovács I (2012) Sleep EEG fingerprints reveal accelerated thalamocortical oscillatory dynamics in Williams syndrome. Res Dev Disabil 33: 153–164.

14

Abnormal Brain Activation in Neurofibromatosis Type 1: A Link between Visual Processing and the Default Mode Network

Inês R. Violante[1], Maria J. Ribeiro[1], Gil Cunha[1], Inês Bernardino[1], João V. Duarte[1], Fabiana Ramos[2], Jorge Saraiva[2], Eduardo Silva[3], Miguel Castelo-Branco[1]*

1 Visual Neuroscience Laboratory, Institute of Biomedical Research in Light and Image, Faculty of Medicine, University of Coimbra, Coimbra, Portugal, **2** Medical Genetic Department, Pediatric Hospital of Coimbra, Coimbra, Portugal, **3** Centre for Hereditary Eye Diseases, Department of Ophthalmology, University Hospital of Coimbra, Coimbra, Portugal

Abstract

Neurofibromatosis type 1 (NF1) is one of the most common single gene disorders affecting the human nervous system with a high incidence of cognitive deficits, particularly visuospatial. Nevertheless, neurophysiological alterations in low-level visual processing that could be relevant to explain the cognitive phenotype are poorly understood. Here we used functional magnetic resonance imaging (fMRI) to study early cortical visual pathways in children and adults with NF1. We employed two distinct stimulus types differing in contrast and spatial and temporal frequencies to evoke relatively different activation of the magnocellular (M) and parvocellular (P) pathways. Hemodynamic responses were investigated in retinotopically-defined regions V1, V2 and V3 and then over the acquired cortical volume. Relative to matched control subjects, patients with NF1 showed deficient activation of the low-level visual cortex to both stimulus types. Importantly, this finding was observed for children and adults with NF1, indicating that low-level visual processing deficits do not ameliorate with age. Moreover, only during M-biased stimulation patients with NF1 failed to deactivate or even activated anterior and posterior midline regions of the default mode network. The observation that the magnocellular visual pathway is impaired in NF1 in early visual processing and is specifically associated with a deficient deactivation of the default mode network may provide a neural explanation for high-order cognitive deficits present in NF1, particularly visuospatial and attentional. A link between magnocellular and default mode network processing may generalize to neuropsychiatric disorders where such deficits have been separately identified.

Editor: Yu-Feng Zang, Hangzhou Normal University, China

Funding: This work was supported by the University of Coimbra [Grant number III/14/2008] and the Portuguese Foundation for Science and Technology [Grant numbers PIC/IC/83155/2007, PTDC_SAU-ORG_118380, PIC/IC/82986/2007,SFRH/BD/41348/2007 to I.R.V., SFRH/BPD/34392/2006 to M.J.R, and SFRH/BD/41401/2007 to I.B.]. The funders had no role in study design, data collection and analysis, decision to publish, or preparation of the manuscript.

Competing Interests: The authors have declared that no competing interests exist.

* E-mail: mcbranco@fmed.uc.pt

Introduction

Neurofibromatosis type 1 (NF1) is a neurodevelopmental disorder, with an incidence of 1 in 3500 individuals [1] and one of the most common autosomal dominant genetic disorders affecting the human nervous system. It is caused by mutations in a single gene (*NF1*) and constitutes therefore a valuable model for understanding genetic, neurochemical and brain-behaviour relationships.

NF1 is commonly associated with cognitive impairment and learning disabilities. The neuropsychological deficits reported include visual perception, motor, visuomotor, language, memory and attention domains [2,3,4,5]. However, the hallmark cognitive deficit of the disorder is visuospatial impairment [6,7], for which a number of studies have provided behavioural ([5,8] see [9,10] for review) and functional magnetic resonance imaging (fMRI) [8,9] evidences.

The fact that performance on visuospatial tasks is impaired in individuals with NF1 suggests that information processing in early visual areas might be deficient.

In the early visual system information is transmitted via three parallel channels: the magnocellular (M), parvocellular (P) and koniocellular pathways. Although these pathways may be difficult to differentiate, one can take advantage of the physiological properties of their constituent neurons [10] to generate stimuli with a preferential bias activation of each pathway. Magnocellular population responses are relatively tuned to achromatic stimuli with low spatial and high temporal frequencies and they provide the dominant input to the dorsal stream, which plays an important role in spatial localization and motion processing. The parvocellular pathway is more sensitive to stimuli with low temporal and high spatial frequencies and projects primarily to the ventral stream, important in object processing. Additionally, at low contrast levels visual information is primarily conveyed via the magnocellular system [11]. The function of the koniocellular pathway is less defined, but it is known to play a role in colour vision [12]. Recently, using psychophysical measures of contrast sensitivity, we showed relative deficits in the M and P channels, with preserved koniocellular function in individuals with NF1 [13].

However, the neural substrates of visual impairments in this condition are still poorly understood.

In the present study, we focused on the activation of the early cortical visual system using stimuli with different contrast and different temporal and spatial frequency properties to provide a relative bias concerning the activation of the M or P pathways. Our aim was to establish the neurofunctional status of the early visual cortex in patients with NF1.

Based upon prior studies [13], we hypothesized that patients with NF1 would show impairments in activation of low-level visual areas, and therefore we conducted confirmatory analysis in retinotopically-defined areas, V1, V2 and V3. Relative to control subjects, patients with NF1 showed reduced activation to both stimuli categories in these areas. This finding corroborates downstream deficits that may lead to the visuospatial impairments characteristic of the cognitive phenotype in patients with NF1. Additionally, we investigated the activation pattern of high-level visual and non visual regions modulated by the different stimuli to examine possible functional consequences of low-level visual impairments. We observed differences between controls and patients with NF1 in mainly, but not only, higher-order visual areas that presented significantly lower blood-oxygen-level-dependent (BOLD)-signal in patients. Importantly, at a high-level processing stage the differences observed between patients and controls depended on the stimulus type, with the response to M activation (low contrast, low spatial, high temporal stimulation) showing an intriguing pattern in the midline default mode network areas, where patients presented higher BOLD-signal than controls.

Materials and Methods

Ethics Statement

The study was conducted in accordance with the Declaration of Helsinki and all procedures were reviewed and approved by the Ethics Commissions of the Faculty of Medicine of the University of Coimbra *(Comissão de Ética da Faculdade de Medicina de Coimbra)* and of the Children's Hospital of Coimbra (*Comissão de Ética do Centro Hospitalar de Coimbra*). Written informed consent was obtained from participants older than 18 years of age and from the parents/guardians in the case of participants younger than 18 years of age. Children and adolescents younger than 18 years of age gave written or oral informed consent.

Participants

Ninety one individuals participated in this study: 25 children and adolescents with NF1, 29 control children and adolescents, 17 adults with NF1 and 20 control adults. Due to the exclusion criteria defined concerning intracranial abnormalities, neuropsychological assessment, performance on the behavioural task and movement within MRI acquisitions (see below), 24 participants were excluded from our analysis. Thus, for analysis, we included: 15 children and adolescents with NF1, 24 chronological age-matched control children and adolescents, 13 female adults with NF1 and 15 chronological age-matched control female adults. Demografic details are shown in Table 1.

Participants with NF1 were recruited and diagnosed in collaboration with the Clinical Genetics Department of the Pediatric Hospital of Coimbra according to the NIH defined diagnostic criteria [14]. For the children/adolescent control group, participants were recruited among unaffected siblings and from a local school. The adult control group was recruited among the unaffected parents or from an adult educational school. These adult schools provide learning programs for adults with low educational levels and many adult participants with NF1 are also attendants.

In order to ensure that participants included in the study had no central nervous system pathology, a FLAIR MRI sequence was performed in addition to the standard structural scan. Neuroradiological assessment was carried out by an experienced neuroradiologist. Participants were excluded from this study if they had a clinically significant intracranial abnormality on MRI ($n = 6$ individuals with NF1, 2 controls) such as intracranial tumor, optic glioma or other imaging abnormalities. UBOs (Unidentified Bright Objects - T2 hyperintensities, commonly found in patients with NF1) were not considered exclusion criteria.

None of the participants had a psychiatric illness, epilepsy or were taking medication for treating depression. Participants were also excluded if they had full-scale IQ below 70, for the children/adolescent groups, or Raven score below 3 ($n = 1$ NF1), in the adult groups. Parents of children on stimulant medication for attention deficit hyperactivity disorder (ADHD) were requested not to give their children the medication on the days of testing ($n = 2$ NF1, 1 control). All the participants had normal or corrected-to-normal visual acuity.

Ophthalmological assessment was performed by an experienced ophthalmologist to rule out eye disorders in the NF1 group. This included best-corrected visual acuity, stereopsis evaluation using Randot, slit lamp examination of anterior chamber structures and fundus examination. No anomalies that could affect vision were found.

Neuropsychological Assessment

Participants younger than 17 years old received the Portuguese adapted version of the Wechsler Intelligence Scale for Children (WISC-III) [15], while 17 years old or older participants performed the first set of the Raven Standard Progressive Matrices [16] as an indication of non-verbal intelligence. Three control children/adolescents and one adolescent with NF1 were unavailable to perform IQ tests. However, their school records were in accordance with their chronological age, indicating adequate intellectual functioning. Neuropsychological details are shown in Table 1. Children with NF1 presented significantly lower full-scale IQ (FSIQ) score than control children ($p = 0.013$). In the adults groups, the average Raven scores between NF1 and the control group were not statistically different.

Stimuli and Task Design

Retinotopic mapping. The boundaries of low-level retinotopic visual areas were defined employing a fast approach using the polar angle of the standard retinotopic mapping procedure [17,18]. Polar angle maps were obtained using a black and white checkerboard wedge flickering at 8 Hz in counterphase (48 s full cycle, 4 cycles per scan and two scans per subject) centred around an orange-coloured fixation point. Polar angle maps provide the information of angle reversion needed to properly delineate both dorsal and ventral visual areas of V1, V2 and V3.

M- and P-biased stimulation. Stimuli were pattern-reversed checkerboards filling the entire screen ($30.3^\circ \times 23.1^\circ$) designed using the Psychophysics Toolbox for Matlab [19]. To bias the activation of the M-pathway we used stimuli with low spatial frequency, 0.25 cycles per degree (cpd) fundamental frequency, and high temporal frequency (18 Hz), with low contrast (18%) that preferentially activates (though not exclusively) the M pathway. This stimulus is similar to the one used by Liu et al [20]. P-biased stimulation was achieved using a higher spatial frequency (2 cpd), lower temporal frequency (2 Hz) and 100% contrast. Stimuli were presented in a block-design composed of 6 blocks for

Table 1. Demographic and neuropsychological characteristics of patients and control groups.

	Children and adolescents		Adults	
	NF1, n = 15	**Controls, n = 24**	**NF1, n = 13**	**Controls, n = 15**
Age (years)				
Mean ± SD	11.7±2.9	12.0±2.3	33.1±4.9	32.7±5.6
Range	7–17	7–16	25–42	26–44
Gender ratio				
Female/Male	9/6	13/11	13/0	15/0
Full-scale IQ (WISC-III)				
Mean ± SD	96.9±16*	113.0±19.7	-	-
Raven score				
Mean ± SD	-	-	6.7±2.4	7.8±2.9

Significant differences between NF1 patients and controls are indicated by *$p<0.05$.

each stimulus (16 seconds per block) randomly presented and interleaved with a rest condition (fixation only, 10 seconds). To maintain subjects engaged and to control for attention and fixation participants were asked to fixate a central dot and report a subtle colour change, from red to pink and the other way around, with a button press. Time intervals between colour changes were chosen randomly from 2, 4, 6, 8 or 10 seconds. The task ran throughout the experiment.

Only participants with a high level of detection (>85%) and a low rate of false alarms (<0.3, calculated as the ratio between the number of false alarms and the number of colour changes) were included in these study. 4 patients with NF1 and 4 control participants were excluded by not meeting these criteria.

Stimuli were projected using an LCD projector (AVOTEC Silent Vision 6011, Florida, USA) onto a screen that participants viewed via a fixed mirror placed on the MRI head coil. Participants' eyes were monitored with a camera placed on the mirror system (Avotec Real Eye 5721, Florida, USA).

Imaging Procedures

Scanning was performed on a 3T Siemens TimTrio scanner at the Portuguese Brain Imaging Network, using a 12-channel birdcage head coil. For each participant we acquired: i) two T_1-weighted (T_1w) MPRAGE sequences, 1×1×1 mm voxel size, repetition time (TR) 2.3 s, echo time (TE) 2.98 ms, flip angle (FA) 9°, field of view (FOV) 256×256, 160 slices; ii) a T_2-weighted (T_2w) FLAIR sequence, 1×1×1 mm voxel size, TR 5 s, TE 2.98 ms, Inversion Time (TI) 1.8 s, FOV 250 250, 160 slices; iii) one run of fMRI scanning for the M/P-biased stimuli and two runs of the polar angle stimuli using single shot echo planar imaging (EPI) acquired in the axial plane orthogonal to the anterior commissure covering the occipital, temporal and frontal cortices, with 2×2×2 mm voxel size, TR 2 s, TE 39 ms with a 128×128 matrix, FA 90°, FOV 256×256, 26 slices.

FLAIR images were used to identify T_2 hyperintensities, a common neuroradiological finding in patients with NF1. A neuroradiologist, who was blind to the participants' clinical history observed the MR structural scans and reported on the distribution and number of UBOs. Twelve of the fifteen (80%) children and seven of the thirteen (53.8%) adults with NF1 had one or more UBOs. The frequency of UBOs is in accordance with published data [21]. None of the control participants had UBOs.

Image Analysis

Image processing and analysis were carried out using BrainVoyager QX 2.1 (Brain Innovation, Maastricht, The Netherlands). Analyses to determine total intracranial volume were performed using Statistical Parametric Mapping 8 (SPM8, http://www.fil.ion.ucl.ac.uk/spm).

Image Processing and Analysis in Retinotopically-defined Areas

Anatomical image processing. High-resolution T_1w anatomical images were averaged, intensity normalized and re-oriented into a space where the anterior and the posterior commissure lie in the same plane (AC-PC). Afterwards, cortex was segmented using automatic segmentation routines [22], mesh representations of each hemisphere were created and inflated for polar angle maps projection.

Functional image processing. We applied slice scan time correction, linear trend removal, temporal high-pass filtering (2 cycles per run), modest spatial smoothing (FWHM 2 mm, yielding a small but clear smoothing effect) and a correction for small interscan head movements. Participants were excluded from further analysis if any within-run movement exceeding 2 mm was detected (n = 2 NF1, 4 controls).

Retinotopic mapping. Polar angle maps were obtained from the average of two runs, created based on linear regression analysis and projected onto the AC-PC anatomical surfaces of each subject. The cross-correlation was calculated for each run, as a function of the time lag (in TR units, 2 seconds per lag). Lag values at each voxel were encoded in pseudocolors, voxels were included into the statistical map if $r > 0.25$, $p<0.05$. Retinotopic areas V1, V2 dorsal (d), V2 ventral (v), V3d and V3v were manually defined for each subject in each hemisphere in the inflated meshes. Obtained regions-of-interest (ROIs) were used as "masks" to the analysis of the blood-oxygen-level-dependent (BOLD) signal elicited by M- and P-biased stimulation.

M- and P-biased stimulation. Statistical analyses were performed on individual and group data using the general linear model (GLM). Predictors for the response to M- and P- biased stimulation were obtained by convolution of a condition box-car time course with a two-gamma function [23]. Retinotopically-defined areas were used as ROIs to perform ROI analysis on each subject in the AC-PC space. Within each ROI, a GLM for the M/P-biased stimuli experiment, corrected for temporal serial correlations, was computed and the individual beta values evoked by each stimulus were retrieved and analysed using PAWS Statistics 18.

Volume-based Processing and Analysis of Cortical Activation

We were interested in effects that could be generalized to children, adults and overall population irrespective of age and thus we compared the NF1 studied group (children, adolescents and adults) with a matched control group.

Since benign macrocephaly is common in NF1, previous fMRI studies were restricted to ROI analysis [8,9,24]. To overcome this methodological difficulty and be able to perform whole-brain analysis we ensured that the total intracranial volume was not statistically different between matched clinical groups.

Total intracranial volume measurements. Total intracranial brain volume for each subject was calculated with the VBM8 toolbox in SPM8. Group comparisons for brain volume were evaluated with independent samples t-tests.

In the children groups, we observed no significant differences in total intracranial volume, which makes it valid to perform normalization procedures and group analysis since it is unlikely that systematic variances in the warping procedure result in false group differences.

Adults, however, presented a significant difference in total intracranial volume. Therefore, for this analysis we excluded the 4 control participants with the smallest brain volumes. We analysed 13 patients with NF1 and 11 controls with no intracranial volume significant group difference. Moreover, the overall control and NF1 groups composed by children and adults (without the 4 previously excluded adult participants) did not present a difference in total intracranial volume.

Cortex-based alignment. Whole-volume statistical comparisons regarding the activation to the M/P-biased stimuli were conducted in the cortical surface space after performing cortex-based alignment. In order to do that, brains previously transformed to AC-PC space were normalized into Talairach standard space [25]. Following normalization we performed the segmentation routine applied in BrainVoyager. The reconstructed folded cortical representations of each subject and hemisphere were morphed into a spherical representation and aligned to all the other subjects' spheres iteratively [26,27]. This procedure was conducted to improve the spatial correspondence mapping between subjects' brains [28]. It has been demonstrated that cortical alignment substantially improves group results by reducing anatomical variability [28,29]. Cortex-based alignment was performed for the children, adult and overall groups separately.

Group comparisons of the neural activity elicited by the M- and P-biased stimuli in aligned cortices. Statistical analysis was performed using Random effects (RFX) analyses in order to generalize findings to the population level [30]. In the first stage, a whole-volume RFX GLM was performed to estimate condition effects (beta values) separately for each subject and stimuli. At the second level, an independent samples t-test was used to compare patients and controls for each stimulus category. Statistical maps were corrected for multiple comparisons using cluster-size thresholding [27,31]. Each map was thresholded at $p<0.01$ uncorrected and, for correction, submitted to cortex-based cluster threshold estimation based on a Monte Carlo simulation with 1000 iterations. This procedure yielded a statistical map with a cluster size of 45 mm^2 for the adults group and 41 mm^2 for the children and overall groups, corresponding to a corrected α value of $p<0.05$.

We examined the BOLD timecourses in voxel clusters with statistical significant differences between the clinical groups, NF1 and control. The functional response profiles for each group were reported after the subtraction of the fixation condition from the timecourse.

Demographic, Neuropsychological, Behavioural and BOLD Activation in Retinotopically Defined Areas Analyses

Statistical analyses were performed with PAWS Statistics 18 (SPSS Inc., Chicago, USA).

First, we verified the normality assumption for the different parameters using the Shapiro Wilk's test. For normally distributed data, we used independent samples t-tests, ANOVA and Pearson's correlation analyses. When the data did not meet assumptions of sphericity, we used the epsilon value to choose the type of correction applied: the Huynh-Feldt (for $\varepsilon >0.75$) or the Greenhouse–Geiser (for $\varepsilon <0.75$). For the non-normal data, we used the Mann-Whitney test for comparison between two independent samples.

Results

Behaviour

There was no between group differences on the performance in the behavioural task, neither for children nor for adults clinical groups. Both NF1 patients and controls responded to the fixation task, which imposed a moderate attentional load, with a high degree of accuracy (above 95% correct trials) and low number of false alarms.

Activity in Retinotopically Defined Areas

The magnitude of activation elicited by the M- and P-biased stimuli was retrieved from low-level visual areas V1, V2d, V2v, V3d and V3v of each subject's hemispheres. Analysis was performed on 15 children with NF1, 24 control children, 13 adults with NF1 and 15 control adults. First, we performed a repeated measures ANOVA using stimuli (M-biased vs P-biased), visual area (V1, V2d, V2v, V3d, V3v) and hemisphere (left vs right) as within subjects variables and clinical group (NF1 vs controls) and age group (children vs adults) as between subjects factors.

We found a highly significant effect of clinical group [$F_{(1,63)}=12.892$, $p<0.001$] and a significant effect of age group [$F_{(1,63)}=5.988$, $p=0.017$] with no interaction between clinical group and age group [$F_{(1,63)}=0.133$, NS], indicating a similar deficit in visual activation in both children and adults with NF1. Besides, we found a significant effect of stimulus type [$F_{(1,63)}=76.818$, $p<0.001$], visual area [$F_{(1,63)}=38.039$, $p<0.001$] and an interaction between stimulus type and visual area [$F_{(4, 236)}=84.595$ $p<0.001$]. Differences between patients and controls were indicated by the overall clinical group effect and also by significant interactions in visual area x clinical group [$F_{(4, 228.3)}=2.445$, $p=0.05$] and stimulus type x visual area x clinical group [$F_{(4,236)}=3.483$, $p=0.01$]. Differences between children and adults were revealed by the overall age group effect and also by significant visual area x age group [$F_{(4, 228.3)}=4.011$, $p=0.005$] and a stimulus type x visual area x clinical group [$F_{(4,236)}=3.483$, $p=0.01$] interactions. Three way interactions involving stimulus type, visual area and groups were explored in subsequent repeated measures ANOVA.

Given that no effect of hemisphere or interaction between hemisphere and group was found we averaged the signal of both hemispheres and performed a repeated measures analysis for each stimulus type using visual areas (V1, V2d, V2v, V3d, V3v) as within subjects variables and clinical group (NF1 vs controls) and age group (children vs adults) as between subjects factors.

Concerning the stimulus with low spatial and high temporal frequency and low contrast (biasing the M pathway), differences between patients with NF1 and controls were evident as an overall significant effect of clinical group [$F_{(1,63)} = 9.914$, $p = 0.003$] and a significant interaction between area and clinical group [$F_{(3.5, 37)} = 6.194$, $p<0.001$]. This interaction was attributable to significantly lower activations from patients with NF1 than controls in visual areas V2d ($t_{(65)} = 3.5$, $p = 0.001$), V2v ($t_{(65)} = 2.5$, $p = 0.017$) and V3d ($t_{(65)} = 3.5$, $p = 0.001$), but not in V1 and V3v, as shown in Figure 1. Differences between children and adults were indicated by a marginally significant effect of age group [$F_{(1,63)} = 3.850$, $p = 0.054$] and a significant visual area x age group interaction [$F_{(3.5, 37)} = 6.194$, $p<0.001$]. This interaction was attributable to adults activating more than children in visual areas V2d ($t_{(65)} = 2.3$, $p = 0.025$) and V3d ($t_{(65)} = 2.5$, $p = 0.014$), Figure 1.

Regarding the stimulus with high contrast, higher spatial and lower temporal frequency (biasing the P pathway), we observed an overall clinical group effect [$F_{(1,63)} = 5.785$, $p = 0.019$] but no visual area x clinical group interaction [$F_{(3.8, 242.3)} = 1.026$, NS], indicating that effects were comparable across visual areas (see Figure 1). Furthermore, for this stimulus type an age group effect was not present [$F_{(1,63)} = 3.285$, NS], neither an interaction between visual area and age group [$F_{(3.8, 242.3)} = 1.321$, NS], indicating that there is no difference in activation between children and adults when responding to the stimulus biasing the P pathway, as shown in Figure 1.

Correspondence between Low-level Visual Deficits in NF1 and Cognitive Abilities

BOLD activation to each stimulus type in each visual area did not correlate with IQ for children and adolescents and Raven scores for adults. The lack of correspondence suggests that abnormal activation of low-level visual areas is not explained by low intellectual abilities.

Volume Based Analysis of Cortical Activation: Random Effects Analysis

To further identify cortical regions showing group differences in brain activation evoked by each of the stimuli used we compared the BOLD activation between clinical groups (NF1 n = 28 and controls n = 35, 4 control adults were not included in this analysis,

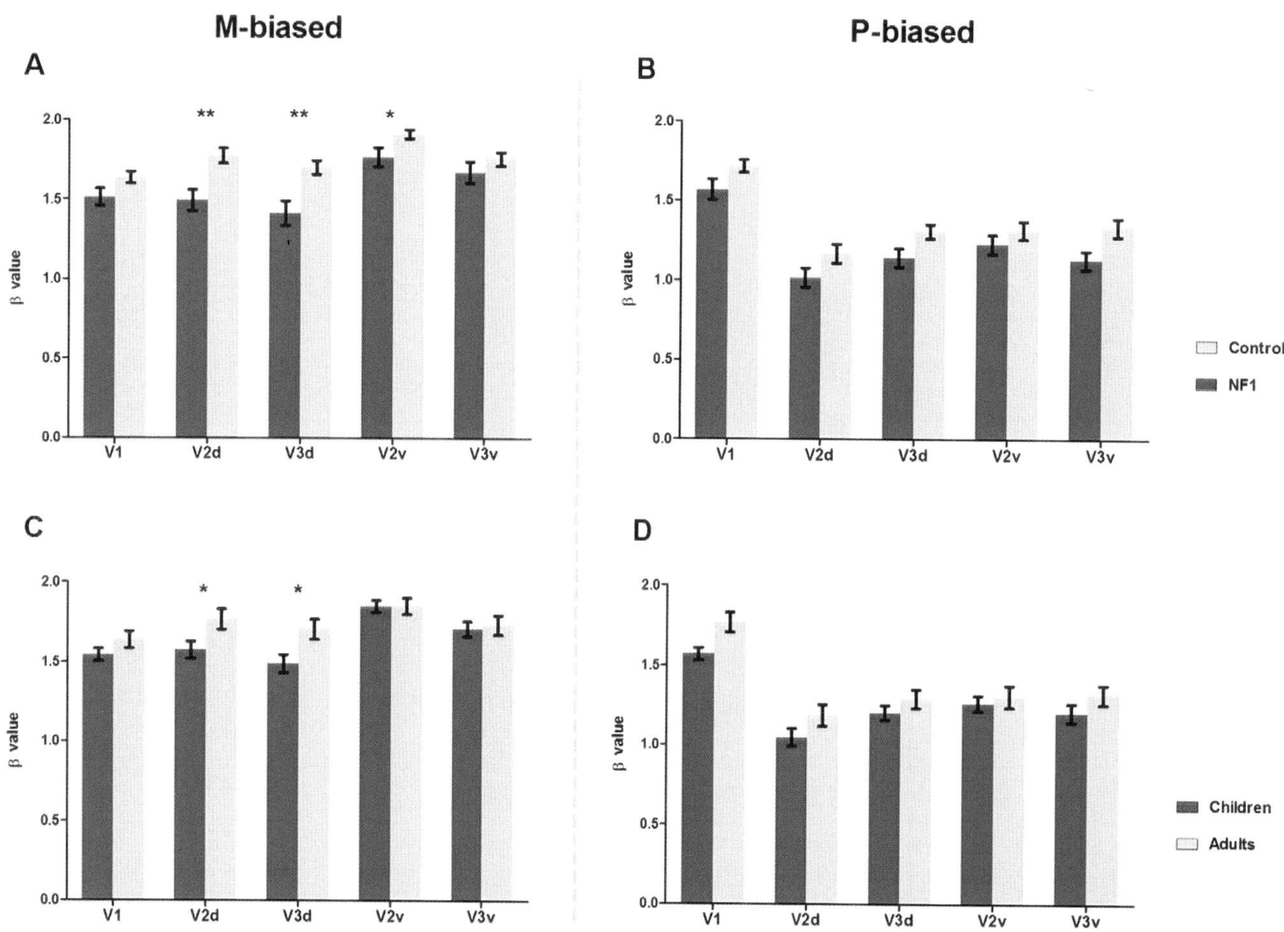

Figure 1. BOLD activity in retinotopically defined areas for M- and P-biased stimuli. A and B depict mean beta values in retinotopically defined areas V1, V2d, V3d, V2v, V3v for patients with NF1 (dark grey; n = 28, 15 children and 13 adults) and controls (light grey; n = 39, 24 children and 15 adults) in the presence of M-biased stimulus (A) and P-biased stimulus (B).C and D depict mean beta values in retinotopically defined areas for children (dark grey; n = 39, 15 with NF1 and 24 controls) and adults (light grey; n = 28, 13 with NF1 and 15 controls) in the presence of M-biased stimulus (C) and P-biased stimulus (D). Significant differences between groups are indicated by *$p<0.05$, **$p<0.01$. Error bars represent SEM.

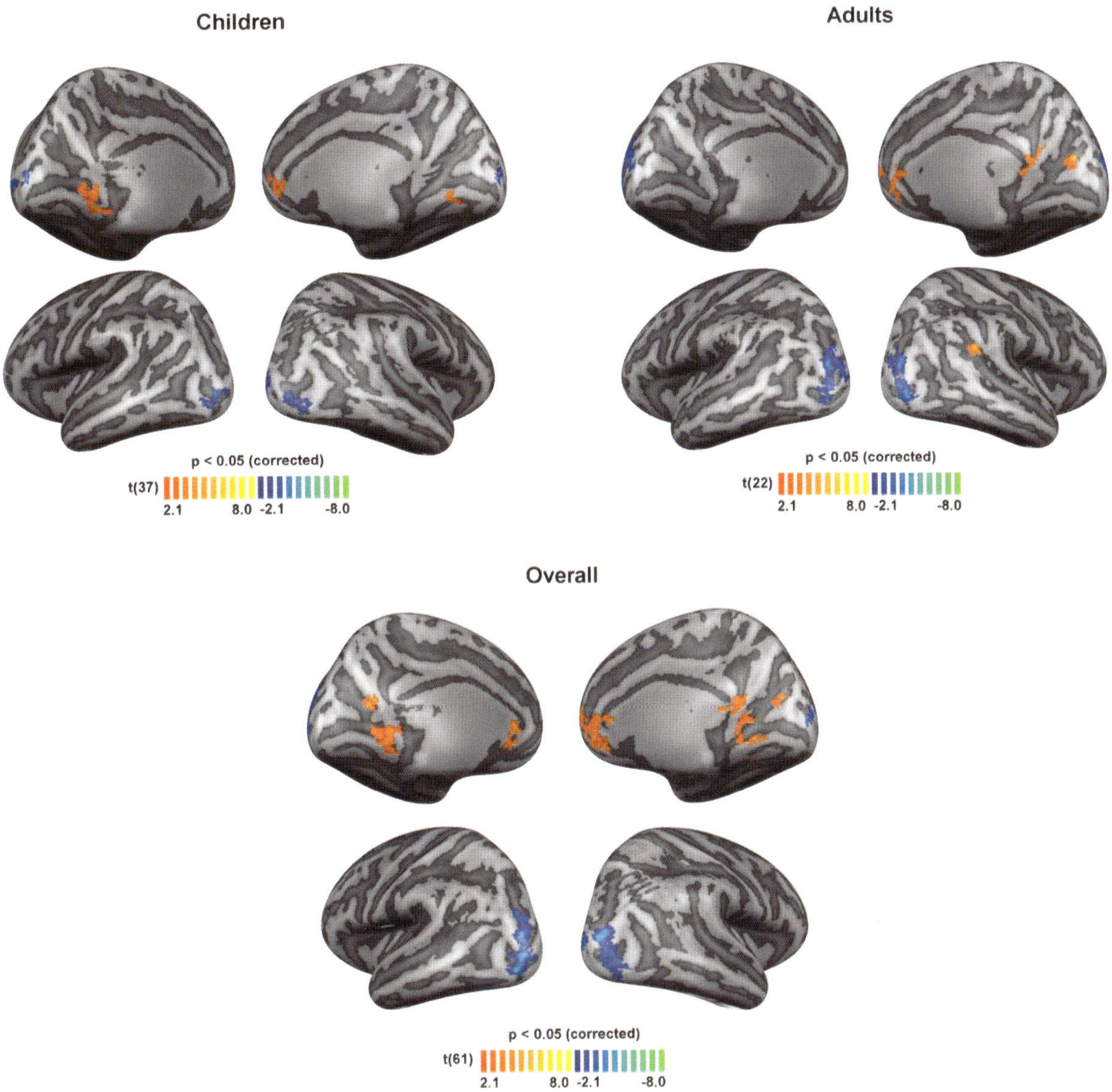

Figure 2. Significant differences in brain activations between patients with NF1 and controls, regarding the M-biased stimulus for children, adults and overall (children and adults) groups. Blue colours depict regions where activation was lower for individuals with NF1 than controls. Orange colours depict regions where activation was higher for individuals with NF1 than controls. Results are shown on views of the left and right hemispheres of cortex-based aligned three-dimensional reconstructions generated from the average anatomical data sets of the subjects in each group (children, adults, overall). Light grey represents gyri, dark grey represents sulci. T-maps thresholded at $p<0.05$ corrected using cortex-based cluster threshold estimation (cluster size 41 mm^2). N = 15 children with NF1, 24 control children, 13 adults with NF1 and 11 control adults.

see Materials and Methods section). Figures 2 and 3 show differences in BOLD activation elicited by the M- and P-biased stimulation, respectively.

Figure 2 shows the differences in activation profiles between patients with NF1 and controls in the presence of the low contrast, low spatial, high temporal frequency stimulus (M-biased). Overall, individuals with NF1 showed significantly lower activations than controls in the middle and superior occipital gyri bilaterally, consistent with the locations for V2d and V3d, as observed in the ROI analysis; differences in V2v were probably not observed due to their lower statistical significance. Surprisingly, clusters of higher activation for patients with NF1 relative to controls were observed in the cingulate gyrus, retrosplenial cortex, medial prefrontal cortex, parieto-occipital sulcus and lingual gyrus. Table 2 summarizes the brain regions with significant differences between groups.

In the presence of the stimulus that biased, although not exclusively, the P pathway, patients with NF1 activated less than controls in regions within the occipital lobe, including the inferior occipital gyrus, occipital pole, the calcarine and occipito-temporal sulci, Figure 3, Table 3.

We further examined the functional response profiles of regions showing significant statistical differences between groups. Brain regions where patients with NF1 presented lower activation than controls (blue clusters in Figures 2 and 3) were due to hypoactivation, i.e. less activation from the individuals

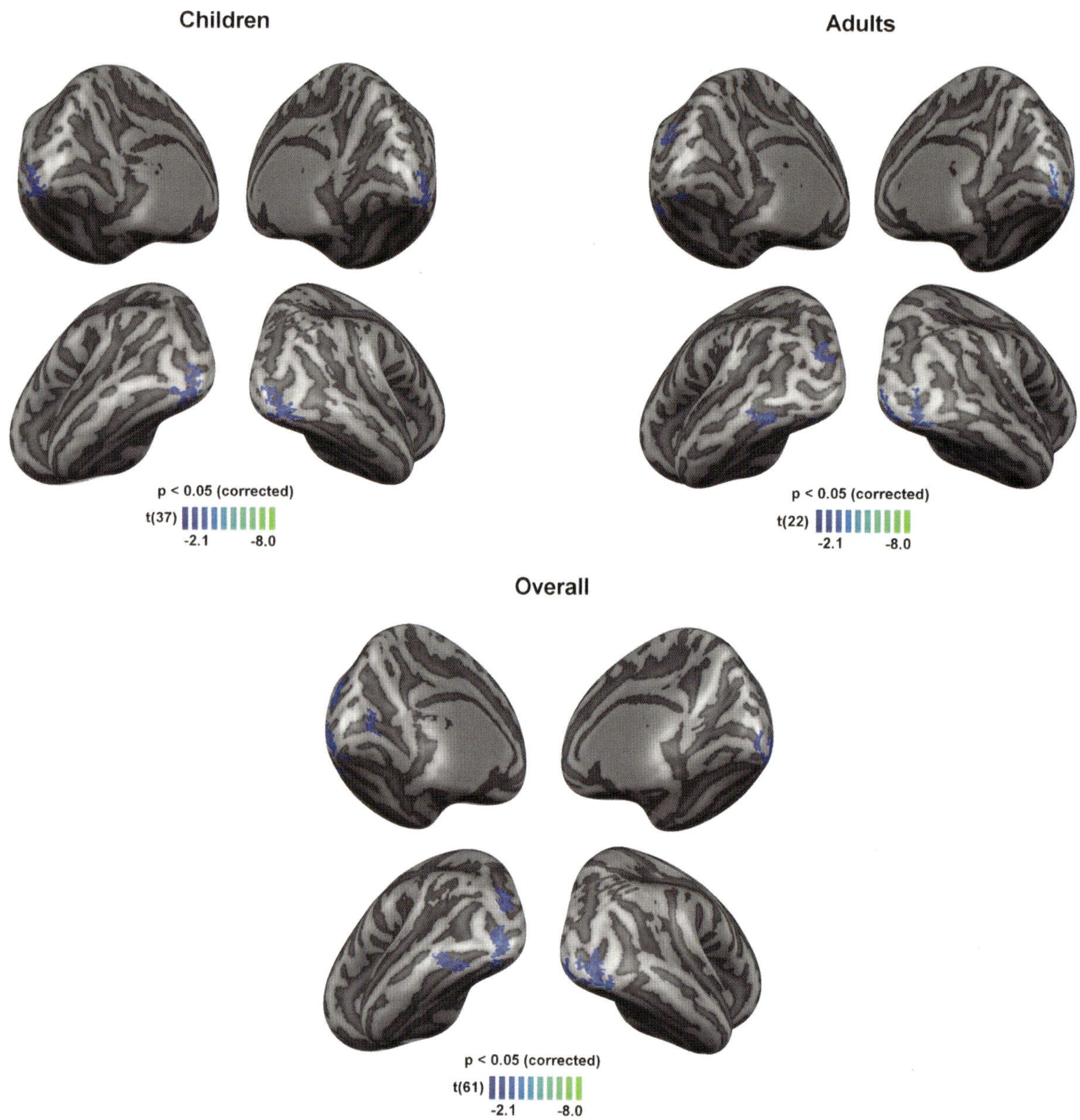

Figure 3. Significant differences in brain activations between patients with NF1 and controls, regarding the P-biased stimulus for children, adults and overall (children and adults) groups. Blue colours depict regions where activation was lower for individuals with NF1 than controls. Results are shown on views of the left and right hemispheres of cortex-based aligned three-dimensional reconstructions generated from the average anatomical data sets of the subjects in each group (children, adults, overall). Light grey represents gyri, dark grey represents sulci. T-maps thresholded at $p<0.05$ corrected using cortex-based cluster threshold estimation (cluster size 41 mm^2). N = 15 children with NF1, 24 control children, 13 adults with NF1 and 11 control adults.

with NF1 (timecourses not shown), as expected. However, the stimulus driving preferentially the M pathway resulted in a number of regions showing significantly higher BOLD signal in individuals with NF1 than controls, as mentioned above. Interestingly, in the retrosplenial cortex, the anterior cingulate cortex and the medial prefrontal cortex, the differences between groups emerged because individuals with NF1 presented positive BOLD activations while controls deactivated, Figure 4. Additionally, in the lingual gyrus, controls showed negative BOLD signals while patients with NF1 did not show activations in this area.

Discussion

The present work provides the first fMRI study on basic visual processing deficits in children, adolescents and adult patients with NF1. We used stimuli that were designed, based on functional properties, to preferentially activate the magnocellular or parvocellular pathways. Regions showing differences between controls and patients with NF1 were either visual or belonging to the default mode network.

Our findings indicate that individuals with NF1 have deficient activation of the visual cortex, as compared to their respective control group, for both types of low-level visual stimulation, in

Table 2. Localization and cluster size of the regions with significant between-group differences in activation during M-biased stimulation for the overall (children and adults) groups.

Region	BA	Center of Mass (T. coord.)			Cluster size (mm^2)
		X	Y	Z	
NF1< Control					
RH middle and superior occipital gyri					
	17/18/19	32.29	–82.61	0.64	300
	18	11.98	–94.96	7.13	41
LH middle and superior occipital gyri	17/18/19	–30.25	–83.29	6.41	374
NF1> Control					
RH anterior cingulate and medial prefrontal	10/32	6.72	41.61	6.68	373
LH anterior cingulate	32	–1.91	24.17	4.06	196
RH retrosplenial and lingual gyrus	17/29/30	11.40	–50.16	2.41	101
RH retrosplenial	30	2.87	–49.67	11.85	83
RH parieto-occipital fissure (cuneus)	18	15.72	–67.72	15.84	42
LH parieto-occipital fissure (cuneus)	17/18	–44.77	–59.94	17.88	59
LH lingual gyrus	17	–14.38	–45.16	–1.68	196

X, Y and Z indicate the center of mass in Talairach coordinates. BA, Brodmann areas. LH, left hemisphere. RH, right hemisphere.
Regions were determined by t-test second level analysis corrected with cluster threshold estimation ($p<0.05$, cluster size 41 mm^2) performed after the group-based RFX GLM analysis. Talairach coordinates are derived from the clusters shown in Figure 2.

agreement with our previous report of impaired contrast sensitivity in the M and P pathways of patients with NF1 [13]. Accordingly, we observed a similar deficit in visual activation both in children and adults with NF1. Such similarity is also reflected in no significant effect in the interaction between clinical group and age group. This finding indicates that low-level visual processing deficits do not ameliorate with age.

In what concerns the stimulus with low contrast, low spatial and high temporal frequency (driving into a larger extent the M pathway), patients with NF1 manifested more pronounced deficits in activating early visual retinotopic areas, V2d, V2v and V3d. The fact that early visual deficits are mainly explained by extrastriate V2/V3 contributions suggests that it is the emergence of early complex (intermediate vision) functional properties that is mostly impaired in NF1. Furthermore, dorsal V2 and V3 areas showed larger extent of hypoactivation than ventral V2 and V3 regions, in accordance with the notion of functional asymmetries in early visual cortex [32,33,34], and with the notion that M input dominates in dorsal regions [35,36].

Regarding the stimulus with high contrast, higher spatial frequency and low temporal frequency (more tuned to the P pathway), patients with NF1 showed an activation deficit that was equally distributed across retinotopically-defined visual areas, and also deficient neural activation in visual areas in the inferior occipital and occipito-temporal regions.

Table 3 Localization and cluster size of the regions with significant between-group differences in activation during P-biased stimulation for the overall (children and adults) groups.

Region	BA	Center of Mass (T. coord.)			Cluster size (mm^2)
		X	Y	Z	
NF1< Control					
RH inferior occipital gyrus	17/18	33.41	–81.66	-11.19	138
LH inferior occipital gyrus					
	18	–31.95	–86.26	–8.20	152
	19	–25.59	–78.34	–17.18	41
LH superior occipital gyrus	18/19	–27.53	–79.18	14.97	144
RH occipital pole	17	–94.25	–10.73	2.09	47
LH calcarine sulcus	17	–8.89	–70.57	6.29	72
LH occipito-temporal sulcus	37	–43.85	–60.40	–10.17	109

X, Y and Z indicate the center of mass in Talairach coordinates. BA, Brodmann areas. LH, left hemisphere. RH, right hemisphere.
Regions were determined by t-test second level analysis corrected with cluster threshold estimation ($p<0.05$, cluster size 41 mm^2) performed after the group-based RFX GLM analysis. Talairach coordinates are derived from the clusters shown in Figure 3.

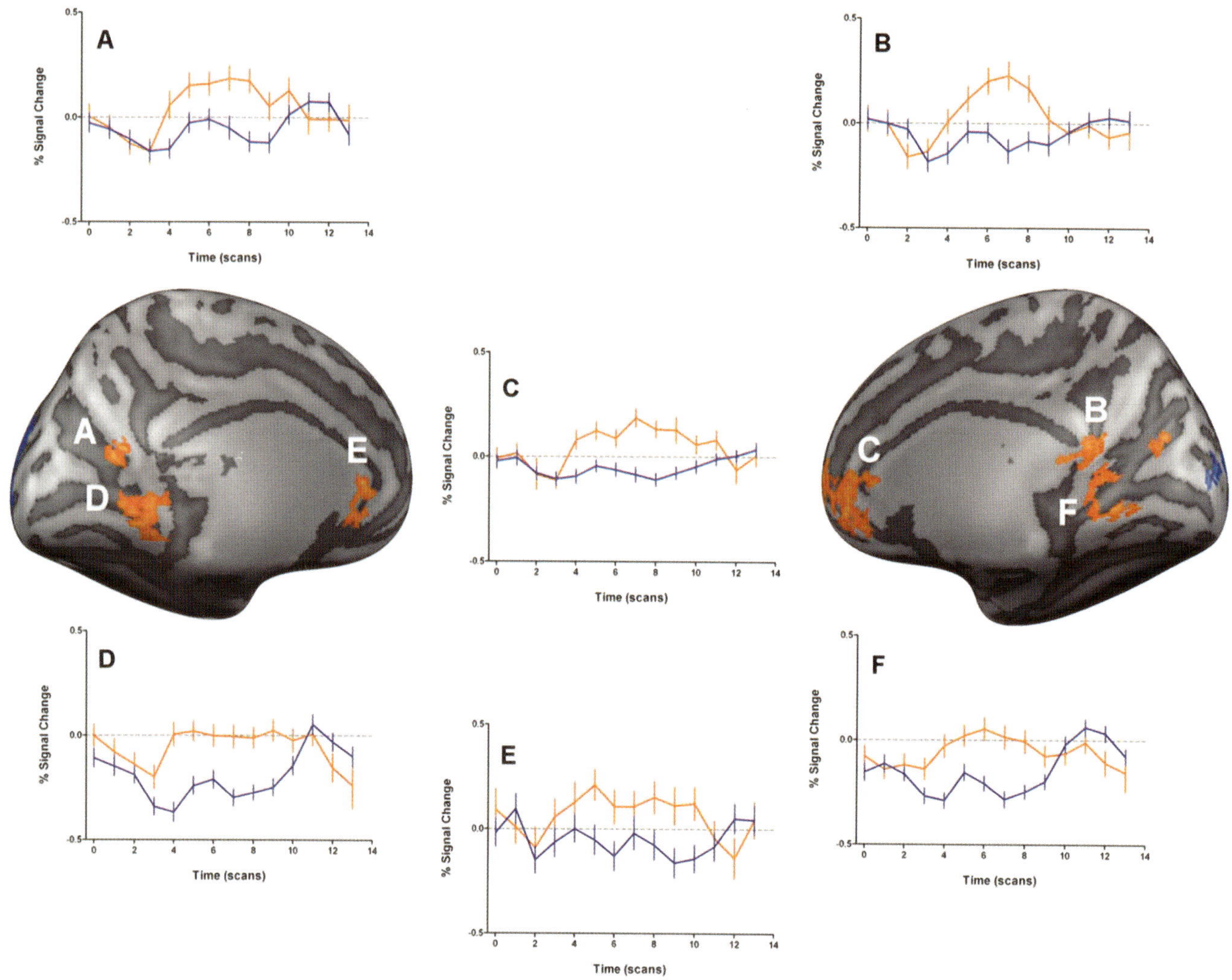

Figure 4. Time course information of the clusters with significantly higher activations for patients with NF1 than controls, regarding the M-biased stimulus for the overall (children and adults) group. Results are shown on lateral views of the left and right hemispheres of cortex-based aligned three-dimensional reconstructions generated from the average anatomical data sets of the subjects. T-maps are thresholded at $p<0.05$ corrected using cortex-based cluster threshold estimation (cluster size 41 mm^2). Plots A to F correspond to the timecourse information for the clusters with the same letter in the cortex representations. Timecourse percent signal change is shown in orange lines for patients with NF1 and blue lines for controls. Error bars reflect mean SEs. N = 28 patients with NF1 and 35 control subjects.

Altered visual processing in lower and higher levels of the dorsal and ventral streams may explain the visuospatial deficits that characterize the cognitive phenotype in NF1. Accordingly, Clements-Stephens et al. [9] reported, en passage, hypoactivation of the occipital cortex in patients with NF1 while performing the judgement of line orientation test. This test is known to be impaired in NF1 and recruits preferentially dorsal stream structures that build-up on information from low-level visual areas [37,38].

Another finding from the present study is the difference in activation between age groups observed for the M-biased stimulation in dorsal areas V2 and V3, with adults showing more activation than children. Recently, functional [39,40] and structural [41] studies focusing on the maturation of the dorsal and ventral streams suggested a slower maturation of the dorsal in relation to the ventral pathway. Our finding is an indication corroborating the late maturation of the dorsal pathway even for low-level visual areas, where ventral and dorsal pathways emerge and bifurcate.

Turning now to the differences between patients with NF1 and controls in the functional response profiles in brain regions outside visual areas, we were intrigued by the specific patterns observed for the M-biased stimulation. While P-biased stimulation did not cause differences outside visual regions, M tuned stimulus induced surprising positive BOLD activity in patients with NF1 while controls deactivated. This pattern was observed in posterior brain regions: parieto-occipital sulcus and retrosplenial cortex, as well as anterior brain regions: anterior cingulate and medial prefrontal cortex. Interestingly, these findings imply an anomalous activation pattern in patients with NF1 in regions belonging to the brain default-mode network (DMN). Regions belonging to the DMN commonly include the medial prefrontal cortex extending to the anterior cingulate, posterior cingulate/retrosplenial cortex and the parietal cortices in the region of the angular gyri. By definition, the DMN brain regions are active during task irrelevant thoughts [42], daydreaming [43] and self-referential thought [44] and deactivate during performance of cognitively demanding or engaging tasks

[42,45,46]. This set of brain regions has intrinsic functional correlation with each other [47,48].

During M-stimulation the NF1 group failed to deactivate the DMN suggesting that during these particular stimulation periods the participants with NF1 had a higher tendency to task-irrelevant thoughts than during the other task conditions. The mechanisms behind this abnormal DMN activation could be related to the attentional deficits known to occur in children with NF1. In that sense, one may hypothesise that activity in the DMN is explained by greater incidence of ADHD related symptoms in patients with NF1, and thus an inability to stay on the task and tendency to daydream. In any case in order to understand the neural mechanisms contributing to DMN activation it is important to account its dependence on stimulus type, given it only occurred during M-biased stimulation. The "magnocellular advantage" theory proposed by Laycock et al. [49,50] suggests an important role for the M pathway in driving attentional mechanisms in higher-order cortical regions. How this relates to abnormal DMN activation is an intriguing aspect to be explored in future studies.

Although our data does not set aside an ultimate explanation of this effect, our finding of paradoxical activation in midline DMN regions (medial prefrontal cortex, anterior cingulate and retrosplenial cortex) might give insightful information that can help in better understanding attentional deficits in patients with NF1 [51], and their implications for abnormal cognitive processing. Taking into account that low level visual impairments can impact high-level cognitive functions, our results provide evidence for a specific and intriguing link between the magnocellular pathway and the default mode network. In fact, it has been observed that in clinical populations with impaired magnocellular processing, as schizophrenia [52,53], autism [54,55], and Fragile X syndrome [56], the midline DMN regions fail to deactivate [57], [58], [59,60]. In summary, this study provides the first functional brain imaging indication that the early visual system is impaired in NF1, providing pathophysiological evidence for a potential impact in the high-level visual cognitive profile of patients with NF1. Moreover, our results provide an intriguing link between impaired magnocellular and default mode network processing, a finding that has been separately observed in autism and schizophrenia. Additional studies will be needed to further define the impact of these impairments in high-level cognitive functions of patients with NF1, particularly the abnormal allocation of neural resources observed in the midline regions of the default mode network.

Acknowledgments

We thank the participants with NF1 and their families, as well as all the control subjects that participated in this study. We also thank Carlos Ferreira and João Marques for help with MRI scanning and José Rebola for assisting in data processing.

Author Contributions

Conceived and designed the experiments: IRV MJR GC MCB. Performed the experiments: IRV. Analyzed the data: IRV GC JVD. Wrote the paper: IRV MJR MCB. Performed the neurophsychological characterization of the participants: IB. Performed the neuroradiological assessment of the participants: GC. Performed the ophtalmologic assessment of patients with NF1: ES. Recruited and diagnosed the patients with NF1: FR JS.

References

1. Kayl AE, Moore BD 3rd (2000) Behavioral phenotype of neurofibromatosis, type 1. Ment Retard Dev Disabil Res Rev 6: 117–124.
2. Riccardi V (1992) Neurofibromatosis: phenotype, natural history and pathogenesis. Baltimore: Johns Hopkins University Press.
3. Friedman JM, Birch P, Greene C (1993) National Neurofibromatosis Foundation International Database. Am J Med Genet 45: 88–91.
4. North K (2000) Neurofibromatosis type 1. Am J Med Genet 97: 119–127.
5. Levine TM, Materek A, Abel J, O'Donnell M, Cutting LE (2006) Cognitive profile of neurofibromatosis type 1. Semin Pediatr Neurol 13: 8–20.
6. Hyman SL, Shores A, North KN (2005) The nature and frequency of cognitive deficits in children with neurofibromatosis type 1. Neurology 65: 1037–1044.
7. Rowbotham I, Pit-ten Cate IM, Sonuga-Barke EJ, Huijbregts SC (2009) Cognitive control in adolescents with neurofibromatosis type 1. Neuropsychology 23: 50–60.
8. Billingsley RL, Jackson EF, Slopis JM, Swank PR, Mahankali S, et al. (2003) Functional magnetic resonance imaging of phonologic processing in neurofibromatosis 1. J Child Neurol 18: 731–740.
9. Clements-Stephens AM, Rimrodt SL, Gaur P, Cutting LE (2008) Visuospatial processing in children with neurofibromatosis type 1. Neuropsychologia 46: 690–697.
10. Leventhal AG (1991) Vision and visual dysfunction. Vol 4, The Neural basis of visual function, edited by A. G. Leventhal: Macmillan.
11. Livingstone M, Hubel D (1988) Segregation of form, color, movement, and depth: anatomy, physiology, and perception. Science 240: 740–749.
12. Hendry SH, Reid RC (2000) The koniocellular pathway in primate vision. Annu Rev Neurosci 23: 127–153.
13. Ribeiro MJ, Violante IR, Bernardino I, Ramos F, Saraiva J, et al. (2012) Abnormal achromatic and chromatic contrast sensitivity in Neurofibromatosis type 1. Invest Ophthalmol Vis Sci 53: 287–293.
14. Neurofibromatosis. Conference statement (1988) National Institutes of Health Consensus Development Conference. Archives of neurology 45: 575–578.
15. Wechsler D (2003) Escala de Inteligência para Crianças - Terceira Edição (WISC-III): Manual. Lisboa: Cegoc-Tea.
16. Raven J, Raven JC, Court JH (1993) Manual for Raven's progressive matrices and vocabulary scales. Oxford: Oxford Psychologists. xii,G60p. p.
17. Engel SA, Rumelhart DE, Wandell BA, Lee AT, Glover GH, et al. (1994) fMRI of human visual cortex. Nature 369: 525.
18. Sereno MI, Dale AM, Reppas JB, Kwong KK, Belliveau JW, et al. (1995) Borders of multiple visual areas in humans revealed by functional magnetic resonance imaging. Science 268: 889–893.
19. Brainard DH (1997) The Psychophysics Toolbox. Spat Vis 10: 433–436.
20. Liu CS, Bryan RN, Miki A, Woo JH, Liu GT, et al. (2006) Magnocellular and parvocellular visual pathways have different blood oxygen level-dependent signal time courses in human primary visual cortex. AJNR Am J Neuroradiol 27: 1628–1634.
21. Payne JM, Moharir MD, Webster R, North KN (2010) Brain structure and function in neurofibromatosis type 1: current concepts and future directions. J Neurol Neurosurg Psychiatry 81: 304–309.
22. Kriegeskorte N, Goebel R (2001) An efficient algorithm for topologically correct segmentation of the cortical sheet in anatomical mr volumes. Neuroimage 14: 329–346.
23. Friston KJ, Josephs O, Rees G, Turner R (1998) Nonlinear event-related responses in fMRI. Magn Reson Med 39: 41–52.
24. Shilyansky C, Karlsgodt KH, Cummings DM, Sidiropoulou K, Hardt M, et al. (2010) Neurofibromin regulates corticostriatal inhibitory networks during working memory performance. Proc Natl Acad Sci U S A 107: 13141–13146.
25. Talairach J, Tornoux P (1988) Co-planar stereotaxic atlas of the human brain : 3-dimensional proportional system : an approach to cerebral imaging. Stuttgart: Georg Thieme. 122 p. p.
26. Formisano E, Esposito F, Di Salle F, Goebel R (2004) Cortex-based independent component analysis of fMRI time series. Magn Reson Imaging 22: 1493–1504.
27. Goebel R, Esposito F, Formisano E (2006) Analysis of functional image analysis contest (FIAC) data with brainvoyager QX: From single-subject to cortically aligned group general linear model analysis and self-organizing group independent component analysis. Hum Brain Mapp 27: 392–401.
28. Fischl B, Sereno MI, Tootell RB, Dale AM (1999) High-resolution intersubject averaging and a coordinate system for the cortical surface. Hum Brain Mapp 8: 272–284.
29. Jo HJ, Lee JM, Kim JH, Shin YW, Kim IY, et al. (2007) Spatial accuracy of fMRI activation influenced by volume- and surface-based spatial smoothing techniques. Neuroimage 34: 550–564.
30. Penny W, Holmes A, Friston K (2003) Random effects analysis. In: Frackowiak R FK, Frith C, Dolan R, Friston K, Price C, Zeki S, Ashburner J, Penny W, editor. Human Brain Function. 2nd ed: Academic Press.
31. Forman SD, Cohen JD, Fitzgerald M, Eddy WF, Mintun MA, et al. (1995) Improved assessment of significant activation in functional magnetic resonance imaging (fMRI): use of a cluster-size threshold. Magn Reson Med 33: 636–647.
32. Liu T, Heeger DJ, Carrasco M (2006) Neural correlates of the visual vertical meridian asymmetry. J Vis 6: 1294–1306.
33. Eickhoff SB, Rottschy C, Kujovic M, Palomero-Gallagher N, Zilles K (2008) Organizational principles of human visual cortex revealed by receptor mapping. Cereb Cortex 18: 2637–2645.

34. Mendola JD, Conner IP, Sharma S, Bahekar A, Lemieux S (2006) fMRI Measures of perceptual filling-in in the human visual cortex. J Cogn Neurosci 18: 363–375.
35. Bullier J, Hupe JM, James AC, Girard P (2001) The role of feedback connections in shaping the responses of visual cortical neurons. Progress in brain research 134: 193–204.
36. Bullier J (2001) Integrated model of visual processing. Brain Res Brain Res Rev 36: 96–107.
37. Tranel D, Vianna E, Manzel K, Damasio H, Grabowski T (2009) Neuroanatomical correlates of the Benton Facial Recognition Test and Judgment of Line Orientation Test. J Clin Exp Neuropsychol 31: 219–233.
38. Kesler SR, Haberecht MF, Menon V, Warsofsky IS, Dyer-Friedman J, et al. (2004) Functional neuroanatomy of spatial orientation processing in Turner syndrome. Cereb Cortex 14: 174–180.
39. Bucher K, Dietrich T, Marcar VL, Brem S, Halder P, et al. (2006) Maturation of luminance- and motion-defined form perception beyond adolescence: a combined ERP and fMRI study. Neuroimage 31: 1625–1636.
40. Klaver P, Lichtensteiger J, Bucher K, Dietrich T, Loenneker T, et al. (2008) Dorsal stream development in motion and structure-from-motion perception. Neuroimage 39: 1815–1823.
41. Loenneker T, Klaver P, Bucher K, Lichtensteiger J, Imfeld A, et al. Microstructural development: organizational differences of the fiber architecture between children and adults in dorsal and ventral visual streams. Hum Brain Mapp 32: 935–946.
42. McKiernan KA, Kaufman JN, Kucera-Thompson J, Binder JR (2003) A parametric manipulation of factors affecting task-induced deactivation in functional neuroimaging. J Cogn Neurosci 15: 394–408.
43. Mason MF, Norton MI, Van Horn JD, Wegner DM, Grafton ST, et al. (2007) Wandering minds: the default network and stimulus-independent thought. Science 315: 393–395.
44. Gusnard DA, Akbudak E, Shulman GL, Raichle ME (2001) Medial prefrontal cortex and self-referential mental activity: relation to a default mode of brain function. Proc Natl Acad Sci U S A 98: 4259–4264.
45. Shulman GL, Corbetta M, Buckner RL, Raichle ME, Fiez JA, et al. (1997) Top-down modulation of early sensory cortex. Cereb Cortex 7: 193–206.
46. Raichle ME, MacLeod AM, Snyder AZ, Powers WJ, Gusnard DA, et al. (2001) A default mode of brain function. Proc Natl Acad Sci U S A 98: 676–682.
47. Greicius MD, Krasnow B, Reiss AL, Menon V (2003) Functional connectivity in the resting brain: a network analysis of the default mode hypothesis. Proc Natl Acad Sci U S A 100: 253–258.
48. Fox MD, Snyder AZ, Vincent JL, Corbetta M, Van Essen DC, et al. (2005) The human brain is intrinsically organized into dynamic, anticorrelated functional networks. Proc Natl Acad Sci U S A 102: 9673–9678.
49. Laycock R, Crewther SG, Crewther DP (2007) A role for the 'magnocellular advantage' in visual impairments in neurodevelopmental and psychiatric disorders. Neurosci Biobehav Rev 31: 363–376.
50. Laycock R, Crewther DP, Crewther SG (2008) The advantage in being magnocellular: a few more remarks on attention and the magnocellular system. Neurosci Biobehav Rev 32: 1409–1415.
51. Huijbregts S, Swaab H, de Sonneville L (2010) Cognitive and motor control in neurofibromatosis type I: influence of maturation and hyperactivity-inattention. Dev Neuropsychol 35: 737–751.
52. Martinez A, Hillyard SA, Dias EC, Hagler DJ Jr, Butler PD, et al. (2008) Magnocellular pathway impairment in schizophrenia: evidence from functional magnetic resonance imaging. J Neurosci 28: 7492–7500.
53. Coleman MJ, Cestnick L, Krastoshevsky O, Krause V, Huang Z, et al. (2009) Schizophrenia patients show deficits in shifts of attention to different levels of global-local stimuli: evidence for magnocellular dysfunction. Schizophr Bull 35: 1108–1116.
54. Sutherland A, Crewther DP (2010) Magnocellular visual evoked potential delay with high autism spectrum quotient yields a neural mechanism for altered perception. Brain 133: 2089–2097.
55. Pellicano E, Gibson L, Maybery M, Durkin K, Badcock DR (2005) Abnormal global processing along the dorsal visual pathway in autism: a possible mechanism for weak visuospatial coherence? Neuropsychologia 43: 1044–1053.
56. Kogan CS, Boutet I, Cornish K, Zangenehpour S, Mullen KT, et al. (2004) Differential impact of the FMR1 gene on visual processing in fragile X syndrome. Brain 127: 591–601.
57. Kennedy DP, Redcay E, Courchesne E (2006) Failing to deactivate: resting functional abnormalities in autism. Proc Natl Acad Sci U S A 103: 8275–8280.
58. Menon V, Leroux J, White CD, Reiss AL (2004) Frontostriatal deficits in fragile X syndrome: relation to FMR1 gene expression. Proc Natl Acad Sci U S A 101: 3615–3620.
59. Pomarol-Clotet E, Salvador R, Sarro S, Gomar J, Vila F, et al. (2008) Failure to deactivate in the prefrontal cortex in schizophrenia: dysfunction of the default mode network? Psychol Med 38: 1185–1193.
60. Salgado-Pineda P, Fakra E, Delaveau P, McKenna PJ, Pomarol-Clotet E, et al. Correlated structural and functional brain abnormalities in the default mode network in schizophrenia patients. Schizophr Res 125: 101–109.

15

Aggregation of PolyQ Proteins Is Increased upon Yeast Aging and Affected by Sir2 and Hsf1: Novel Quantitative Biochemical and Microscopic Assays

Aviv Cohen, Liron Ross, Iftach Nachman, Shoshana Bar-Nun*

Department of Biochemistry and Molecular Biology, George S. Wise Faculty of Life Sciences, Tel Aviv University, Tel Aviv, Israel

Abstract

Aging-related neurodegenerative disorders, such as Parkinson's, Alzheimer's and Huntington's diseases, are characterized by accumulation of protein aggregates in distinct neuronal cells that eventually die. In Huntington's disease, the protein huntingtin forms aggregates, and the age of disease onset is inversely correlated to the length of the protein's polyglutamine tract. Using quantitative assays to estimate microscopically and capture biochemically protein aggregates, here we study in *Saccharomyces cerevisiae* aging-related aggregation of GFP-tagged, huntingtin-derived proteins with different polyQ lengths. We find that the short 25Q protein never aggregates whereas the long 103Q version always aggregates. However, the mid-size 47Q protein is soluble in young logarithmically growing yeast but aggregates as the yeast cells enter the stationary phase and age, allowing us to plot an "aggregation timeline". This aging-dependent aggregation was associated with increased cytotoxicity. We also show that two aging-related genes, *SIR2* and *HSF1*, affect aggregation of the polyQ proteins. In Δ*sir2* strain the aging-dependent aggregation of the 47Q protein is aggravated, while overexpression of the transcription factor Hsf1 attenuates aggregation. Thus, the mid-size 47Q protein and our quantitative aggregation assays provide valuable tools to unravel the roles of genes and environmental conditions that affect aging-related aggregation.

Editor: Anne C. Hart, Brown University, United States of America

Funding: Initial stages of this study were supported by a grant from the Chief Scientist Office of the Ministry of Health, Israel (grant no. 3-3211 to SB) and later by a grant from The Israel Science Foundation (grant no. 384/11 to SB). IN is supported in part by the Edmond J. Safra Center for Bioinformatics at Tel Aviv University. The funders had no role in study design, data collection and analysis, decision to publish, or preparation of the manuscript.

Competing Interests: The authors have declared that no competing interests exist.

* E-mail: shoshbn@tauex.tau.ac.il

Introduction

Huntington's disease (HD) is a progressive neurodegenerative disorder manifested by dysfunction and cell death mainly in the striatal and cortical brain regions [1–3]. HD patients experience deteriorating symptoms including chorea, progressive dementia, psychiatric manifestations, and death within 15 years of symptoms onset. Currently there is neither cure nor treatment to postpone the onset of HD or to slow its progression [4–6]. HD is an autosomal dominant genetic disease, caused by mutations in the first exon of the huntingtin gene, *Htt*, that increase the number of CAG repeats to generate expanded polyglutamine (polyQ) tracts in the N-terminal region of the huntingtin protein [7].

It is still unclear why the ubiquitously expressed huntingtin has a distinctive neurological phenotype and if huntingtin's loss-of-function leads to HD [8;9]. The widely accepted notion is that HD is caused by a harmful gain-of-function of expanded polyQ since mice models with mutated huntingtin exon 1 recapitulate HD symptoms, including neuronal dysfunction and death [10]. Hence, although CAG repeat RNA was recently proposed as an auxiliary toxic agent in polyQ disorders [11], it appears that the deleterious effects in HD are mostly related to the tendency of the mutated huntingtin protein to misfold and aggregate. This property is observed with purified proteins and in neurons, where cellular aggregates are mainly composed of huntingtin [12]. *In vivo* and *in vitro* studies of polyQ fibrillogenesis indicate that aggregation is an intrinsic feature of long polyQ tracts and this tendency increases with the length of the polyQ repeat [13;14]. Indeed, HD is one of nine known polyQ repeat autosomal dominant disorders, all of which result from mutations that expand the polyQ tract within different but specific proteins [15–18]. Although the mutated proteins have no shared qualities beside the polyQ mutation, all these disorders are characterized by progressive neurodegeneration as well as the formation of polyQ protein aggregates.

The common risk factor of all aggregation diseases is aging [19–21] and, in HD, the combination of aging and genetic mutations is manifested by inverse correlation between the age of disease onset and the number of CAG repeats. Repeats shorter than 35Q are asymptomatic, whereas repeats exceeding the 40Q threshold ensure HD development such that 40–50Q give rise to the normal adult-onset of HD while longer repeats result in juvenile cases [22–27]. Although various statistical models strongly correlate the mean age of HD onset with the length of the CAG repeat [28;29], patients with the same polyQ length exhibit very different ages of onset. Hence, modifiers of HD and aggregation, apart from the length of the polyQ, must be implicated [5]. Based on screening HD patients or model organisms, combinations of genetic and environmental factors clearly affect the age of HD onset [22].

Cellular aging is considered as a progressive decline in the proteostasis machinery and the response to changing environment.

Aging is caused partly by genetic factors accompanied by metabolic, environmental and stochastic factors [30;31]. Progress in cellular aging research is driven by single-celled eukaryotes such as the budding yeast *Saccharomyces cerevisiae*. In this organism, genetic modulators of replicative lifespan (RLS) are being identified, and chronological lifespan (CLS) is considered useful for understanding the aging process in non-dividing mammalian cells such as neurons [32;33]. Importantly, a subset of pathways that influence longevity in yeast is conserved in other eukaryotes, including mammals. A genome-wide screen in *S. cerevisiae* has identified CLS-affecting genes that are highly conserved in other species, suggesting that longevity is a fundamental process conserved in evolution [34]. Finally, the stationary phase model of aging in yeast recapitulates many pathological alterations observed during neuronal aging, highlighting the power of yeast as a model system to explore the molecular basis of aging–related diseases of the central nervous system [35].

Among the conserved genes implicated in determining lifespan are the sirtuins, a family of class III NAD+-dependent protein deacetylases. In their unique lysine deacetylation reaction, NAD+ is cleaved, 29-O-acetyl-ADP-ribose is generated and nicotinamide (NAM) is released. Silent information regulator 2 (Sir2) in yeast or its closest mammalian homolog Sirt1 are conserved from yeast to mammals and are shown to regulate metabolism and longevity [36–38]. RLS in yeast is extended when Sir2 is overexpressed and decreases upon *SIR2* deletion [39]. Also, lifespan extension associated with dietary restriction (DR) requires Sir2 and NAD+ since it is annulled by deletion of either *SIR2* or *NPT1* (a gene in the NAD^+ biosynthetic pathway). However, the role of sirtuins in DR-mediated lifespan extension is controversial; in yeast at stationary phase, Sir2 actually blocks extreme CLS extension mediated by DR [40].

Heat shock factor 1 (Hsf1), a master regulator of transcription, is another highly conserved protein that plays an important role in longevity as well as in maintaining proteostasis and adequate response to proteotoxic stresses. In *Caenorhabditis elegans*, Hsf1 is required for enhanced thermotolerance and suppression of proteotoxicity and was also shown to regulate aging [41;42] and to affect lifespan extension by DR [43]. Hsf1 is a regulator of lifespan also in yeast, as the CLS extender Ecl2 in *Schizosaccharomyces pombe* and its functional homolog YGR146C in *S. cerevisiae* are direct targets of Hsf1 and overexpression of Hsf1 in fission yeast extends CLS [44]. Hsf1 is activated by heat-shock, oxidative, metabolic or environmental stresses, although our understanding of Hsf1 regulation remains incomplete. In yeast, under normal growth conditions, Hsf1 is a constitutively phosphorylated homotrimer but inactive. Upon exposure to stress, Hsf1 is hyperphosphorylated and adopts an active conformation. Hsf1 binds to heat shock response elements (HSE) in the promoter region of its target genes and activates their expression [45–48]. Among the many Hsf1 target genes are the molecular chaperones, which resolve damaged/misfolded and aggregated proteins generated by heat stress or metabolism [49;50]. Interrelations between Hsf1 and Sirt1, the closest mammalian homolog of Sir2, may underlie their effects on proteostasis. Sirt1 phosphorylation is required for cell survival under stress, and mammalian Hsf1 is one of the substrates that phosphorylated Sirt1 deacetylates and co-activates, allowing the deacetylated Hsf1 to bind to HSE and activate the molecular chaperones network [51–53].

Among the genetically manipulatable model organisms for studying aggregation and toxicity of polyQ proteins, *S. cerevisiae* provides unsurpassed tools to decipher disease-associated cellular processes and identify novel therapeutic targets [54]. Although this unicellular eukaryote neither resembles neurons nor expresses endogenous huntingtin, the relevant cellular pathways appear to be highly conserved between humans and yeast. Hence, yeast is an established system for studying the causes and consequences of polyQ aggregation, and to address aging, DR and oxidative stress at the cellular and molecular levels [33;35;55–67]. Here we follow the effects of aging and altered expression or activity of *SIR2* and *HSF1* on the aggregation of polyQ proteins in *S. cerevisiae*. Our most interesting results are with the 47Q that harbors a mid-size polyQ tract characteristic of the threshold of HD onset. We find that 47Q is non-toxic and soluble in growing yeast, but aggregates as cells age. Upon *SIR2* deletion, the aging-dependent aggregation is aggravated, while overexpression of Hsf1 attenuates aggregation. Hence, Sir2 and Hsf1 appear to affect aggregation-related processes during aging.

Results

Quantitative measurements of polyQ proteins aggregation in yeast cells

Aggregates of polyQ proteins and their distribution in live cells are usually detected by fluorescence microscopy, owing to a fluorescent tag attached to the polyQ proteins [55;56]. Although aggregation patterns differ from cell to cell, images are usually evaluated qualitatively and any quantitative analysis merely determines how many cells in a population contain aggregates of polyQ proteins [56]. In this study we express in yeast, under galactose induction, GFP- and FLAG-tagged polyQ proteins harboring 25, 47 or 103 glutamine residues (referred to as 25Q, 47Q and 103Q), to demonstrate the basic characteristics conferred by the different polyQ lengths (Figure 1A, B). Among them, aggregation-prone polyQ proteins are toxic to different organisms, including yeast [57]. Indeed, upon galactose induction, expression of the 103Q inhibits cell growth, whereas 25Q expression does not (Figure 1C). A calculated duplication time of less than 2 hrs for cells harboring polyQ plasmids when grown in glucose was extended to around 4 hrs for cells expressing 25Q and to around 10 hrs for cells expressing 103Q when grown in galactose.

Aggregates of polyQ proteins are formed in cells under different circumstances and are correlated with cytotoxicity. To gain insights into the various factors that affect aggregation, we developed a reproducible, quantitative and linear method to measure the amount of aggregates in yeast cells. This method takes advantage of the insolubility of polyQ aggregates in sodium dodecyl sulfate (SDS) [13]. Briefly, following cell lysis, samples are divided into two aliquots. One aliquot is adsorbed directly onto a nitrocellulose membrane to estimate total amounts of polyQ proteins, whereas SDS up to 2% (w/v) is added to the other aliquot that is filtered through a SDS-soaked membrane to capture the polyQ aggregates. While high concentration of SDS that denatures and charges proteins prevents their adsorption, aggregates are resistant to SDS and are retarded on the membrane. By immunoblotting we quantify the amounts of total polyQ proteins adsorbed to the untreated membrane (Figure 2A) and the aggregates retarded on the SDS-treated membrane (Figure 2B). These amounts are linear over a 10-fold range of cell lysates applied, thus allow calculating an "aggregation index" as the ratio of the aggregates to the total polyQ proteins (Figure 2C). Clearly, while both 25Q and 103Q are expressed (Figures 1B and 2A), aggregates are detected only for 103Q and not for 25Q (Figure 2B, C).

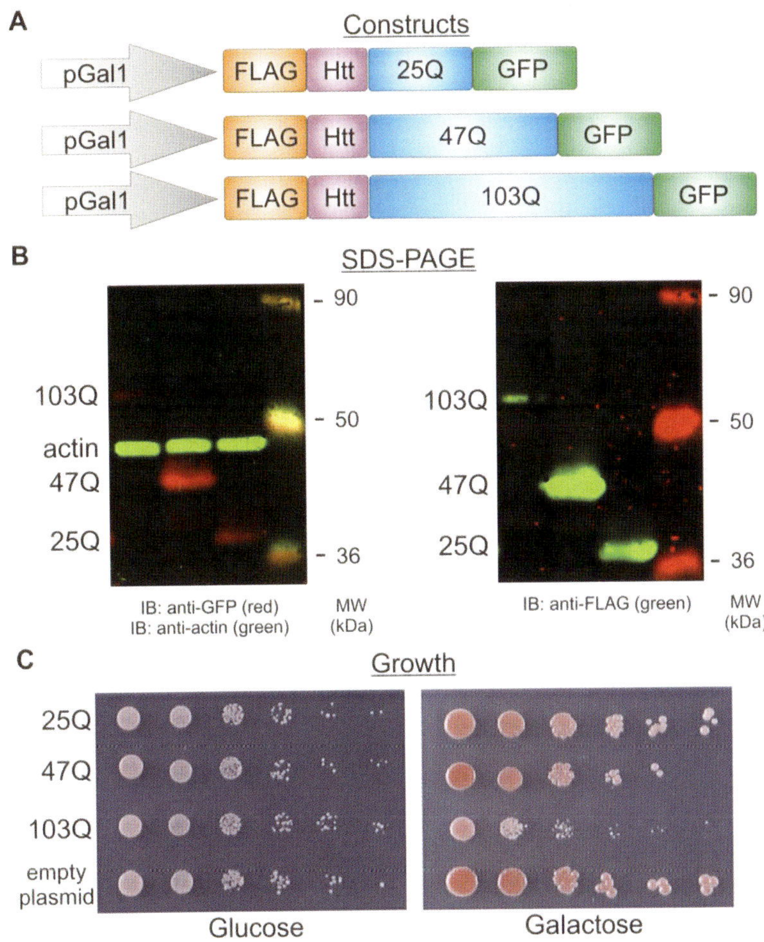

Figure 1. Proteins with polyQ of different lengths show different characteristics. A Schematic representation of the constructs used to express polyQ proteins. Each contains a FLAG tag at its N-terminus, followed by huntingtin's exon 1 encoding the first 17 amino acids (Htt), a polyQ tract of different length, and GFP at the C-terminus. Expression of all polyQ proteins is driven by the pGal1 promoter that is induced by galactose and repressed by glucose. B Wild-type cells (W303–1b) expressing the 25Q, 47Q or 103Q were grown logarithmically (0.6–1 A_{600}) for 8 hours under galactose induction. Cell lysates were resolved by SDS-PAGE and polyQ proteins were detected by immunoblotting (IB) with a mouse anti-FLAG antibody followed by IRDye 800CW-conjugated goat anti-mouse IgG (right panel) or a rabbit anti-GFP followed by Dylight 680-labeled goat anti-rabbit IgG (left panel, red). A mouse anti-actin followed by IRDye 800CW-conjugated goat anti-mouse IgG was used as a loading control (left panel, green). Blots were visualized by the Odyssey Infrared Imaging System. C Wild-type cells (W303–1b) expressing the 25Q, 47Q, 103Q or an empty plasmid were grown logarithmically in glucose and 10-fold serial dilutions (starting with 7.5×10^6 cells) were spotted on glucose or galactose plates.

Increased aggregation of long and mid-size polyQ protein is observed upon aging

The quantitative analysis allows us to monitor the aggregation of the various polyQ proteins during cell aging and draw a timeline for the aggregation process. Aggregate formation of the long 103Q occurs very early and it somewhat increases as the cells age, while the short 25Q does not aggregate at any age (Figure 3B, C). Importantly, the mid-size 47Q does not aggregate in logarithmically growing young cells, but its aggregation is markedly increased as the cells age (Figure 3B, C). The 47Q aggregation starts when the cells enter the stationary phase and stop dividing and progresses with age (Figure 3C).

This aggregation of the various polyQ proteins and especially the aging-dependent change in 47Q aggregation is strongly corroborated by our quantitative fluorescence microscopy. To quantify the aggregation level within individual cells, we analyze in hundreds of cells per sample the ratio R between the GFP fluorescence in the brightest focus and the average GFP fluorescence in the whole cell (Figure 4 A, B and Figures S1, S2 and S3). In 25Q-expressing cells with no aggregates this ratio is close to 1 (Figures 4B and S1), 103Q-expressing cells with aggregates show ratio values higher than 1 (Figures 4B and S3), and in 47Q-expressing cells the ratio increases upon aging (Figures 4B and S2). When R is plotted along the yeast aging process (Figure 4C), this ratio is in striking agreement with the Aggregation Index determined by filtration (Figure 3C). By defining cells with R above a cutoff of 1.5 as having aggregates, we calculated the fraction of cells with aggregates (Figure 4D). Both quantitative approaches reflect the aging-dependent aggregation of the 47Q, with no aggregation of the 25Q and immediate onset of aggregation of the 103Q. While this manuscript was under revision, a study in *C. elegans* reported the *in vivo* dynamics of polyQ aggregation using fluorescence microscopy, fluorescence recovery after photobleaching and fluorescence correlation spectroscopy [68]. Also in that study, the brightest foci represented aggregates, as they were immobile. The decline in R of 103Q at late time points stems from an age-dependant decline of total GFP fluorescence in these cells, as shown in Figures 4B and S3. Since

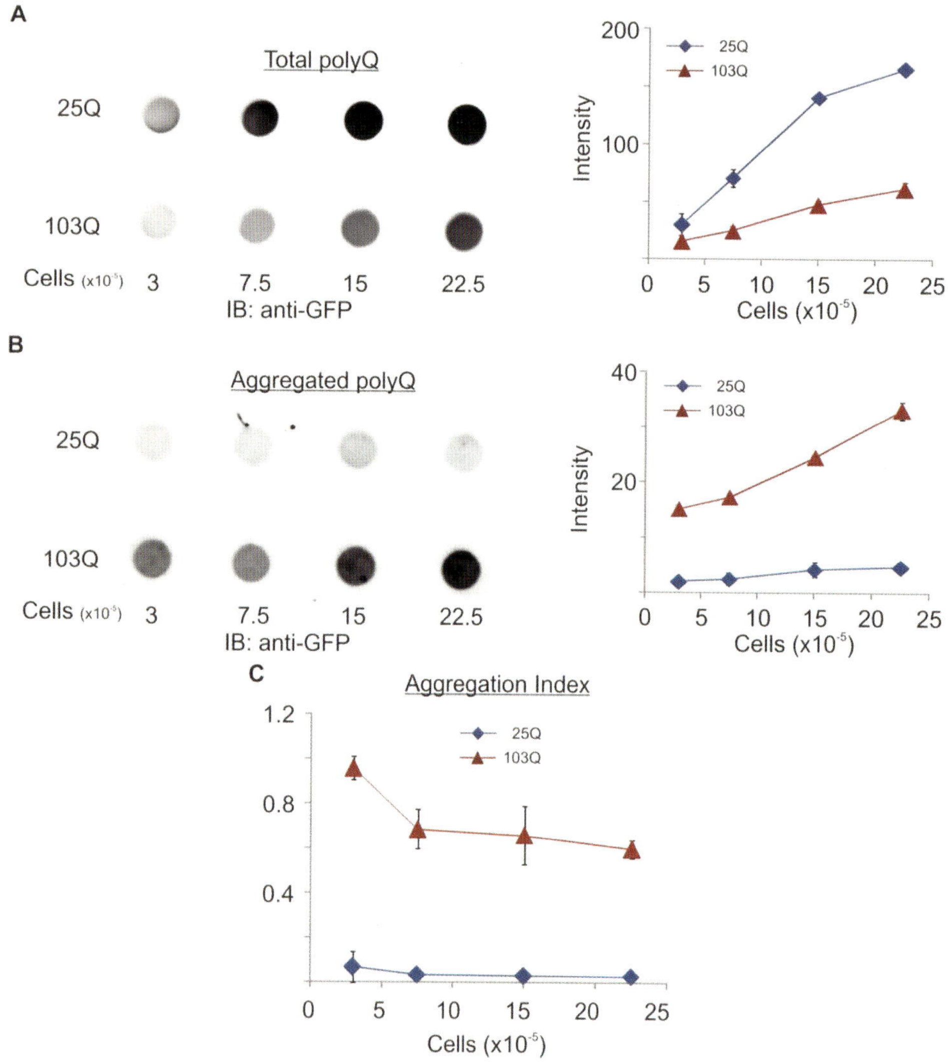

Figure 2. Quantitative filter retardation assay for polyQ proteins aggregates. Wild-type cells (KFY100) expressing 25Q or 103Q were grown for 3 days under galactose induction. Cells were lysed and lysates from the indicated number of cells were A adsorbed onto untreated nitrocellulose to estimate the total amount of polyQ proteins, or B SDS was added and lysates were filtered through SDS-soaked membranes to capture polyQ aggregates. On both membranes, polyQ proteins were quantified by immunoblotting (IB) with a rabbit anti-GFP antibody followed by Dylight 680-labeled goat anti-rabbit IgG and visualized (only one set of transformants is presented) and quantified by the Odyssey Infrared Imaging System. C Aggregation Index (in arbitrary units) was calculated as the ratio between the filtered (panel B) and absorbed (panel A) polyQ proteins. Data from 3 independent transformants are presented as mean ± SE.

this decline is not observed in the filter retardation assay (Figure 3), it is likely not the consequence of aggregates loss. Combined, our two quantitative analyses indicate that the mid-size 47Q is soluble in growing yeast and aggregates progressively as the yeast age.

Upon *SIR2* deletion, the aging-dependent aggregation is aggravated, while overexpression of Hsf1 attenuates aggregation

One of the proteins that are firmly linked to aging is the NAD+-dependent protein deacetylase Sir2. Thus, we next followed the aggregation of polyQ proteins in a mutant lacking the *SIR2* gene. When compared to wild-type cells (Figure 3C), it is evident that despite similar expression level of the polyQ proteins, the aggregation of both 47Q and 103Q is increased remarkably in aging Δ*sir2* cells (Figure 5A, squares and triangles, respectively), and irrespective of *SIR2* deletion, 25Q still does not aggregate (Figure 5A, diamonds). Being a class III deacetylase that cleaves NAD^+ for its activity, Sir2 releases nicotinamide (NAM), which is reported to be a noncompetitive inhibitor of Sir2 [69]. Indeed, in the presence of NAM, 47Q aggregation increases in aged cells (Figure 5B) in a concentration-dependent manner (Figure 5C). Even the highest concentration of NAM (40 mM) affects neither the already highly aggregated 103Q nor the never aggregated 25Q (Figure 5C).

Another aging-related protein, whose activity and content are critical for the cellular response to proteotoxic stresses, is Hsf1 [41;43;44]. When *HSF1* is overexpressed from a plasmid in wild-type cells, we find attenuated aging-dependent aggregation of the mid-size 47Q and the long 103Q, as compared to cells expressing an empty plasmid (pRS314) instead of p*HSF1* (Figure 5D). Our results indicate that Hsf1 is involved in aggregation of polyQ proteins in aging cells.

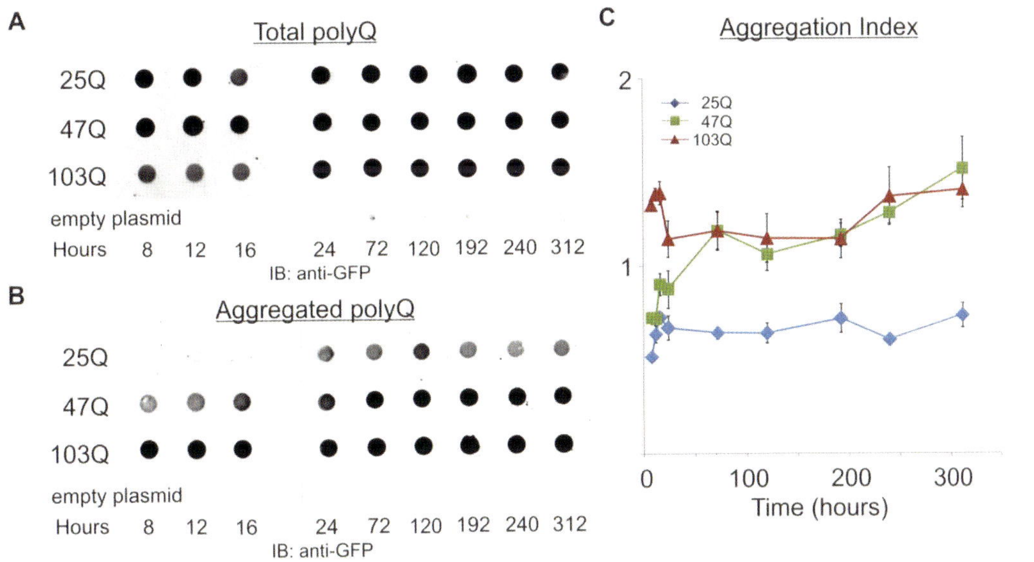

Figure 3. Quantitative retardation assay reveals that aggregation of 47Q increases upon aging. Wild-type cells (W303–1b) expressing 25Q, 47Q or 103Q were grown under galactose induction for the indicated time, and at each time point 11.25×10^5 cells (within the linear range; see Figure 2) were lysed. Early time points (8–16 hrs) were done separately from later time points. Total amounts A and captured aggregates B of polyQ proteins were quantified and Aggregation Index C was calculated as described in and in Figure 2. Data from 3 independent transformants, 3 triplicates each, are presented as mean ± SE. Statistical significance between the different polyQ was calculated by split-plot ANOVA. We found $p<0.0001$ between 25Q and 47Q; $p<0.001$ between 47Q and 103Q; and no significance between experiments of each polyQ.

Discussion

Neurodegeneration and aging, intimately interrelated processes, are the subject of intensive clinical research. The complexity of both processes, let alone when combined, makes it extremely difficult to elucidate the mechanisms that underlie aging-dependent neurodegeneration. Aging is poorly defined at the molecular level and the effects of aging on cellular processes are not fully understood. Nevertheless, many key genes implicated in longevity are highly conserved in evolution, suggesting that they operate in fundamental mechanisms. Neurodegenerative diseases are also diverse but one of their major hallmarks is the deposition of specific aggregation-prone proteins. To date neither the basis for the toxicity of these aggregates, nor their formation or the cellular processes affected by them is fully explained. Because of the close links between the two processes, models in mice, flies, worms and yeast were developed to study the effects of aging on protein aggregation and neurodegeneration.

In this study we expressed GFP-tagged proteins with different polyQ lengths in *S. cerevisiae* and followed their fate as a function of aging. We show that the short 25Q protein never aggregates and remains soluble at all times. The long 103Q protein is already aggregated very early after induction of its expression and levels of aggregates only slightly increase as the cells age. Our most interesting finding, shown in yeast for the first time, is that the mid-size 47Q protein is soluble and evenly dispersed in logarithmically growing yeast but begins to aggregate as the yeast cells enter the stationary phase. As the yeast cells aging progresses, the Aggregation Index (Figure 3) and the number of cells visualized with aggregates (Figure 4) increase further and sometimes even exceed the aggregation level of 103Q. Similar aging-dependent aggregation of mid-size polyQ proteins was also reported in *C. elegans* [19;68]. Our results demonstrate that the ability of yeast cells to maintain mid-size polyQ proteins in solution declines upon their aging. The sharp threshold in the onset of HD when huntingtin's polyQ tract contains around 45 residues (45Q) [22] suggests that our results with the near-threshold mid-size 47Q in aging yeast closely simulate the situation in humans. Thus, aging yeast may serve a reliable model system to study the dependence of aggregation on aging, a hallmark of many neurodegenerative disorders.

We show that yeast aging affects the aggregation of polyQ proteins and implicate aging-related genes in this phenomenon (Figures 3,4,5). Clearly, *HSF1* overexpression decreases aggregation of 47Q or 103Q (Figure 5D). These results may reflect an aging-dependent functional decline in Hsf1 and/or its many targets, mostly the chaperone network. Indeed, upregulation of chaperones increases longevity and enhances aging-related stress resistance in various models [70]. In particular, overexpression of Hsp70 extends the lifespan of *C. elegans* [71] and *Drosophila melanogaster* [72]. Likewise, a very recent screen of ~900,000 small molecules has identified new classes of proteostasis regulators that induce HSF-1-dependent chaperone expression and restore protein folding in multiple conformational disease models [73]. It appears that proteostasis diseases are aggravated when the capacity of the chaperone network to cope with inherited misfolding-prone proteins, aging, or metabolic/environmental stresses declines [74].

Another major gene that has been implicated in aging in several organisms, including yeast where it was first discovered, is the class-III deacetylase Sir2, although its role in aging remains controversial. As noted above, there are two models of aging in yeast, RLS and CLS [75]. Whereas replicative aging may be a useful model for mitotically active cells, chronological aging represents more faithfully postmitotic cells, such as neurons. Interestingly, Sir2 is beneficial for RLS, whereas Δ*sir2* cells show higher CLS and better resistance to different stress conditions [40]. Here we find in aging Δ*sir2* cells increased aggregation (Figure 5A) that is also detected when Sir2 activity is blocked by NAM (Figure 5B, C).

Although further investigation is required to understand the role of Sir2 in aggregates formation in aging yeast, this phenomenon

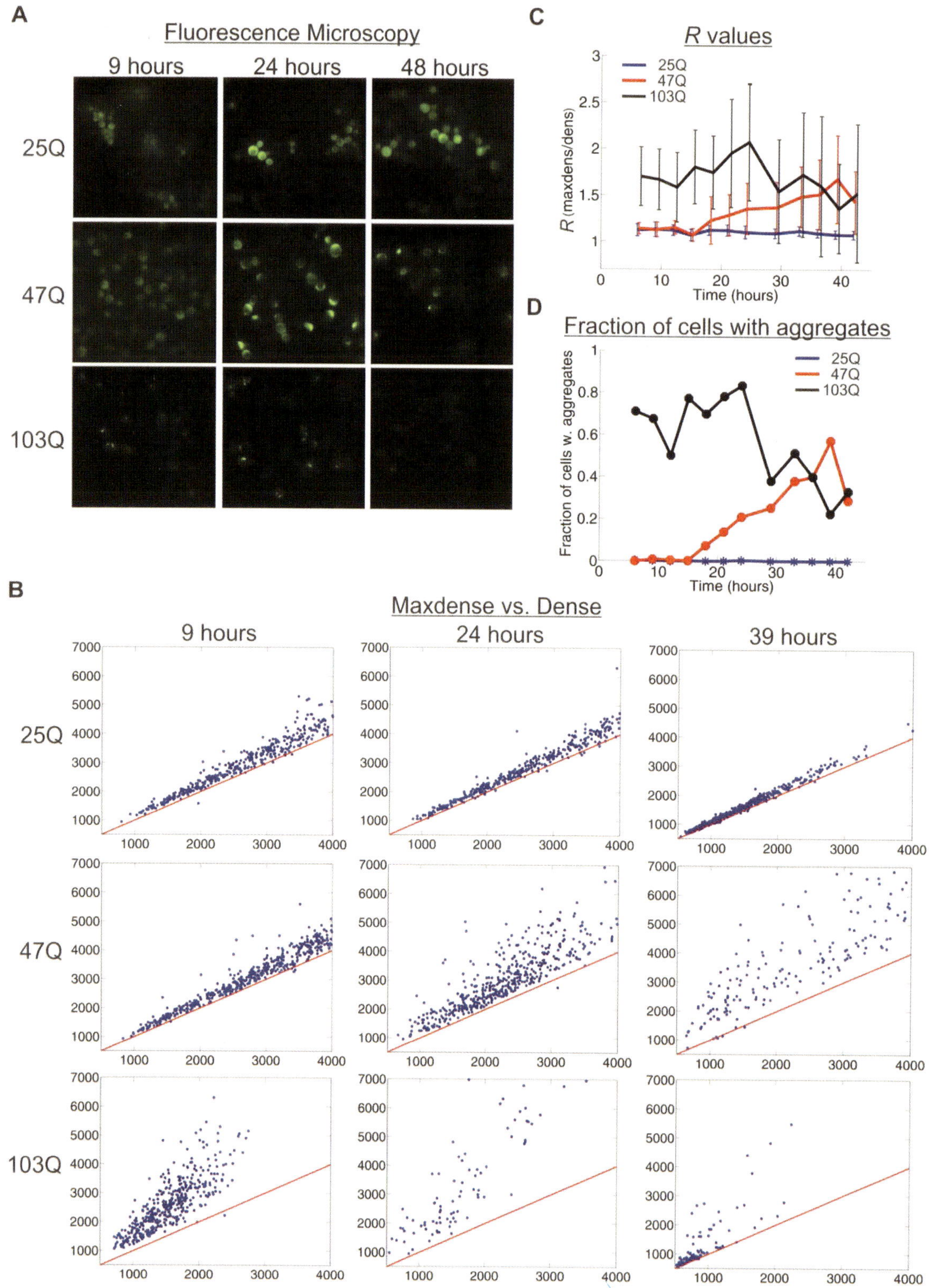

Figure 4. Quantitative microscopic assay reveals that aggregation of 47Q increases upon aging. A Wild-type cells (W303–1b) expressing 25Q, 47Q or 103Q were grown under galactose induction for up to 42 hrs. At each time point hundreds of cells were imaged by fluorescence microscopy. Images of 3 representative time points are presented. B Microscopic images from a similar experiment were analyzed for the presence of aggregates in individual cells as presented by the ratio between the maximal density (y axis) and the density (x axis) and 3 representative time points are presented (for all time points, see Figures S1, S1 and S3). C The ratio *R* between the maximal density and the density throughout the experiment plotted over time. At each time point the mean values ± SD are shown and the error bars reflect the variability between individual cells. D The fraction of cells with aggregates (defined as cells with *R* above a cutoff of 1.5) plotted over time.

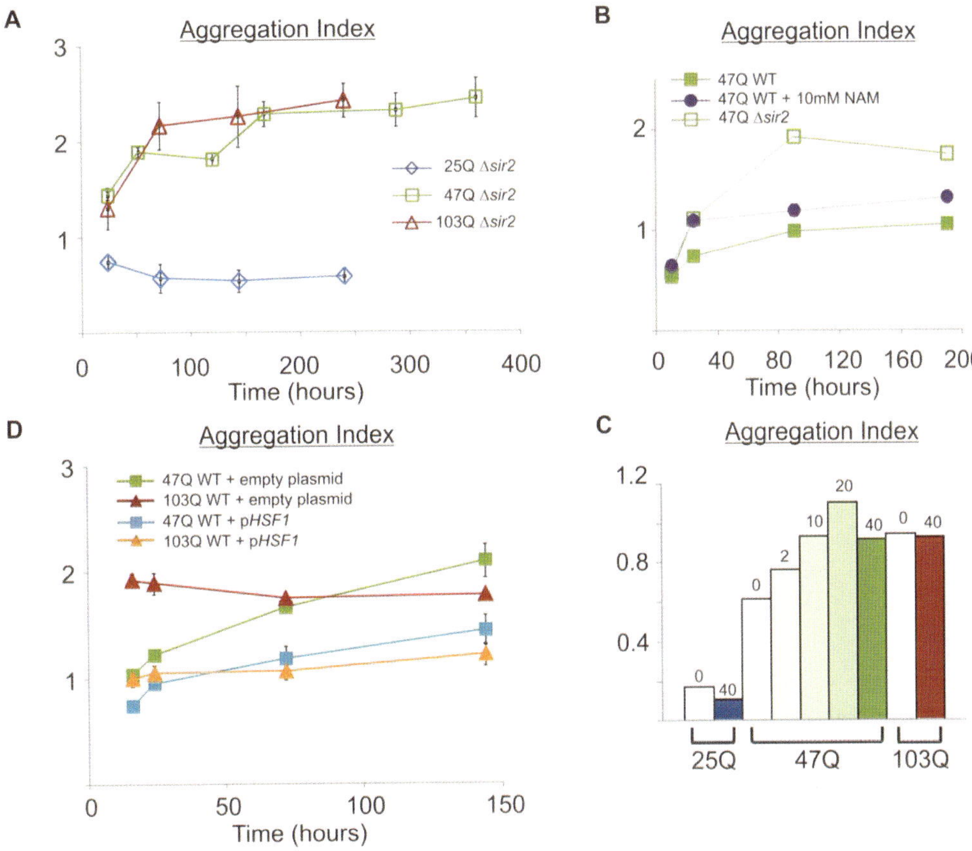

Figure 5. Sir2 and Hsf1 are involved in the aging-dependent aggregation of polyQ proteins. A Δ*sir2* (RS1717; W303–1b *sir2*Δ::*his5*$^{+}$) cells expressing 25Q, 47Q or 103Q were grown under galactose induction for the indicated time, collected, lysed, and Aggregation Index was calculated for each time point, as described in Figure 3. Data from 3 independent transformants, 3 triplicates each, are presented as mean ± SE. B Wild-type (WT, W303–1b) or Δ*sir2* cells expressing 47Q were grown for the indicated time under galactose induction. Wild-type cells were also exposed to 10mM nicotinamide (NAM). Cells were, collected and lysed and Aggregation Index for each time point was calculated as described in Figure 3. C Wild-type cells (W303–1b) expressing the indicated polyQ proteins were grown under galactose induction for 72 hours with the indicated concentration (mM) of NAM. Cells were collected, lysed and Aggregation Index was calculated as described in Figure 3. D Wild-type (W303–1b) cells expressing the indicated polyQ proteins and harboring either an empty (pRS314) or p*HSF1* plasmid were grown under galactose induction for the indicated time. Cells were collected, lysed and Aggregation Index was calculated for each time point as described in Figure 3. Data from 3 independent transformants, 3 triplicates each, are presented as mean ± SE.

may reflect accelerated aging and failure to segregate damaged proteins in Sir2 mutants [76], possibly due to Sir2 involvement in maintaining the activity of the TRiC/CCT complex [77]. The ongoing debate of whether aggregates are protective or harmful to cells is still open. Uncoupling between aggregation and toxicity was recently reported from RNA interference genetic screens in *C. elegans* that have identified novel regulators of the proteostasis network [78]. Indeed, aggregates are observed in affected cells and serve as a hallmark of Alzheimer's, Parkinson's and HD. Also, in HD, polyQ aggregates are detected before the onset of clinical symptoms [79]. Yet, the formation of polyQ aggregates was reported to improve neurons survival compared to cells that had more diffuse distribution of huntingtin [80]. Moreover, analysis of polyQ structural changes showed that a soluble monomeric beta-sheet conformer of the expanded polyQ was a major cause of cytotoxicity [81]. Therefore, large aggregates may be the result of an active mechanism that has evolved to protect the cell by sequestering the toxic species, either the misfolded proteins and/or their oligomers [82;83]. It remains to be established how Sir2 and Hsf1 affect, directly or indirectly, the aggregation of polyQ proteins. Interestingly, deacetylation by Sirt1 (the closest mammalian homolog of Sir2) is reported to be one of the activation modes of the mammalian Hsf1 [51]. If yeast Hsf1 activity is also regulated by Sir2, this suggests a coordinated mechanism designed to handle aggregation-prone proteins.

The filter retardation aggregation assay we describe here (Figure 2) is simple, reproducible, and linear within a wide range of concentrations. Supported by the fluorescence microscopy (Figure 4), these assays allow monitoring the level of protein aggregation throughout the life of yeast populations in a quantitative fashion. Both assays can be easily applied to other cells and organisms. By these methods, and capitalizing on the ease and speed of genetic screening in yeast, this model system is particularly amenable to study the effects of genetic and environmental factors on aging and aging-dependent aggregation and determine their consequences on cytotoxicity and cell survival.

Materials and Methods

Yeast strains and plasmids

The yeast strains of *Saccharomyces cerevisiae* employed in this study are W303–1b (*MATα ura3-52 trp1Δ2 leu2–3,112 his3–11 ade2–1 can1–100*) and KFY100 (*MATa his4–619 leu2–3,112 ura3–52*). Δ*sir2* (RS1717; W303–1b *sir2*Δ::*his5*$^{+}$) was generously provided by

Prof. R. Sternglanz, Stony Brook University, USA [84]. The pRS314-*HSF1* plasmid was kindly provided by Prof. DJ Thiele, University of Michigan Medical School, USA.

The polyQ constructs used in this study were previously described [56]. They were generously provided by Prof. M. Sherman, Boston University, USA. The cDNAs encode the first 17 N-terminal amino acids of Huntingtin exon 1 (Htt_{17}), followed by alternating CAG/CAA repeats of different lengths (encoding 25, 47 or 103 glutamine residues). These were fused in frame with a FLAG tag at the N-terminus, and green fluorescent protein (GFP) at the C-terminus, generating FLAG-Htt_{17}-Q_{25}-GFP (25Q), FLAG-Htt_{17}-Q_{47}-GFP (47Q) and FLAG-Htt_{17}-Q_{103}-GFP (103Q) (Figure 1A). The constructs were subcloned into the *URA3*-containging pYES2 vector, so the regulated expression of the polyQ proteins is under the galactose-inducible pGal1 promoter.

Growth conditions

Yeast were regularly grown in minimal media which contained 0.67% (w/v) yeast nitrogen base, the appropriate nutrients required for selection of transformants, and 2% (w/v) glucose. For galactose induction, cells were transferred to medium containing 4% (w/v) galactose only, or 2% (w/v) galactose and 2% (w/v) fructose. Stationary phase cells that stopped dividing and reached 3.0–6.0 A_{600} (starting from 1.5×10^6 cells/ml of glucose starters; cell number was calculated as $1A_{600} = 1.5 \times 10^7$cells/ml) were grown for up to 15 days. All cells undergoing galactose induction were grown in 10 ml medium in 100 ml loosely-capped bottles, unless indicated otherwise.

For growth experiments, cells were grown logarithmically (0.6–1 A_{600}) diluted to equal cell density (0.5 A_{600}) and spotted as 10-fold serial dilutions on plates containing 2% (w/v) agar, 0.67% (w/v) yeast nitrogen base, the appropriate nutrients required for selection, and 2% (w/v) glucose or 4% (w/v) galactose. Alternatively, yeast cells were grown in glucose- or galactose-containing minimal liquid media, starting at 0.05 A_{600} and following their growth up to 0.8 A_{600}, for calculating the duplication time.

Quantitative fluorescence microscopy

Yeasts grown to logarithmic or stationary phase were viewed under the DMRBE fluorescence microscope (Leica). GFP was viewed using Chroma 41017 filter (excitation 470/40) and snapshots were taken using Magnafire 12-bit color CCD camera (Figure 4A). For aggregate quantification (Figure 4B), yeasts grown to logarithmic or stationary phase were imaged on a Nikon TiE fluorescent microscope with a 100X/1.49NA objective. GFP images of hundreds of cells were taken with 480/20 excitation filter, 525/40 emission filter (Chroma) using an Andor Clara 16-bit CCD camera. Images were processed using custom Matlab code [85]. Briefly, cells were segmented using the DIC channel. Fluorescence densities were computed by dividing total cell fluorescence by cell area. Independently, fluorescent foci were identified in the GFP channel using local adaptive thresholding, and then mapped to cells by location. Maximal density was computed from the fluorescence of the brightest focus in the cell divided by the focus area. The ratio R between the maximal density and the density is used as a measure for aggregation.

Sample collection and alkaline lysis

Cell samples were collected at different times throughout the experiments, as indicated. Cell density was determined as A_{600}, identical numbers of cells were collected by centrifugation (13,000 rpm, 1 minute, 4°C), washed with 0.01 M NaN_3 in phosphate-buffered saline (PBS), and frozen (−20°C), to allow simultaneous lysis. Importantly, aggregates and protein levels were not affected by freezing (data not shown). Cells were lyzed by incubation for 30 minutes on ice in lysis buffer containing 0.2 M NaOH and 0.5% (v/v) β-mercaptoethanol, pH was adjusted to 8.0 with 5N HCl and samples were boiled for 5 minutes.

Filter retardation and blotting assays

The protocol for measuring aggregation levels is based on modified versions of previously described methods: aggregates filtration [86] and total protein dot blotting. Equal amounts of boiled lysates were diluted 5-fold in either PBS or PBS supplemented with 2% (w/v) SDS (PBS/SDS). Samples in PBS were applied to PBS-soaked nitrocellulose membranes (0.2 μ; Protran Whatman) to absorb all proteins. Samples in PBS/SDS were filtered through nitrocellulose membrane soaked in PBS/SDS to retard only the aggregates. At least three independent transformants were analyzed and triplicate samples from each (total of 9 samples) were tested for absorbance and retardation assays. The data are presented as mean ± SE. All samples were applied to a 96-well dot blotter (Biorad). Membranes were blocked with 10% skim milk in PBS and polyQ proteins were detected by immunoblotting.

Immunoblotting

The polyQ proteins were detected by a mouse anti-FLAG antibody (clone M2, Sigma). The secondary antibody used was IRDye 800CW-conjugated goat anti-mouse (LI-COR Biosciences). Alternatively, rabbit anti-GFP (ab290, Abcam) was used as a primary antibody followed by goat anti-rabbit IgG DyLight 680-labled (072-06-15-06, KPL). Secondary antibodies were visualized and quantified by the Odyssey Infrared Imaging System (LI-COR Biosciences).

Supporting Information

Figure S1 Quantitative microscopic assay reveals that 25Q never aggregates. Wild-type cells (W303-1b) expressing 25Q were grown under galactose induction for up to 42 hrs. At each time point hundreds of cells were imaged by fluorescence microscopy. Images were analyzed for the presence of aggregates in individual cells as presented by the ratio between the maximal density (y axis) and the density (x axis).

Figure S2 Quantitative microscopic assay reveals that aggregation of 47Q increases upon aging. Wild-type cells (W303-1b) expressing 47Q were grown under galactose induction for up to 42 hrs. At each time point hundreds of cells were imaged by fluorescence microscopy. Images were analyzed for the presence of aggregates in individual cells as presented by the ratio between the maximal density (y axis) and the density (x axis).

Figure S3 Quantitative microscopic assay reveals that 103Q is always aggregated. Wild-type cells (W303-1b) expressing 103Q were grown under galactose induction for up to 42 hrs. At each time point hundreds of cells were imaged by fluorescence microscopy. Images were analyzed for the presence of aggregates in individual cells as presented by the ratio between the maximal density (y axis) and the density (x axis).

Acknowledgments

We are indebted to Prof. R Sternglanz Stony Brook University USA, Prof. DJ Thiele University of Michigan Medical School USA and Prof. M Sherman Boston University USA, for their generous gifts of plasmids and strains. We are grateful to Noa Alumot and Daria Riabov for their valuable contribution. We thank Joseph Roitelman, Eran Bosis and members of our laboratory for critical reading of the manuscript.

Author Contributions

Conceived and designed the experiments: AC LR IN SB. Performed the experiments: AC LR. Analyzed the data: AC LR IN SB. Contributed reagents/materials/analysis tools: IN. Wrote the paper: AC IN SB.

References

1. Harper PS (1991) Aspects of Huntington's Disease. In: Harper PS (ed) Huntington Disese Major Problems in Neurology. W.B. Sanders Co., London, 281 315.
2. Myers RH, MacDonald ME, Koroshetz WJ, Duyao MP, Ambrose CM, et al. (1993) De novo expansion of a (CAG)n repeat in sporadic Huntington's disease. Nat Genet 5: 168–173.
3. Hedreen JC, Folstein SE (1995) Early loss of neostriatal striosome neurons in Huntington's disease. J Neuropathol Exp Neurol 54: 105–120.
4. Vonsattel JP, DiFiglia M (1998) Huntington disease. J Neuropathol Exp Neurol 57: 369–384.
5. Wexler NS, Lorimer J, Porter J, Gomez F, Moskowitz C, et al. (2004) Venezuelan kindreds reveal that genetic and environmental factors modulate Huntington's disease age of onset. Proc Natl Acad Sci U S A 101: 3498–3503.
6. Novak MJ, Tabrizi SJ (2010) Huntington's disease. BMJ 340: c3109.
7. The Huntington's Disease Collaborative Research Group (1993) A novel gene containing a trinucleotide repeat that is expanded and unstable on Huntington's disease chromosomes. Cell 72: 971–983.
8. Cattaneo E, Zuccato C, Tartari M (2005) Normal huntingtin function: an alternative approach to Huntington's disease. Nat Rev Neurosci 6: 919–930.
9. Suopanki J, Gotz C, Lutsch G, Schiller J, Harjes P, et al. (2006) Interaction of huntingtin fragments with brain membranes – clues to early dysfunction in Huntington's disease. J Neurochem 96: 870–884.
10. Davies SW, Turmaine M, Cozens BA, DiFiglia M, Sharp AH, et al. (1997) Formation of neuronal intranuclear inclusions underlies the neurological dysfunction in mice transgenic for the HD mutation. Cell 90: 537–548.
11. Wojciechowska M, Krzyzosiak WJ (2011) Cellular toxicity of expanded RNA repeats: focus on RNA foci. Hum Mol Genet 20: 3811–3821.
12. DiFiglia M, Sapp E, Chase KO, Davies SW, Bates GP, et al. (1997) Aggregation of huntingtin in neuronal intranuclear inclusions and dystrophic neurites in brain. Science 277: 1990–1993.
13. Scherzinger E, Lurz R, Turmaine M, Mangiarini L, Hollenbach B, et al. (1997) Huntingtin-encoded polyglutamine expansions form amyloid-like protein aggregates in vitro and in vivo. Cell 90: 549–558.
14. Saunders HM, Gilis D, Rooman M, Dehouck Y, Robertson AL, et al. (2011) Flanking domain stability modulates the aggregation kinetics of a polyglutamine disease protein. Protein Sci 20: 1675–1681.
15. Zoghbi HY, Orr HT (1999) Polyglutamine diseases: protein cleavage and aggregation. Curr Opin Neurobiol 9: 566–570.
16. Fischbeck KH (2001) Polyglutamine expansion neurodegenerative disease. Brain Res Bull 56: 161–163.
17. Ross CA, Poirier MA, Wanker EE, Amzel M (2003) Polyglutamine fibrillogenesis: the pathway unfolds. Proc Natl Acad Sci U S A 100: 1–3.
18. Landles C, Bates GP (2004) Huntingtin and the molecular pathogenesis of Huntington's disease. Fourth in molecular medicine review series. EMBO Rep 5: 958–963.
19. Morley JF, Brignull HR, Weyers JJ, Morimoto RI (2002) The threshold for polyglutamine-expansion protein aggregation and cellular toxicity is dynamic and influenced by aging in Caenorhabditis elegans. Proc Natl Acad Sci U S A 99: 10417–10422.
20. Morimoto RI (2008) Proteotoxic stress and inducible chaperone networks in neurodegenerative disease and aging. Genes Dev 22: 1427–1438.
21. Ben Zvi A, Miller EA, Morimoto RI (2009) Collapse of proteostasis represents an early molecular event in Caenorhabditis elegans aging. Proc Natl Acad Sci U S A.
22. Gusella JF, MacDonald ME (2009) Huntington's disease: the case for genetic modifiers. Genome Med 1: 80.
23. Telenius H, Kremer HP, Theilmann J, Andrew SE, Almqvist E, et al. (1993) Molecular analysis of juvenile Huntington disease: the major influence on (CAG)n repeat length is the sex of the affected parent. Hum Mol Genet 2: 1535 1540.
24. Andrew SE, Goldberg YP, Kremer B, Telenius H, Theilmann J, et al. (1993) The relationship between trinucleotide (CAG) repeat length and clinical features of Huntington's disease. Nat Genet 4: 398–403.
25. Snell RG, MacMillan JC, Cheadle JP, Fenton I, Lazarou LP, et al. (1993) Relationship between trinucleotide repeat expansion and phenotypic variation in Huntington's disease. Nat Genet 4: 393–397.
26. Stine OC, Pleasant N, Franz ML, Abbott MH, Folstein SE, et al. (1993) Correlation between the onset age of Huntington's disease and length of the trinucleotide repeat in IT-15. Hum Mol Genet 2: 1547–1549.
27. Kremer B, Goldberg P, Andrew SE, Theilmann J, Telenius H, et al. (1994) A worldwide study of the Huntington's disease mutation. The sensitivity and specificity of measuring CAG repeats. N Engl J Med 330: 1401–1406.
28. Langbehn DR, Hayden MR, Paulsen JS (2010) CAG-repeat length and the age of onset in Huntington disease (HD): a review and validation study of statistical approaches. Am J Med Genet B Neuropsychiatr Genet 153B: 397–408.
29. Langbehn DR, Brinkman RR, Falush D, Paulsen JS, Hayden MR (2004) A new model for prediction of the age of onset and penetrance for Huntington's disease based on CAG length. Clin Genet 65: 267–277.
30. Sohal RS, Mockett RJ, Orr WC (2002) Mechanisms of aging: an appraisal of the oxidative stress hypothesis. Free Radic Biol Med 33: 575–586.
31. Taylor RC, Dillin A (2011) Aging as an event of proteostasis collapse. Cold Spring Harb Perspect Biol 3:
32. Fontana L, Partridge L, Longo VD (2010) Extending healthy life span – from yeast to humans. Science 328: 321–326.
33. Parrella E, Longo VD (2008) The chronological life span of Saccharomyces cerevisiae to study mitochondrial dysfunction and disease. Methods 46: 256–262.
34. Fabrizio P, Hoon S, Shamalnasab M, Galbani A, Wei M, et al. (2010) Genome-wide screen in Saccharomyces cerevisiae identifies vacuolar protein sorting, autophagy, biosynthetic, and tRNA methylation genes involved in life span regulation. PLoS Genet 6: e1001024.
35. Chen Q, Ding Q, Keller JN (2005) The stationary phase model of aging in yeast for the study of oxidative stress and age-related neurodegeneration. Biogerontology 6: 1–13.
36. Haigis MC, Guarente LP (2006) Mammalian sirtuins – emerging roles in physiology, aging, and calorie restriction. Genes Dev 20: 2913–2921.
37. Frye RA (2000) Phylogenetic classification of prokaryotic and eukaryotic Sir2-like proteins. Biochem Biophys Res Commun 273: 793–798.
38. Schwer B, Verdin E (2008) Conserved metabolic regulatory functions of sirtuins. Cell Metab 7: 104–112.
39. Kaeberlein M, McVey M, Guarente L (1999) The SIR2/3/4 complex and SIR2 alone promote longevity in Saccharomyces cerevisiae by two different mechanisms. Genes Dev 13: 2570–2580.
40. Fabrizio P, Gattazzo C, Battistella L, Wei M, Cheng C, et al. (2005) Sir2 blocks extreme life-span extension. Cell 123: 655–667.
41. Hsu AL, Murphy CT, Kenyon C (2003) Regulation of aging and age-related disease by DAF-16 and heat-shock factor. Science 300: 1142–1145.
42. Garigan D, Hsu AL, Fraser AG, Kamath RS, Ahringer J, et al. (2002) Genetic analysis of tissue aging in Caenorhabditis elegans: a role for heat-shock factor and bacterial proliferation. Genetics 161: 1101–1112.
43. Steinkraus KA, Smith ED, Davis C, Carr D, Pendergrass WR, et al. (2008) Dietary restriction suppresses proteotoxicity and enhances longevity by an hsf-1-dependent mechanism in Caenorhabditis elegans. Aging Cell 7: 394–404.
44. Ohtsuka H, Azuma K, Murakami H, Aiba H (2011) hsf1 (+) extends chronological lifespan through Ecl1 family genes in fission yeast. Mol Genet Genomics 285: 67–77.
45. Sorger PK (1991) Heat shock factor and the heat shock response. Cell 65: 363–366.
46. Yamamoto A, Mizukami Y, Sakurai H (2005) Identification of a novel class of target genes and a novel type of binding sequence of heat shock transcription factor in Saccharomyces cerevisiae. J Biol Chem 280: 11911–11919.
47. Akerfelt M, Morimoto RI, Sistonen L (2010) Heat shock factors: integrators of cell stress, development and lifespan. Nat Rev Mol Cell Biol 11: 545–555.
48. Sorger PK, Pelham HR (1988) Yeast heat shock factor is an essential DNA-binding protein that exhibits temperature-dependent phosphorylation. Cell 54: 855–864.
49. Hahn JS, Hu Z, Thiele DJ, Iyer VR (2004) Genome-wide analysis of the biology of stress responses through heat shock transcription factor. Mol Cell Biol 24: 5249–5256.
50. Eastmond DL, Nelson HC (2006) Genome-wide analysis reveals new roles for the activation domains of the Saccharomyces cerevisiae heat shock transcription factor (Hsf1) during the transient heat shock response. J Biol Chem 281: 32909–32921.
51. Westerheide SD, Anckar J, Stevens SM Jr., Sistonen L, Morimoto RI (2009) Stress-inducible regulation of heat shock factor 1 by the deacetylase SIRT1. Science 323: 1063–1066.
52. Gidalevitz T, Prahlad V, Morimoto RI (2011) The stress of protein misfolding: from single cells to multicellular organisms. Cold Spring Harb Perspect Biol 3:
53. Monteiro JP, Cano MI (2011) SIRT1 deacetylase activity and the maintenance of protein homeostasis in response to stress: an overview. Protein Pept Lett 18: 167–173.
54. Swinnen E, Buttner S, Outeiro TF, Galas MC, Madeo F, et al. (2011) Aggresome formation and segregation of inclusions influence toxicity of alpha-synuclein and synphilin-1 in yeast. Biochem Soc Trans 39: 1476–1481.
55. Krobitsch S, Lindquist S (2000) Aggregation of huntingtin in yeast varies with the length of the polyglutamine expansion and the expression of chaperone proteins. Proc Natl Acad Sci U S A 97: 1589–1594.
56. Meriin AB, Zhang X, He X, Newnam GP, Chernoff YO, et al. (2002) Huntington toxicity in yeast model depends on polyglutamine aggregation mediated by a prion-like protein Rnq1. J Cell Biol 157: 997–1004.

57. Duennwald ML, Jagadish S, Giorgini F, Muchowski PJ, Lindquist S (2006) A network of protein interactions determines polyglutamine toxicity. Proc Natl Acad Sci U S A 103: 11051–11056.
58. Kaeberlein M, Burtner CR, Kennedy BK (2007) Recent developments in yeast aging. PLoS Genet 3: e84.
59. Sherman MY, Muchowski PJ (2003) Making yeast tremble: yeast models as tools to study neurodegenerative disorders. Neuromolecular Med 4: 133–146.
60. Willingham S, Outeiro TF, DeVit MJ, Lindquist SL, Muchowski PJ (2003) Yeast genes that enhance the toxicity of a mutant huntingtin fragment or alpha-synuclein. Science 302: 1769–1772.
61. Outeiro TF, Muchowski PJ (2004) Molecular genetics approaches in yeast to study amyloid diseases. J Mol Neurosci 23: 49–60.
62. Giorgini F, Guidetti P, Nguyen Q, Bennett SC, Muchowski PJ (2005) A genomic screen in yeast implicates kynurenine 3-monooxygenase as a therapeutic target for Huntington disease. Nat Genet 37: 526–531.
63. Giorgini F, Muchowski PJ (2006) Screening for genetic modifiers of amyloid toxicity in yeast. Methods Enzymol 412: 201–222.
64. Duennwald ML, Jagadish S, Muchowski PJ, Lindquist S (2006) Flanking sequences profoundly alter polyglutamine toxicity in yeast. Proc Natl Acad Sci U S A 103: 11045–11050.
65. Ehrnhoefer DE, Duennwald M, Markovic P, Wacker JL, Engemann S, et al. (2006) Green tea (−)-epigallocatechin-gallate modulates early events in huntingtin misfolding and reduces toxicity in Huntington's disease models. Hum Mol Genet 15: 2743–2751.
66. Duennwald ML, Lindquist S (2008) Impaired ERAD and ER stress are early and specific events in polyglutamine toxicity. Genes Dev 22: 3308–3319.
67. Giorgini F, Muchowski PJ (2009) Exploiting yeast genetics to inform therapeutic strategies for Huntington's disease. Methods Mol Biol 548: 161–174.
68. Beam M, Silva MC, Morimoto RI (2012) Dynamic imaging by fluorescence correlation spectroscopy identifies diverse populations of polyglutamine oligomers formed in vivo. J Biol Chem.
69. Imai S, Armstrong CM, Kaeberlein M, Guarente L (2000) Transcriptional silencing and longevity protein Sir2 is an NAD-dependent histone deacetylase. Nature 403: 795–800.
70. Voisine C, Pedersen JS, Morimoto RI (2010) Chaperone networks: tipping the balance in protein folding diseases. Neurobiol Dis 40: 12–20.
71. Yokoyama K, Fukumoto K, Murakami T, Harada S, Hosono R, et al. (2002) Extended longevity of Caenorhabditis elegans by knocking in extra copies of hsp70F, a homolog of mot-2 (mortalin)/mthsp70/Grp75. FEBS Lett 516: 53–57.
72. Tatar M, Khazaeli AA, Curtsinger JW (1997) Chaperoning extended life. Nature 390: 30.
73. Calamini B, Silva MC, Madoux F, Hutt DM, Khanna S, et al. (2012) Small-molecule proteostasis regulators for protein conformational diseases. Nat Chem Biol 8: 185–196.
74. Powers ET, Morimoto RI, Dillin A, Kelly JW, Balch WE (2009) Biological and chemical approaches to diseases of proteostasis deficiency. Annu Rev Biochem 78: 959–991.
75. Muller I, Zimmermann M, Becker D, Flomer M (1980) Calendar life span versus budding life span of Saccharomyces cerevisiae. Mech Ageing Dev 12: 47–52.
76. Erjavec N, Larsson L, Grantham J, Nystrom T (2007) Accelerated aging and failure to segregate damaged proteins in Sir2 mutants can be suppressed by overproducing the protein aggregation-remodeling factor Hsp104p. Genes Dev 21: 2410–2421.
77. Liu B, Larsson L, Caballero A, Hao X, Oling D, et al. (2010) The polarisome is required for segregation and retrograde transport of protein aggregates. Cell 140: 257–267.
78. Silva MC, Fox S, Beam M, Thakkar H, Amaral MD, et al. (2011) A genetic screening strategy identifies novel regulators of the proteostasis network. PLoS Genet 7: e1002438.
79. Weiss A, Klein C, Woodman B, Sathasivam K, Bibel M, et al. (2008) Sensitive biochemical aggregate detection reveals aggregation onset before symptom development in cellular and murine models of Huntington's disease. J Neurochem 104: 846–858.
80. Arrasate M, Mitra S, Schweitzer ES, Segal MR, Finkbeiner S (2004) Inclusion body formation reduces levels of mutant huntingtin and the risk of neuronal death. Nature 431: 805–810.
81. Nagai Y, Inui T, Popiel HA, Fujikake N, Hasegawa K, et al. (2007) A toxic monomeric conformer of the polyglutamine protein. Nat Struct Mol Biol 14: 332–340.
82. Caughey B, Lansbury PT (2003) Protofibrils, pores, fibrils, and neurodegeneration: separating the responsible protein aggregates from the innocent bystanders. Annu Rev Neurosci 26: 267–298.
83. Cohen E, Bieschke J, Perciavalle RM, Kelly JW, Dillin A (2006) Opposing activities protect against age-onset proteotoxicity. Science 313: 1604–1610.
84. Wang CL, Landry J, Sternglanz R (2008) A yeast sir2 mutant temperature sensitive for silencing. Genetics 180: 1955–1962.
85. Nachman I, Regev A, Ramanathan S (2007) Dissecting timing variability in yeast meiosis. Cell 131: 544–556.
86. Wanker EE, Scherzinger E, Heiser V, Sittler A, Eickhoff H, et al. (1999) Membrane filter assay for detection of amyloid-like polyglutamine-containing protein aggregates. Methods Enzymol 309: 375–386.

When Cytokinin, a Plant Hormone, Meets the Adenosine A_{2A} Receptor: A Novel Neuroprotectant and Lead for Treating Neurodegenerative Disorders?

Yi-Chao Lee[1 ❡], Ying-Chen Yang[2 ❡], Chuen-Lin Huang[3,4], Tsun-Yung Kuo[2,5], Jung-Hsin Lin[6,7,8], De-Ming Yang[9,10], Nai-Kuei Huang[10,11*]

1 Ph.D. Program for Neural Regenerative Medicine, College of Medical Science and Technology, Taipei Medical University, Taipei, Taiwan, Republic of China, **2** Department of Animal Science, National Ilan University, Ilan, Taiwan, Republic of China, **3** Medical Research Center, Cardinal Tien Hospital, Hsintien, New Taipei City, Taiwan, Republic of China, **4** Graduate Institute of Physiology and Department of Physiology and Biophysics, National Defense Medical Center, Taipei, Taiwan, Republic of China, **5** Institute of Biotechnology, National Ilan University, Ilan, Taiwan, Republic of China, **6** School of Pharmacy, National Taiwan University, Taipei, Taiwan, Republic of China, **7** Division of Mechanics, Research Center for Applied Sciences, Academia Sinica, Taipei, Taiwan, Republic of China, **8** Institute of Biomedical Sciences, Academia Sinica, Nankang, Taipei, Taiwan, Republic of China, **9** Department of Medical Research and Education, Taipei Veterans General Hospital, Taipei, Taiwan, Republic of China, **10** Institute of Biophotonics, National Yang-Ming University, Taipei, Taiwan, Republic of China, **11** National Research Institute of Chinese Medicine, Taipei, Taiwan, Republic of China

Abstract

It is well known that cytokinins are a class of phytohormones that promote cell division in plant roots and shoots. However, their targets, biological functions, and implications in mammalian systems have rarely been examined. In this study, we show that one cytokinin, zeatin riboside, can prevent pheochromocytoma (PC12) cells from serum deprivation-induced apoptosis by acting on the adenosine A_{2A} receptor (A_{2A}-R), which was blocked by an A_{2A}-R antagonist and a protein kinase A (PKA) inhibitor, demonstrating the functional ability of zeatin riboside by mediating through A_{2A}-R signaling event. Since the A_{2A}-R was implicated as a therapeutic target in treating Huntington's disease (HD), a cellular model of HD was applied by transfecting mutant huntingtin in PC12 cells. By using filter retardation assay and confocal microscopy we found that zeatin riboside reversed mutant huntingtin (Htt)-induced protein aggregations and proteasome deactivation through A_{2A}-R signaling. PKA inhibitor blocked zeatin riboside-induced suppression of mutant Htt aggregations. In addition, PKA activated proteasome activity and reduced mutant Htt protein aggregations. However, a proteasome inhibitor blocked both zeatin riboside-and PKA activator-mediated suppression of mutant Htt aggregations, confirming mediation of the A_{2A}-R/PKA/proteasome pathway. Taken together, zeatin riboside might have therapeutic potential as a novel neuroprotectant and a lead for treating neurodegenerative disorders.

Editor: Kari Hoyt, Ohio State University, United States of America

Funding: This work was supported by Cardinal Tien Hospital (CTH-98-1-2A18), the National Research Institute of Chinese Medicine (NRICM99-DBCM-07), and the National Science Council, R.O.C. (NSC99-2320-B-077-006). The funders had no role in study design, data collection and analysis, decision to publish, or preparation of the manuscript.

Competing Interests: The authors have declared that no competing interests exist.

* E-mail: andrew@nricm.edu.tw

❡ These authors contributed equally to this work.

Introduction

Cytokinins are plant hormones that play essential roles in regulating various aspects of plant growth and development, such as *de novo* bud formation, release of buds from apical dominance, leaf expansion, chloroplast formation, delay of senescence, promotion of seed germination, and control of the cell cycle [1,2]. Naturally occurring cytokinins are mainly adenine derivatives, such as isopentyladenine and *trans*-zeatin, and synthetic cytokinins include some adenine analogues, such as 6-benzyladenine and kinetin. In plants, the cytokinin signaling pathway is similar to bacterial and yeast two-component signal transduction pathways; it is specifically similar to histidine-aspartate multi-step phosphorelays, which are comprised of sensor kinases, histidine phosphotransfer proteins, and response regulators [3]. In animal cells, cytokinins are also of interest for their antioxidative, antitumorigenic, and anti-aging activities [4–7].

Previously, cytokinin-binding proteins were found in mammalian sera [8], demonstrating the existence of mammalian targeting proteins for plant hormones. Later, Froldi et al. [9] showed that 6-benzyladenine could act on a purinergic type-2 receptor that induces calcium mobilization in rat atria, suggesting a membrane-bound protein for cytokinins in animal cells. In addition, since cytokinins are important at specific phases of the plant cell cycle [10], in parallel, their anticancer effects were attributed to mediation by cyclins [11] or cyclin-dependent kinases [12,13], suggesting the potential for cytokinins as anticancer drugs [7]. Thus, cytokinin might be used as a plant hormone and also could possibly serve as a candidate for treating human diseases. However, most of the targeting sites and mechanisms are still mostly unknown.

On the other hand, purinoreceptors can be subdivided into P1 receptors, which bind adenosine as a natural ligand, and P2 receptors, which bind ATP, ADP, and adenine dinucleotides, but also pyrimidines like UTP and UDP [14]. On the basis of cloning, pharmacology, and transduction mechanisms, the P1 receptor family is divided into four subtypes (A_1, A_{2A}, A_{2B}, and A_3), while the P2 receptor family is divided into P2X ionotropic receptors ($P2X_{1-7}$) and P2Y metabotropic G protein-coupled receptors ($P2Y_{1,\ 2,\ 4,\ 6,}$ and $_{11-14}$) [15]. These receptors are involved in regulating health and disease [16], including neuroprotection and neurodegeneration [17–20], such as ischemia, epilepsy, depression, Alzheimer's disease (AD), Parkinson's disease (PD), and Huntington's disease (HD). Therefore, due to the close connections of these purinoreceptors in regulating diverse physiological and pathological neuronal functions, recent advances in therapies using purinergic-related drugs in a wide range of pathological conditions have occurred [18,21–23]. In addition, 6-benzyladenine can act on the P2 receptor [9], and almost all cytokinins are present in plants as both a free base and corresponding nucleosides and nucleotides [24] which have similar adenosine-based structures as agonists of P1 receptors. We thus questioned if cytokinins (with or without ribosides) can act on P1 receptors. Among them, the adenosine A_{2A} receptor (A_{2A}-R) has drawn attention as a potential therapeutic drug target in HD because it is highly prevalent in the striatum where mutant huntingtin (Htt) causes selective neural cell loss and atrophy. Therefore, A_{2A}-R-related drugs were suggested for treating HD [25,26].

HD is an autosomal dominant neurodegenerative disorder caused by the expansion of a glutamine repeat in the Htt with a distinct phenotype characterized by chorea, dystonia, incoordination, cognitive decline, and behavioral difficulties [27]. Mutant Htt results from a CAG trinucleotide expansion in exon 1 leading to an expanded polyglutamine (polyQ) strand at the N terminus and a putative toxic gain of function. Normally, the *Htt* gene has 35 or fewer CAG repeats in its N-terminal region, whereas that of HD patients is associated with 36 or more repeats. The numbers of CAG repeats is negatively correlated with the onset age of HD [28]. During disease progression, concentration and short-term memory diminish, and involuntary movements of the head, trunk, and limbs increase. Finally, death results from complications such as choking, infection, and heart failure. Currently, therapeutic strategies for treating HD patients are mostly for symptom relief, and some treatments have unfavorable side effects [29]. Therapeutic drugs to treat HD are urgently needed to be developed.

Collectively, in this study, we found that cytokinin can act on the A_{2A}-R and prevent mutant Htt aggregations suggesting that cytokinin could possibly be applied as a lead or a novel neuroprotectant for treating neurodegenerative disorders.

Results

Zeatin Riboside Activates the A_{2A}-R Signaling and Prevents Serum Deprivation-induced Apoptosis

Kinetin riboside and zeatin riboside, but not kinetin, zeatin, or N^6-benzyladenine, significantly prevented serum deprivation-induced cell death (Fig. 1A). As the positive controls, NGF (Fig. 1A) and CGS 21680 (CGS; a commercially available A_{2A}-R agonist) also prevented serum deprivation-induced cell death (Fig. 1B) [30]. Since zeatin riboside at 100 μM exerted the highest protection with the exception of that by kinetin riboside, 100 μM zeatin riboside was used throughout the following experiments. Zeatin riboside also reversed H_2O_2–induced cell death (Fig. 1A). Pharmacologically, two commercially available A_{2A}-R-specific antagonists [ZM 241385 (ZM) and SCH 58218 (SCH)] and a PKA inhibitor (H-89) dose-dependently blocked the protection by zeatin riboside (Fig. 1B). The blockade of zeatin riboside protection by ZM was re-confirmed by trypan blue exclusion assay (Fig. 1B). In addition, zeatin riboside prevented serum deprivation-induced increased fluorescence of Annexin V-FITC (a marker of apoptotic events) (Fig. 1C). As expected, ZM and SCH blocked the protective effect of zeatin riboside as revealed by imaging (Fig. 1C, upper panels) and flow cytometry studies (Fig. 1C, lower panels). Further, during the differential time course of serum deprivation, zeatin riboside significantly attenuated serum deprivation-induced cleavage of poly (ADP-ribose) polymerase (PARP) and caspase-3 at 24 h (Fig. 1D).

Zeatin Riboside Targets the A_{2A}-R and Decreases Mutant Htt Aggregations which Impair Proteasome Activity

The filter retardation assay and confocal microscopic study revealed that zeatin riboside significantly decreased mutant Htt (109Q) aggregations (Fig. 2A–C). CGS also prevented mutant Htt aggregations (Fig. 2A). However, in the absence and presence of zeatin riboside treatment, normal Htt (25Q) failed to induce any significant aggregations (Fig. 2A–C). ZM or H-89 pretreatment significantly reversed the zeatin riboside-induced decrease in mutant Htt aggregations (Fig. 2B–D). Alternatively, as revealed by contransfection with pZsProsensor, mutant Htt, but not normal Htt, resulted in an increased intensity of green fluorescent proteins (GFPs) (Fig. 2D). Zeatin riboside significantly blocked this phenomenon, which was also reversed by ZM pretreatment (Fig. 2D).

Inhibition of Proteasome Exacerbates Htt Aggregations

MG 132, a proteasome inhibitor, significantly induced intense green fluorescence in normal Htt-overexpressed cells (Fig. 3A). In addition, MG 132 exacerbated mutant Htt-induced protein aggregations and reversed zeatin riboside-induced suppression of Htt aggregations (Fig. 3A and 3B). Compared to Htt-25Q overexpression, that of Htt-109Q significantly reduced proteasome activity (Fig. 3C). MG 132 drastically inhibited proteasome activity in both Htt-25Q- and Htt-109Q-overexpressing cells (Fig. 3C). ZM significantly attenuated zeatin riboside-induced increased proteasome activity in both Htt-25Q- and Htt-109Q-overexpressing cells (Fig. 3C).

Activation of PKA Results in a Decrease in Mutant Htt Aggregations

Forskolin (FK) and dibutyl-cyclic AMP (db-cAMP) (two known PKA activators) significantly attenuated mutant Htt-induced protein aggregations, while H-89 reversed this phenomenon (Fig. 4A, B). In addition, FK also blocked mutant Htt-induced increases in GFPs (Fig. 4B). H-89 blocked this phenomenon afforded by FK (Fig. 4B). MG 132 not only blocked the protection by FK but also exacerbated Htt aggregations in both 25Q- and 109Q-overexpressing cells (Fig. 4B). FK had no effect on normal Htt or GFP expressions (Fig. 4B). FK significantly increased proteasome activity in both normal and mutant Htt-overexpressed cells; however, H-89 pretreatment blocked the effects of FK (Fig. 4C). Additionally, overexpression of mutant Htt decreased proteasome activity (Fig. 4C). In addition, FK and zeatin riboside significantly increased the ratio of YFP/CFP in AKAR1-transfected cells; however, H-89 pretreatment blocked the effects of both FK and zeatin riboside (Fig. 4D).

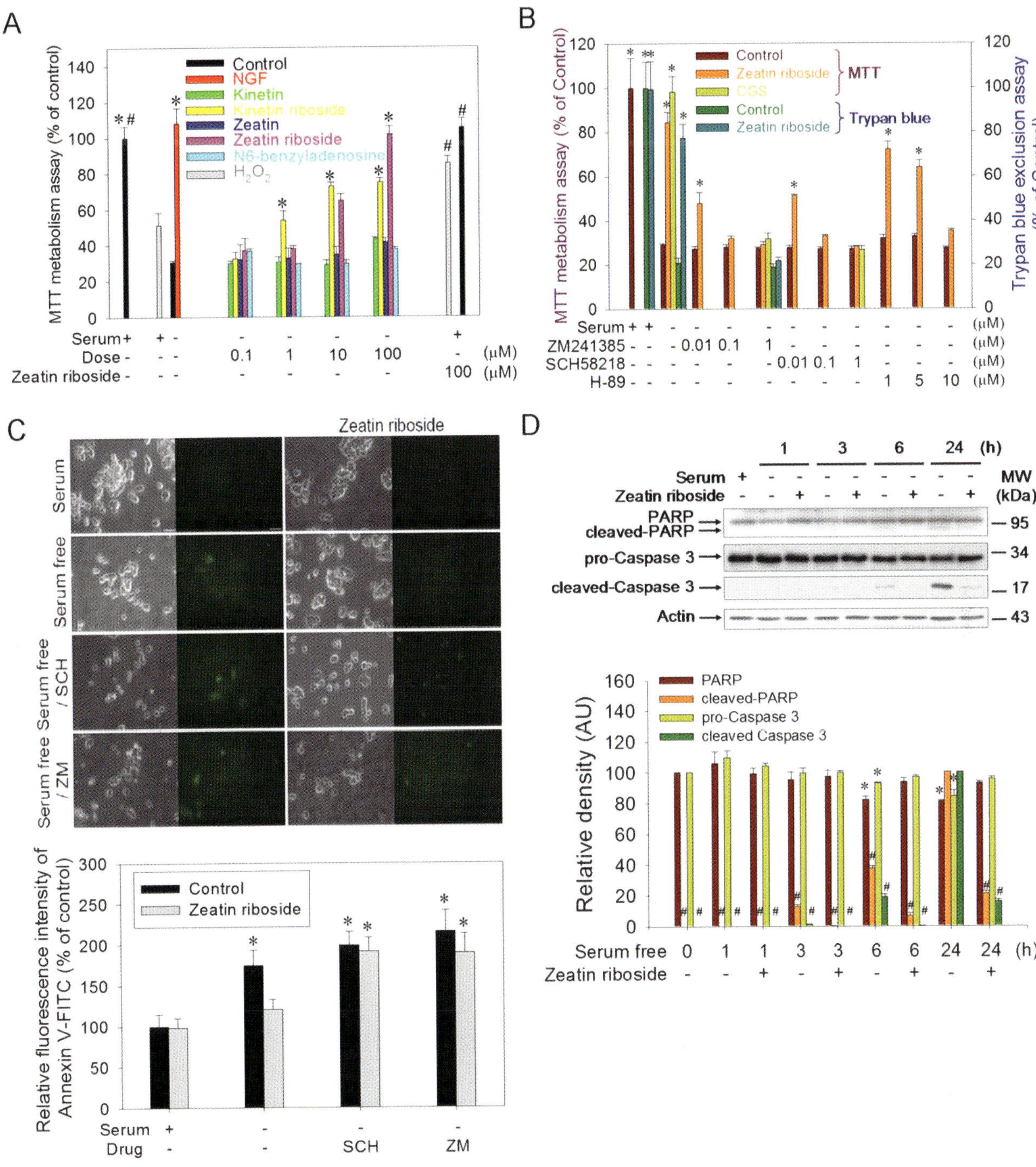

Figure 1. Cytokinins acting on the A_{2A}-R prevent serum deprivation-induced PC12 cell apoptosis. (A) Serum-contained and serum-deprived cells were treated with or without the indicated reagent(s) for 24 h. NGF were treated in 100 ng/ml. Besides, cells pretreated with zeatin riboside (100 μM) for 3 h were treated with or without H_2O_2 (25 μM) for 24 h. Cell viability was expressed as a percentage of the results from the MTT assay with respect to the mean value of the serum-contained control group. Data points represent the mean ± SEM ($n = 3\sim6$). $^*p < 0.05$, compared to its serum-deprived group. $\#p < 0.05$, compared to the H_2O_2-treated group. (B) Serum-deprived cells were pretreated with or without the indicated reagents for 30 min. Zeatin riboside or CGS (0.1 μM) was added for another 24 h. Cell viability was expressed as a percentage of the results from the MTT and trypan blue exclusion assays with respect to the mean value of the serum-contained control group. Data points represent the mean ± SEM ($n = 3\sim6$). $^*p < 0.05$, compared to its serum-deprived group. (C) Serum-deprived cells were pretreated with or without 1 μM ZM or 1 μM SCH for 30 min. Zeatin riboside was added for 24 h and followed by Annexin V-FITC staining. Cells were subjected to image and cytometry analysis. Bar represents 50 μm. Data points represent the mean ± SEM ($n = 3\sim6$). $^*p < 0.05$, compared to the serum-contained control group. (D) Serum-contained or -deprived cells in the presence or absence of zeatin riboside were harvested and subjected to a Western blot analysis. The relative optical density of the bands were quantified by densitometry relative to actin and normalized to the levels in serum-contained control group or in serum-deprived for 24 h group. Data points (mean ± SEM) represent one out of three independent experiments that gave similar results. $^*p < 0.05$, compared to its serum-containing control group. $\#p < 0.05$, compared to its 24 h serum-deprived group. AU represents arbitrary unit.

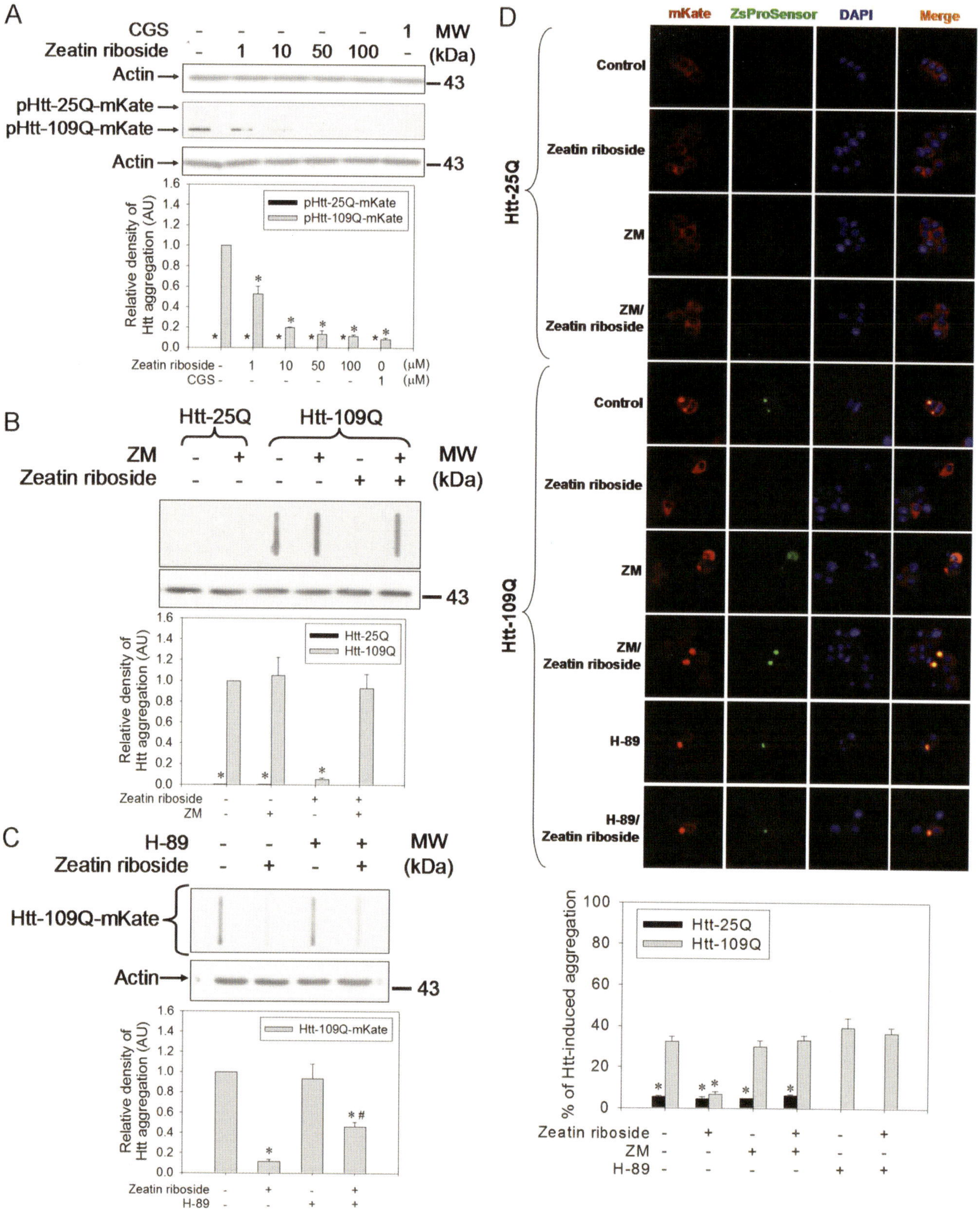

Figure 2. Zeatin riboside acting on the A_{2A}-R attenuates mutant Htt aggregations. (A) pHtt-25Q-mKate- or pHtt-109Q-mKate-transfected cells were treated with 1 μM CGS or zeatin riboside for 24 h. Cells were harvested and subjected to a filter retardation assay and Western blot analysis. (B) The transfected cells were pretreated with or without 1 μM ZM for 30 min and treated with zeatin riboside for another 24 h. Cells were harvested and subjected to a filter retardation assay and Western blot analysis. (C) The transfected cells were pretreated with or without 5 μM H-89 for 30 min and treated with zeatin riboside for another 24 h. Cells were harvested and subjected to a filter retardation assay and Western blot analysis. The relative optical density of the bands (A~C) were quantified by densitometry relative to actin and normalized to the levels under the Htt-109Q-overexpressed control condition. Data points represent the mean ± SEM. *$p<0.05$, compared to the mutant Htt control group. #$p<0.05$,

compared to the zeatin riboside-treated mutant Htt group. (D) After 1 μM ZM pretreatment for 30 min, pHtt-25Q-mKate- or pHtt-109Q-mKate-transfected and pZsProSensor-co-transfected cells were treated with or without zeatin riboside for another 24 h and subjected to a confocal microscopic analysis. Bar represents 5 μm. In each group, the mKate-aggregated cells in proportion to the transfected cells were counted (100~150 cells) These data points (mean ± SEM) represent one out of three independent experiments that gave similar results. $^{*}p<0.05$, compared to the mutant Htt control group.

Discussion

Zeatin Riboside Mediates the A_{2A}-R Signalings and Prevents Serum Deprivation-induced Apoptosis

According to our recently published pharmacophore models of the A_{2A}-R [31], the *Ki* of some cytokinins were ranged from 2.9 to 46 μM (Supplement S1). We next tested their biological functions using a serum deprivation-induced cell death model that highlighted the functional role of the A_{2A}-R [30]. Among these cytokinins, only kinetin and zeatin with riboside were protective in this model (Fig. 1A). The inabilities of other cytokinins in preventing cell death were not clear. Further works were required to be done to reveal if they could act as antagonists. The protection by zeatin riboside was blocked by two A_{2A}-R antagonists, ZM and SCH (Fig. 1B), indicating an A_{2A}-R-mediated effect. The protections of NGF and CGS (Fig. 1A B) were also consisted with the previously published article [30]. Besides, except serum deprivation-induced cell death, zeatin riboside also prevented H_2O_2-induced cell death (Fig. 1A), further confirming the protections of zeatin riboside. Annexin V-FITC staining confirmed that ZM and SCH could block the protection by zeatin riboside in antagonizing serum deprivation-induced apoptosis (Fig. 1C). A time course study of serum deprivation-induced cleavage of PARP and caspase 3 which was blocked by zeatin riboside (Fig. 1D) also confirmed that serum deprivation induces apoptosis [30]. Furthermore, the above identified protectants (CGS and NGF) and other known protectants (db-cAMP and FK) [30] were also confirmed to prevent serum deprivation-induced cleavage of PARP (Supplement S2). Although serum deprivation-induced apoptosis is well documented, there are still different forms of death events should be concerned, for instance, serum deprivation-induced autophagic cell death [32,33] or a new form of death (parthanatos) which is triggered by the nuclear translocation of mitochondrial apoptosis inducing factor resulting in caspase-independent cell death [34]. Thus, the involvement of zeatin riboside in antagonizing other form of cell death is currently unknown and requires further investigation.

Normally, signaling of the A_{2A}-R sequentially couples with $G_s\alpha$ and involves activation of adenylyl cyclase, formation of cAMP, stimulation of PKA, and phosphorylation activation of the CREB at Ser133 [30,35,36], which plays a pivotal role in neuronal survival [37] and genetic models of HD [38]. We further examined and found that zeatin riboside did induce CREB phosphorylation which could also be blocked by ZM and H-89 (Supplement S3A). Besides, CREB overexpression blocked mutant Htt aggregations (Supplement S3B) may further confirm the importance of A_{2A}-R signalings in this system. Therefore, since the A_{2A}-R has implicated as a therapeutic target in treating HD [25,26,39], we thus tested if zeatin riboside could be a candidate to treat HD.

Zeatin Riboside Targets the A_{2A}-R and Decreases Mutant Htt Aggregations that Impair Proteasome Activity

In order to study HD outside of animal models, several cell models were established and examined [40,41]. In this study, plasmid which harbors the exon 1 region of the Htt gene with 25 or 109 CAG repeats conjugating with the red fluorescent protein (mKate) as a reporter were transiently transfected (Supplement S4). The filter assay revealed that zeatin riboside dose-dependently attenuated mutant Htt aggregations (Fig. 2A). CGS also prevented Htt aggregates in this system (Fig. 2A), consistent with previous findings [26]. Further, ZM (Fig 2B) and H-89 (Fig. 2C) attenuated zeatin riboside-induced suppression of mutant Htt aggregations, demonstrating that zeatin riboside targets the A_{2A}-R and the subsequent PKA to prevent mutant Htt aggregations. Alternatively, the imaging study revealed that 109Q, not 25Q, induced highly condensed and punctuated red and green fluorescent proteins (Fig. 2D), indicating decreased proteasome activity. However, zeatin riboside alleviated all of these phenomena which could be reversed by ZM or H-89 pretreatment (Fig.2D), consistent with the filter assay data. These data indicated that zeatin riboside by acting on the A_{2A}-R prevents Htt aggregates and Htt aggregates impair proteasome activity [42,43]. Therefore, it is possible that zeatin riboside could elevate proteasome activity to degrade Htt aggregates.

Zeatin Riboside Elevates Proteasome Activity and Proteasome Inhibition Exacerbates Htt Aggregations

The ubiquitin-proteasome system (UPS) plays an essential role in degrading misfolded and damaged proteins that are poly-ubiquitinated by ubiquitin ligases and targeted to proteasomes for degradation, such as mutant Htt [44]. We thus examined the importance of proteasomes in degrading Htt aggregates. MG 132, a proteasome inhibitor, was applied, and found that MG 132 exacerbated Htt aggregations with both 109Q and 25Q (Fig. 3A), consistent with previous findings [45]. MG 132 also blocked zeatin riboside-induced suppression of mutant Htt aggregates (Fig. 3A & 3B), confirming the functional role of proteasomes in degrading Htt aggregates in this system. In addition to the imaging study, proteasome activity was also detected. Our data revealed that mutant Htt overexpression downregulated proteasome activity (Fig. 3C). However, zeatin riboside respectively elevated and reversed the proteasome activity in normal and mutant Htt-overexpressed cells. MG 132 drastically inhibited proteasome activity in normal and mutant Htt-overexpressed cells (Fig. 3C). Consequently, our data demonstrated that zeatin riboside elevated proteasome activity and then promoted mutant Htt degradation by acting on the A_{2A}-R.

PKA Activation Increases Proteasome Activity and Mutant Htt Degradation

Since PKA is the downstream target of A_{2A}-R, we subsequently examined if PKA was also involved in mediating Htt aggregates in this system. Indeed, both FK- and db-cAMP-induced suppression of mutant Htt aggregates were reversed by H-89 (Fig. 4A), which indicates a positive role of PKA in suppressing mutant Htt aggregations. Alternatively, the inhibition by H-89 of FK-induced suppression of Htt aggregates (Fig. 4B) and the increase in proteasome activity (Fig. 4C) could also be reproduced using a confocal study and activity assay, further confirming PKA-mediated activation of proteasome activity and degradation of Htt aggregates. Besides, in order to demonstrate whether zeatin riboside resulted in PKA activation, a genetically encoded reporter (AKAR1) of PKA activity was used [46]. As expected, H-89

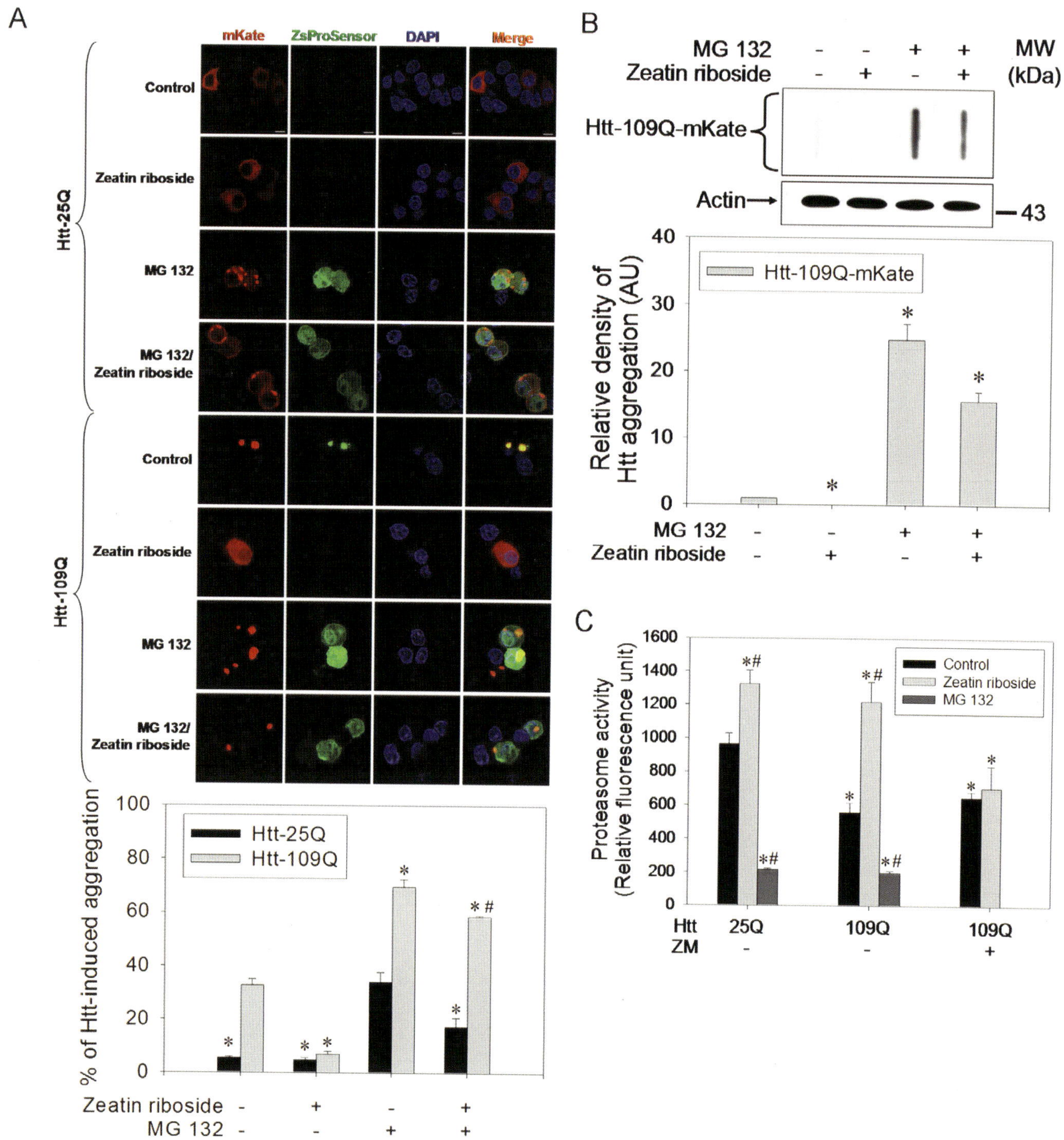

Figure 3. Zeatin riboside attenuates mutant Htt aggregations through increasing proteasome activity. (A) With or without 1 μM MG 132 pretreatment for 30 min and following the presence or absence of zeatin riboside for 24 h, pHtt-25Q-mKate- or pHtt-109Q-mKate-transfected and pZsProSensor-co-transfected cells were subjected to a confocal microscopic analysis. Bar represents 5 μm. In each group, the mKate-aggregated cells in proportion to the transfected cells were counted (100~150 cells). Data points represent the mean ± SEM. *$p<0.05$, compared to the mutant Htt control group. #$p<0.05$, compared to the MG 132-treated mutant Htt group. (B) With or without 1 μM MG 132 pretreatment for 30 min, pHtt-109Q-mKate-transfected cells were treated with or without zeatin riboside for 24 h and subjected to a filter retardation assay and Western blot analysis. The relative optical density of the bands were quantified by densitometry relative to actin and normalized to the levels under the Htt-109Q-overexpressed control condition which was set as 1.0. Data points represent the mean ± SEM. *$p<0.05$, compared to the mutant Htt control group. AU represents arbitrary unit. (C) pHtt-25Q-mKate-transfected cells were treated with or without zeatin riboside or 1 μM MG 132. pHtt-109Q-mKate-transfected cells were pretreated with or without 1 μM ZM for 30 min and then supplemented with or without zeatin riboside or 1 μM MG 132 for 24 h and subjected to a proteasome activity assay. *$p<0.05$, compared to the Htt-25Q control group. #$p<0.05$, compared to the Htt-109Q control group. These data represent one out of three independent experiments that gave similar results.

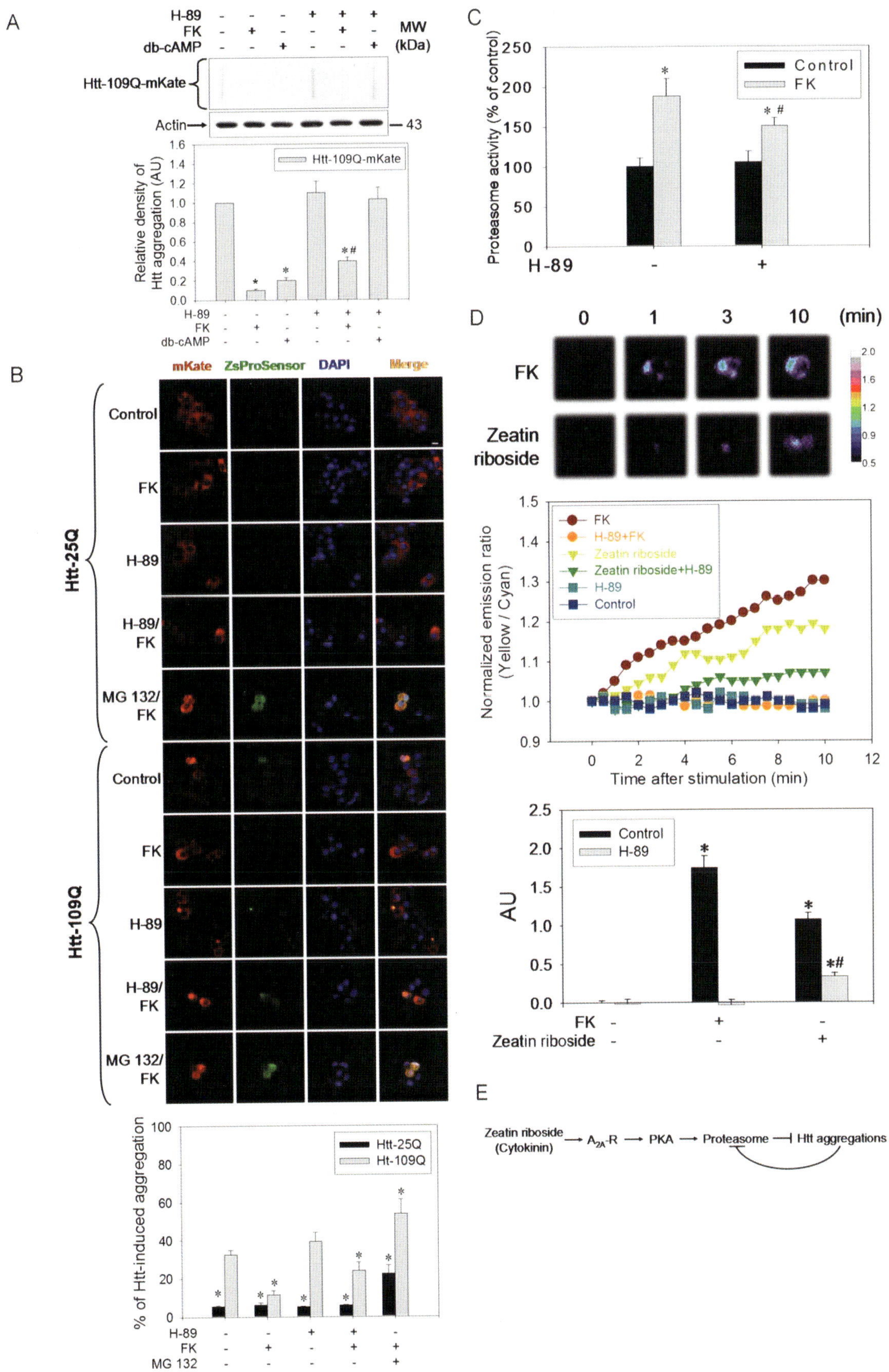

Figure 4. PKA attenuates mutant Htt aggregations through increasing proteasome activity. (A) With or without 1 μM H-89 pretreatment for 30 min, pHtt-109Q-mKate-transfected cells were treated with or without 10 μM FK or 100 μM db-cAMP for 24 h and subjected to a filter

retardation assay and Western blot analysis. The relative optical density of the bands were quantified by densitometry relative to actin and normalized to the levels under the Htt-109Q-overexpressed control condition which was set as 1.0. Data points represent the mean ± SEM. *$p<0.05$, compared to the mutant Htt control group. #$p<0.05$, compared to the FK-treated mutant Htt group. AU represents arbitrary unit. (B) After 5 μM H-89 or 1 μM MG 132 pretreatment for 30 min, pHtt-25Q-mKate- or pHtt-109Q-mKate-transfected and pZsProSensor-co-transfected cells were treated with or without 10 μM FK for 24 h and subjected to a confocal microscopic analysis. In each group, the mKate-aggregated cells in proportion to the transfected cells were counted (100~150 cells). Data points represent the mean ± SEM. *$p<0.05$, compared to the mutant Htt control group. (C) With or without 5 μM H-89 pretreatment for 30 min, pHtt-109Q-mKate-transfected cells were supplemented with or without zeatin riboside or 10 μM FK for 24 h and subjected to a proteasome activity assay. *$p<0.05$, compared to the control group. #$p<0.05$, compared to the FK-treated but without H-89-pretreated group. (D) With or without 10 μM H-89 pretreatment for 30 min, AKAR1-transfected cells were added with or without 10 μM FK or zeatin riboside and the FRET images (upper panel) were acquired and analyzed (middle panel). Bar represents 5 μm. In each group, the area under the curve (AUC) subtracting with the background level was calculated and plotted in arbitrary unit (AU) (lower panel). Data represents the mean ± SEM ($n=3\sim6$). *$p<0.05$, compared to the control group. (E) Zeatin riboside-mediated suppression of mutant Htt aggregations involves activation of the adenosine A_{2A} receptor (A_{2A}-R), PKA, and proteasome. Mutant Htt aggregations in turn inhibit proteasome activity. These data represent one out of three independent experiments that gave similar results.

blocked both zeatin riboside- and FK-induced FRET responses, (Fig. 4D), demonstrating that zeatin riboside does mediate PKA. Therefore, zeatin riboside-induced suppression of Htt aggregations is mediated by the A_{2A}-R and subsequent PKA-dependent pathways (Fig. 4E). Currently, the mechanism of mutant Htt-induced impairment of the UPS is not clear [43,47]; although it was proposed that polyQ peptides may be transiently retained in the proteolytic core, thus impairing proteasome activity. However, it is also possible that mutant Htt aggregates are difficult to recognize by proteasomes. Further investigations are required to answer these questions.

Implications of Cytokinins

Recently, biomedical implications of cytokinins have gradually garnered attention. For instance, kinetin was found to alleviate some messenger (m)RNA splicing diseases, such as familial dysautonomia [48]. It was also shown to delay the onset and decrease the extent of aging characteristics in cultured human skin fibroblasts [6] and is widely marketed today in a variety of skin-care products. Although kinetin was reported to protect against oxidative damage to both DNA and proteins [5,49], the molecular mechanism for the anti-aging properties is unknown. Since kinetin is currently used only for topical applications, toxicity studies are currently underway to assess its potential as a treatment for familial dysautonomia. On the other hand, zeatin has been found to prevent scopolamine-induced memory impairment in mice [50] and β-amyloid-induced PC12 cell neurotoxicity [51], suggesting the therapeutic potential of cytokinins in treating neurodegeneration.

In this study, for the first time, we pharmacologically demonstrated that zeatin riboside can target the A_{2A}-R to prevent serum deprivation-induced apoptosis and mutant Htt aggregations, suggesting a therapeutic potential in treating neuronal injury and neurodegeneration. In addition, our previously published articles show that a novel compound, N-(4-hydroxybenzyl)adenosine purified from *Gastrodia elata* [52], had A_{2A}-R-binding potency that exerted protection in treating R6/2 mice (an HD animal model) [53]. This compound may be a novel therapeutic drug and lead to the development of new drugs to treat other neurodegenerative diseases [31]. Therefore, regarding plant hormones, cytokinins, the application of zeatin riboside or others with A_{2A}-R-binding affinities may also be possibly implicated as novel neuroprotectants and leads for alternative treatments of neurodegeneration [25,54].

Taken together, in this study, we showed that zeatin riboside could prevent serum deprivation-induced apoptosis and mutant Htt aggregations through activation of the A_{2A}-R and subsequent PKA-dependent pathways. These findings also indicate the therapeutic potential of zeatin riboside in treating neuronal injury, HD, and other polyQ diseases, such as spinocerebellar ataxias.

Materials and Methods

Reagents and Cell Culture

All reagents were purchased from Sigma Chemical (St. Louis, MO, USA) except where otherwise specified. Nerve growth factor (NGF) was purchased from Alomone Labs Ltd (Jerusalem, Israel). 4-[2-[[6-Amino-9-(*N*-ethyl-β-D-ribofuranuronamidosyl)-9*H*-purin-2-yl]amino]ethyl] benzene pro-panoic acid (CGS 21680), 2-(2-furanyl)-7-(2-phenylethyl)-7*H*-pyrazolo[4,3-*e*][1,2,4] triazolo[1,5-*c*]pyrimidin-5-amine (SCH 58261), and 4-(2-[7-amino-2-(2-furyl)[1,2,4] triazolo[2,3-*a*][1,3,5] triazin-5-ylamino]ethyl)phenol (ZM 241385) were purchased from Tocris (Bristol, UK). H-89 was purchased from Biomol (Plymouth Meeting, PA, USA). All antibodies were purchased from Millipore (Bedford, MA, USA) except where otherwise specified. The anti-PARP antibody was purchase from Epitomics (1078; Burlingame, CA, USA). The anti-cleaved caspase 3 antibody was purchase from Cell Signaling (9664; Danvers, MA, USA). Plasmids including the proteasome sensor vector (pZsProSensor-1) were purchased form Clontech (Mountain View, CA, USA). Restriction enzymes were purchased from Fermantas (Vilnius, Lithuania). The AKAR1 plasmid was obtained from Dr. Roger Y. Tsien (Department of Pharmacology, Department of Chemistry & Biochemistry, University of California, San Diego, CA, USA). Dulbecco's modified Eagle's medium (DMEM), fetal bovine serum (FBS), and horse serum were purchased from HyClone (Logan, UT, USA). Rat PC12 cells purchased from American Type Culture Collection (ATCC; Manassas, VA, USA) were maintained in DMEM supplemented with 10% horse serum and 5% FBS and incubated in a CO_2 incubator (5%) at 37°C. pHtt-25Q-mKate and pHtt-109Q-mKate were prepared as described previously [55].

MTT and Trypan Blue Exclusion Assays

Survival was assessed by the 3-(4,5-dimethylthiazol-2-yl)-2,5-diphenyl tetrazolium bromide (MTT) metabolism assay as described previously [56]. In brief, after treatment, MTT was added to the medium (0.5 mg/ml) and incubated at 37°C for 2~3 h. The plating number was 10^4 cells/well in a 96-well plate. After discarding the medium, DMSO was applied to the well to dissolve the formazan crystals, and the absorbances at 570 and 630 nm in each well were measured on a micro-enzyme-linked immunosorbent assay (ELISA) reader. In addition, after different treatments, cells growing on 6-well (4×10^5 cells/well) plate were scraped and counted using a hemacytometer after trypan blue staining (0.3%).

Transient Transfection

Lipofectamine™ 2000 (Invitrogen) was used as a vehicle to transfer plasmids into cells as described by the protocol. Normally, 5 μg of DNA combined with 5 μl of Lipofectamine™ 2000 was applied to each well of 6-well plates. The plating number was $(1\sim1.5)\times10^6$ cells/well. After transfections for 6 h, cells were treated with reagents for another 24 h. Images were then taken with a Zeiss Axiovert 200 M inverted fluorescence microscope (Göttingen, Germany).

Annexin V-FITC Staining and Analysis

An Annexin V (FITC-conjugated) apoptosis kit (K101–400; BioVision, Mountain View, CA, USA) was used to analyze apoptotic cells. The experimental protocol followed the manufacturer's instructions. In brief, after a 24-h treatment, cells growing on 12-well plates at $(3\sim4)\times10^5$ cells/well were loaded with 0.5 ml binding buffer and 5 μl Annexin V-FITC. After incubation for 5 min in the dark, cells were washed once with 1 ml of culture medium (without phenol red) to take phase contrast and fluorescent micrographs. Besides, the stained-cells could also be used for flow cytometry analysis (FACScan®, Becton Dickinson, Franklin Lakes, NJ). The mean values of the fluorescent intensities of FITC were collected using an FL-1 channel ($488/530^{Ex/Em}$ nm). Five thousand live cells were analyzed per sample.

Western Blot Analysis

Equal amounts of cell lysates (20 μg/well) derived from the filtered assay were separated by SDS-polyacrylamide gel electrophoresis (PAGE) and then electroblotted onto Immobilon polyvinylidene difluoride (PVDF) membranes (Millipore). Membranes were blocked with 5% skim milk in TBST (100 mM Tris-HCl and 150 mM NaCl; pH 7.4, containing 0.05% Tween 20) for 1 h at room temperature and then incubated with the first antibody (1/1000~2000) at 4°C for overnight. The anti-PARP antibody was used to probe pro- and cleaved-form of PARP. The anti-caspase 3 (9662; Cell Signaling, Danvers, MA, USA) and anti-cleaved caspase 3 antibodies were respectively used to probe pro- and cleaved-form of caspase 3. Actin was used as an internal control and probed with anti-actin (MAB1501) antibody. After three washes with TBST, the blot was incubated with a second antibody (1:5000) conjugated to horseradish peroxidase for 1 h, processed for visualization using an enhanced chemiluminescence system (Pierce, Rockford, IL, USA), and exposed to Kodak XAR-5 film (Rochester, New York, USA) to obtain the fluorographic images. The freeware ImageJ (http://imagej.nih.gov/ij/download.html) was used to measure the required image density.

Filter Retardation Assay

This method followed that described by Wanker et al. [57] with a few modifications. In brief, harvested cells were resuspended in lysis buffer (50 mM Tris-HCl (pH 8.8), 100 mM NaCl, 5.0 mM $MgCl_2$, 1 mM EDTA, and 0.5% (w/v) IPGEAL containing 1× protease inhibitor cocktail (Roche Diagnostics, Indianapolis, IN, USA)) and sonicated for 10 s (1 pulse/s). Equal protein concentrations (15~20 μg/well) in each group were filtered through a 2% sodium dodecylsulfate (SDS)-pre-equilibrated cellulose-acetate membrane (0.2 μm; Whatman, Maidstone, Kent, UK) using the Bio-Dot SF Apparatus (Bio-Rad, Hercules, CA, USA). During suction, each well was washed with 200 μl 0.1% SDS twice. The blot was blocked in TBS (100 mM Tris-HCl and 150 mM NaCl; pH 7.4) containing 3% nonfat dried milk for 1 h at room temperature and then incubated with the anti-polyglutamine (1:5000; MAB1574) antibody in 3% bovine serum albumin (BSA) with 0.02% NaN_3 (4°C overnight) to probe normal and mutant Htts. The subsequent methods were the same as those described above.

Proteasome Activity Assay

Proteasome activity was indirectly studied by transfecting pZsProSensor-1 (Clontech), a eukaryotic expression vector designed to express ZsGreen fused to the mouse ornithine decarboxylase degradation domain which is highly susceptible to proteasome degradation. Therefore, this vector was used to monitor proteasome activity in living cells. Normally, if proteasomes are active in living cells, the protein does not accumulate. However, when proteasome activity decreases, such as the addition of a proteasome inhibitor, the fusion protein accumulates in cells resulting in increased green fluorescence. Therefore, proteasome activity is inversely correlated with the green fluorescence. Alternatively, a 20S Proteasome Activity Assay kit (APT280; Millipore, Billerica, MA, USA) was used to measure the proteasome activity according to the protocol.

PKA Activity Assay

This method was carried out as described by Zhang et al. [46]. In brief, after AKAR1 transfection for 24 h, cells were imaged on a Zeiss Axiovert 200 M microscope with a 40×/1.3NA oil-immersion objective lens and a cooled CCD camera (CoolSNAP HQ^2; Photometrics, Tucson, AZ, USA). Dual-emission ratio imaging was acquired with a 420DF20 excitation filter, a 450DRLP dichroic mirror, and two emission filters (475DF40 for cyan and 535DF25 for yellow (Chroma Technology, Bellows Falls, VT, USA)) altered by a filter changer (Lambda DG-4; Sutter Instruments, San Rafael, CA, USA). Fluorescence images were background-corrected. Exposure times were 50~200 ms, and images were taken every 30~60 s.

Confocal Microscopy

Transfected cells growing on poly-L-lysine-coated cover slides were fixed with 4% paraformaldehyde at room temperature for 10 min, and DAPI (1 μg/ml) stain was applied for another 10 min. After three washes with PBS, cover slides were mounted onto glass slides with Aqua Poly-Mount (Polysciences, Warrington, PA, USA). Images of cells were visualized with a Leica TSC SP confocal laser scanning microscope (Wetzlar, Germany).

Statistical Analysis

Results were analyzed by one- or two-way analysis of variance (ANOVA) according to which was appropriate. Two-way ANOVA with repeated measurements were used to analyze the differences in PKA activity assay. Differences between means were assessed by the Student-Newman-Keuls method and were considered significant at $p<0.05$.

Supporting Information

Supplement S1 The Ki of cytokinin on molecular modeling of A_{2A}-R. Purple and cyan circles respectively represent hydrogen and bond donor.

Supplement S2 CGS, db-cAMP, FK, and NGF prevent serum deprivation-induced PARP cleavage. Serum-contained or -deprived cells in the presence or absence of CGS (0.1 μM), db-cAMP (100 μM), FK (10 μM), or NGF (50 ng/ml) were harvested and subjected to the Western blot analysis.

Supplement S3 Zeatin riboside activates the cAMP response element-binding protein (CREB) through a protein kinase A (PKA)-dependent pathway. (A) Cells deprived of serum were pretreated with 5 μM H-89 or 1 μM ZM for 30 min and then treated in the presence or absence of zeatin riboside or 10 μM FK for 1 h. Cells were harvested and subjected to a Western blot analysis. (B) Cells transfected with pHtt-109Q-mKate were also co-transfected with or without pCMV-CREB or promoter-less pEGFP for 24 h. Cells were harvested and subjected to the filter retardation assay and Western blot analysis.

Supplement S4 Zeatin riboside prevents mutant Htt (109Q)-induced aggregations. (A) After pretreatment with ZM or H-89 for 30 min, cells over-expressing normal Htt-25Q-mKate and mutant Htt-109Q-mKate were treated with or without 100 μM zeatin riboside for 24 h. The images of cells in red fluorescence (mKate) and bright field (BF) were taken by a fluorescence microscope. Bar represents 50 μm.

Acknowledgments

We thank Mr. D.P. Chamberlin for critically editing the manuscript.

Author Contributions

Conceived and designed the experiments: N-KH C-LH. Performed the experiments: N-KH Y-CL. Analyzed the data: Y-CY T-YK. Contributed reagents/materials/analysis tools: J-HL D-MY. Wrote the paper: N-KH.

References

1. Mok DW, Mok MC (2001) Cytokinin Metabolism and Action. Annu Rev Plant Physiol Plant Mol Biol 52: 89–118.
2. Havlicek L, Hanus J, Vesely J, Leclerc S, Meijer L, et al. (1997) Cytokinin-derived cyclin-dependent kinase inhibitors: synthesis and cdc2 inhibitory activity of olomoucine and related compounds. J Med Chem 40: 408–412.
3. Ferreira FJ, Kieber JJ (2005) Cytokinin signaling. Curr Opin Plant Biol 8: 518–525.
4. Honma Y, Ishii Y (2002) Differentiation of human myeloid leukemia cells by plant redifferentiation-inducing hormones. Leuk Lymphoma 43: 1729–1735.
5. Verbeke P, Siboska GE, Clark BF, Rattan SI (2000) Kinetin inhibits protein oxidation and glycoxidation in vitro. Biochem Biophys Res Commun 276: 1265–1270.
6. Rattan SI, Clark BF (1994) Kinetin delays the onset of ageing characteristics in human fibroblasts. Biochem Biophys Res Commun 201: 665–672.
7. Bifulco M, Malfitano AM, Proto MC, Santoro A, Caruso MG, et al. (2008) Biological and pharmacological roles of N6-isopentenyladenosine: an emerging anticancer drug. Anticancer Agents Med Chem 8: 200–204.
8. Jayabaskaran C, Senapathy P, Jacob TM (1981) Cytokinin binding proteins from mammalian sera. J Biosci: 269–274.
9. Froldi G, Gallo U, Ragazzi E, Caparrotta L (1999) 6-Benzylaminopurine: a plant derived cytokinin inducing positive inotropism by P2-purinoceptors. Planta Med 65: 245–249.
10. Hartig K, Beck E (2006) Crosstalk between auxin, cytokinins, and sugars in the plant cell cycle. Plant Biol (Stuttg) 8: 389–396.
11. Tiedemann RE, Mao X, Shi CX, Zhu YX, Palmer SE, et al. (2008) Identification of kinetin riboside as a repressor of CCND1 and CCND2 with preclinical antimyeloma activity. J Clin Invest 118: 1750–1764.
12. Vieira HL, Boya P, Cohen I, El Hamel C, Haouzi D, et al. (2002) Cell permeable BH3-peptides overcome the cytoprotective effect of Bcl-2 and Bcl-X(L). Oncogene 21: 1963–1977.
13. Spichal L, Krystof V, Paprskarova M, Lenobel R, Styskala J, et al. (2007) Classical anticytokinins do not interact with cytokinin receptors but inhibit cyclin-dependent kinases. J Biol Chem 282: 14356–14363.
14. Ralevic V, Burnstock G (1998) Receptors for purines and pyrimidines. Pharmacol Rev 50: 413–492.
15. Burnstock G (2007) Purine and pyrimidine receptors. Cell Mol Life Sci 64: 1471–1483.
16. Gessi S, Merighi S, Varani K, Borea P (2011) Adenosine Receptors in Health and Disease. In: Jacobson K, Linden J, editors. Pharmacology of Purine and Pyrimidine Receptors. San Diego, CA: Academic Press. pp 41–75.
17. Stone T, Ceruti S, Abbracchio M (2009) Adenosine Receptors and Neurological Disease: Neuroprotection and Neurodegeneration. In: Stone T, Ceruti S, Abbracchio M, editors. Adenosine Receptors in Health and Disease. Berlin Heidelberg: Springer-Verlag. pp 535–587.
18. Burnstock G (2006) Pathophysiology and therapeutic potential of purinergic signaling. Pharmacol Rev 58: 58–86.
19. Burnstock G (2007) Physiology and pathophysiology of purinergic neurotransmission. Physiol Rev 87: 659–797.
20. Gomes CV, Kaster MP, Tome AR, Agostinho PM, Cunha RA (2011) Adenosine receptors and brain diseases: neuroprotection and neurodegeneration. Biochim Biophys Acta 1808: 1380–1399.
21. Williams M, Jarvis MF (2000) Purinergic and pyrimidinergic receptors as potential drug targets. Biochem Pharmacol 59: 1173–1185.
22. Kaiser SM, Quinn RJ (1999) Adenosine receptors as potential therapeutic targets. Drug Discov Today 4: 542–551.
23. Simons C, Wu Q, Htar TT (2005) Recent advances in antiviral nucleoside and nucleotide therapeutics. Curr Top Med Chem 5: 1191–1203.
24. Haberer G, Kieber JJ (2002) Cytokinins. New insights into a classic phytohormone. Plant Physiol 128: 354–362.
25. Blum D, Hourez R, Galas MC, Popoli P, Schiffmann SN (2003) Adenosine receptors and Huntington's disease: implications for pathogenesis and therapeutics. Lancet Neurol 2: 366–374.
26. Chou SY, Lee YC, Chen HM, Chiang MC, Lai HL, et al. (2005) CGS21680 attenuates symptoms of Huntington's disease in a transgenic mouse model. J Neurochem 93: 310–320.
27. Walker FO (2007) Huntington's disease. Lancet 369: 218–228.
28. Wellington CL, Brinkman RR, O'Kusky JR, Hayden MR (1997) Toward understanding the molecular pathology of Huntington's disease. Brain Pathol 7: 979–1002.
29. Brusa L, Orlacchio A, Moschella V, Iani C, Bernardi G, et al. (2009) Treatment of the symptoms of Huntington's disease: preliminary results comparing aripiprazole and tetrabenazine. Mov Disord 24: 126–129.
30. Huang NK, Lin YW, Huang CL, Messing RO, Chern Y (2001) Activation of protein kinase A and atypical protein kinase C by A(2A) adenosine receptors antagonizes apoptosis due to serum deprivation in PC12 cells. J Biol Chem 276: 13838–13846.
31. Chen JB, Liu EM, Chern TR, Yang CW, Lin CI, et al. (2011) Design and synthesis of novel dual-action compounds targeting the adenosine A(2A) receptor and adenosine transporter for neuroprotection. ChemMedChem 6: 1390–1400.
32. Guillon-Munos A, van Bemmelen MX, Clarke PG (2005) Role of phosphoinositide 3-kinase in the autophagic death of serum-deprived PC12 cells. Apoptosis 10: 1031–1041.
33. Uchiyama Y (2001) Autophagic cell death and its execution by lysosomal cathepsins. Arch Histol Cytol 64: 233–246.
34. Andrabi SA, Dawson VL, Dawson TM (2008) Mitochondrial and nuclear cross talk in cell death: parthanatos. Ann N Y Acad Sci 1147.
35. Fredholm BB, Chen JF, Cunha RA, Svenningsson P, Vaugeois JM (2005) Adenosine and brain function. Int Rev Neurobiol 63: 191–270.
36. Johannessen M, Moens U (2007) Multisite phosphorylation of the cAMP response element-binding protein (CREB) by a diversity of protein kinases. Front Biosci 12: 1814–1832.
37. Mantamadiotis T, Lemberger T, Bleckmann SC, Kern H, Kretz O, et al. (2002) Disruption of CREB function in brain leads to neurodegeneration. Nat Genet 31: 47–54.
38. Choi YS, Lee B, Cho HY, Reyes IB, Pu XA, et al. (2009) CREB is a key regulator of striatal vulnerability in chemical and genetic models of Huntington's disease. Neurobiol Dis 36: 259–268.
39. Mievis S, Blum D, Ledent C (2011) A2A receptor knockout worsens survival and motor behaviour in a transgenic mouse model of Huntington's disease. Neurobiol Dis 41: 570–576.
40. Lunkes A, Mandel JL (1998) A cellular model that recapitulates major pathogenic steps of Huntington's disease. Hum Mol Genet 7: 1355–1361.
41. Igarashi S, Morita H, Bennett KM, Tanaka Y, Engelender S, et al. (2003) Inducible PC12 cell model of Huntington's disease shows toxicity and decreased histone acetylation. Neuroreport 14: 565–568.
42. Fukui H, Moraes CT (2007) Extended polyglutamine repeats trigger a feedback loop involving the mitochondrial complex III, the proteasome and huntingtin aggregates. Hum Mol Genet 16: 783–797.
43. Finkbeiner S, Mitra S (2008) The ubiquitin-proteasome pathway in Huntington's disease. TheScientificWorldJournal 8: 421–433.
44. Chen PJ, Hsieh CL, Su KP, Hou YC, Chiang HM, et al. (2009) Rhizomes of Gastrodia elata B(L) possess antidepressant-like effect via monoamine modulation in subchronic animal model. Am J Chin Med 37: 1113–1124.
45. Li X, Wang CE, Huang S, Xu X, Li XJ, et al. (2010) Inhibiting the ubiquitin-proteasome system leads to preferential accumulation of toxic N-terminal mutant huntingtin fragments. Hum Mol Genet 19: 2445–2455.
46. Zhang J, Ma Y, Taylor SS, Tsien RY (2001) Genetically encoded reporters of protein kinase A activity reveal impact of substrate tethering. Proc Natl Acad Sci U S A 98: 14997–15002.
47. Li XJ, Li S (2011) Proteasomal dysfunction in aging and Huntington disease. Neurobiol Dis 43: 4–8.
48. Axelrod FB, Liebes L, Simson GG, Mendoza S, Mull J, et al. (2011) Kinetin Improves IKBKAP mRNA Splicing in Patients With Familial Dysautonomia. Pediatr Res 70: 480–483.

49. Olsen A, Siboska GE, Clark BF, Rattan SI (1999) N(6)-Furfuryladenine, kinetin, protects against Fenton reaction-mediated oxidative damage to DNA. Biochem Biophys Res Commun 265: 499–502.
50. Kim MJ, Choi SJ, Lim ST, Kim HK, Kim YJ, et al. (2008) Zeatin supplement improves scopolamine-induced memory impairment in mice. Biosci Biotechnol Biochem 72: 577–581.
51. Choi SJ, Jeong CH, Choi SG, Chun JY, Kim YJ, et al. (2009) Zeatin prevents amyloid beta-induced neurotoxicity and scopolamine-induced cognitive deficits. J Med Food 12: 271–277.
52. Huang NK, Chern Y, Fang JM, Lin CI, Chen WP, et al. (2007) Neuroprotective principles from Gastrodia elata. J Nat Prod 70: 571–574.
53. Huang NK, Lin JH, Lin JT, Lin CI, Liu EM, et al. (2011) A new drug design targeting the adenosinergic system for Huntington's disease. PLoS One 6: e20934.
54. Popoli P, Blum D, Martire A, Ledent C, Ceruti S, et al. (2007) Functions, dysfunctions and possible therapeutic relevance of adenosine A2A receptors in Huntington's disease. Prog Neurobiol 81: 331–348.
55. Huang CL, Yang JM, Wang KC, Lee YC, Lin YL, et al. (2011) Gastrodia elata prevents huntingtin aggregations through activation of the adenosine A(2A) receptor and ubiquitin proteasome system. J Ethnopharmacol 138: 162–168.
56. Mosmann T (1983) Rapid colorimetric assay for cellular growth and survival: application to proliferation and cytotoxicity assays. J Immunol Methods 65: 55–63.
57. Wanker EE, Scherzinger E, Heiser V, Sittler A, Eickhoff H, et al. (1999) Membrane filter assay for detection of amyloid-like polyglutamine-containing protein aggregates. Methods Enzymol 309: 375–386.

Comprehensive Behavioral and Molecular Characterization of a New Knock-In Mouse Model of Huntington's Disease: zQ175

Liliana B. Menalled[1], Andrea E. Kudwa[1], Sam Miller[1], Jon Fitzpatrick[1], Judy Watson-Johnson[1], Nicole Keating[1], Melinda Ruiz[1], Richard Mushlin[1], William Alosio[1], Kristi McConnell[1], David Connor[1], Carol Murphy[1], Steve Oakeshott[1], Mei Kwan[1], Jose Beltran[1], Afshin Ghavami[1], Dani Brunner[1], Larry C. Park[2], Sylvie Ramboz[1], David Howland[2]*

1 PsychoGenics Inc., Tarrytown, New York, United States of America, **2** CHDI Management/CHDI Foundation, Princeton, New Jersey, United States of America

Abstract

Huntington's disease (HD) is an autosomal dominant neurodegenerative disorder characterized by motor, cognitive and psychiatric manifestations. Since the mutation responsible for the disease was identified as an unstable expansion of CAG repeats in the gene encoding the huntingtin protein in 1993, numerous mouse models of HD have been generated to study disease pathogenesis and evaluate potential therapeutic approaches. Of these, knock-in models best mimic the human condition from a genetic perspective since they express the mutation in the appropriate genetic and protein context. Behaviorally, however, while some abnormal phenotypes have been detected in knock-in mouse models, a model with an earlier and more robust phenotype than the existing models is required. We describe here for the first time a new mouse line, the zQ175 knock-in mouse, derived from a spontaneous expansion of the CAG copy number in our CAG 140 knock-in colony [1]. Given the inverse relationship typically observed between age of HD onset and length of CAG repeat, since this new mouse line carries a significantly higher CAG repeat length it was expected to be more significantly impaired than the parent line. Using a battery of behavioral tests we evaluated both heterozygous and homozygous zQ175 mice. Homozygous mice showed motor and grip strength abnormalities with an early onset (8 and 4 weeks of age, respectively), which were followed by deficits in rotarod and climbing activity at 30 weeks of age and by cognitive deficits at around 1 year of age. Of particular interest for translational work, we also found clear behavioral deficits in heterozygous mice from around 4.5 months of age, especially in the dark phase of the diurnal cycle. Decreased body weight was observed in both heterozygotes and homozygotes, along with significantly reduced survival in the homozygotes. In addition, we detected an early and significant decrease of striatal gene markers from 12 weeks of age. These data suggest that the zQ175 knock-in line could be a suitable model for the evaluation of therapeutic approaches and early events in the pathogenesis of HD.

Editor: Hitoshi Okazawa, Tokyo Medical and Dental University, Japan

Funding: CHDI Foundation is a not-for-profit biomedical research organization exclusively dedicated to discovering and developing therapeutics that slow the progression of Huntington's disease. The research described was conducted by PsychoGenics under a fee-for-service agreement for CHDI Foundation in collaboration with and funded by CHDI Foundation. The funder, through CHDI Management, fully participated in study design, data collection and analysis, the decision to publish, and preparation of the manuscript. CHDI Foundation has recently provided financial support to the Public Library of Science for PLOS Currents: Huntington Disease.

Competing Interests: PsychoGenics conducted the research through a fee-for-service agreement for CHDI Foundation. LP and DH are employed by CHDI Management, Inc., as advisors to CHDI Foundation, Inc. LM, AK, SM, JF, JWJ, NK, MR, RM, WA, KM, DC, CM, SO, MK, JB, AG, DB, and SR are/were employed by PsychoGenics. There are no patents, products in development or marketed products to declare. The authors fully adhere to all the PLOS ONE policies on sharing data and materials, as detailed online in the guide for authors.

* E-mail: David.Howland@CHDIFoundation.org

Introduction

Huntington's disease (HD) is a progressive, inherited neurodegenerative disorder characterized by involuntary movements, cognitive impairment and psychiatric manifestations. The onset of symptoms typically occurs in midlife, although it can range from early childhood to over 70 years of age [2]. While the pathological hallmark of the disease is the loss of medium spiny neurons in the striatum, neurodegeneration in the cortex and other brain areas is also observed [3]. HD is caused by an unstable expansion within the trinucleotide poly(CAG) tract located in exon 1 of the *huntingtin* gene leading to the production of a huntingtin protein with an expanded polyglutamine stretch near the N terminus [4]. Since the identification of the mutation responsible for the disease, numerous mouse models have been generated to investigate disease pathogenesis and therapeutic approaches preclinically, with all these models carrying an abnormal expansion of the CAG-repeat stretch derived from the human *huntingtin* gene.

Existing mouse models can be divided into 2 groups based on their genetics, described as transgenic or knock-in (KI) models. Transgenic mouse models have been generated by inserting into the complete murine genome either a fragment (e.g. R6/2 and N171-82Q models) or a full-length copy (BAC HD and YAC HD models) of the human *huntingtin* gene carrying an abnormal expansion of the CAG repeat tract [5,6]. In contrast, KI mouse models carry expanded CAG repeats contained within the native murine *huntingtin* gene [7,8] such that KI models more closely mimic the genetic context of patients with HD. KI models may contain either expanded CAG repeats within an unmodified murine gene (e.g. $Hdh^{(CAG(150))}$) or a chimeric human/mouse exon 1 carrying the expanded CAG repeat region and the human polyproline region (e.g. CAG 71, CAG 94, CAG 140, and the zQ175 model described here).

The first KI models generated, with relatively low CAG repeat numbers, displayed either a mild or no behavioral phenotype [9,10]. Subsequent models carrying longer expansions, however, showed behavioral abnormalities, with the $Hdh^{(CAG(150))}$ and CAG 140 models receiving the most attention in behavioral testing. Motor deficits like poor rotarod performance, abnormal locomotion and exploratory behavior and abnormal gait have been consistently observed in homozygous mice of both lines, with the onset and severity of those abnormalities varying depending on the line examined, the specifics of the protocol used, and the strain background of the test mice [7,8,11–14]. In addition, cognitive and senory gating deficits have been reported in the $Hdh^{(CAG(150))}$ line [15].

Given that homozygosity is very rare in humans, efforts have also been made to examine heterozygous mice. These efforts have met with limited success, with only relatively mild behavioral deficits observed with a late age of onset [11–13].

Given the inverse relationship between age of HD onset and CAG repeat length [16], an increase in the CAG repeat length of a KI mouse model would be expected to produce a more robust and earlier abnormal phenotype in both the heterozygotes and homozygotes. This would be beneficial for the evaluation of therapeutic approaches as well as for the examination of the early steps involved in HD pathogenesis.

We present here a detailed behavioral examination of a new mouse line carrying around 188 CAG repeats, the zQ175 KI, which was derived from the CAG 140 KI mouse model [1]. Our behavioral battery included both standard (rotarod, open field, procedural 2-choice swim test, and grip strength) and novel (PhenoCube) tests to comprehensively evaluate these novel mice. We also examined whether changes in the striatal gene markers that are affected in HD could be detected in these mice, and whether behavioral and transcriptional abnormalities would progress as the animals' aged.

Materials and Methods

A spontaneous expansion of the CAG repeat number was identified in a litter from our CAG 140 KI colony [1]. Founder mice from this litter were used to establish a novel colony, providing the animals used in this work. The first animals obtained carried around 175 CAG repeats, leading to the name zQ175, with the letter z used to identify that the line was derived from a line created by Scott Zeitlin. However, due to instability of the mutation, by the time the colony was stabilized the line carried around 188 CAG repeats. For tracking purposes, the CHDI nomenclature for this new KI line is CHDI-81003003.

Subjects

Homozygous, heterozygous and wild type (WT) mice were generated by crossing heterozygous zQ175 mice on a C57B/l6J background. Animals were ear notched at around 10–15 days. Mice were weaned and implanted with RFID electronic chips (DataMars, OH) for identification at around 21 days. The average CAG repeat length in the primary test cohort was 186.2±15 (SEM = 1.4) for the heterozygous and 188.7±12 (SEM = 1.0) for the homozygous animals. Genotyping and CAG repeat count were determined by Laragen Inc. (Culver City, CA), from PCR of tail snips taken at 10–15 days of age. CAG repeat length and range in the other cohorts examined were comparable.

Three cohorts of mice were evaluated in the behavioral work described here, a primary test group (n = 9–12/sex/genotype) which underwent a full battery of testing and two secondary groups of animals (each: 7–16/sex/genotype) evaluated in the PhenoCube and swim tank (see Table 1 below for details).

Tissue was collected at three timepoints, at 12, 18 and 41 weeks of age, with an n = 5–12 per group. Tissue from the 12 and 18 week timepoints was collected from behaviorally naïve satellite groups, while the 41 week collection was taken from animals evaluated in the PhenoCube at 37 weeks (see cohort 3 in Table 1).

Animal care was in accordance with the United States Public Health Service Policy on Humane Care and Use of Laboratory Animals, and procedures were approved by the Institutional Animal and Use Committee of Psychogenics, Inc. (PHS OLAW animal welfare assurance number A4471-01), an AAALAC International accredited institution (Unit #001213).

Husbandry

Mice from the primary test and satellite cohorts were housed in mixed genotype groups of 3–4 animals in OptiMICE® cages (Animal Care Systems, CO) with beta chip bedding (Northeastern Products Corp., NY). The PhenoCube test cohorts were instead housed in genetically homogenous groups of 6 to 10 in larger optiRAT® cages (Animal Care Systems, CO). All animals had *ad libitum* access to food (Purina 5001) and water except where noted. The cage environment was enriched with the addition of plastic bones, shredded paper and play tunnels. Temperature (68–76C), humidity (30–70%) and the light-dark cycle (6:00–18:00 EST) were controlled and monitored daily.

Body Weight and Survival

In the main test cohort, body weight was measured weekly and all mice were examined daily for survival analysis. At 47 weeks of age, the animals underwent scheduled food restriction and were maintained at 85% of their free feeding weights by daily administration of limited quantities of food. At 75 weeks of age, these mice were returned to *ad libitum* feeding conditions and survival analysis and measurement continued.

The PhenoCube and tissue collection cohorts received *ad libitum* food at all times, but body weight data are not included here.

Behavioral Testing (Primary Test Cohort)

Researchers were blind to the genotypes of the mice during testing. Mice were transported from their colony room in their home cages to the behavioral testing room, where they were allowed to acclimate for at least one hour prior to the beginning of the experiment.

Rotarod. Mice were tested over 3 consecutive days. Each daily session included a single training trial of 5 min at 4 RPM on the rotarod apparatus (Rotamex, OH). One hour later, the animals were tested for 3 consecutive accelerating trials of 5 min with the rotarod speed changing from 0 to 40 RPM over 300 s, with an inter-trial interval of at least 30 min. The latency to fall from the rod was recorded for each trial, with mice remaining on the rod for more than 300 sec removed and scored at 300 s.

Open field. Activity chambers (Med Associates Inc, St Albans, VT; 27×27×20.3 cm) were equipped with infrared (IR) beams. Mice were placed in the center of the chamber and their behavior was recorded for 30 min, with analysis performed on the

Table 1. Test ages for behavioral work, broken down by test cohort.

	Age (weeks)																					
	4	5	8	9	12	13	16	17	20	21	22	24	25	28	29	30	32	33	36	37	38	58
Cohort 1																						
Open field in the light phase	√		√		√		√		√			√		√			√		√			
Open field in the dark phase	√		√		√		√		√				√	√			√		√			
Rearing/climbing in the light phase	√		√		√		√		√			√					√					
Rearing/climbing in the dark phase													√					√				
Grip Strength in the light phase	√		√		√		√		√			√					√					
Grip Strength in the dark phase													√					√				
Rotarod in the light phase		√		√		√		√		√					√					√		
Rotarod in the dark phase											√					√					√	
Cohort 2																						
PhenoCube							√															
Procedural 2 choice swim tank test																						√
Cohort 3																						
PhenoCube																				√		

following five measures: total locomotion, locomotion in the center of the open field, rearing rate in the center, total rearing frequency and velocity. Testing was carried out in both the light and dark phase of the diurnal cycle (see Table 1 below for details), in all cases at least 1 hour after the light change; testing in the dark phase was performed under red light, while testing in the light phase was performed in normal white light.

Grip strength. Mice were scruffed by the lower back and tail and lowered towards a mesh grip piece attached to a force gauge (Chatillion Force Gauge, San Diego Instruments, San Diego, CA) until the animal grabbed with both front paws. The animal was then lowered toward the platform and gently pulled straight back with consistent force until it released its grip. The forelimb grip force was recorded on the strain gauge.

Rearing-climbing. The rearing climbing chamber consisted of a metal wire mesh pencil holder placed upside down over a balance and a test mouse, such that the test animals' weight was removed from the balance once it began to climb the mesh (modified from Hickey et al., 2005). Weight data was collected for 300 sec and latency to climb was automatically extracted.

Neurological assessment. Mice were examined for 1–2 minutes at 33 and 93 weeks of age. Scores for the following parameters were evaluated by simple observation of the test mice: head tremor, head twitch, head bobbing, head searching, body tremor, body twitch, tail tremor, tail twitch, straub tail, piloerection, shallow respiration, flattened body posture, swollen face, ptosis, irritability, seizure, urine staining, lacrimation, salivation, limb splay, catalepsy, abnormal gait, tip toe walking, slow careful movements, excessive grooming, circling, sniffing, chewing, state of dehydration, presence of an abnormal level of locomotor activity, and any observed seizures. In addition, tests of the startle, tail pinch and righting reflexes were carried out by direct manipulation of the test animals. To test the startle reflex, a small hand clicker was used to generate a loud popping noise and the following behaviors scored in the immediate aftermath: jumping, freezing, and rapid eye blinks. For the air righting reflex, each mouse was removed from the home cage and dropped from ~30 cm to the arena floor, with the animals' posture in the air scored. To measure the tail pinch reflex, forceps were used to gently squeeze the end of the tail.

Overall assessment for all these measures was scored as follows: A score of 0 was assigned for normal behavior (e.g. standard locomotor activity) or for the absence of abnormal features (e.g. the absence of piloerection); a score of 1 was given when mild abnormalities were observed and a score of 2 was given when severe abnormalities were observed. Rectal body temperature was also measured.

Behavioral Testing (Secondary Cohorts)

Procedural 2-Choice swim test. Testing was carried out using a modified version of the rectangular swim tank described by Lione [17], with the tank measuring 76 cm×30.5 cm×30.5 cm, filled with opaque water to a depth of 6″ and maintained at 25±1°C. An escape platform was located 0.5 cm below the surface of the water at one end of the tank. On each test trial, mice were released from a set location relative to the platform in the middle of the tank, facing the tank wall closest to the experimenter and equidistant from either end of the tank, and were allowed to swim freely for up to 60 s. If an animal successfully reached the hidden platform within 60 s, it was allowed to remain there for 5 s and then removed from the tank. If an animal failed to find the platform within 60 s it would be manually placed onto the platform and allowed to remain there for 5 s. No spatial cues were provided within the tank environment, such that the animals were required to learn a procedural strategy to approach the platform, by turning in a particular direction.

Mice were given 4 blocks of 2 training trials each day with a 30–45 min inter-block interval. Entry point for each mouse alternated between trials within a block, along with the side of the tank in which the platform was placed, to eliminate any possible contribution of room cues to the choice of swim direction. The location of the platform was counterbalanced across groups. A correct choice was scored if the animal turned in the direction of the platform and successfully mounted the platform. An incorrect choice was scored if the animal swam in the direction opposite the platform. No choice was scored if the animal either did not make a choice, by swimming in the middle of the tank, or turned initially toward the platform but did not mount the platform.

Phenocube®. Animals were evaluated in the PhenoCube® system in 72 h-test sessions, following a 16 h- water deprivation period in the home cage. Within the PhenoCube® environment, behavior was automatically monitored at all times. The cages were maintained on a 12:12 light/dark cycle, with white light during the day and red light during the night, maintaining a low subjective light level for the subjects during the night period. While inside the cage, water was only available from within the PhenoCube® corners, while food was freely available on the cage floor at all times. Where possible, mice were left undisturbed during the course of experimental sessions. Two cohorts of mice were tested in the PhenoCube, one at 16 and one at 36 weeks of age, with all animals naïve to the PhenoCube environment at the start of testing.

The PhenoCube® system was based on extensively customized Intellicage boxes (New Behavior AG) fitted with proprietary video analysis equipment. In all test sessions, the test animals initially received magazine training through a simple magazine training protocol, allowing them to freely retrieve water from any of the PhenoCube® corners. Early in the light period on day 2, after a full night in the cage, the protocol was switched to a more stringent training protocol requiring the animals to visit specific locations to retrieve water and to alternate between potentially reinforced locations.

Quantification of Transcripts

Tissue collection. At each specified age, striatal tissues were dissected and frozen on dry ice until they were processed for RNA extraction.

Total RNA extraction. Tissues were homogenized 2×1 min at 25 Hz in 750 µL of QIAzol Lysis Reagent (Cat # 79306, Qiagen, Valencia, CA) with TissueLyser (Qiagen, Valencia, CA) and 5 mm stainless steel beads (Cat # 69989, Qiagen, Valencia, CA). Once tissues were disrupted, samples were allowed to incubate at room temperate for 5 minutes. For the RNA extraction procedure, the manufacturer's protocol for RNeasy 96 Universal Tissue Kit (Cat # 74881, Qiagen, Valencia, CA) for RNA isolation was followed. Briefly, 150 µL of Chloroform (Cat # C2432, Sigma-Aldrich, St. Louis, MO) was added and samples were shaken vigorously for 15 seconds followed by 3 minutes incubation at room temperature. The aqueous phase was separated from the organic phase by centrifugation at 6,000×g (Beckman Coulter Avanti J-30I), at 4°C for 15 minutes. The aqueous phase was then transferred to a new 96-well block and total RNA was precipitated with an equal volume of 70% ethanol. Total volume was then transferred to an RNeasy 96-well plate, followed by centrifuging at 6,000×g (Beckman Coulter Avanti J-30I), at room temperature for 4 minutes. Total RNA bound to column membranes was then treated with RNase-Free DNase set (Cat # 79254, Qiagen, Valencia, CA) for 30 minutes, followed by 3 washing steps with RW1 and RPE buffers (provided with RNeasy 96 Universal Tissue Kit). RNA was eluted with RNase-Free water (25 µL for striatum samples).

Total RNA quantification and reverse transcription. To ensure integrity, 2 µL of total RNA in conjunction with NorthernMax -Gly Sample Loading Dye (Cat # AM8551, Applied BioSystems, Foster City, CA) were subjected to electrophoresis in 1% agarose in NorthernMax -Gly 1× Gel Prep/Running Buffer (Cat # AM8678, Applied Biosystems, Foster City, CA). Good RNA integrity was determined by visualization of intact 16S and 23S ribosomal RNAs and the absence of any smearing. Furthermore, RNA was quantified using Quan-iT RiboGreen RNA Kit (Cat # R11490, Invitrogen, Carlsbad, CA) and analyzed with the SpectraMax Gemini XPS fluorescent plate reader (Molecular Devices, Sunnyvale, CA). One microgram of total RNA was reverse transcribed into cDNA with 3.2 µg random hexamers (Cat # 11034731001, Roche Applied Science, Indianapolis, IN), 1 mM each dNTP (Cat # 11814362001), Roche Applied Science, Indianapolis, IN), 20U Protector RNase Inhibitor (Cat # 03335402001, Roche Applied Science, Indianapolis, IN), 1X Transcriptor Reverse Transcription reaction buffer and 10U Transcriptor Reverse Transcriptase (Cat # 03531287001, Roche Applied Science, Indianapolis, IN) in 20 µL total volume. The reactions were allowed to proceed at room temperature for 10 minutes, at 55°C for 30 minutes, then were inactivated at 85°C for 5 minutes in GeneAmp PCR Systems 9700 thermal cycler (Applied Biosystems, Foster City, CA). cDNA samples were diluted 10 to 100 fold with RNase-Free water for qPCR analysis.

Quantitative PCR (qPCR). Five microliters of the diluted cDNA were amplified with 12.5 µL 2× FastStart Universal Probe Master Rox (Cat # 04914058001, Roche Applied Science, Indianapolis, IN), 0.5 µL Universal Probe Library Probe (Roche Applied Science, Indianapolis, IN), 200 nM of gene specific primer- HPLC purified (Sigma-Aldrich, St. Louis, MO) in 25 µL reaction volume. The reactions were run on the ABI 7900HT Sequence Detection System (Applied Biosystems, Foster City, CA). qPCR conditions were initially set at 95°C for 10 minutes in order to activate the FastStart Taq DNA Polymerase followed by 40 cycles of 95°C for 15 seconds and 60°C for 1 minute. Primers and Universal Probe Library information are listed in Table 2.

qPCR data analysis. Total RNA from whole brain of C57BL6 mice was reverse transcribed as described above. cDNA samples from multiple reverse transcription reactions were pooled together and used to create qPCR standard curves for the genes of interest and also served as the calibrator, diluted just as the sample cDNA, to normalize plate to plate variations. To generate the standard curve, pooled cDNA was serial diluted from 1:5 to 1:1000 in RNase-free water and assayed in triplicate in each qPCR assay. The Ct values (number of cycles required for the PCR amplicon detection to reach threshold) were plotted against the logarithm value of dilution samples and a linear trend line was obtained for each gene. PCR efficiencies were calculated using the equation of PCR efficiency $= 10^{(1/-\text{slope})}$. Note that a PCR efficiency of 2 is the value for ideal PCR amplification where the amplicons double in quantity per PCR cycle.

Each sample of cDNA (diluted 1:10) was assayed in triplicate and the Ct values averaged. Values which lay greater than 0.5 standard deviations from the average were discarded. The relative quantity of the PCR product (relative to the calibrator) is calculated as follows:

Relative Quantity of Target gene = $(\text{PCR Efficiency}_{\text{Target}})^{(\text{Ct calibrator-Ctsample})}$.

Relative Quantity of Housekeeping Gene 1 = $(\text{PCR Efficiency}_{\text{housekeeping1}})^{(\text{Ct calibrator-Ctsample})}$.

Relative Quantity of Housekeeping Gene 2 = $(\text{PCR Efficiency}_{\text{housekeeping2}})^{(\text{Ct calibrator-Ctsample})}$.

Relative Quantity of Housekeeping Gene 3 = $(\text{PCR Efficiency}_{\text{housekeeping3}})^{(\text{Ct calibrator-Ctsample})}$.

The geometric mean for the three housekeeping genes is calculated as follows:

Geometric mean = (relative quantity of housekeeping gene 1 * relative quantity of housekeeping gene 2 * relative quantity of housekeeping gene 3)$^{(1/3)}$.

The relative level of the target gene is calculated as follows:

Relative Quantity of Target gene/Geometric mean of housekeeping genes.

Table 2. Qualitative Polymerase Chain Reaction (qPCR) information.

Mouse Gene	Mouse Gene ID	Gene Bank Accession Number	5′ Primer Sequence	3′ Primer Sequence	Universal Probe Library Number
ATP synthase subunit beta	ATP5b	NM_016774.3	GGCACAATGCAGGAAAGG	TCAGCAGGCACATAGATAGCC	77
Eukaryotic initiation factor 4A-II	EIF4A2	NM_013506.2, NM_001123037.1, NM_001123038.1	GCCAGGGACTTCACAGTTTC	TTCCCTCATGATGACATCTCTTT	93
Ubiquitin B	Ubc	NM_019639.4	GACCAGCAGAGGCTGATCTT	CCTCTGAGGCAGAAGGACTAA	11
Dopamine Receptor D2	Drd2	NM_010077.2	TGAACAGGCGGAGAATGG	CTGGTGCTTGACAGCATCTC	17
Dopamine- and cAMP-regulated neuronal phosphoprotein	DARPP32	NM_0144828.1	CCACCCAAAGTCGAAGAGAC	GCTAATGGTCTGCAGGTGCT	98
Cannabinoid receptor type 2	Cnr1	NM_007726.3	GGGCAAATTTCCTTGTAGCA	GGCTCAACGTGACTGAGAAA	79
cAMP and cAMP-inhibited cGMP 3′,5′-cyclic phosphodiesterase 10a	PDE10a	NM_011866.2	GAAGGCTGACCGAGTGTTTC	GGGATGGAGAGAAAGATAGGC	45
Glutamate transporter 1	GLT1	NM_001077515.2 NM_001077514.3 NM_011393.2	GGTCATCTTGGATGGAGGTC	ATACTGGCTGCACCAATGC	83

The 3 striatal housekeeping genes used in this study were: *ATP5b*, *Eif4a2* and *Ubc*. The relative level of the target gene (*Drd2*, *DARPP32*, *Cnr1*, *PDE10a* and *GLT1*) was then normalized to age and gender matched wild type control animals.

Data Analysis

An alpha level of.05 was selected for all inferential statistics. Repeated measures analysis (age as dependent factor) was carried out with SAS (SAS Institute Inc.) using Mixed Effect Models. This approach was based on likelihood estimation which was more robust to missing values than moment estimation. The models were fitted using the procedure PROC MIXED [18]. For parametric analyses, genotype, gender, age and their interactions were considered in all the models and significant genotype × age, genotype × gender and genotype × age × gender interactions were followed up with simple main effects to determine at which age the genotype differences reached significance.

For PhenoCube® testing, data were summarized across the two full day/night periods obtained after the mice had fully acclimated to the PhenoCube® environment. Data collapsed from these two test periods was then evaluated via ANOVA as outlined above, though line graphs are also presented describing the full experimental sessions in shorter time bins, to provide a visual representation of the animals' behavioral patterns. For these PhenoCube analyses, an additional factor of day/night cycle was included, capturing activity differences across the animals' activity cycles.

Rearing and climbing data were analyzed using Chi square analysis (StatView), seperately comparing the WT group to homozygous and to heterozygous animals. The proportion of mice to reach the acquisition criterion in the swim test task was assessed using Kaplan-Meier event analysis over the entire acquisition test period, followed up with Chi square analysis of the effects of genotype on performance on individual test days.

The neurological assessment data were analyzed using Chi square analysis.

Survival data were analyzed with Kaplan–Meier analysis, with the p values derived from the Mantel–Cox Log-rank statistic.

Results

Behavioral Evaluation

General health and neurological abnormalities. At 33 weeks of age, body tremor was observed in 68% of the homozygous mice but in only 4% in the WT group (χ^2 test, $p<0.05$). 21% of homozygous mice were found to be hypoactive, while locomotor activity was normal in all WT mice at this age (χ^2 test, $p<0.05$). In contrast to homozygous mice, tremors were observed in only 13% of the heterozygous mice, not differing significantly from the WT controls, with no apparent hypoactivity observed at this age (χ^2 tests, $ps>0.05$). When body temperature was evaluated, homozygous mice presented a significantly lower body temperature than WT animals ($p<0.05$), with no difference detected between heterozygous and WT animals (Mean values ± SEM: WT, 36.12°C ±0.54; heterozygous, 35.76°C ±0.64; homozygous: 35.60°C ±0.75; Genotype effect $F(2,63)=3.784$, $p<0.05$).

At 93 weeks of age, neurological assessment revealed that a high percentage (between 80 and 100%) of the surviving homozygous mice presented with loss of air righting reflex, body tremor, abnormal gait, limb splay, hunched posture, flattened body posture and piloerection, differing significantly from WT controls (χ^2 test, $ps<0.05$). Interestingly, features of pre-seizure activity, such as body twitches, straub tail and partial praying seizure activity without rearing, were observed in most of the homozygous mice (>80% of animals). An abnormal startle response and poor grooming were observed in 66% and 50% of the homozygous mice examined (χ^2 test, $ps<0.05$). Heterozygous mice at 93 weeks also presented significantly abnormal body tremor (70% of mice), startle response (~80%), piloerection (85%) and abnormal gait (including limb splay and hunched posture; 90–100% of mice) relative to WT control animals (χ^2 test, $ps<0.05$). Overall neurological abnormalities appeared more severe in the homozygous than in the heterozygous animals. As at 33 weeks, the

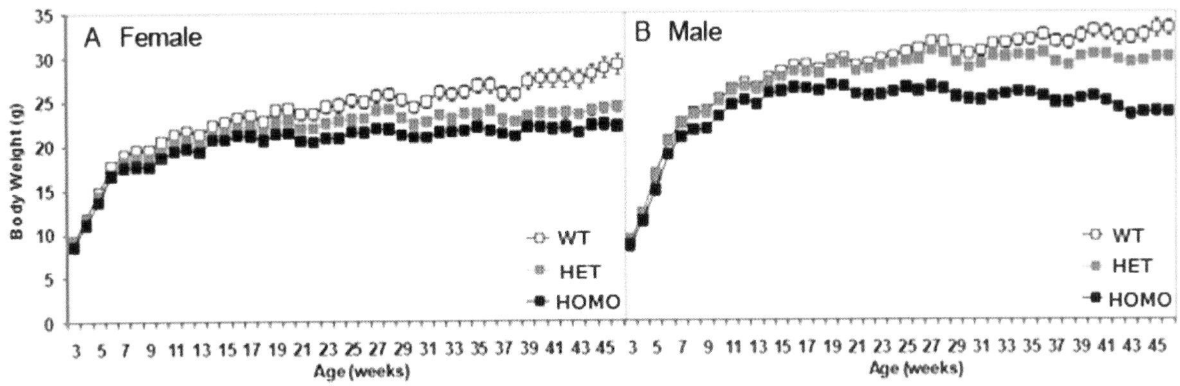

Figure 1. Body weight (mean ± SEM) of wild type, heterozygous and homozygous mice as a function of age for female (A) and male (B) mice.

homozygous mice again presented a significantly lower body temperature at 93 weeks of age than either WT or heterozygous mice animals (*ps* <0.05), with no difference in body temperature detected between heterozygous and WT animals (WT: 36.78°C ±0.56; heterozygous: 36.49°C ±0.92; homozygous: 35.45°C ±0.72; $F(2,44) = 7.04$, $p<0.05$). No seizures were observed at any age either spontaneously or during handling/behavioral testing.

Loss of body weight in both heterozygous and homozygous zQ175 KI mice. Homozygous female and male mice gained body weight at the same rate as WT mice up to 7 and 5 weeks of age, respectively. Subsequently, the homozygous animals were significantly lighter then WT controls. While the body weight of female homozygous mice remained constant during the evaluation period, male homozygous body weight first plateaued and then progressively decreased with increasing age. Homozygous mice were also significantly lighter than heterozygous mice from 4 weeks onward in the male group and from 19 to 32, from 34 to 36 and at 38 weeks of age in the female group.

Heterozygous zQ175 mice were also significantly lighter than WT controls, but this phenotype was observed at later ages than in the homozygous mice, being apparent only at 26 and from 28 weeks of age onwards in the male group and at 10, 13 and from 15 weeks of age onwards in the female group (Figure 1, genotype main effect, $F_{(2,61)} = 41.60$, $p<0.0001$; age main effect, $F_{(8,2294)} = 212.59$, $p<0.0001$; genotype × age interaction, $F_{(76,2294)} = 2.37$, $p<0.0001$; genotype × age × gender interaction, $F_{(114,2294)} = 3.04$, $p<0.0001$; simple main effects $ps<0.05$).

Reduced survival in zQ175 homozygous mice. Survival differences began to appear relative to WT controls in the homozygous group at around 76 weeks of age (see Figure 2), with all homozygous mice dead by 104 weeks of age with a median survival of 90.1 weeks (WT vs. homozygous Kaplan-Meier Mantel-Cox: $p<0.0001$). At this age (104 weeks), only around 25% of the heterozygous mice and 8% of the WT mice had died, with no analysis performed on the WT vs. heterozygous comparison.

Hypoactivity in the dark phase is seen in open field testing: Total distance. Mice were evaluated during the light and dark phase of the diurnal cycle in open field to assess motor function, general activity, reaction to a novel environment, and exploration mice. In the testing during the dark phase of the diurnal cycle, homozygous mice presented a decreased total distance travelled relative to WT controls from 8 weeks of age. While the same phenotype was observed in heterozygous animals, onset was much later, with hypoactivity seen only from 20 weeks of age onwards. In addition, the homozygous mice were significantly more hypoactive than were heterozygous mice at 8, 12, 16, 25 and 36 weeks of age (genotype main effect, $F_{(2,61)} = 29.01$, $p<0.0001$; age main effect, $F_{(8,483)} = 142.32$, $p<0.0001$; genotype × age interaction, $F_{(16,483)} = 3.74$, $p<0.0001$; simple main effects $ps<0.05$, Figure 3).

Hypoactivity in the dark phase is seen in open field testing: Rearing. Homozygous mice reared significantly less than WT mice during the dark phase of the diurnal cycle at all ages except at 4 and 28 weeks of age. While there was an evident decrease in locomotor and rearing activity of the homozygous mice as they aged, this was paralleled by decreases in the activity of the WT control group, producing an overall genotype effect and precluding evaluation of the progression of motor deficits using those parameters. Heterozygous mice reared significantly less than WT controls at 16 and 32 weeks of age and more than homozygous mice at 12, 16, 25 and 32 weeks of age (genotype main effect, $F_{(2,61)} = 11.02$, $p<0.0001$; age main effect, $F_{(8,483)} = 52.82$, $p<0.0001$; genotype × age interaction, $F_{(16,483)} = 2.60$, $p<0.0008$; simple main effects $ps<0.05$, Figure 4).

Hypoactivity is also seen in the light phase in open field testing: Total distance. Similarly, testing in the light phase of the diurnal cycle revealed robust hypoactivity in the female

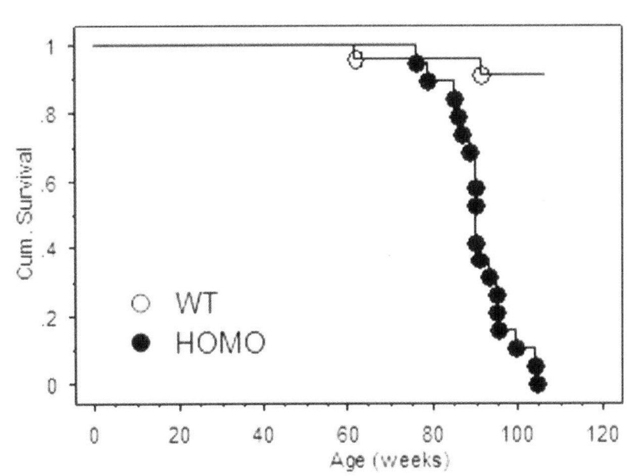

Figure 2. Kaplan-Meier survival curve in WT vs. homozygous mice as a function of genotype and age.

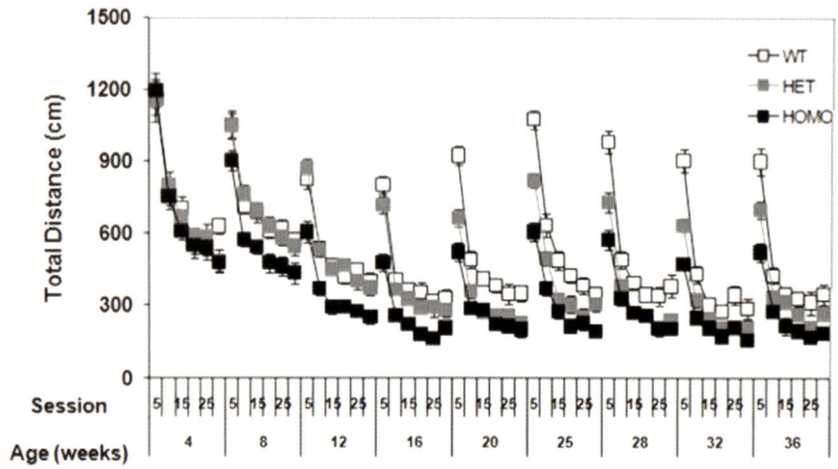

Figure 3. Total distance covered in the Open Field per 5 minute bin (mean ± SEM) of wild type, heterozygous and homozygous mice as a function of age and test time during the dark phase of the diurnal cycle.

homozygous mice relative to WT controls starting at 8 weeks of age. However, in the light period, no significant differences were observed between the heterozygous female and WT female animals, though homozygous female mice were hypoactive relative to the heterozygous female mice at 8, 12, 20, 28 and 32 weeks of age. In the male group, homozygous and heterozygous mice both presented significantly decreased locomotor activity relative to WT males only at 20 weeks of age (Figures S1A and S1B, genotype main effect, $F_{(2,61)} = 9.75$, $p < 0.0003$; age main effect, $F_{(8,482)} = 86.79$, $p < 0.0001$; genotype × age interaction, $F_{(16,482)} = 2.02$, $p < 0.02$; genotype × gender × age interaction, $F_{(24,482)} = 2.82$, $p < 0.0001$; simple main effects $ps < 0.05$).

Hypoactivity is also seen in the light phase in open field testing: Rearing. Homozygous mice reared significantly less than did WT controls mice during the light phase of the diurnal cycle at all ages, regardless of gender (Figure S2, genotype main effect, $F_{(2,61)} = 3.58$, $p < 0.04$; age main effect, $F_{(8,482)} = 42.0$, $p < 0.0001$). No significant differences were detected when comparing the heterozygous animals to either homozygous or WT mice.

Motor deficits are seen in both homozygous and heterozygous mice: Rotarod performance. To assess motor coordination, mice were tested using the accelerating rotator protocol. During the diurnal dark period, both homozygous and heterozygous mice showed a reduced latency to fall from the rotarod relative to WT control mice at 30 and 38 weeks of age (Figure 5, genotype main effect, $F_{(2,60)} = 5.13$, $p < 0.01$; age main effect, $F_{(2,120)} = 9.69$, $p < 0.0001$; genotype × age interaction, $F_{(4,120)} = 6.28$, $p < 0.0001$; simple main effects $ps < 0.05$). No significant deficits were detected in the light phase (data not shown).

Deficits in grip strength performance were detected in homozygous mice. To assess muscle strength, mice were tested in the grip strength test.At all ages and genotypes, female mice showed weaker grip strength than did males. The homozygous mice presented a decreased grip strength performance than did

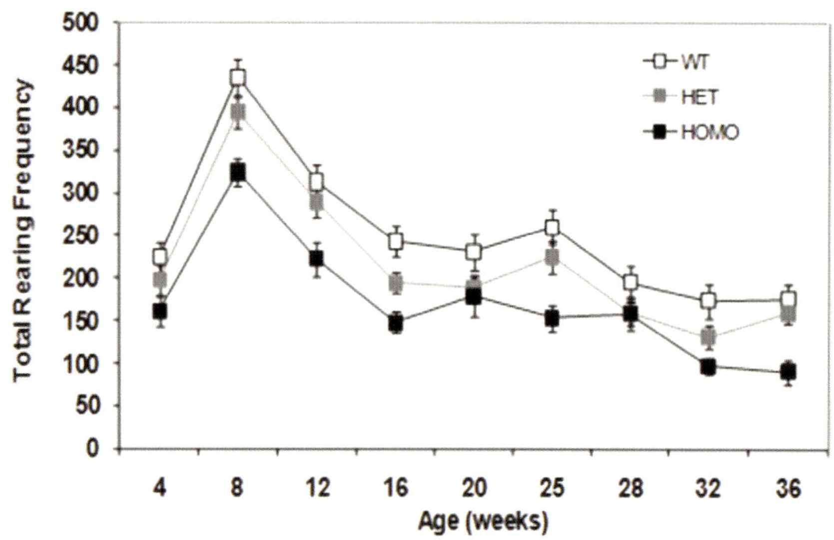

Figure 4. Rearing frequency in the Open Field (mean ± SEM) of wild type, heterozygous and homozygous mice as a function of age during the dark phase of the diurnal cycle.

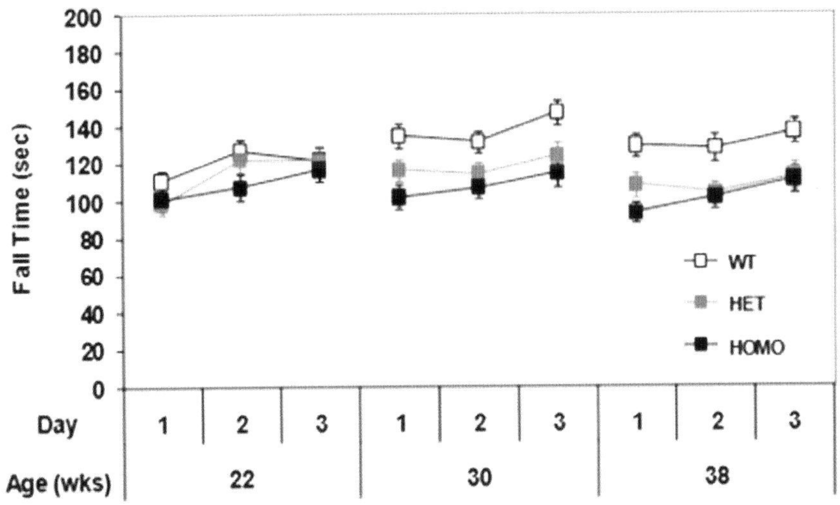

Figure 5. Latency to fall from the rotarod (mean ± SEM) of wild type, heterozygous and homozygous mice as a function of age during the dark phase of the diurnal cycle.

WT controls at all the ages evaluated in both the light and dark phases of the diurnal cycle, with testing starting at 4 weeks of age (light phase data not shown: genotype main effect, $F_{(2,61)} = 9.39$, $p<0.0005$; gender main effect, $F_{(1,61)} = 28.12$, $p<0.05$, age main effect, $F_{(6,363)} = 218.42$, $p<0.0001$; simple main effects, *ps* <0.05, Figure 6: dark period data: genotype main effect, $F_{(2,60)} = 6.56$, $p<0.005$; gender main effect, $F_{(1,60)} = 5.49$, $p<0.04$, age main effect, simple main effects, *ps* <0.05, Figure S3).

Decreased climbing activity was observed in homozygous mice. To assess climbing activity mice were evaluated in the rearing-climbing assay. A smaller proportion of mice in the homozygous group climbed during the dark phase of the diurnal cycle at 33 weeks of age (Figure 7, χ^2 test, $p<0.05$) but not at 25 weeks of age. Decreased climbing activity relative to WT mice was observed in the homozygous animals during testing in the light phase at 32 weeks of age, but not at younger ages(data not shown). No deficits were detected in the heterozygous mice.

Cognitive deficits in homozygous mice. To assess learning and memory, mice were tested in the procedural two-choice swim test, a simple left-right discrimination task. Homozygous mice performed significantly less well than either heterozygous or WT mice in overall acquisition of the procedural swim tank task at 58 weeks, with a significantly lower percentage of correct choices recorded during acquisition (genotype main effect: $F_{(2,58)} = 9.15$, $p<0.001$; simple main effects $ps<0.05$; Figure 8) as well as a significantly higher level of incorrect choices (genotype main effect: $F_{(2,58)} = 8.89$, $p<0.001$; simple main effects *ps* <0.05, data not shown). Choice latencies were also significantly higher in homozygous mice than in either heterozygous or WT mice (genotype main effect: $F_{(2,58)} = 58.60$, $p<0.0001$; genotype × day interaction: $F_{(16,464)} = 3.28$, $p<0.0001$; simple main effects $ps<0.05$, data not shown).

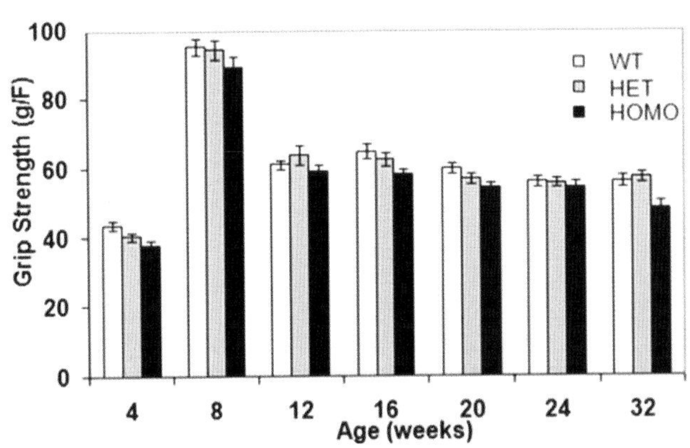

Figure 6. Grip strength (mean ± SEM) of wild type, heterozygous and homozygous mice as a function of age during the light phase of the diurnal cycle.

PhenoCube®. PhenoCube is a high-throughput platform that assesses circadian, cognitive and motor behavior exhibited by group-housed mice. Data are presented here from two separate cohorts of naïve animals. The initial cohort was tested at 16 weeks of age, while the second cohort was tested first at 36 weeks of age. Prior to testing, animals were minimally disturbed, living in their testing groups in the colony rooms. In some cases, animals failed to record licks within the PhenoCube® corners and consequently were removed from testing – no data from these mice are presented.

PhenoCube® – visit frequency. Inspection of these data indicated that all mice show markedly increased activity in the night vs. the day periods, with genotype differences consequently became more apparent during the night time. There appeared to be clear differences between all three genotypes at both ages, though the effects were clearer in the 16 week test age (Figure 9, than at 37 week of age (Figure 10) as the WT animals become less active with age. Consistently, there were significant main effects of both test age and day/night cycle, smaller $F_{(1,\ 119)} = 12.9$, along with a significant overall effect of genotype, $F_{(2,\ 119)} = 23.3$, all *ps* *<0.0001*. There were also significant interactions amongst these factors, with a significant genotype × test age and a significant genotype × day/night cycle interaction, smaller $F_{(2,\ 119)} = 5.44$, along with a significant three way interaction between genotype, test age and day/night cycle, $F_{(3,\ 119)} = 9.18$, all *ps* *<0.01*. Follow-up analysis confirmed that all three genotypes were statistically distinct in the night period at both ages, with the zQ175 heterozygous mice less active than WT controls but more active than zQ175 KI homozygous mice, smallest $t_{(119)} = 2.00$, *ps* *<0.05*.

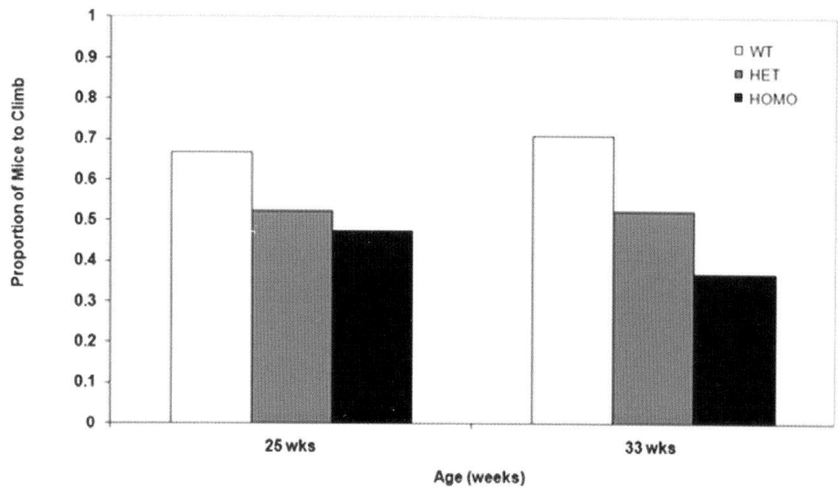

Figure 7. Proportion of mice climbing in the rearing climbing assay in the wild type, heterozygous and homozygous group during the dark phase of the diurnal cycle.

More detailed breakdown of these statistics is presented in Appendix S1, below.

Level of expression of striatal transcripts. To evaluate whether striatal mRNA expression was affected by zQ175 genotype, the mRNA expression levels of dopamine D2 receptor (*Drd2*), phosphodiesterase-10a (*PDE10a*), cannabinoid receptor-1 (*Cnr1*), dopamine-and cyclic-AMP-regulated phosphoprotein (*DARPP32*), and glutamine transporter-1 (GLT1) were assessed. Striatal samples from homozygous and heterozygous mice were examined at 12 (males and females), 18 (male only), and 41 (males and females) weeks of age. The geometric mean of three housekeeping genes, *ATP5B*, *EIF4A2*, and *Ubc*, as has been previously described [19] was used to normalize the transcripts of interest. In order to better evaluate the validity of the disease marker changes, we decided to first examine the degree of housekeeping gene variability by normalizing each housekeeping gene to the geometric mean of itself and two other housekeeping genes (data not shown). This exercise allowed us to better interpret whether changes obtained with the genes of interest are to the same extent or superior to those of normalized housekeeping genes. It is important to note that in most cases, housekeeping genes did not show either genotypic or age related changes (data not shown).

Transcript abnormalities were seen in both heterozygous and homozygous mice. We detected transcript level differences between the genotypes and sexes. In 12 weeks old female heterozygous mice, only *DARPP32* mRNA level was significantly reduced (post hocs, $ps < 0.05$; Figure 11; Table S1 presents the F and p values for the significant main effects and interactions for the different gene markers examined for male and female mice), whereas in 12 week-old female homozygous mice a significant reduction in expression level of all transcripts reported in this study was observed ($ps < 0.05$). In males, however, transcript downregulation in both homozygous and heterozygous mice occurred around 18 weeks of age with a significant downregulation of *Drd2*, *DARPP32*, *Cnr1* and *PDE10A* mRNA levels ($ps < 0.05$). At this age, GLT1was the only transcript that showed genotype differences since a significant reduction of expression was detected in 18 weeks old male homozygous but not in heterozygous mice ($ps < 0.05$). An age dependent decrease of mRNA expression level has been also been noted. At 41 weeks of age, *Drd2*, *DARPP32*, *Cnr1* and *PDE10a* transcriptional levels were significantly reduced in both males and females of heterozygous and homozygous mice, with the greatest reduction (about 50%) seen in homozygous mice relative to their WT littermates ($ps < 0.05$). In addition at 41 weeks of age, *GLT1* mRNA expression level was not only reduced in female

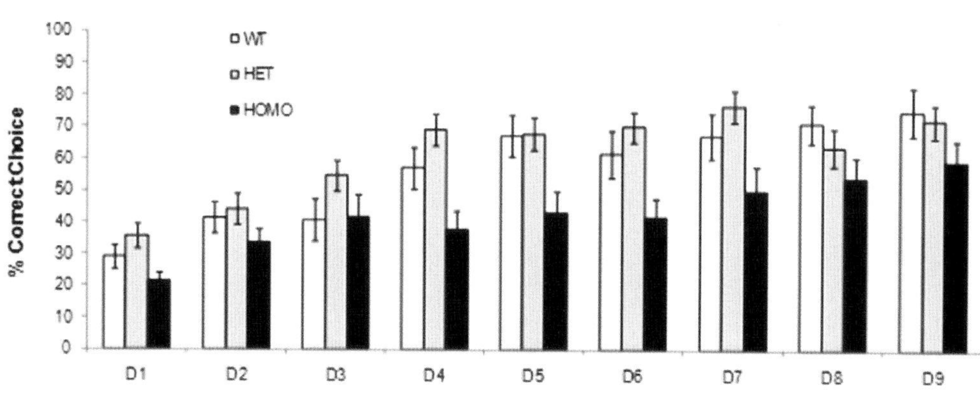

Figure 8. Percent correct choices for WT, heterozygous and homozygous mice per test day during acquisition of the procedural swim tank at 58 weeks of age.

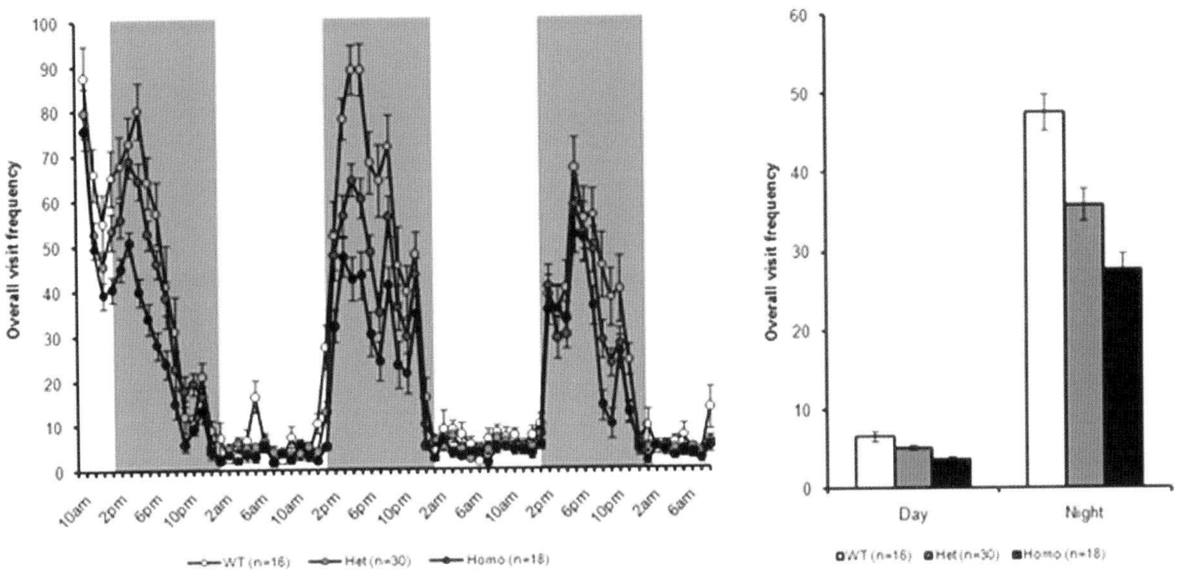

Figure 9. Overall visit frequency during PhenoCube testing at 16 weeks, broken down into 1 hour bins (A) and summarized across the two complete light/dark periods from lights-on on day 2 (B).

homozygous, but at this age a significant downregulation was also noted in both homozygous male and heterozygous female mice.

Discussion

Novel HD mouse models that present a more robust and earlier onset of phenotype and that more closely mimic human HD are required. We present here a behavioral and molecular characterization of a new KI HD mouse model, the zQ175 KI line, that carries around 188 CAG repeats. This line arose spontaneously in a litter carrying around 175 CAG repeats in our CAG 140 mouse colony (Menalled, Sison et al. 2003); due to the instability of the mutation and multiple rounds of breeding, we developed a colony carrying around 188 CAG repeats. Careful selection from a large pool of potential breeder animals thereafter allowed us to maintain the line with around 188 CAG repeats, as in the cohorts used here. We show that homozygous mice present robust motor and cognitive abnormalities, many of them with an earlier onset than reported in other KI models. Data from the PhenoCube® platform confirm that motor abnormalities detected in both homozygous and heterozygous mice were not related to handling stress, since clear hypoactivity was observed when the animals were spontaneously active. Decreased body weight was detected in both heterozygotes and homozygotes, along with reduced lifespan in the homozygotes. Abnormalities were also observed in striatal mRNA expression. Critically, both the behavioral and transcriptional phenotype observed in these mice appeared at younger ages than

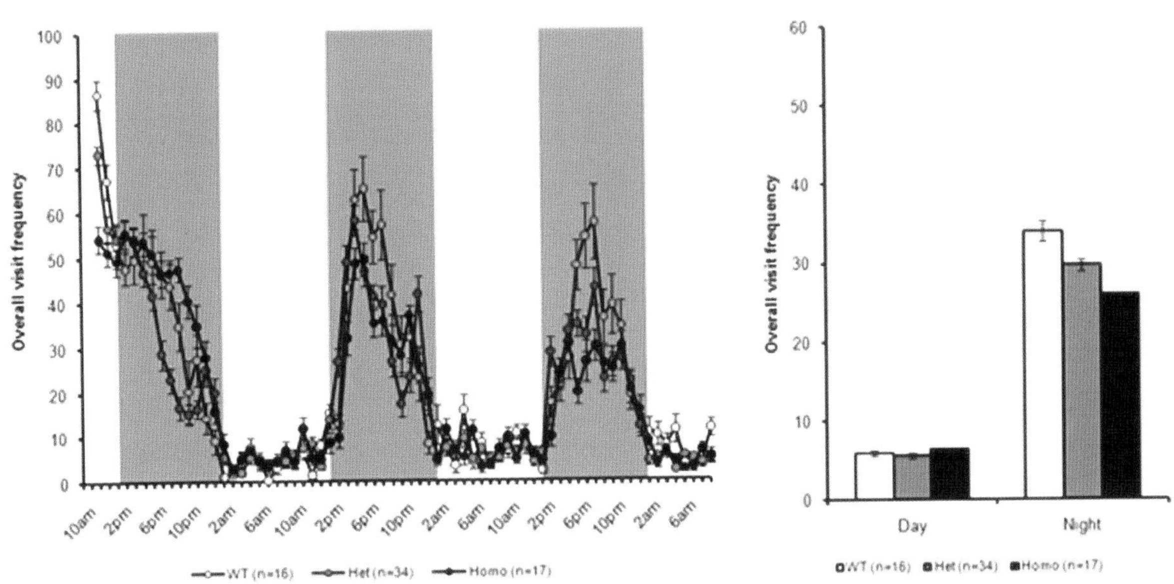

Figure 10. Overall visit frequency during PhenoCube testing at 37 weeks, broken down into 1 hour bins (A) and summarized across the two complete light/dark periods from lights-on on day 2 (B).

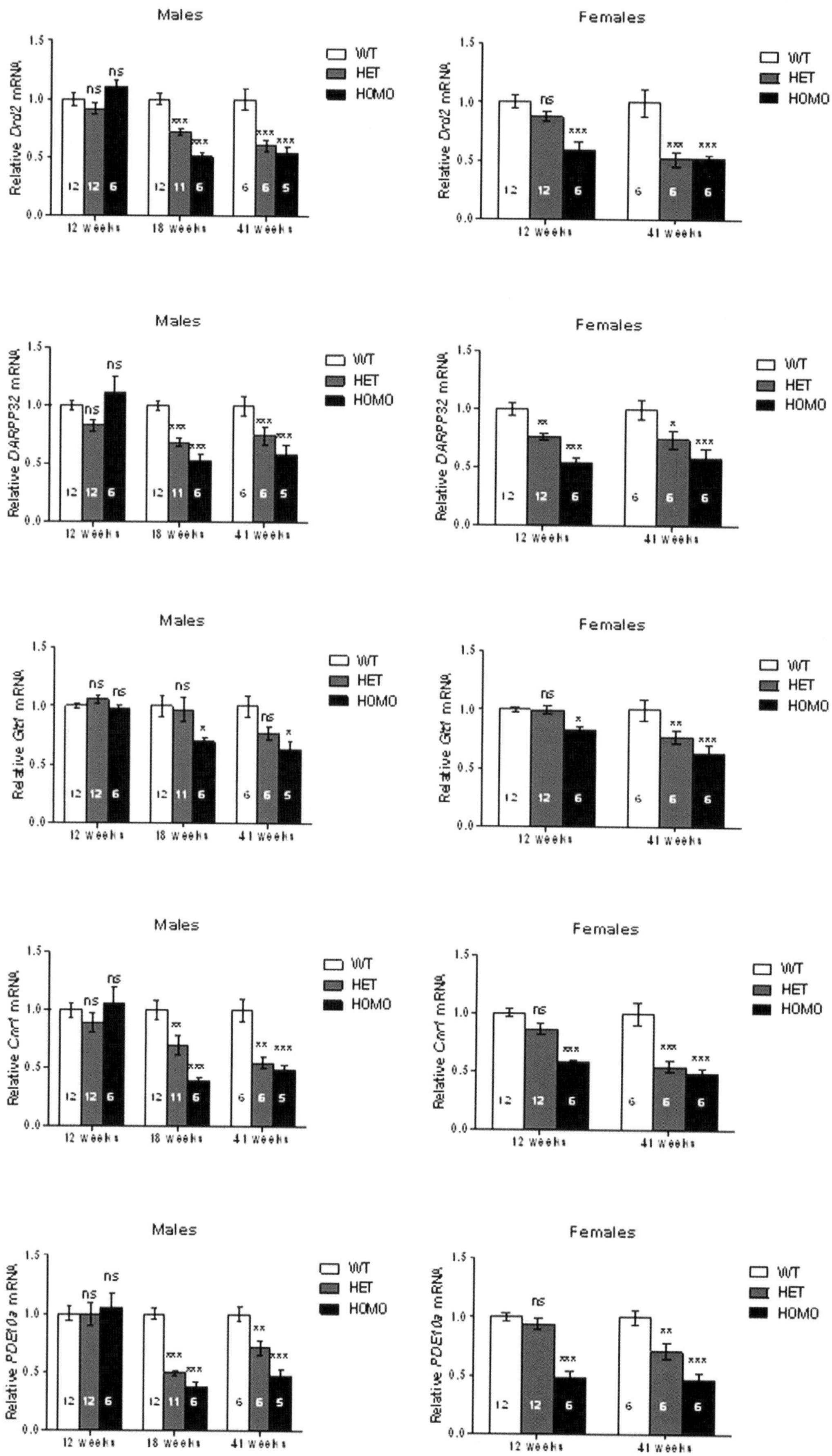
Males
Females
Relative Drd2 mRNA
Relative DARPP32 mRNA
Relative Gtf1 mRNA
Relative Cnr1 mRNA
Relative PDE10a mRNA
WT
HET
HOMO
12 weeks
18 weeks
41 weeks
ns
1.5
1.0
0.5
0.0

Figure 11. The relative striatal mRNA expression level of wildtype (WT), heterozyous (HET) and homozygous (HOMO) zQ175 mice at 12, 18 and 41 weeks of age, analyzed by qPCR. Relative mRNA levels are normalized to age matched and gender matched wild type controls. For normalization, the geometric mean of UBbc, Eif4a2 and ATP5B was used. Gender separation was performed with the 12 and 41 week groups. *, $p<0.05$; **, $p<0.01$; ***, $p<0.001$. The number on each bar graph represents "n" for each group.

in previously described models, particularly in the heterozygotes. Importantly, power analysis shows that group sizes of 4–15 mice for most of the transcripts analyzed are sufficient to detect a 50% improvement (final number needed depends on age, genotype and sex of interest; $\alpha = 0.05$, 80% power, see Table S2 for details). A sample size of 15 animals also allows the evaluation of potential therapies in HOM mice using a general heath and motor behavioral battery and of 35 to include the cognitive domain (for more details see Table S3). Deficits in the HET mice are not as pronounced compared to the deficits detected in the HOM group. Sample sizes of 5–22 HET mice are sufficient to detect a 50% improvement in most of the transcripts analyzed (Table S2). A sample size of 37 HET mice allows us to detect an effect size of at least 50% in body weight and in the total distance in the open field test (first 5 min) when performed during the dark phase of the diurnal cycle (Table S3). Together, our data indicate that these zQ175 KI mice represent a valuable new preclinical model of HD.

General Health Abnormalities

Loss of body weight is a progressive and characteristic symptom of HD [20]. Decreased body weight has been observed in numerous mutant mouse and rat models of HD [21,22] and was recapitulated in the new model described here. Significantly, the body weight of the heterozygous zQ175 mice was intermediate between that of the homozygous and WT mice, in a manner consistent with previous findings that lower levels of WT full-length huntingtin are associated with decreased body weight (Van Raamsdonk et al., 2006).

Given the inverse relationship typically seen between the age of onset of HD phenotype and the CAG repeat length, it is perhaps surprising that these zQ175 mice present a significantly earlier onset of body weight abnormalities than were recently reported in a KI mouse line carrying 200 CAG repeats, the HdhQ200 model [8]. Since the CAG repeat length of the zQ175 and HdhQ200 lines are comparable, our results highlight that differences in age of onset of body weight phenotype in KI HD mouse models are not exclusively influenced by CAG repeat length, but are also affected by background strain, colony conditions, and genetic construct used [23]. A progressive decline in the animals' general health was detected in both the homozygous and heterozygous zQ175 KI mice. Specifically tremors, hypoactivity, abnormal gait, and flattened body posture were more prevalent as the animals aged. While these abnormalities are consistent with those seen in other KI mice expressing similarly long CAG repeats, none of those models presented these type of deficits at such an early age (from 33 weeks) [8,11,14,24]. Furthermore, these zQ175 homozygous mice are the first KI animals in which a significantly reduced lifespan has been reported [1,8,14]. Given that the mice described here were food restricted from 47 to 75 weeks of age, some caveats might exist with these survival data, but it is worth noting that the survival curve observed here up to 58 weeks is very similar to that of a second cohort evaluated in our laboratory that did not undergo food restriction (unpublished observation).

Reduced grip strength is seen in HD patients and also in a number of HD mouse models [25,26]. Decreased forelimb grip strength was detected from 4 weeks of age in these homozygous zQ175 mice and has previously been reported at around the same age in the $Hdh^{(CAG(150))}$ homozygous KI mouse (Woodman, Butler et al. 2007).

Motor Abnormalities

Motor abnormalities, cardinal features of the human condition, are also apparent in many HD mouse models [1,8,12,14,15,27]. We used four behavioral methods to evaluate motor decline; rotarod performance, open field activity, climbing behavior, and the PhenoCube® system. Testing in the diurnal dark phase when spontaneous activity was higher (illustrated by the PhenoCube data) showed genotype-dependent deficits that otherwise might not have been observed. Whilst the basic locomotor and rearing abnormalities detected in this new line have an early onset and are robust, especially in the homozygotes, the deficits in those parameters did not seem to progress with age (at least as examined, up to 36 weeks). It is possible that these mice might progress at older ages, though age-related decline in performance of the WT mice may complicate analysis.

Similarly, rotarod deficits were observed both in the heterozygous and homozygous zQ175 mice from 30 weeks of age, but no progression of these deficits was observed with age, again as with previous observations in CAG 140 mice [13,14]. Our results warrant further examination in, for example, a beam test and running wheels that have shown progression in other KI mouse models [8].

In PhenoCube® testing, significant hypoactivity was detected in both heterozygotes and homozygotes at the ages tested (16 and 36 weeks), with significantly reduced activity also observed in homozygotes relative to heterozygotes.

A moderately-enriched environment is part of the regular housing conditions for HD mouse models in our facility, and such environments can ameliorate HD phenotypes in mouse models as well as patients [28–30]. The early phenotype we detected in this new KI line (relative to other KI lines) occurred despite this enriched environment, again highlighting the robustness of the phenotype in the zQ175 line.

Cognitive Abnormalities

Cognitive decline is a key feature of HD, with a very specific pattern of progressive deficits predominantly related to damage to the frontal-striatal circuitry, and this damage is recapitulated in many HD mouse models. We trained zQ175 mice in a simple procedural response learning that should be impaired by striatal dysfunction and which had previously revealed very substantial deficits in the R6/2 mouse (unpublished observations). We found that zQ175 homozygotes presented deficits in this task at 58 weeks, while there were no differences between the heterozygous and WT mice. Previous accounts of cognitive deficits in $Hdh^{(CAG(150))}$ homozygous KI mice indicated impairments in demanding tasks (i.e. reversal learning and extradimensional shifts) apparent as early as 4–6 months of age while no deficits were detected in simple response learning tasks [15,31].Work in our laboratory has revealed significant deficits in zQ175 heterozygous mice in a more complex visual discrimination reversal task with a touchscreen [32,33]. Furthermore, work in the R6/2 transgenic HD mouse has similarly demonstrated that more complex learning deficits (e.g. reversal) can be identified at earlier ages than simpler learning deficits (e.g. acquisition) [17]. The significant deficit in simple procedural response learning in zQ175 mice at 58 weeks of age may therefore be the result of either their advanced age or their higher CAG repeat expansion, and warrants further evaluation of younger zQ175 cohorts in this and other cognitive assays to better define the nature and breadth of impairment.

Transcriptional Dysfunction

Previous studies in both humans and mouse models of HD indicated that transcript levels of specific genes in the striatum are reduced [34–44]. We also show here that expression levels of previously reported striatal transcripts such as dopamine D2 receptor (*Drd2*), phosphodiesterase-10a (*PDE10a*), cannabinoid receptor-1 (*Cnr1*), dopamine-and cyclic-AMP-regulated phosphoprotein (*DARPP32*), and glutamine transporter-1 (*GLT1*), were also reduced in zQ175 mice. Further study will determine whether this downregulation is due to neuronal loss or dysfunction; it is unlikely that loss is the only cause since the expression of housekeeping genes was unaltered.

In general, behavioral deficits in zQ175 mice emerge at about the same age as do transcriptional abnormalities, with homozygotes showing a phenotype earlier than heterozygotes. It is important to note that the differential onset of the phenotype in heterozygotes vs. homozygotes in this report and a previous study [13] do not translate to observations in HD patients; patients either homozygous or heterozygous for the mutant huntingtin gene typically have a similar onset of disease symptoms and differentiate only later in disease progression [45]. Interestingly, the onset of transcript downregulation in male mice is the same for both the homozygotes and heterozygotes (18 weeks).

Summary

In summary, we describe here a new zQ175 KI mouse model that closely mimics the human genetic lesion and presents robust and early behavioral and molecular alterations in both homozygous and heterozygous mice. Further characterization will determine its utility as a suitable model for the study of HD pathogenesis, as well as for the evaluation of therapeutic approaches.

Supporting Information

Figure S1 Total distance travelled (mean ± SEM) of wild type, heterozygous and homozygous zQ175 mice as a function of age for female (A) and male (B) mice during the light phase of the diurnal cycle.

Figure S2 Rearing frequency (mean ± SEM) of wild type, heterozygous and homozygous mice as a function of age during the light phase of the diurnal cycle.

Figure S3 Average grip strength (mean ± SEM) of wild type, heterozygous and homozygous mice as a function of age during the dark phase of the diurnal cycle.

Table S1 F and p value table for the significant main effects and interactions for the different gene markers examined for male and female mice.

Table S2 Summarizes the sample size needed to detect a 50% effect in the transcripts evaluated with an alpha of 0.05 and a power of 0.8 for the HET and HOM mice.

Table S3 Summarizes the sample size needed to detect a 50% effect in the behavioral measures evaluated with an alpha of 0.05 and a power of 0.8 for the HET and HOM mice. Longitudinal power analyses were run with Age as a factor (day for the P-2CST test), in addition to Genotype. In the analysis all the ages described in the Result Section were included when applicable.

Appendix S1 Detailed PhenoCube® statistics.

Acknowledgments

Michael Olson, Justin Torello and Russell Port for technical support. Ethan Signer, Allan Tobin and Simon Noble for helpful discussions and comments on an initial draft of this manuscript.

Author Contributions

Conceived and designed the experiments: LM SR DH DB SO CM AK AG LP. Performed the experiments: SM JF JWJ NK MR WA KMC DC MK JB. Analyzed the data: LM AK SO AG MK DC RM. Wrote the paper: LM SO SR DH AG.

References

1. Menalled LB, Sison JD, Dragatsis I, Zeitlin S, Chesselet MF (2003) Time course of early motor and neuropathological anomalies in a knock-in mouse model of Huntington's disease with 140 CAG repeats. J Comp Neurol 465: 11–26.
2. Roos RA, Hermans J, Vegter-van der Vlis M, van Ommen GJ, Bruyn GW (1993) Duration of illness in Huntington's disease is not related to age at onset. J Neurol Neurosurg Psychiatry 56: 98–100.
3. Vonsattel JP, Myers RH, Stevens TJ, Ferrante RJ, Bird ED, et al. (1985) Neuropathological classification of Huntington's disease. J Neuropathol Exp Neurol 44: 559–577.
4. The Huntington's Disease Collaborative Research Group (1993) A novel gene containing a trinucleotide repeat that is expanded and unstable on Huntington's disease chromosomes. The Huntington's Disease Collaborative Research Group. Cell 72: 971–983.
5. Gray M, Shirasaki DI, Cepeda C, Andre VM, Wilburn B, et al. (2008) Full-length human mutant huntingtin with a stable polyglutamine repeat can elicit progressive and selective neuropathogenesis in BACHD mice. J Neurosci 28: 6182–6195.
6. Hickey MA, Chesselet MF (2003) The use of transgenic and knock-in mice to study Huntington's disease. Cytogenet Genome Res 100: 276–286.
7. Menalled LB (2005) Knock-in mouse models of Huntington's disease. NeuroRx 2: 465–470.
8. Heng MY, Duong DK, Albin RL, Tallaksen-Greene SJ, Hunter JM, et al. (2010) Early autophagic response in a novel knock-in model of Huntington disease. Hum Mol Genet 19: 3702–3720.
9. White JK, Auerbach W, Duyao MP, Vonsattel JP, Gusella JF, et al. (1997) Huntingtin is required for neurogenesis and is not impaired by the Huntington's disease CAG expansion. Nat Genet 17: 404–410.
10. Wheeler VC, White JK, Gutekunst CA, Vrbanac V, Weaver M, et al. (2000) Long glutamine tracts cause nuclear localization of a novel form of huntingtin in medium spiny striatal neurons in HdhQ92 and HdhQ111 knock-in mice. Hum Mol Genet 9: 503–513.
11. Lin CH, Tallaksen-Greene S, Chien WM, Cearley JA, Jackson WS, et al. (2001) Neurological abnormalities in a knock-in mouse model of Huntington's disease. Hum Mol Genet 10: 137–144.
12. Heng MY, Tallaksen-Greene SJ, Detloff PJ, Albin RL (2007) Longitudinal evaluation of the Hdh(CAG)150 knock-in murine model of Huntington's disease. J Neurosci 27: 8989–8998.
13. Rising AC, Xu J, Carlson A, Napoli VV, Denovan-Wright EM, et al. (2011) Longitudinal behavioral, cross-sectional transcriptional and histopathological characterization of a knock-in mouse model of Huntington's disease with 140 CAG repeats. Exp Neurol 228: 173–182.
14. Hickey MA, Kosmalska A, Enayati J, Cohen R, Zeitlin S, et al. (2008) Extensive early motor and non-motor behavioral deficits are followed by striatal neuronal loss in knock-in Huntington's disease mice. Neuroscience 157: 280–295.
15. Brooks S, Higgs G, Jones L, Dunnett SB (2010) Longitudinal analysis of the behavioural phenotype in Hdh((CAG)150) Huntington's disease knock-in mice. Brain Res Bull.

16. Andrew SE, Goldberg YP, Kremer B, Telenius H, Theilmann J, et al. (1993) The relationship between trinucleotide (CAG) repeat length and clinical features of Huntington's disease. Nat Genet 4: 398–403.
17. Lione LA, Carter RJ, Hunt MJ, Bates GP, Morton AJ, et al. (1999) Selective discrimination learning impairments in mice expressing the human Huntington's disease mutation. J Neurosci 19: 10428–10437.
18. Singer J (1998) Using SAS PROC MIXED to fit multilevel models,hierarchical models, and individuals growth models. Journal of Educational and Behavioral Statistics 24: 323–355.
19. Benn CL, Fox H, Bates GP (2008) Optimisation of region-specific reference gene selection and relative gene expression analysis methods for pre-clinical trials of Huntington's disease. Mol Neurodegener 3: 17.
20. Sanberg PR, Fibiger HC, Mark RF (1981) Body weight and dietary factors in Huntington's disease patients compared with matched controls. Med J Aust 1: 407–409.
21. Menalled LB, Chesselet MF (2002) Mouse models of Huntington's disease. Trends Pharmacol Sci 23: 32–39.
22. von Horsten S, Schmitt I, Nguyen HP, Holzmann C, Schmidt T, et al. (2003) Transgenic rat model of Huntington's disease. Hum Mol Genet 12: 617–624.
23. Lloret A, Dragileva E, Teed A, Espinola J, Fossale E, et al. (2006) Genetic background modifies nuclear mutant huntingtin accumulation and HD CAG repeat instability in Huntington's disease knock-in mice. Hum Mol Genet 15: 2015–2024.
24. Woodman B, Butler R, Landles C, Lupton MK, Tse J, et al. (2007) The Hdh(Q150/Q150) knock-in mouse model of HD and the R6/2 exon 1 model develop comparable and widespread molecular phenotypes. Brain Res Bull 72: 83–97.
25. Fellows S, Schwarz M, Schaffrath C, Domges F, Noth J (1997) Disturbances of precision grip in Huntington's disease. Neurosci Lett 226: 103–106.
26. Gordon AM, Quinn L, Reilmann R, Marder K (2000) Coordination of prehensile forces during precision grip in Huntington's disease. Exp Neurol 163: 136–148.
27. Menalled L, El-Khodor BF, Patry M, Suarez-Farinas M, Orenstein SJ, et al. (2009) Systematic behavioral evaluation of Huntington's disease transgenic and knock-in mouse models. Neurobiol Dis 35: 319–336.
28. Hockly E, Cordery PM, Woodman B, Mahal A, van Dellen A, et al. (2002) Environmental enrichment slows disease progression in R6/2 Huntington's disease mice. Ann Neurol 51: 235–242.
29. Trembath MK, Horton ZA, Tippett L, Hogg V, Collins VR, et al. (2010) A retrospective study of the impact of lifestyle on age at onset of Huntington disease. Mov Disord 25: 1444–1450.
30. van Dellen A, Blakemore C, Deacon R, York D, Hannan AJ (2000) Delaying the onset of Huntington's in mice. Nature 404: 721–722.
31. Brooks SP, Betteridge H, Trueman RC, Jones L, Dunnett SB (2006) Selective extra-dimensional set shifting deficit in a knock-in mouse model of Huntington's disease. Brain Res Bull 69: 452–457.
32. Murphy C, Paterson N, Oakeshott S, He D, Alosio B, et al. (In preparation) Impairments in simple discrimination reversal and intra-dimensional shift in the BAC HD and z_Q175 mouse models of Huntington's disease.
33. Morton AJ, Skillings E, Bussey TJ, Saksida LM (2006) Measuring cognitive deficits in disabled mice using an automated interactive touchscreen system. Nat Methods 3: 767.
34. Albin RL, Qin Y, Young AB, Penney JB, Chesselet MF (1991) Preproenkephalin messenger RNA-containing neurons in striatum of patients with symptomatic and presymptomatic Huntington's disease: an in situ hybridization study. Ann Neurol 30: 542–549.
35. Augood SJ, Faull RL, Emson PC (1997) Dopamine D1 and D2 receptor gene expression in the striatum in Huntington's disease. Ann Neurol 42: 215–221.
36. Bibb JA, Yan Z, Svenningsson P, Snyder GL, Pieribone VA, et al. (2000) Severe deficiencies in dopamine signaling in presymptomatic Huntington's disease mice. Proc Natl Acad Sci U S A 97: 6809–6814.
37. Chan EY, Luthi-Carter R, Strand A, Solano SM, Hanson SA, et al. (2002) Increased huntingtin protein length reduces the number of polyglutamine-induced gene expression changes in mouse models of Huntington's disease. Hum Mol Genet 11: 1939–1951.
38. Denovan-Wright EM, Robertson HA (2000) Cannabinoid receptor messenger RNA levels decrease in a subset of neurons of the lateral striatum, cortex and hippocampus of transgenic Huntington's disease mice. Neuroscience 98: 705–713.
39. Hebb AL, Robertson HA, Denovan-Wright EM (2004) Striatal phosphodiesterase mRNA and protein levels are reduced in Huntington's disease transgenic mice prior to the onset of motor symptoms. Neuroscience 123: 967–981.
40. Hu H, McCaw EA, Hebb AL, Gomez GT, Denovan-Wright EM (2004) Mutant huntingtin affects the rate of transcription of striatum-specific isoforms of phosphodiesterase 10A. Eur J Neurosci 20: 3351–3363.
41. Luthi-Carter R, Strand A, Peters NL, Solano SM, Hollingsworth ZR, et al. (2000) Decreased expression of striatal signaling genes in a mouse model of Huntington's disease. Hum Mol Genet 9: 1259–1271.
42. McCaw EA, Hu H, Gomez GT, Hebb AL, Kelly ME, et al. (2004) Structure, expression and regulation of the cannabinoid receptor gene (CB1) in Huntington's disease transgenic mice. Eur J Biochem 271: 4909–4920.
43. Menalled L, Zanjani H, MacKenzie L, Koppel A, Carpenter E, et al. (2000) Decrease in striatal enkephalin mRNA in mouse models of Huntington's disease. Exp Neurol 162: 328–342.
44. Richfield EK, Maguire-Zeiss KA, Cox C, Gilmore J, Voorn P (1995) Reduced expression of preproenkephalin in striatal neurons from Huntington's disease patients. Ann Neurol 37: 335–343.
45. Squitieri F, Gellera C, Cannella M, Mariotti C, Cislaghi G, et al. (2003) Homozygosity for CAG mutation in Huntington disease is associated with a more severe clinical course. Brain 126: 946–955.

18

Mapping Genetically Controlled Neural Circuits of Social Behavior and Visuo-Motor Integration by a Preliminary Examination of Atypical Deletions with Williams Syndrome

Fumiko Hoeft[1,2¤], Li Dai[3], Brian W. Haas[1,4], Kristen Sheau[1], Masaru Mimura[2], Debra Mills[5], Albert Galaburda[6], Ursula Bellugi[7], Julie R. Korenberg[3*❡], Allan L. Reiss[1,8*❡¤]

1 Center for Interdisciplinary Brain Sciences Research (CIBSR), Stanford University School of Medicine, Stanford, CA, United States of America, **2** Department of Neuropsychiatry, Keio University, School of Medicine, Tokyo, Japan, **3** Department of Pediatrics & The Center for Integrated Neuroscience and Human Behavior, The Brain Institute, University of Utah, Salt Lake City, UT, United States of America, **4** Department of Psychology, University of Georgia, Athens, GA, United States of America, **5** School of Psychology, Bangor University, Gwynedd, United Kingdom, **6** Department of Neurology, Beth Israel-Deaconess Medical Center, Harvard Medical School, Cambridge, MA, United States of America, **7** Laboratory for Cognitive Neuroscience, Salk Institute for Biological Studies, La Jolla, CA, United States of America, **8** Departments of Radiology and Pediatrics, Stanford University School of Medicine, Stanford, CA, United States of America

Abstract

In this study of eight rare atypical deletion cases with Williams-Beuren syndrome (WS; also known as 7q11.23 deletion syndrome) consisting of three different patterns of deletions, compared to typical WS and typically developing (TD) individuals, we show preliminary evidence of dissociable genetic contributions to brain structure and human cognition. Univariate and multivariate pattern classification results of morphometric brain patterns complemented by behavior implicate a possible role for the chromosomal region that includes: 1) GTF2I/GTF2IRD1 in visuo-spatial/motor integration, intraparietal as well as overall gray matter structures, 2) the region spanning ABHD11 through RFC2 including LIMK1, in social cognition, in particular approachability, as well as orbitofrontal, amygdala and fusiform anatomy, and 3) the regions including STX1A, and/or CYLN2 in overall white matter structure. This knowledge contributes to our understanding of the role of genetics on human brain structure, cognition and pathophysiology of altered cognition in WS. The current study builds on ongoing research designed to characterize the impact of multiple genes, gene-gene interactions and changes in gene expression on the human brain.

Editor: Carlos Penha-Goncalves, Instituto Gulbenkian de Ciência, Portugal

Funding: This study was funded by NICHD P01 HD033113 and NICHD R01 HD049653-S1. FH was funded by NICHD K23 HD054720. The funders had no role in study design, data collection and analysis, decision to publish, or preparation of the manuscript.

Competing Interests: The authors have declared that no competing interests exist.

* Email: reiss@stanford.edu (ALR); Julie.korenberg@hsc.utah.edu (JK)

❡ The laboratories of ALR and JK contributed equally to the findings presented in this manuscript.

¤ Current address: Division of Child and Adolescent Psychiatry, Department of Psychiatry, University of California San Francisco (UCSF), San Francisco CA, United States of America

Introduction

Imaging genetics research provides an unprecedented opportunity for studying interactions among genes, brain and behavior in humans. For example, studies have explored associations of common genetic polymorphisms, including those related to catechol-*O*-methyl transferase (*COMT*), monoamine oxidase A (*MAOA*) and serotonin transporter length polymorphism (*5-HTTLPR/SLC6A4*), with brain structure and function [1]. Similarly, examination of rare, atypical duplications and deletions associated with disorders such as Williams-Beuren syndrome (WS) can further illuminate our understanding of gene-brain-behavior relationships [2].

WS is a neurodevelopmental disorder caused by a hemizygous deletion of approximately 28 genes on 7q11.23 [3]. WS is associated with poor visuo-spatial construction and increased social drive [4]. The existence of this well delineated profile and known genetic architecture of WS offers unique opportunities to investigate the neurogenetic basis of cognition in humans [5]. Using this approach comparing WS to typically developing (TD) controls, studies have found the genes deleted in WS to be important for intraparietal sulcus (IPS) morphology, which in turn mediates visuo-spatial construction [6], and amygdala-orbitofrontal (OFC)-fusiform circuitry as related to socio-emotional abilities [7–9]. These studies suggest genetically controlled neural circuitries for regulating human behavior, and show how brain imaging data may serve as ideal intermediate endophenotypes mediating gene and behavior.

To further gain a better understanding of the neurogenetic basis of human behavior using this 'model disease' approach, the current study undertook a targeted investigation of persons with WS having rare atypical deletions (AWSdel) by comparing these individuals to WS and TD groups. While most individuals with WS exhibit the full 'classic deletion,' there are rare cases (~2%) where relatively smaller deletions occur [10]. It is currently unknown how smaller WS deletions impact brain structure in WS. By investigating AWSdel, new insights into the role of specific genes on brain and behavior can be obtained. To accomplish this goal, we collected brain imaging data and behavioral data from samples of AWSdel, WS and TD. There were three types of deletions among the AWSdel cases; i.e., one where the genes *GTF2I and GTF2IRD1* were spared, another where the region from *TRIM50/FKBP6* to (but not including) *STX1A* was spared, and a third where small deletions occurred between *ABHD11* through *RFC2* including *LIMK1* (**Figure 1**). We focused on visuo-spatial and social cognition, two key phenotypes of WS and examined whether each AWSdel case resembled WS or TD. The overarching objective of this investigation was to deduce gene-brain-behavior associations by examining genes that are commonly deleted in those with similar neuroanatomical and behavioral profiles among individuals comprising our AWSdel sample (**Figure 1**).

Material and Methods

Ethics Statement

All procedures were approved by the Institutional Review Boards of Stanford University and Salk Institute. All participants provided written informed consent or assent. Parents or guardians provided written consent in addition to written assent if the participants were minors.

Subjects

Participants included a total of 72 with WS, 54 with TD, and 8 individuals with AWSdel (**Table 1, 2**). The 8 individuals with AWSdel had previously received a clinical diagnosis of WS. In each case, one or more genes commonly deleted in WS were spared (AWSdel-01 [ID#: 5623; spared for *GTF2I and GTF2IRD1*], AWSdel-02 [ID#: 5657; spared from *FKBP6/FZD9* up to *WBSCR22*, deletion includes *STX1A*], AWSdel-03 family i-vi [ID#s: 5882, 5884-5888; small deletions from *ABHD11* through *RFC2* including *LIMK1*) on chromosome 7q11.23 (**Figure 1**).

Exclusion criteria included a history of significant medical and neurological conditions or symptoms not known to be associated with WS such as cerebral palsy, stroke, multiple sclerosis, Parkinson's disease or head trauma resulting in loss of consciousness. Epilepsy occurs in WS but does not have as high a rate as in other neurodevelopment conditions such as autism, fragile X and tuberous sclerosis. Thus, these were exclusions for WS (typical AND atypical) as well as for controls. All WS and AWSdel participants received cognitive-behavioral, genetic and imaging assessments as part of a multi-site program project grant on genetics, neuroanatomy, neurophysiology, and cognition.

Healthy control participants (with no history of major psychiatric, neurological, or cognitive impairment) were recruited at both the Salk Institute and Stanford University. TD control participants were further screened to rule out any history of learning, language, or behavioral disorder over the phone using a screening form as in our prior studies of WS and other neurogenetic conditions (e.g. [25]).

Genetic Testing

In order to confirm the extent of each participant's deletion (typical WS and AWSdel), a series of genetic analyses were performed. Specifically, deletions in all the typical WS were confirmed by the use of Fluorescence in Situ Hybridization (FISH) with bacterial artificial chromosomes (BACs) including in all cases, probes for ELN and in addition, subsets of probes marking the ends of the typically deleted region (1008H17 for FKBP6, FZD9; 592D8 for ELN, LIMK1; and 1184P14 for GTF2I), for the typically non-deleted single copy gene, CALN1 (815K3) located upstream of the centromeric duplicated region. Probes for the duplicated regions flanking the common deletion were employed along with ELN as a screen for the common deletion [16]. For atypical participants AWSdel-01 and AWSdel-02, further FISH analyses used a total of twenty-one sequenced linked DNAs isolated from either BACs [16] or cosmids [17] to cover the region defining the deletion breakpoints as described in [18]. Quantitative PCR was performed using probes spanning from CALN1 to

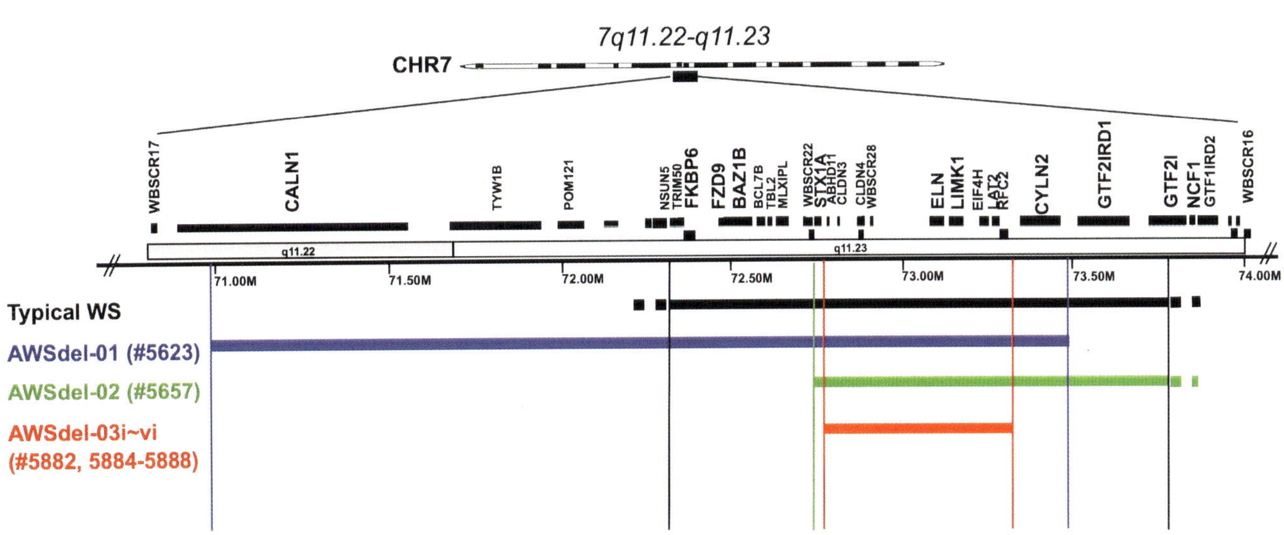

Figure 1. Schematic diagram of deleted genes in WS and in partial deletion participants (AWSdel). Genes listed in the figure are either ones known to be expressed in the brain and are important for neurodevelopment, synaptic plasticity and neuronal reorganization: *LIMK1* [54], *FZD9* [55], *STX1A* [56], *CYLN2* [57], *GTF2 I*[58] and *GTF2IRD1* [59], or are break-points.

Table 1. Demographic information. WS and TD groups.

	1.5T Data (matching AWSdel-01 & AWS-del02 data)						3.0T Data (matching AWSdel-03i-vi data)					
	WS (N=42)		TD (N=40)		T/Chi-square tests		WS (N=30)		TD (N=14)		T/Chi-square tests	
	mean	SD	mean	SD	T/chi	P	mean	SD	mean	SD	T/chi	P
Age	29.20	9.00	27.47	7.36	0.95	0.35	30.01	10.23	30.77	10.00	0.21	0.65
Gender	M 19 F 23		M 16 F 24		0.07	0.79	M 13 F 17		M 7 F 7		0.01	0.92
Full-Scale IQ (ss)	68.55	8.34	104.25	12.42	12.51	<0.001	63.61	11.35	116.17	13.76	12.60	<0.001
Verbal IQ (ss)	71.90	7.43	103.31	11.03	12.37	<0.001	63.14	11.00	113.25	14.39	12.02	<0.001
Performance IQ (ss)	67.55	8.55	104.56	12.72	12.65	<0.001	68.25	11.13	115.08	11.98	11.93	<0.001
Beery VMI (ss)	49.81	7.86	91.07	9.91	15.92	<0.001	51.50	8.03				
Benton JLO (crpr)	11.54	6.64	26.18	2.35	12.36	<0.001	9.92	7.22				
Block Design (ss)	4.32	1.68	12.25	2.32	14.11	<0.001	3.34	1.80				
Approachability (raw)	17.62	7.77	7.81	7.47	4.34	<0.001	15.04	6.59				
Lt Amygdala Volume (ml)	1.80	0.34	1.60	0.33	2.72	0.008	1.85	0.34	2.10	0.28	2.53	0.02
Rt Amygdala Volume (ml)	1.65	0.26	1.46	0.29	3.12	0.003	1.77	0.32	1.88	0.25	1.22	0.23

See also Figure 2B.
F: female, M: male, VMI: Visuo-Motor Integration, JLO: Judgement of Line Orientation, ss: standard score, crps: raw score adjusted for age and gender, raw: non-normed raw score. Amygdala gray matter volumes adjusted for total cranium gray matter volumes.

Table 2. Demographic information. Atypical deletion cases and their deviations from WS and TD groups.

	AWSdel-01			AWSdel-02			AWSdel-03i			AWSdel-03ii	AWSdel-03iii	AWSdel-03iv	AWSdel-03v	AWSdel-03vi
	mean	**vs. WS (Z)**	**vs. TD (Z)**	**mean**	**vs. WS (Z)**	**vs. TD (Z)**	**mean**	**vs. WS (Z)**	**vs. TD (Z)**					
Age	41.0	1.31	**1.84**	29.9	0.08	0.33	38.8	1.06	1.54	15.8	14.6	12.9	10.6	9.4
Gender	M			M			M			F	F	F	F	M
Verbal IQ (ss)	90	**2.44**	-1.21	84	1.63	**−1.75**	88	**2.17**	−1.39	74	74	84	76	85
Performance IQ (ss)	87	**2.27**	−1.38	78	1.22	**−2.09**	82	**1.69**	**−1.77**	80	73	94	81	75
Full-Scale IQ (ss)	88	**2.33**	−1.31	79	1.25	**−2.03**	84	**1.85**	−1.63	75	71	87	77	78
Beery VMI (ss)	75	**3.21**	−1.62	54	0.53	**−3.74**	81	**3.97**	−1.02	88	72	93	83	80
Benton JLO (crpr)	25	**2.03**	−0.50	15	0.52	**−4.75**	17	0.82	**−3.90**					
Block Design (ss)	9	**2.79**	−1.40	10	**3.39**	−0.97	7	1.60	**−2.26**					
Approachability (raw)	21	0.44	**1.77**	26	1.08	**2.44**	28	1.34	**2.70**					
Lt Amygdala Volume - adjusted (ml)	2.26	1.34	**1.98**	2.27	1.36	**2.01**	2.33	1.55	**2.21**					
Rt Amygdala Volume - adjusted (ml)	1.67	0.08	0.72	2.19	**2.08**	**2.51**	1.77	0.46	1.06					

See also Figure 2B.
F: female, M: male, VMI: Visuo-Motor Integration, JLO: Judgement of Line Orientation, ss: standard score, crps: raw score adjusted for age and gender, raw: non-normed raw score. Amygdala gray matter volumes adjusted for total cranium gray matter volumes. Bold values are those that are significant.

WBSCR16 and template DNA isolated from blood and/or lymphoblast cell lines, to determine the deleted region of atypical participants AWSdel-01, AWSdel-02, AWSdel-03i-vi [18]. Finally, a custom high resolution genomic NimbleGen array [15] spanning a 13 Mb region that included the typical deletion, flanking repeats and surrounding single copy DNA, was used to define the deletion structures in atypical participants AWSdel-01, AWSdel-02, AWSdel-03-i, iv, v [15,19]. A schematic diagram showing atypical deletions of these 8 cases is presented in **Figure 1.**

Cognitive/Behavioral Testing

Participants were given a standard battery of measures that included the Wechsler Adult Intelligence Scale (WAIS) [20] and Wechsler Intelligence Scale for Children (WISC) [21] to measure verbal, performance and full-scale IQ. IQ was available for all but 5 WS and 2 TD. There were no significant differences between the participants with and without IQ in level of cognitive function on any measure listed in **Table 1** (all p's >0.1).

Participants also completed a series of tasks designed to assess visuo-spatial functioning. This included the Block Design subtest of the IQ tests (a timed test where the participant arranges the blocks with white and/or red sides according to a pattern), Beery Visuo-Motor Integration [22] (the participant reproduces simple line drawings) and non-normed Benton Judgment of Line Orientation test [23] (the participant identifies the slope of the presented lines on the display of 11 lines).

Lastly we used a non-normed test to measure social approachability in each participant [24]. This task involves participants reporting how likely they would approach a person depicted in a photograph.

WS individuals showed significantly reduced IQ and visuo-spatial abilities, and significantly higher social approachability scores (all p's<0.05). Please see **Table 2** for mean scores, statistics, and scores of partial deletion cases. Analyses of cognitive profiles were performed in parallel to the anatomical brain measures described below with a cut-off score of z = 1.65 (1-tailed) instead of z = 1.96 that was used for brain measures.

Acquisition of Anatomical Brain Measures

MRI data were collected on two scanners (1.5 T and 3.0 T, respectively). Data from 2 of the AWSdel (AWSdel-01, AWS-del02), 42 WS and 40 TD individuals were obtained using a 1.5T MRI scanner. Data from AWSdel-03i ~ AWSdel03vi (father and 5 adolescent children), 30 WS and 14 TD individuals were obtained at a subsequent time using a 3.0T MRI scanner. The **Main Text** reports findings comparing AWSdel (including AWSdel-03 data obtained from a 3.0T) to WS and TD data from 1.5T. The results were unchanged when 3.0T reference data from individuals with WS and TD MRI served as the reference to which MRI data from individuals with AWS (acquired from both 1.5T and 3.0T scanners) were compared (see **Supporting Results**).

All 1.5T data (42 WS, 40 TD, AWSdel-01, AWSdel-02) were acquired with a GE-Signa 1.5T scanner (General Electric, Milwaukee, WI) located at one of three sites: University of California, San Diego Medical Center Magnetic Resonance Imaging Institute (N = 59), Scripps Clinic, San Diego (N = 53), or Stanford University (N = 5). Across all locations and in all cases, sagittal brain images were acquired with the same three-dimensional (3D) volumetric radio frequency spoiled gradient echo (spoiled gradient-recalled acquisition in a steady state) pulse sequence using the following scan parameters: repetition time, 24 msec; echo time, 5 msec; flip angle, 45°; number of excitations, 2; matrix size, 256 × 192; field of view, 24 cm; slice thickness, 1.2 mm; 124 contiguous slices.

The remaining participants (30 WS, 14 TD, AWSdel-03i~vi) underwent MRI on a GE-Signa 3.0 T scanner (General Electric, Milwaukee, WI) at Stanford University. In these cases, coronal brain images were acquired with a three-dimensional enhanced fast gradient echo (EFGRE3D) pulse sequence using the following scan parameters: repetition time, 6 msec; echo time, 1.5 msec; flip angle, 15°; number of excitations, 3; matrix size, 256 × 256; field of view, 24 cm; slice thickness, 1.5 mm; 124 contiguous slices.

Voxel Based Morphometry (VBM) Processing

VBM analyses of 42 WS and 40 TD MR images from the 1.5T scanners were performed using SPM5 (http://www.fil.ion.ucl.ac.uk/spm) and VBM5.1 (http://dbm.neuro.uni-jena.de/vbm). After bias correction, T1 images were segmented into gray matter, white matter and cerebral spinal fluid. Hidden Markov Random Field (prior probability weight 0.3) was used to encode spatial information through spatial constraints of neighboring voxels. Normalization was performed using both adult and custom templates created from the 42 individuals with WS and 40 with TD. Both Jacobian modulated (non-linear warping only; reflecting regional gray matter volume) and nonmodulated (reflecting gray matter density) images were smoothed with an isotropic Gaussian kernel with full-width at half-maximum (FWHM) of 8 mm. Analyses of gray matter density were performed to compare with our previous report on WS individuals [25]. Segmentation and normalization for each participant was confirmed by manual inspection of the images. These steps were repeated for the 30 WS and 14 TD MR images collected using 3.0T.

Regions of Interest (ROIs)

ROIs were restricted to brain regions that showed significant differences between WS and TD individuals in gray matter images processed using VBM (**Figure S1, Table S1**). Results comparing WS and TD are reported in **Supporting Results** and not in the **Main Text** because the results (from 1.5T) have been reported previously (e.g. [25]) and results from 3.0T are used to replicate our findings. Our particular interest was in the intraparietal sulcus (IPS; right more than left), thought to be critical for visuo-spatial processing, and the amgydala, orbitofrontal cortex and fusiform gyri (right more than left) thought to be critical for social cognition and face processing. While the amygdala did not reach significance comparing WS and TD with VBM, based on evidence that the amygdala is structurally and functionally abnormal in WS and its importance in socio-emotional functioning [25,26], this region was manually delineated as described below.

Volumetric Measures of the Amygdala

Amygdala volumes were obtained from delineation based on anatomical landmarks by trained research staff who followed a detailed protocol [25]. Briefly, the amygdala delineation was initiated on the coronal slice where the anterior commissure was best distinguished and proceeded in the posterior direction until both the amygdala and hippocampus were clearly visible on the same slice. Superior, inferior and lateral boundaries were each designated by prominent white matter tracks, while the medial boundary was designated by either white matter or cerebral spinal fluid. Inter-rater reliabilities for all volumes described in this study were ≥ 0.90 as determined by the intraclass correlation coefficient.

Univariate Analyses

Brain images of each AWSdel case processed using VBM were compared to the WS and TD datasets (see **Supporting Methods**). We generated two voxel-wise z-score maps per AWSdel case that indicated how each AWSdel's brain image deviated from WS and TD groups (thresholded at $z>1.96$ and $z<-1.96$, p's<0.05). For example, if a partial deletion case showed $|z|>1.96$ from one group and $|z|<1.96$ from the other, then it was determined that the partial deletion case resembled the latter group. In the case of the AWSdel-03 family (father and 5 children with same atypical WS deletion), after creating these thresholded z-score maps for each family member AWSdel-03i~vi, we further created probabilistic maps using the thresholded images to examine the proportion of family members that showed $z>1.96$ or $z<-1.96$. These z-score and probabilistic images allowed us to visualize whether each AWSdel case showed a relative propensity for WS-like versus TD-like neuroanatomical patterns.

Results comparing WS and TD groups utilizing standard SPM5 and custom templates (**Figure S1, Table S1**), gray matter volume and density (**Figure S1**), and 1.5T and 3.0T scanners (**Figure S2**) are also reported in **Supporting Results**. AWSdel results comparing standard gray matter volume and density (**Figure S3**) and 1.5T and 3.0T scanners (**Figure S4**), are also reported in **Supporting Results**. There were no observable differences in results obtained from different templates, measures (volume vs. density) and magnet strength that appeared to influence the current findings. Further, though age and gender were corrected for all imaging analyses, the results did not change; hence we report findings without these covariates.

Multivariate Pattern Classification Analyses (MVPA)

Cross-validated linear support vector machine (SVM) was utilized as the primary method of performing MVPA to accomplish two objectives. First, these analyses were conducted as a complementary approach to univariate analyses described above for investigating whether voxels in brain regions related to visuo-spatial functioning and social cognition would classify each AWSdel individual as belonging to either the WS or TD group. Second, MVPA was used to investigate whether each AWSdel individual would be classified as WS or TD when the entire population of either gray matter or white matter voxels were considered.

Voxels included in the MVPA were segmented using one of two approaches: 1) bilateral superior parietal lobules (SPL), orbitofrontal cortices (OFC), amygdalae and fusiform gyri were defined using the WFU PickAtlas (http://fmri.wfubmc.edu/cms/software#PickAtlas) and Automated Talairach Atlas Label (AAL) (http://www.cyceron.fr/freeware/), then coregistered to the modulated VBM gray matter images, and 2) masks comprising all brain gray or white matter voxels were obtained from the SPM5 generated segmentation. Non-smoothed images were down-sampled to 4mm voxels and voxel-by-subject matrices were created for each (set) of these brain regions. Linear support vector machine (SVM) analyses were performed (regularization parameter C = 1), with leave-one-out cross-validation using an in-house toolbox used in previous studies [27–33]. Feature reduction was performed using leave-one-out recursive feature elimination (RFE), recursively eliminating 30% of the voxels to identify the optimal performance [34,35]. A classifier from each of the leave-one-out cross-validation steps was applied to each AWSdel individual, allowing us to calculate the probability of each AWSdel individual being classified as an individual with WS or TD. As reference, visuo-spatial regions classified WS from TD at 100% accuracy, social regions at 95.1% accuracy, gray matter at 97.6% accuracy and white matter at 98.8% accuracy. These references indicate that MVPA is capable of classifying WS and TD controls and serves as a basis for performing further MVPA on AWSdel cases.

Results

Neuroanatomical and Behavioral Abnormalities Associated with Visuo-Spatial Function in Atypical WS Deletion Cases (AWSdel)

Results from the IPS, a region that plays a central role in visuo-spatial processing [36] and in which a specific cluster was defined from the between-group WS vs. TD comparison (see **Supporting Results, Figure S1**, and **Figure S2**), are shown in **Figure 2A and Table 3** (see also **Figure S3, Figure S4**). AWSdel-01 showed voxels with values exceeding $z>1.96$ compared to WS, but no voxels with values that were $|z|>1.96$ when compared to TD, indicating that AWSdel-01 shows IPS volumes within the distribution of TD. In AWSdel-02, voxels with values $z<-1.96$ compared to TD were found in the IPS, but no voxels with values that were $|z|>1.96$ when compared to WS, indicating that AWSdel-02 shows IPS volumes comparable to WS. Further, in AWSdel-03, all family members showed voxels with values within the range of TD ($|z|<1.96$) and greater than WS (all members showed $z>1.96$), indicating that AWSdel-03 shows IPS volumes similar to TD. Since MRI data of the AWSdel-03 family were collected from 3.0T rather than the 1.5T reference data from 42 WS and 40 TD participants, AWSdel-03 cases were also compared to the 3.0T reference dataset of 30 WS and 14 TD participants. Results from this 3.0T scanner comparison (**Figure S4**) were essentially identical to the 1.5T results in **Figure 2A**.

We created a classifier (model) designed to optimally discriminate between WS and TD using permutation-based MVPA.

Table 3. Z-scores of each WS atypical deletion case (AWSdel) from the WS or TD group in each brain region of interest: Left/right (Lt/Rt intraparietal sulcus (IPS), Rt orbitofrontal cortex (OFC), and Lt/Rt fusiform gyrus (FG).

	Lt IPS	Rt IPS	Rt OFC	Lt FG	Rt FG
AWSdel-01	6.00	5.28	7.79	8.02	9.74
AWSdel-02	−2.03	−2.65	2.15	3.20	2.26
AWSdel-03	3.41(2.12)	2.86(2.09)	3.28(1.36)	4.18(2.43)	2.55(0.77)

Numbers indicate # of Z scores above the TD group with the exception of AWSdel-02 Lt/Rt IPS which indicate Z scores below the WS group. When compared to WS, $Z<1.96$ except AWSdel-02 Rt Amyg was $Z=2.08$ compared to the WS group. AWSdel-03 family (03i ~ 03vi) are listed as the mean average of the 6 members and standard deviation in brackets.

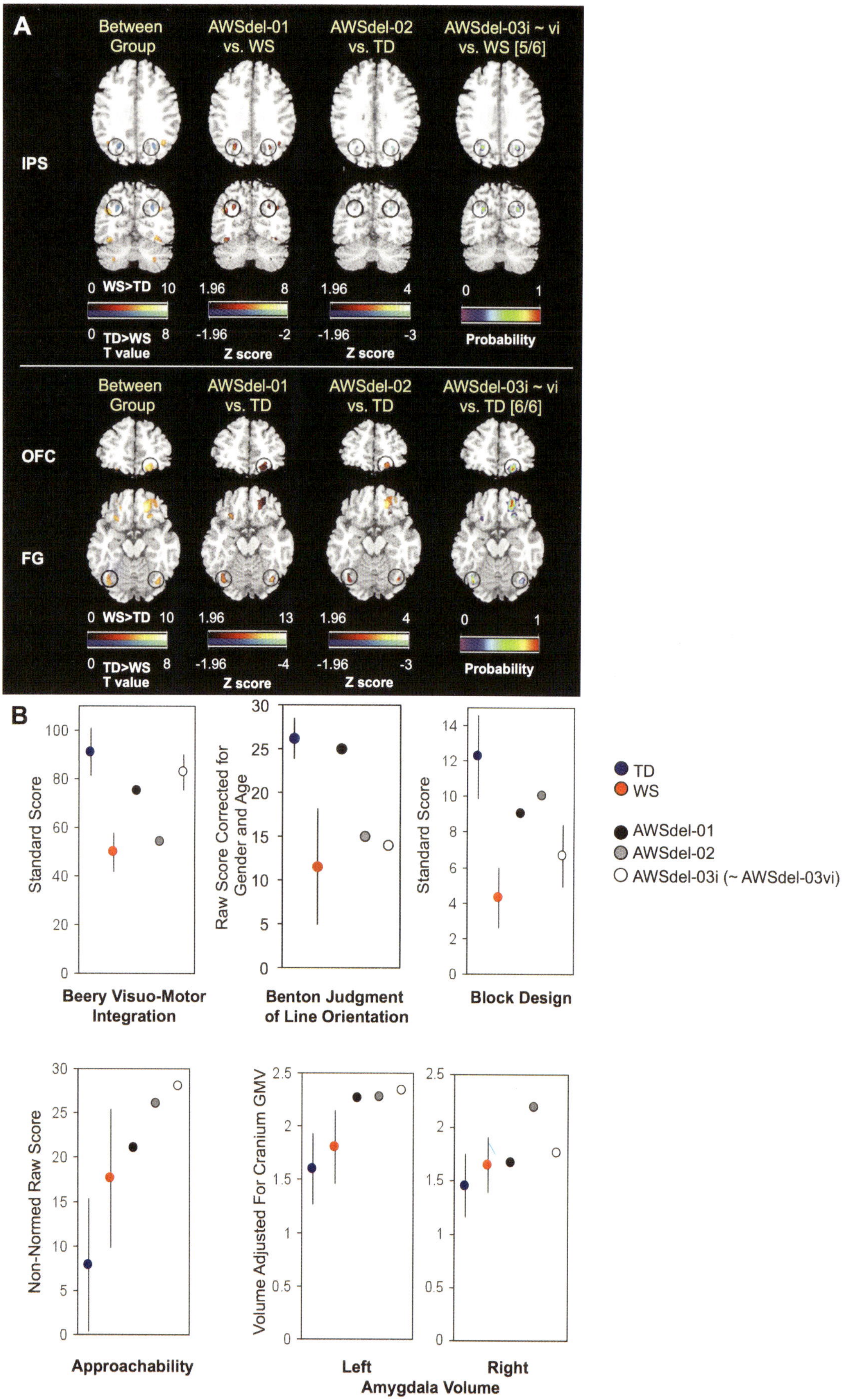
A
Between Group
AWSdel-01 vs. WS
AWSdel-02 vs. TD
AWSdel-03i ~ vi vs. WS [5/6]
IPS
0 WS>TD 10
0 TD>WS 8
T value
1.96 8
-1.96 -2
Z score
1.96 4
-1.96 -3
Z score
0 1
Probability
Between Group
AWSdel-01 vs. TD
AWSdel-02 vs. TD
AWSdel-03i ~ vi vs. TD [6/6]
OFC
FG
0 WS>TD 10
0 TD>WS 8
T value
1.96 13
-1.96 -4
Z score
1.96 4
-1.96 -3
Z score
0 1
Probability
B
Standard Score
Beery Visuo-Motor Integration
Raw Score Corrected for Gender and Age
Benton Judgment of Line Orientation
Standard Score
Block Design
TD
WS
AWSdel-01
AWSdel-02
AWSdel-03i (~ AWSdel-03vi)
Non-Normed Raw Score
Approachability
Volume Adjusted For Cranium GMV
Left
Right
Amygdala Volume

Figure 2. Gray matter volumes and cognitive profiles of typical WS, TD, and atypical deletion (AWSdel) individuals. A. Gray matter deviation maps in AWSdel individuals. First column represents VBM between group differences between WS (N = 42) and TD (N = 40). Second and third columns represent the degree to which atypical cases AWSdel-01 and AWSdel-02 deviated from the comparison group (thresholded at [z]> 1.96). The fourth column represents probability maps of how many participants showed positive deviation of z > 1.96 in AWSdel-03i~vi. Numbers in square-brackets in the fourth column indicate how many participants out of the total of 6 AWSdel-03 participants showed this deviation in its peak voxel. **B.** Cognitive measures and amygdala volumes (from manual volumetric measurements) are plotted for WS, TD and AWSdel groups. See **Table 1** for detailed statistics. Benton judgment of line and Social approachability scores are not plotted for the AWSdel-03 children (WSdel-03ii~vi) as age-adjusted normed scores are not available. IPS: intraparietal sulcus, OFC: orbitofrontal cortex, FG: fusiform gyrus, Lt: left, Rt: right. Error bars represent standard deviation. Left hemisphere is shown on the left side in the brain maps.

MVPA was performed using voxel intensity measures from objectively and anatomically defined left and right superior parietal lobules (SPL) within VBM processed images. Consistent with VBM results, using permutation-based analyses, AWSdel-01 and all AWSdel-03 family members were categorized as TD with 100% probability, and AWSdel-02 was categorized as WS with 100% probability.

Behavioral performance on visuo-spatial functions (Beery Visuo-Motor Integration, Benton Judgment of Line Orientation and Wechsler Block Design tasks) for each AWSdel case compared to that of WS and TD individuals generally paralleled the neuroanatomical results (**Table 1, 2, Figure 2B**). The results of this analysis showed that AWSdel-01 was within or closer to (for visuo-motor integration and block design) the range of TD, AWSdel-02 was within the range of WS (clearly for visuo-motor integration and judgment of line orientation, though not for block design), and AWSdel-03 was within the range of TD (though in this case only for visuo-motor integration and not for judgment of line orientation or block design). Overall, these results implicate *GTF2I* and/or *GTF2IRD1* as candidate genes contributing to altered IPS volumes and visuo-spatial function, in particular visuo-motor integration as consistent with previous animal [37] and human behavioral research [15,38] (**Figure 3**).

Neuroanatomical and Behavioral Abnormalities Associated with Social Cognitive Function in Atypical WS Deletion Cases (AWSdel)

Next, we examined morphometric patterns related to social cognitive function in AWSdel. All AWSdel cases showed increased volumes in bilateral fusiform gyri and the right orbitofrontal cortex (OFC) compared to TD ($z>1.96$); this profile was similar to typical WS participants ($|z|<1.96$) (**Figure 2A, Table 3, Figure S3, Figure S4**). In the manually delineated amygdala, we found that WS showed significantly greater gray matter volume in bilateral amygdala compared to TD (**Table 1**). In the left amygdala, all AWSdel cases showed increased volume compared to TD ($z>1.96$), which was similar to WS ($|z|<1.96$) (**Figure 2B**). Using permutation-based MVPA, we observed that a combination of objectively defined amygdala, OFC and fusiform gyrus regions of interest showed 100% probability (using permutation-based analysis) that all AWSdel cases would be categorized as WS.

Subject performance on social behavior (Adolph's social approachability test) for each AWSdel case was compared to average social behavior scores in WS and TD groups. The results of this analysis showed that all AWSdel cases exhibited increased sociability relative to TD controls, again paralleling the neuroanatomical findings (**Table 2, Figure 2B**). Each case was more similar to the WS group relative to the TD group. There are several genes commonly deleted in our typical WS and AWSdel groups (genes located between *ABHD11* and *RFC2*). However, one gene in particular, *LIMK1*, is known to affect brain development [39], thus suggesting that haploinsufficiency of *LIMK1* as one potential explanation for aberrant OFC, fusiform and amygdala volumes, as well as abnormalities of social approachability in WS (**Figure 3**).

Neuroanatomical Abnormalities of Overall Gray and White Matter Patterns in Atypical WS Deletion Cases (AWSdel)

In our final analyses, we applied cross-validated MVPA to investigate gene(s) that potentially contribute to distinct patterns as derived from voxel-by-voxel volumes comprising the entire gray matter and white matter compartments. Using permutation-based analyses, gray matter results showed that, similar to visuo-spatial processing, AWSdel-01 was categorized as TD with 89.0% probability (and hence as WS with 11% probability), AWSdel-02 as WS with 100% probability and all AWSdel-03 family members as TD with 100% probability. White matter results indicated that AWSdel-01 was categorized as WS with 98.9% probability, AWSdel-02 as WS with 100% probability and AWSdel-03 family members as TD with 100% probability. These results suggest that gray matter structure varies with the presence or absence of *GTF2I/GTF2IRD1*, while white matter structure is most related to the status of genes in the region of *STX1A* and *CYLN2* which are common to AWSdel-01 and AWSdel-02 but outside the deletion in AWSdel-03 (**Figure 3**). Deleted genes in WS that are particularly important in the regulation of cytoskeletal dynamics and possibly in white matter development are *LIMK1*, *STX1A*, *CYLN2 and* possibly *FZD9* [4,40]. Among these genes, *STX1A* and *CYLN2* are deleted in AWSdel-01 and AWSdel-02 and are spared in AWSdel-03 raising the possibility that *STX1A* and *CYLN2* may be among the genes involved in white matter development in WS.

Discussion

Our results provide evidence implicating particular genes in the development of brain structures involved in visuo-spatial function and social cognition in humans. If the contribution of single genes is measureable and related to the characteristic pattern that we observe in this study, the findings indicate a role for *GTF2I* and/or *GTF2IRD1* in IPS volumes known to be involved in visuo-spatial function, and more generally, in patterns of gray matter structure; the *LIMK1* region (and possibly other genes located between *ABHD11* through *RFC2*) in the volumes of the amygdala, OFC and fusiform gyrus, which are known to be involved in social approachability; and *CYLN2/STX1A* in white matter development.

The right IPS has been consistently shown to be involved in visuo-spatial constructions, including visuo-motor integration [36]. Evidence suggests that visuo-motor deficits may be one of the most characteristic features of WS [41], and the IPS results in our 8 atypical cases (with 3 different patterns of atypical deletions) point to *GTF2I* and/or *GTF2IRD1* as critical for the performance of these tasks, as suggested previously [15,38]. The way by which these genes affect the anatomy and behavior demonstrated in this study is not known. *GTF2I* encodes a multifunctional phospho-

A

	Neuroanatomical Measures					Neuropsychological Measures		
VISUO-SPATIAL RELATED NEUROANATOMY								
	Left IPS	**Right IPS**	MVPA			**VMI**	**JLO**	**Block Des.**
Typical WS	Reduced	Reduced	Class. as WS			Reduced	Reduced	Reduced
AWSdel-01 (#5623)	Normal	Normal	Class. as TD			Normal	Normal	Normal
AWSdel-02 (#5657)	Reduced	Reduced	Class. as WS			Reduced	Reduced	Normal
AWSdel-03i~vi (#5882, 5884-5888)	Normal	Normal	Class. as TD			Normal	Reduced	Reduced
Summary	Strongly suggestive of association with AWS-del-02 specific deletion.							
SOCIABILITY RELATED NEUROANATOMY								
	Lt Amyg	**Rt Amyg**	**OFC**	**FG**	MVPA	**Approach.**		
Typical WS	Increased	Increased	Increased	Increased	Class. as WS	Increased		
AWSdel-01 (#5623)	Increased	Increased	Increased	Increased	Class. as WS	Increased		
AWSdel-02 (#5657)	Increased	Increased	Increased	Increased	Class. as WS	Increased		
AWSdel-03i~vi (#5882, 5884-5888)	Increased	Increased	Increased	Increased	Class. as WS	Increased		
Summary	Strongly suggestive of association with deletion common to all AWS.							
GREY MATTER (GM) PATTERN								
	GM MVPA							
Typical WS	Class. as WS							
AWSdel-01 (#5623)	Class. as TD							
AWSdel-02 (#5657)	Class. as WS							
AWSdel-03i~vi (#5882, 5884-5888)	Class. as TD							
Summary	Strongly suggestive of association with AWS-del-02 specific deletion.							
WHITE MATTER (WM) PATTERN								
	WM MVPA							
Typical WS	Class. as WS							
AWSdel-01 (#5623)	Class. as WS							
AWSdel-02 (#5657)	Class. as WS							
AWSdel-03i~vi (#5882, 5884-5888)	Class. as TD							
Summary	Strongly suggestive of association with AWS-del-01 & 02 specific deletion.							

B

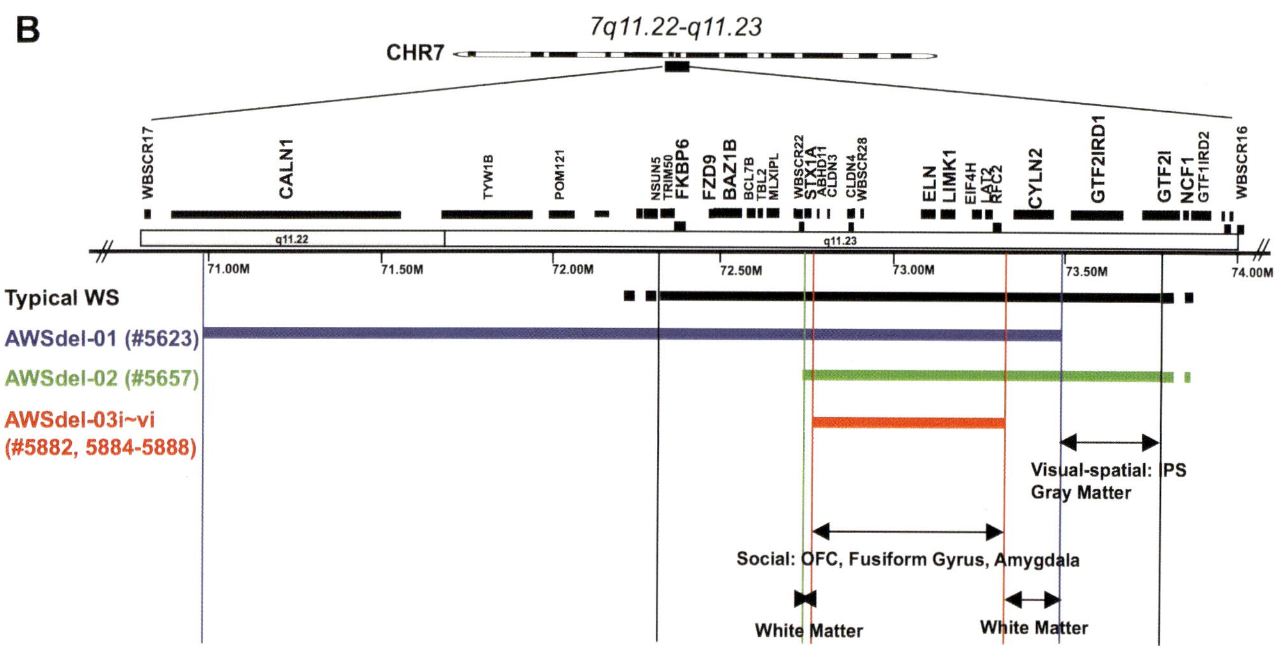

Figure 3. Schematic table (A) and diagram (B) that represent summary of findings.

protein with roles in transcription and signal transduction [42]. The protein encoded by *GTF2IRD1* contains five GTF2I-like repeats and functions as a transcription factor or as a positive transcriptional regulator under the control of the Retinoblastoma protein. Both *Gtf2i* and *Gtf2ird1* are widely expressed in the brain during the embryonic stages of mouse development [43]. In adult mice, they are present exclusively in neurons, but the two proteins play nonredundant, differentially regulated roles, despite their similar structure. At present, the specific genes whose expression are most affected by these regulatory genes are not known. Nor is it known how, and to what extent, *Gtf2i* and *Gtf2ird1* are explicitly involved in IPS morphometric variability, although converging evidence from our previous behavioral study [15] suggests *GTF2IRD1* to be principally responsible.

The cognitive profiles examined here, though partially consistent with the anatomical findings, showed some discrepancies. Visuo-motor integration was consistent with IPS volume findings throughout all cases, but judgment of line orientation and block design results were inconsistent in the AWSdel-03 family (i.e., judgment of line orientation and block design showed more WS-like patterns even though IPS and visuo-motor integration showed TD-like patterns). However, this is not altogether surprising, since behavior is downstream to genetics and neuroanatomy, and hence may be influenced in many different ways that are difficult to reliably assess (as opposed to the more upstream neuroanatomical measure) [1]. Alternatively, it may be that in WS, *GTF2I/GTF2IRD1* have greater involvement in IPS and visual construction and motor components (represented by visuo-motor integration) than visual perceptual functions (represented by judgment of line orientation and block design). In addition, multiple WS genes could contribute to decreased visual perceptual functions.

There is limited behavioral research on WS with partial deletions [11–15]. The current findings replicate our previous report showing the important role of *GTF2IRD1* in visuo-spatial abilities [15]. However, our study results contradict other behavioral studies of visuo-spatial abilities [11–15]. Karmiloff-Smith et al. [11] reported an atypical deletion case with a deletion from *FKBP6* to *GTF2IRDI* and showed this case to be associated with relatively spared visual-spatial functioning and abnormal social behavior. Antonell et al. [13] reported that the deletion of *GTF2I* and *GTF2IRD1* may contribute to the global intellectual deficit and some aspects of the cognitive profile but not visuo-spatial ability. Tassabehji et al. [12] and Gray et al. [14] showed an association between *LIMK1* and visual-spatial construction.

One of the most striking features of WS is gregariousness, reduced fear for strangers, and relative preservation of a subset of face processing skills. The amygdala is known to be an important component of the neural systems involved in retrieving socially relevant knowledge on the basis of facial features, in particular approachability and trustworthiness [24], probably through its role in regulating fear. Further, the OFC is known to regulate amygdala reactivity through a frontal-amygdala-insular circuit that provides feedback about somatic state activation, which aids in social decision-making [44,45] and empathy [46,47]. Finally, the (right) fusiform gyrus is considered to be a face processing region that is particularly important for normal social interactions, and provides input to the anterior limbic regions [48]. Typical WS and all AWSdel participants in this study who have deletions of genes from *ABHD11* through *RFC2* including *LIMK1*, showed developmental anomalies of the amygdala, OFC and/or fusiform cortex. *LIMK1* is a particularly a strong candidate among the deleted genes for playing a role in the anomalous neuroanatomical pattern described above because of its known role in brain function and dendritic spine architecture [39],

LIMK1 is thought to be a component of an intracellular signaling pathway involved in brain development. In particular, *LIMK1* controls actin dynamics via phosphorylation of cofilin, and has been implicated in the control of growth cone motility in cultured neurons [49] and in white matter development [50]. It is difficult to disentangle from our study which neurobiological pathways or neural structures are more directly influenced by *LIMK1* and which brain regions are affected by a combination of interactions among genes in the deleted regions. Nevertheless, it is attractive to propose *LIMK1*, as one gene contributing to abnormal social cognitive profiles in WS, either via impaired input from higher-level visual (fusiform face) areas or through interactions between the OFC and amygdala. It is important to note that these effects may derive from both pre- and post-natal effects on brain development or adult function. Future studies examining the causal relationship of brain activation patterns within these structures in the context of social-affective processing will be of interest.

There are several genes that have been implicated in WS social cognition. Although *LIMK1* was an attractive target, there is only one animal study to date that has suggested a role for *LIMK1* in social cognition (fear responses) and this finding was interpreted within the context of impaired learning and hippocampal function [39]. In other studies, *LIMK1* has only been implicated in visuo-spatial function [51]. In contrast, recent literature on social cognition in WS points to a potential role for *GTF2I/GTF2IRD1* [15,43,52], regions between *LIMK1* and *GTF2I/GTF2IRD1* [53], or regions between *FKBP6* and *GTF2IRD1* [11]. These genes are further implicated by mice with heterozygous or homozygous disruption of *Gtf2ird1* who exhibit decreased fear, aggression and anxiety and increased social behaviors as well as increased levels of serotonin metabolites in the amygdala and frontal cortex [43]. Future studies using multiple standardized and non-standardized behavioral measures, in larger samples in conjunction with heterozygous animal models, which can examine single genes at a time, and examining both brain structure and cognitive and social profiles, are warranted.

Finally, *LIMK1*, *CYLN2* and possibly *FZD9* have been implicated in WM development. For example, *LIMK1* and *CYLN2* are known to regulate cytoskeletal dynamics, axon guidance and neuronal migration, and *FZD9* may be critical for dendritic development and axon guidance [4,40]. Our results suggested that genes, including *STX1A* and/or *CYLN2*, may contribute to WM development in WS.

Mice with heterozygous and homozygous disruptions of particular genes are potentially ideal models to study gene-brain-behavior associations, but the behavioral tests available can be limited depending on the behavior/cognitive function of interest. Further, the same genes in humans may not have the same regulatory pathways and expression patterns as that occurring in the brains of non-humans [11]. Some animal studies showing statistical differences between wild-type and homozygous knockout mice fail to demonstrate comparable differences when using heterozygous mice, the genetic state most applicable to WS. Further, the scarcity of AWSdel cases have resulted in only one or two cases described in each report [11–15]. These factors have made it difficult to attribute specific cognitive functions to particular sets of genes. Our study attempted to overcome some of these limitations by examining eight individuals with three types of varying atypical deletions, while also assessing brain structure for the first time in AWSdel cases.

A major limitation is that our current level of analysis only allows attribution of subsets of genes to neuroanatomical and cognitive findings. It is likely that there is more than one contributory gene, gene-gene interactions within and outside the WS deletion, as well as environmental influences and stochastic processes that could contribute to neuroanatomical variations. Another limitation is that, similar to typical controls, individuals with WS demonstrate inter-individual differences in neuropsychological and behavioral function and hence future studies employing more sensitive experimental behavioral measures are warranted. Further, while this is the first study to utilize AWSdel to examine gene-brain-behavior relationships, the small sample-size (8 cases with 3 patterns of deletions) will necessitate replication in future studies. Finally, in contrast to neuroanatomical volumes that are more readily quantified, pinpointing a relationship of these to behavior or cognition is limited by the extent to which a given paradigm mirrors the function of the structure. Therefore, as a first step, we have focused on demonstrating that individuals with AWSdel exhibit structural brain patterns or cognitive profiles that are either consistent or inconsistent with typical WS or TD. Future studies will be useful in refining structure-function relationships in, as well as interactions/connectivity amongst these regions; such studies can help to narrow gene candidates that alter the development or function of specific functional human brain circuits.

In summary, we show that the current preliminary study in individuals with rare, atypical deletions associated with WS provide new insights into the neural mechanisms of cognitive function and putative genetic underpinnings. These studies of intermediate endophenotypes should prompt future research into the relevance of variation in these genes, gene-gene interactions, and developmental and individual differences in gene expression, for regional brain development and normal visuo-spatial function and social behavior.

Supporting Information

Figure S1 Gray matter volume and density differences between WS (N = 42) and TD (N = 40) groups in 1.5T MRI data. Either a custom template created including all WS and TD participants or a standard template provided by SPM5 was used. $p = 0.05$ family-wise error (FWE), extent threshold (ET) = 100.

Figure S2 Gray matter volume measures from the two separate scan parameters (1.5T WS: N = 42, TD: N = 40; 3.0T WS: N = 30, TD = 14) in the regions of interest (ROIs) are plotted and compared. See Main Text Methods for definition of ROIs and how bilateral intraparietal sulcus (IPS), right orbitofrontal cortex (OFC) and right fusiform gyrus (FG) were defined. The results are very similar between the two datasets (~*: $0.05 < p < 0.10$, **: $0.01 < p < 0.05$, ***: $p < 0.001$).

Figure S3 Gray matter density deviation maps of WS atypical deletion (AWSdel) cases. Identical to Figure 2A, but examining gray matter density rather than volume.

Figure S4 Probabilistic maps of participants AWSdel-03i~vi (collected on a 3.0T scanner). Identical to Figure 2A 4th column (which is for gray mater volume) and Figure S3 4th column, with the exception that Figure S4 uses WS and TD data from 3.0T MRI as comparison groups to match scan parameters with AWSdel-03i~vi.

Table S1 Gray matter volume differences between WS (N = 42) and TD (N = 40) groups. A custom template was used. $p = 0.05$ family-wise error (FWE), extent threshold (ET) = 100.
(DOCX)

File S1 Textual supporting information.

Author Contributions

Conceived and designed the experiments: JK DM AG UB AR. Performed the experiments: FH JK UB AR AR LD AG. Analyzed the data: FH JK AR LD MM BH KS. Contributed reagents/materials/analysis tools: FH LD JK. Wrote the paper: FH AR JK LD.

References

1. Meyer-Lindenberg A, Weinberger DR (2006) Intermediate phenotypes and genetic mechanisms of psychiatric disorders. Nat Rev Neurosci 7: 818–827.
2. Korbel JO, Tirosh-Wagner T, Urban AE, Chen XN, Kasowski M, et al. (2009) The genetic architecture of Down syndrome phenotypes revealed by high-resolution analysis of human segmental trisomies. Proc Natl Acad Sci U S A 106: 12031–12036.
3. Hillier LW, Fulton RS, Fulton LA, Graves TA, Pepin KH, et al. (2003) The DNA sequence of human chromosome 7. Nature 424: 157–164.
4. Meyer-Lindenberg A, Mervis CB, Berman KF (2006) Neural mechanisms in Williams syndrome: a unique window to genetic influences on cognition and behaviour. Nat Rev Neurosci 7: 380–393.
5. Jabbi M, Kippenhan JS, Kohn P, Marenco S, Mervis CB, et al. (2012) The Williams syndrome chromosome 7q11.23 hemideletion confers hypersocial, anxious personality coupled with altered insula structure and function. Proc Natl Acad Sci U S A 109: E860–866.
6. Meyer-Lindenberg A, Kohn P, Mervis CB, Kippenhan JS, Olsen RK, et al. (2004) Neural basis of genetically determined visuospatial construction deficit in Williams syndrome. Neuron 43: 623–631.
7. Meyer-Lindenberg A, Hariri AR, Munoz KE, Mervis CB, Mattay VS, et al. (2005) Neural correlates of genetically abnormal social cognition in Williams syndrome. Nat Neurosci 8: 991–993.
8. Golarai G, Hong S, Haas BW, Galaburda AM, Mills DL, et al. (2010) The fusiform face area is enlarged in Williams syndrome. J Neurosci 30: 6700–6712.
9. Haas BW, Hoeft F, Barnea-Goraly N, Golarai G, Bellugi U, et al. (2012) Preliminary evidence of abnormal white matter related to the fusiform gyrus in Williams syndrome: a diffusion tensor imaging tractography study. Genes Brain Behav 11: 62–68.
10. Pober BR (2010) Williams-Beuren syndrome. N Engl J Med 362: 239–252.
11. Karmiloff-Smith A, Broadbent H, Farran EK, Longhi E, D'Souza D, et al. (2012) Social cognition in williams syndrome: genotype/phenotype insights from partial deletion patients. Front Psychol 3: 168.
12. Tassabehji M, Metcalfe K, Karmiloff-Smith A, Carette MJ, Grant J, et al. (1999) Williams syndrome: use of chromosomal microdeletions as a tool to dissect cognitive and physical phenotypes. Am J Hum Genet 64: 118–125.
13. Antonell A, Del Campo M, Magano LF, Kaufmann L, de la Iglesia JM, et al. (2010) Partial 7q11.23 deletions further implicate GTF2I and GTF2IRD1 as the main genes responsible for the Williams-Beuren syndrome neurocognitive profile. Journal of medical genetics 47: 312–320.
14. Gray V, Karmiloff-Smith A, Funnell E, Tassabehji M (2006) In-depth analysis of spatial cognition in Williams syndrome: A critical assessment of the role of the LIMK1 gene. Neuropsychologia 44: 679–685.
15. Dai L, Bellugi U, Chen XN, Pulst-Korenberg AM, Jarvinen-Pasley A, et al. (2009) Is it Williams syndrome? GTF2IRD1 implicated in visual-spatial construction and GTF2I in sociability revealed by high resolution arrays. Am J Med Genet A 149A: 302–314.
16. Korenberg JR, Chen XN, Hirota H, Lai Z, Bellugi U, et al. (2000) VI. Genome structure and cognitive map of Williams syndrome. J Cogn Neurosci 12 Suppl 1: 89–107.
17. Osborne LR, Campbell T, Daradich A, Scherer SW, Tsui LC (1999) Identification of a putative transcription factor gene (WBSCR11) that is commonly deleted in Williams-Beuren syndrome. Genomics 57: 279–284.
18. Mills DL, Dai L, Yam A, Fishman I, Bellugi U, et al. (in revision) Genetic mapping of brain activity in Williams Syndrome: ERP markers of face and language processing are stable across development. Developmental Neuropsychology.
19. Korenberg JR, Dai L, Bellugi U, Järvinen-Pasley A, Mills DL, et al. (2008) Deletion of 7q11.23 Genes and Williams Syndrome. In: Epstein CJ, Erickson RP, Wynshaw-Boris A, editors. Inborn Errors of Development. 2nd ed. Oxford, U.K.: Oxford University Press. pp. 1544–1555.
20. Wechsler D (1997) Wechsler Adult Intelligence Scale. San Antonio, TX USA: The Psychological Corporation.
21. Wechsler D (1991) Wechsler intelligence scale for children. New York: The Psychological Corporation.
22. Beery KE, Bulktenica NA (1997) Developmental test of Visual-Motor Integration, revised. Parsippany, NJ USA: Modern Curriculum Press.
23. Benton AL, Hamsher KD, Varney NR, Spreen O (1983) Contributions to neuropsychological assessment: A clinical manual. New York, NYC: Oxford University Press.
24. Adolphs R, Tranel D, Damasio AR (1998) The human amygdala in social judgment. Nature 393: 470–474.
25. Reiss AL, Eckert MA, Rose FE, Karchemskiy A, Kesler S, et al. (2004) An experiment of nature: brain anatomy parallels cognition and behavior in Williams syndrome. J Neurosci 24: 5009–5015.
26. Haas BW, Mills D, Yam A, Hoeft F, Bellugi U, et al. (2009) Genetic influences on sociability: heightened amygdala reactivity and event-related responses to

positive social stimuli in Williams syndrome. Journal of Neuroscience 29: 1132–1139.
27. Tanaka H, Black JM, Hulme C, Stanley LM, Kesler SR, et al. (2011) The brain basis of the phonological deficit in dyslexia is independent of IQ. Psychol Sci 22: 1442–1451.
28. Marzelli MJ, Hoeft F, Hong DS, Reiss AL (2011) Neuroanatomical spatial patterns in Turner syndrome. Neuroimage 55: 439–447.
29. Hoeft F, Walter E, Lightbody AA, Hazlett HC, Chang C, et al. (2011) Neuroanatomical differences in toddler boys with fragile x syndrome and idiopathic autism. Arch Gen Psychiatry 68: 295–305.
30. Hoeft F, McCandliss BD, Black JM, Gantman A, Zakerani N, et al. (2011) Neural systems predicting long-term outcome in dyslexia. Proc Natl Acad Sci U S A 108: 361–366.
31. Hoeft F, Lightbody AA, Hazlett HC, Patnaik S, Piven J, et al. (2008) Morphometric spatial patterns differentiating boys with fragile X syndrome, typically developing boys, and developmentally delayed boys aged 1 to 3 years. Arch Gen Psychiatry 65: 1087–1097.
32. Gothelf D, Hoeft F, Ueno T, Sugiura L, Lee AD, et al. (2011) Developmental changes in multivariate neuroanatomical patterns that predict risk for psychosis in 22q11.2 deletion syndrome. J Psychiatr Res 45: 322–331.
33. Etkin A, Prater KE, Hoeft F, Menon V, Schatzberg AF (2010) Failure of anterior cingulate activation and connectivity with the amygdala during implicit regulation of emotional processing in generalized anxiety disorder. Am J Psychiatry 167: 545–554.
34. De Martino F, Valente G, Staeren N, Ashburner J, Goebel R, et al. (2008) Combining multivariate voxel selection and support vector machines for mapping and classification of fMRI spatial patterns. Neuroimage 43: 44–58.
35. Formisano E, De Martino F, Bonte M, Goebel R (2008) "Who" is saying "what"? Brain-based decoding of human voice and speech. Science 322: 970–973.
36. Jackson SR, Husain M (2006) Visuomotor functions of the posterior parietal cortex. Neuropsychologia 44: 2589–2593.
37. Edelmann L, Prosnitz A, Pardo S, Bhatt J, Cohen N, et al. (2007) An atypical deletion of the Williams-Beuren syndrome interval implicates genes associated with defective visuospatial processing and autism. J Med Genet 44: 136–143.
38. Hirota H, Matsuoka R, Chen XN, Salandanan LS, Lincoln A, et al. (2003) Williams syndrome deficits in visual spatial processing linked to GTF2IRD1 and GTF2I on chromosome 7q11.23. Genet Med 5: 311–321.
39. Meng Y, Zhang Y, Tregoubov V, Janus C, Cruz L, et al. (2002) Abnormal spine morphology and enhanced LTP in LIMK-1 knockout mice. Neuron 35: 121–133.
40. Marenco S, Siuta MA, Kippenhan JS, Grodofsky S, Chang WL, et al. (2007) Genetic contributions to white matter architecture revealed by diffusion tensor imaging in Williams syndrome. Proc Natl Acad Sci U S A 104: 15117–15122.
41. Hocking DR, Bradshaw JL, Rinehart NJ (2007) Fronto-parietal and cerebellar contributions to motor dysfunction in Williams syndrome: A review and future directions. Neurosci Biobehav Rev.
42. Caraveo G, van Rossum DB, Patterson RL, Snyder SH, Desiderio S (2006) Action of TFII-I outside the nucleus as an inhibitor of agonist-induced calcium entry. Science 314: 122–125.
43. Young EJ, Lipina T, Tam E, Mandel A, Clapcote SJ, et al. (2007) Reduced fear and aggression and altered serotonin metabolism in Gtf2ird1-targeted mice. Genes Brain Behav.
44. Bar-On R, Tranel D, Denburg NL, Bechara A (2003) Exploring the neurological substrate of emotional and social intelligence. Brain 126: 1790–1800.
45. Davidson RJ, Putnam KM, Larson CL (2000) Dysfunction in the neural circuitry of emotion regulation—a possible prelude to violence. Science 289: 591–594.
46. Blair RJ (2001) Neurocognitive models of aggression, the antisocial personality disorders, and psychopathy. J Neurol Neurosurg Psychiatry 71: 727–731.
47. Fine C, Lumsden J, Blair RJ (2001) Dissociation between 'theory of mind' and executive functions in a patient with early left amygdala damage. Brain 124: 287–298.
48. Kanwisher N, Yovel G (2006) The fusiform face area: a cortical region specialized for the perception of faces. Philos Trans R Soc Lond B Biol Sci 361: 2109–2128.
49. Proschel C, Blouin MJ, Gutowski NJ, Ludwig R, Noble M (1995) Limk1 is predominantly expressed in neural tissues and phosphorylates serine, threonine and tyrosine residues in vitro. Oncogene 11: 1271–1281.
50. Sparrow N, Manetti ME, Bott M, Fabianac T, Petrilli A, et al. (2012) The actin-severing protein cofilin is downstream of neuregulin signaling and is essential for Schwann cell myelination. J Neurosci 32: 5284–5297.
51. Frangiskakis JM, Ewart AK, Morris CA, Mervis CB, Bertrand J, et al. (1996) LIM-kinase1 hemizygosity implicated in impaired visuospatial constructive cognition. Cell 86: 59–69.
52. Sakurai T, Dorr NP, Takahashi N, McInnes LA, Elder GA, et al. (2011) Haploinsufficiency of Gtf2i, a gene deleted in Williams Syndrome, leads to increases in social interactions. Autism Res 4: 28–39.
53. Li HH, Roy M, Kuscuoglu U, Spencer CM, Halm B, et al. (2009) Induced chromosome deletions cause hypersociability and other features of Williams-Beuren syndrome in mice. EMBO Mol Med 1: 50–65.
54. Bernard O, Ganiatsas S, Kannourakis G, Dringen R (1994) Kiz-1, a protein with LIM zinc finger and kinase domains, is expressed mainly in neurons. Cell Growth Differ 5: 1159–1171.
55. Wang YK, Sporle R, Paperna T, Schughart K, Francke U (1999) Characterization and expression pattern of the frizzled gene Fzd9, the mouse homolog of FZD9 which is deleted in Williams-Beuren syndrome. Genomics 57: 235–248.
56. Fujiwara T, Mishima T, Kofuji T, Chiba T, Tanaka K, et al. (2006) Analysis of knock-out mice to determine the role of HPC-1/syntaxin 1A in expressing synaptic plasticity. J Neurosci 26: 5767–5776.
57. Hoogenraad CC, Eussen BH, Langeveld A, van Haperen R, Winterberg S, et al. (1998) The murine CYLN2 gene: genomic organization, chromosome localization, and comparison to the human gene that is located within the 7q11.23 Williams syndrome critical region. Genomics 53: 348–358.
58. Wang YK, Perez-Jurado LA, Francke U (1998) A mouse single-copy gene, Gtf2i, the homolog of human GTF2I, that is duplicated in the Williams-Beuren syndrome deletion region. Genomics 48: 163–170.
59. Palmer SJ, Tay ES, Santucci N, Cuc Bach TT, Hook J, et al. (2007) Expression of Gtf2ird1, the Williams syndrome-associated gene, during mouse development. Gene Expr Patterns 7: 396–404.

Neurofibromatosis Type 2 Tumor Suppressor Protein, NF2, Induces Proteasome-Mediated Degradation of JC Virus T-Antigen in Human Glioblastoma

Sarah Beltrami[1,2], Emanuela Branchetti[1], Ilker K. Sariyer[1], Jessica Otte[1], Michael Weaver[3], Jennifer Gordon[1]*

1 Department of Neuroscience and Center for Neurovirology, Temple University School of Medicine, Philadelphia, Pennsylvania, United States of America, **2** Biomedical Neuroscience Graduate Program, Temple University School of Medicine, Philadelphia, Pennsylvania, United States of America, **3** Department of Neurosurgery, Temple University School of Medicine, Philadelphia, Pennsylvania, United States of America

Abstract

Neurofibromatosis type 2 protein (NF2) has been shown to act as tumor suppressor primarily through its functions as a cytoskeletal scaffold. However, NF2 can also be found in the nucleus, where its role is less clear. Previously, our group has identified JC virus (JCV) tumor antigen (T-antigen) as a nuclear binding partner for NF2 in tumors derived from JCV T-antigen transgenic mice. The association of NF2 with T-antigen in neuronal origin tumors suggests a potential role for NF2 in regulating the expression of the JCV T-antigen. Here, we report that NF2 suppresses T-antigen protein expression in U-87 MG human glioblastoma cells, which subsequently reduces T-antigen-mediated regulation of the JCV promoter. When T-antigen mRNA was quantified, it was determined that increasing expression of NF2 correlated with an accumulation of T-antigen mRNA; however, a decrease in T-antigen at the protein level was observed. NF2 was found to promote degradation of ubiquitin bound T-antigen protein via a proteasome dependent pathway concomitant with the accumulation of the JCV early mRNA encoding T-antigen. The interaction between T-antigen and NF2 maps to the FERM domain of NF2, which has been shown previously to be responsible for its tumor suppressor activity. Co-immunoprecipitation assays revealed a ternary complex among NF2, T-antigen, and the tumor suppressor protein, p53 within a glioblastoma cell line. Further, these proteins were detected in various degrees in patient tumor tissue, suggesting that these associations may occur *in vivo*. Collectively, these results demonstrate that NF2 negatively regulates JCV T-antigen expression by proteasome-mediated degradation, and suggest a novel role for NF2 as a suppressor of JCV T-antigen-induced cell cycle regulation.

Editor: Joseph S. Pagano, The University of North Carolina at Chapel Hill, United States of America

Funding: This investigation was sponsored by the National Institutes of Health under a Ruth L. Kirchstein National Research Service Award (1T32MH079785) providing support to Sarah Beltrami. This study utilized services offered by core facilities of the Comprehensive NeuroAIDS Center (CNAC NIMH Grant Number P30MH092177) at Temple University School of Medicine. The funders had no role in study design, data collection and analysis, decision to publish, or preparation of the manuscript.

Competing Interests: The authors have declared that no competing interests exist.

* E-mail: jennifer.gordon@temple.edu

Introduction

Disruption of the Neurofibromatosis type 2 (*NF2*) gene, on human chromosome 22, leads to the development of the autosomal dominant disorder Neurofibromatosis type 2, characterized by the development of schwannomas, meningiomas, and ependymomas [1]. Though these tumors are typically benign, NF2 loss has been implicated in the progression of many malignant tumors including highly aggressive mesothelioma tumors in humans [2,3] and mice with heterozygous loss of NF2 are prone to the formation of multiple highly metastatic tumors, predominantly osteosarcomas and fibrosarcomas [4]. Loss of NF2 in glial cultures can lead to hyperproliferation, and formation of tumors in animal models [5–7]. Expression of NF2 has been shown to be absent in certain human glioblastomas and reintroduction can greatly suppress their growth [8–10].

The NF2 tumor suppressor protein is a member of the ERM family of proteins, which primarily facilitate cell to cell adhesion [11–13]. NF2 is responsive to cell confluence and growth factor availability [14–16]. Consequently, NF2 aides in the maintenance of contact inhibition of cell growth and anchorage dependence, whereby loss of NF2 facilitates invasion and mobility of transformed cells [6,17,18,28]. NF2 is different from prototypical tumor suppressor proteins, such as p53, in that it is not known to directly affect the cell cycle, but rather acts as a crucial link between the extracellular environment and cell signaling pathways [14,19]. Theories on the tumor suppressive roles of NF2 have largely been restricted to its actions as a scaffolding protein, however NF2 can be found in the nucleus, where its nuclear localization appears to be mediated by the cell cycle [20–22].

Previously, we have discovered the interaction of NF2 with the major regulatory protein of the human polyomavirus, JC virus (JCV), large tumor antigen (T-antigen), in malignant peripheral nerve sheath tumors (mpnsts) derived from JCV T-antigen transgenic mice [23]. JCV persistently infects the majority of individuals worldwide and is the causative agent of the rare but fatal demyelinating disease, progressive multifocal leukoencephalopathy, PML [24]. In addition to its role in PML pathogenesis,

JCV has exhibited oncogenic potential in cell culture and experimental animal models where T-antigen expression leads to a broad range of CNS malignancies, most notably the formation of neuronal and glial origin tumors including medulloblastomas, astrocytomas, and primitive neuroectodermal tumors. JCV DNA or T-antigen protein expression has been detected in a similarly broad range of human tumors including medulloblastomas, astrocytomas, ependymomas, as well as CNS lymphomas and tumors of the gastrointestinal tract [25].

Potential mechanisms of JCV T-antigen induced oncogenesis have focused on the ability of T-antigen to disrupt the activity of cell cycle regulatory proteins including p53 and Rb [26], T-antigen's enhancement of oncogenic signaling through the Wnt pathway by stabilizing key members, such as β-catenin, LEF-1, and *c-myc* [27], and its interaction with DNA repair proteins [28,29], to name a few. Surprisingly, few mechanisms have been identified that can repress T-antigen-mediated oncogenesis and attention has mainly focused on transcriptional regulation of the JCV promoter (for review see [25]). In addition, many polyomaviruses, including JCV, encode a conserved miRNA targeting the viral early mRNA as an autoregulatory mechanism [30]. Other potential negative regulators of T-antigen expression include SF2/ASF, which inhibits alternative splicing of the JCV early transcript [31], and CBP which partners with p53 to enhance acetylation of T-antigen, affecting its stability [32,33].

In this study, we provide a new mechanism of tumor suppression by NF2 and demonstrate inhibition of JCV T antigen expression. Here, we show that NF2, specifically its FERM domain, negatively regulates JCV T-antigen protein levels via a proteasome-mediated pathway in U-87 MG human glioblastoma cells. Our findings also extend to clinically obtained human glioblastomas, where T-antigen, NF2, and p53, can be detected. Taken together, these results provide new insights into the function of NF2, and provide a potential pathway for inhibiting T-antigen function in glial cells.

Results

NF2 Suppresses T-antigen Protein Expression and JCV Promoter Activity

We previously reported that NF2 colocalizes with the JCV early regulatory protein, T-antigen, in the nucleus of malignant peripheral nerve sheath tumors found in JCV T-antigen transgenic mice [23]. Other tumor suppressor proteins, such as p53 and Rb, also share T-antigen as a nuclear binding partner. Typically these interactions inhibit p53 and Rb from acting as negative regulators of the cell cycle. However, p53 can also act as a negative regulator of JCV replication, via its interaction with the JCV promoter [34]. Here, we set out to examine if NF2 may have an effect on the expression of JCV T-antigen protein. To this end, human U-87 MG glioblastoma cells were transiently transfected with plasmids encoding JCV T-antigen and increasing amounts of HA tagged NF2 (HA-NF2). Immunoblotting of these cellular extracts revealed a dose-dependent decline of T-antigen protein expression occurring with increasing expression of NF2 (Figures 1A and 1B). However, when the reciprocal experiment was conducted in this cell culture system, NF2 expression was unaffected in the presence of increasing amounts of T-antigen (data not shown).

In parallel, we investigated the functional effect this decline of T-antigen protein would have on the activity of the JCV promoter. The JCV promoter is bidirectional, with the early promoter (JCV_E) encoding the regulatory genes for large and small T-antigens, and the late promoter (JCV_L) encoding capsid and accessory genes. Luciferase constructs containing the JCV promoter in either the early or late orientation were co-transfected into U-87 MG cells, along with expression plasmids for T-antigen and HA-NF2. The presence of increasing amounts of NF2 resulted in retention of basal promoter activity of the JCV_E promoter (Figure 1C) and minor suppression of JCV_L activity (Figure 1D). Since T-antigen activates its own promoter, supplementation with T-antigen enhanced the activity of both early and late promoters; however this effect was ameliorated in the presence of NF2.

To confirm whether the effect of NF2 on JCV promoter activity is due to the decrease in T-antigen levels rather than NF2 acting directly upon the viral promoter, we conducted a chromatin immunoprecipitation (ChIP) assay. For this assay, BSB8 cells, derived from a JCV T-antigen induced primitive neuroectodermal tumor in transgenic mice were utilized [35]. Immunoprecipitation of DNA:protein complexes with antibodies to HA-NF2 and T-antigen, followed by PCR amplification using primers specific for the JCV promoter, detected T-antigen in complex with the JCV promoter. However, HA-NF2 failed to precipitate this DNA region, indicating that NF2 does not directly bind the JCV promoter (data not shown). This result is consistent with a previous study whereby NF2 could not be detected in the chromatin containing fraction of the nucleus [22]. Cumulatively, this data suggests that NF2 downregulates JCV transcription via an indirect mechanism, by reducing T-antigen protein expression, so that T-antigen cannot subsequently enhance viral promoter activity.

NF2 Facilitates the Accumulation of JCV T-antigen mRNA

To date, only a few proteins are capable of suppressing the typically robust expression of JCV T-antigen in tumor cells. One of these proteins, p53, can suppress T-antigen expression through suppression of the viral promoter [34]. However, based on our findings above we ruled out the possibility of NF2 acting as a negative viral transcriptional regulator. As mentioned earlier, the alternative splicing factor, SF2, has been shown to inhibit the splicing of JCV T-antigen pre-mRNA thus reducing expression of both large and small T-antigens [36]. In order to determine if NF2 functions as an inhibitor of splicing, we utilized primers that can discriminate among JCV T-antigen pre-mRNA, and large and small T-antigen mRNAs, as previously described (Figure 2A, and [36]). We detected large and small T-antigen mRNAs, but not their shared pre-mRNA, in cDNA derived from JCV T-antigen expressing BSB8 cells (Figure 2B). As shown previously, T-antigen pre-mRNA accumulated with co-transfection of T7 tagged SF2 (T7-SF2) (Figure 2B, lane 4), but not with HA-NF2 in U-87 MG cells (Figure 2C, compare lanes 6–9), suggesting that the mechanism by which NF2 suppresses T-antigen protein occurs downstream of alternative splicing events. In addition, the relative amount of mature T-antigen mRNA in U-87 MG cells co-transfected with T-antigen and HA-NF2 was determined using large T-antigen specific primers (Figure 2A) by quantitative real time PCR (qRT-PCR) analysis. We observed a positive correlation between NF2 overexpression and T-antigen mature mRNA levels (Figure 2B). This accumulation of untranslated T-antigen mRNA combined with a reduction in T-antigen at the protein level as seen above (Figure 1) suggests a blockage of T-antigen expression by NF2 through post transcriptional intervention.

The FERM Domain of NF2 is Responsible for its Binding and Degradation of T-antigen

To establish the region of NF2 responsible for its interactions with T-antigen, we utilized two truncations mutants of full length NF2, one containing the amino terminal FERM (Band 4.1, ezrin, radixin, moesin) domain (HA-FERM) and the other representing the C terminal half of the NF2 protein (HA-

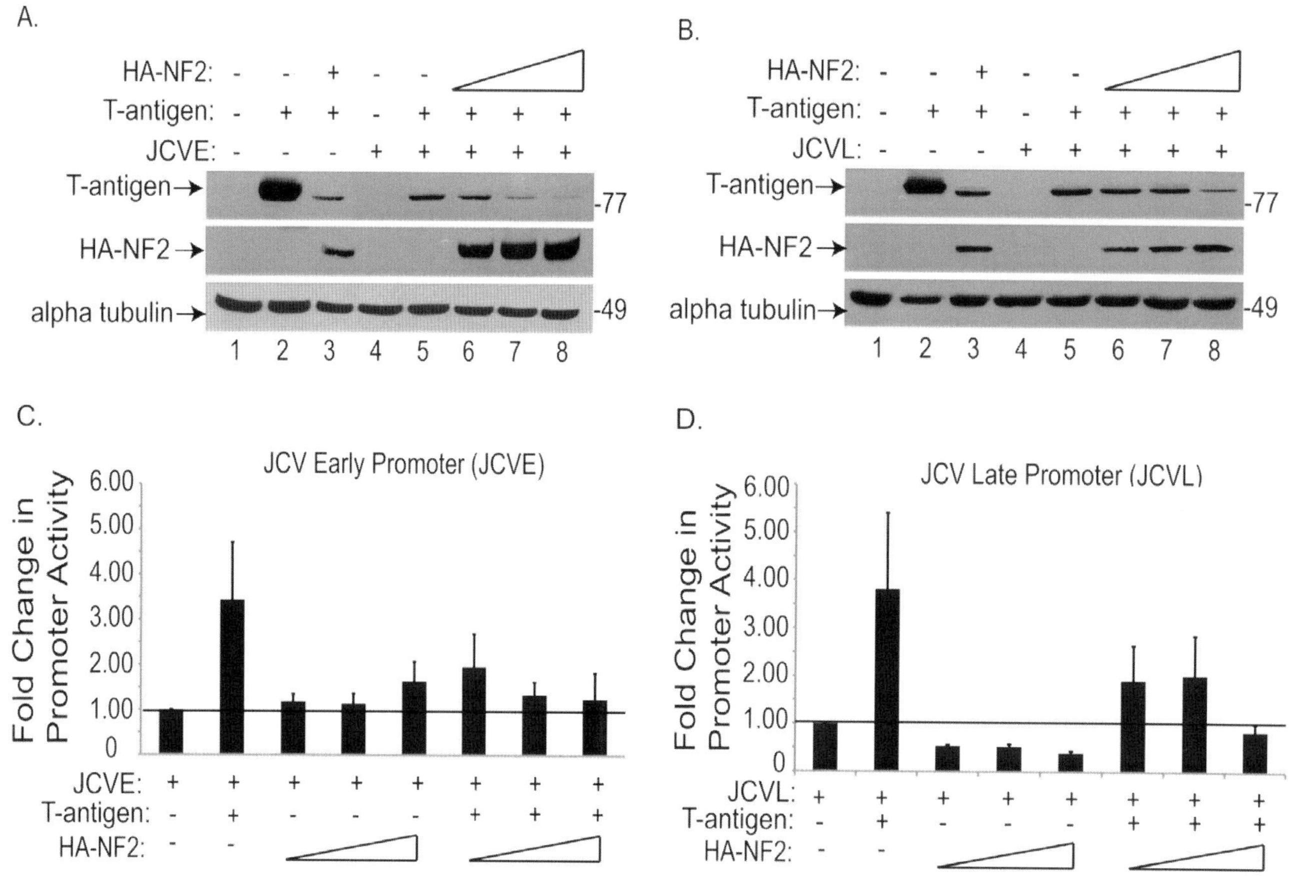

Figure 1. NF2 suppresses T-antigen protein expression and T-antigen mediated activation of JCV_E and JCV_L promoters. U-87 MG glioblastoma cells were transiently transfected with luciferase reporter constructs encoding either the JCV_E (a, c) or JCV_L (b, d) promoters, and plasmids encoding JCV T-antigen or HA tagged NF2 (HA-NF2). Immunoblotting of protein lysates revealed a dose-dependent decline in the expression of T-antigen, in the presence of increasing amounts of HA-NF2 (a, b lanes 5–8). Extracts were also used to conduct luciferase assays to determine JCV_E (c) or JCV_L (d) activation in response to these various transfection conditions. Results are shown here as fold change in luciferase activity, relative to the activity of the promoter alone. NF2 does not appreciably affect the activities of either promoter, while T-antigen greatly enhances the activity of both promoters. In combination, NF2 does prevent T-antigen from enhancing the activities of JCV_E and JCV_L.

ΔFERM). The FERM domain of NF2 is responsible for its anchorage to the plasma membrane and actin binding [37–39]. Further, this domain is suggested to be the tumor suppressive region of NF2 in that it is necessary to prevent cellular proliferation in response to mitogenic signaling, as demonstrated by reductions in growth factor receptor signaling, MTT conversion, and colony formation in soft agar [22,38,40,41]. Co-transfection of these NF2 mutants into U-87 MG cells along with T-antigen, revealed a dose-dependent decline in T-antigen levels with the HA-FERM mutant, similar to full length NF2 (Figure 3A, lanes 1–3), while T-antigen expression remained unaltered in the presence of the HA-ΔFERM mutant (Figure 3A, lanes 4–6). Further, co-immunopreciptation (Co-IP) assays in lysates from these cells revealed that T-antigen binds to the FERM, but not ΔFERM region of NF2 (Figure 3C, compare lanes 5 and 10). These studies further suggest that the FERM domain of NF2 is required for its tumor suppressive capabilities, specifically in T-antigen mediated malignancies.

NF2 Promotes Proteasomal-mediated Degradation of T-antigen

NF2 interacts with a wide array of cellular proteins, including the ubiquitin ligases Mdm2 and DCAF1 [22,42] to promote the degradation of targeted proteins via the proteasome. To determine whether NF2 functions through the proteasome to regulate T-antigen expression, we exposed U-87 MG cells, transfected with T-antigen and HA-NF2 constructs, to the proteasomal inhibitor, MG132. Increasing amounts of NF2 led to a decline in T-antigen protein in samples treated with vehicle alone (Figure 4A, left), while treatment with MG132 ameliorated these affects, such that T-antigen expression was unaltered in the presence of NF2 (Figure 4A, right). Increasing amounts of MG132 led to an accumulation of p21, another protein known to be regulated by this pathway (Figure 4B), indicating the stabilization of proteins subjected to proteasomal degradation. To date, this is the first evidence of proteasomal involvement in the stability of any polyomavirus tumor antigen. A key post-translational modification involved in the targeting of a protein to the proteasome is ubiquitination. To evaluate the ability of JCV T-antigen to bind ubiquitin we conducted a Co-IP assay with T-antigen and an HA-tagged ubiquitin construct (HA-Ub). Using p53 as a protein known to bind ubiquitin, we were able to demonstrate the binding of T-antigen to ubiquitin (Figure 4C, lane 7). Together this data implicates that T-antigen may be subjected to destruction via the ubiquitin-proteasome and that NF2 can enhance this process.

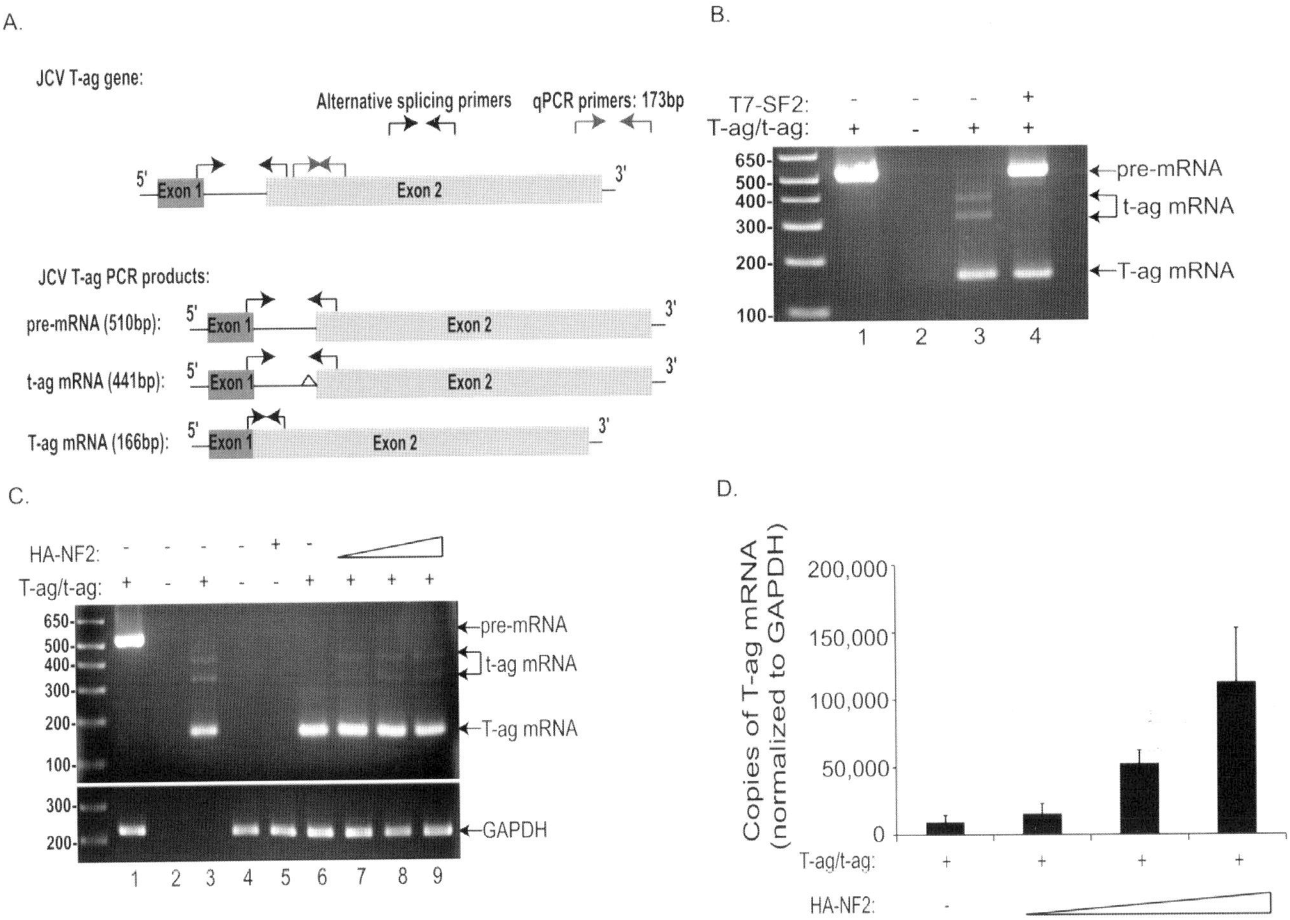

Figure 2. NF2 leads to accumulation of T-antigen mRNA, but does not affect its alternative splicing. Schematic showing all alternatively spliced forms of JCV T-antigen, including the pre-mRNA and both large and small T-antigen mRNAs, and location of primers used for PCR analysis are shown (A, black primers). PCR amplification of cDNA derived from T-antigen expressing BSB8 cells (B, lane 3), detected both large and small T-antigen mRNAs, but not pre-mRNA. Co-transfection of U-87 MG cells with expression plasmids for T-antigen and T7-SF2, an inhibitor of splicing, resulted in an accumulation of pre-mRNA and a reduction in large and small T-antigen mRNAs (B, lane 4). Co-transfection with T-antigen and increasing amounts of HA-NF2 plasmids did not alter the pattern of mRNAs detected (C, compare lanes 6 to 7–9). Q-PCR analysis was also conducted for T-antigen copy number (A, grey primers), expressed as copies of T-antigen mRNA per copy number of the control mRNA GAPDH*, with standard deviations of the mean shown here (D). This assay revealed a dose dependent accumulation of T-antigen mRNA in the presence of NF2. *Note that GAPDH primers used in Panel C only detect human and not mouse GAPDH, therefore a band representing GAPDH from the BSB8 mouse cell line was not detected (C, lane 3).

NF2, T-antigen, and p53 Interact in Human Glioblastomas

NF2, T-antigen, and p53 were previously shown to form a ternary complex in T-antigen positive tumors derived from JCV T-antigen transgenic mice [23]. Yet, it has not been determined if these proteins interact in human tumors or if NF2 and p53 can bind together in the absence of T-antigen. To this end, Co-IP assays were conducted using antibodies against both T-antigen and Myc-tagged p53 (Myc-p53) in extracts from transfected U-87 MG glioblastoma cells. T-antigen was observed to bind to both NF2 and p53, individually (Figure 5A, lanes 4 and 6 respectively) and in complex (Figures 5A and 5B, lane 7). Interestingly, binding between NF2 and p53 independent of T-antigen was not observed (Figure 5B, compare lane 5 to 7), although there is mounting evidence of a tumor suppressive synergy that exists between them [4,43,44].

We then assayed human high grade gliomas resected from patients for the presence of these proteins. Using immunoblotting of fresh tumor tissue, we observed the presence of significant levels of NF2 in three of four high grade glioma tumors analyzed while p53 levels were more variable (Figure 5C). In addition, we detected T-antigen protein in one anaplastic oligodendroglioma (AO812B) and one grade IV glioblastoma (Gli1105). Interestingly, high levels of NF2 and p53 were detected in another glioblastoma sample (Gli906A) in the absence of T-antigen (Figure 5C). Immunohistochemical analysis of parallel sections from one of the T-antigen positive samples (Gli1105) revealed a predominantly cytoplasmic pattern for NF2, while T-antigen and p53 were detected in the nuclei of a subset of tumor cells (Figure 5D–F). NF2 is typically examined in tumor tissues at the gene level to screen for gene deletion, i.e. LOH or mutational inactivation. However, here we examine the role of the NF2 protein as a tumor suppressor, rather than its loss of function. We were able to detect NF2 by immunohistochemistry and Western blotting in Gli1105, and as shown in Figure 5C, varying levels of NF2 are seen in the tumor tissues including some with a more prominent upper band likely representing the phosphorylated form of the protein, suggesting that total levels, as well as phosphorylation status may affect its function in human tumors.

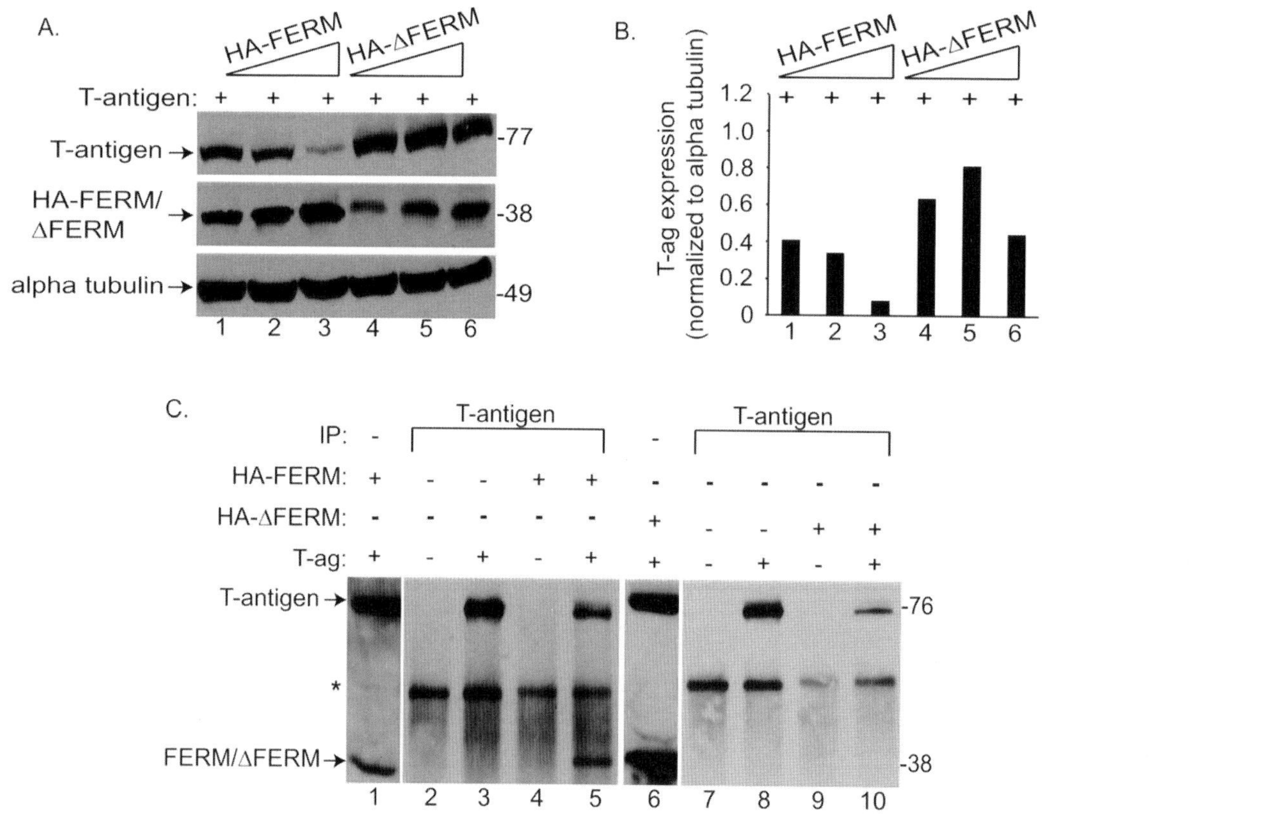

Figure 3. NF2 utilizes a proteasomal-dependent mechanism to promote the degradation of ubiquitin-bound T-antigen. To determine if NF2 utilizes the proteasome to enhance T-antigen protein turnover, U-87 MG cells, transfected with HA-NF2 and T-antigen, were treated with the general proteasome inhibitor, MG132 (A, right), or vehicle (A, left). As shown earlier (Figures 1A and 1B), enhanced expression of NF2, suppresses that of T-antigen (A, left top and bottom). However, this affect was abolished with the addition of MG132 (A, right top and bottom). Band intensity representing T-antigen expression was quantified, normalized to its loading control, and shown as fold change relative to lane 1 (A, bottom left and right). p21, a protein known to be subjected to proteasomal degradation, was immunoblotted for in extracts of untransfected U-87 MG cells or those transfected with HA-NF2 or T-antigen alone, exposed to increasing concentrations of MG132 (B). Expression of this protein increased with drug exposure (B, compare lanes 1, 4, and 7 to subsequent lanes), indicating the effectiveness of MG132 to inhibit degradation of proteins subjected to proteasomal degradation. The ability of T-antigen to bind to ubiquitin, a key post-translational protein attached to proteasome targeted proteins, was assessed by Co-IP. U-87 MG cells were transfected with combinations of Myc tagged p53 (Myc-p53), T-antigen, and HA tagged ubiquitin (HA-Ub), protein complexes were immunoprecipitated with an anti HA antibody or normal mouse serum. Subsequent immunoblotting demonstrated that p53 and T-antigen were not precipitated by the HA antibody alone (C, lanes 2 and 6), but did when co-transfected with HA-Ub (C, lanes 3–4 and 7). Collectively, these results provide the first evidence that T-antigen can bind ubiquitin and suggest that T-antigen is subjected to proteasome-mediated degradation.

Discussion

NF2 is a putative tumor suppressor for glioblastoma growth, in that it is lost in many patient samples and cell lines. Reintroduction of NF2 in these cells can significantly inhibit cell proliferation, cellular transformation, and tumorigenesis [8–10]. While NF2 is not solely localized in the cytoplasm, the potential functions of nuclear NF2 remain unclear. Previous studies from our group indicate that the JCV regulatory protein, T-antigen, binds to NF2, but the functional significance of this interaction had not been elucidated [23]. Here, we provide evidence for a novel role of NF2 as an inhibitor of oncogenic JCV T-antigen expression in glioblastoma cells.

NF2 joins a list of only two other proteins, including p53 and SF2, that downregulate the expression of JCV T-antigen. P53 does so by binding to the JCV bidirectional promoter and preventing the transcription of T-antigen [34]. Since we could not detect NF2 interaction with the JCV promoter by ChIP assay (data not shown) nor observe an impact on promoter activity in the absence of T-antigen (Figures 1D and 1E), regulation of T-antigen by NF2 at the level of the JCV promoter appears unlikely. SF2, on the other hand, inhibits the processing of T-antigen pre-mRNA into its mature form needed for protein translation [36]. The ability for NF2 to serve in a similar capacity is also unlikely as we were unable to observe an accumulation of T-antigen pre-mRNA upon overexpression of NF2 (Figure 2C). Instead, our data suggests that NF2, specifically its tumor suppressive FERM domain, facilitates the proteasomal degradation of ubiquitin bound T-antigen. However, the accumulation of T-antigen mRNA that we observed in the presence of NF2 (Figure 2D), suggests the possibility that NF2 may also inhibit T-antigen at the level of translation. NF2 has been previously implicated to act as an inhibitor of translation [41,45,46]. Conversely, expression of SV40 T-antigen can activate cap-dependent protein translation [47]. Both large and small T-antigens appear to be downregulated by NF2 (Beltrami et al, unpublished observations) suggesting a common mechanism for their inhibition and, indeed, they do share a portion of their 5′ mRNA sequences and amino termini (Beltrami, unpublished observation). Further defining

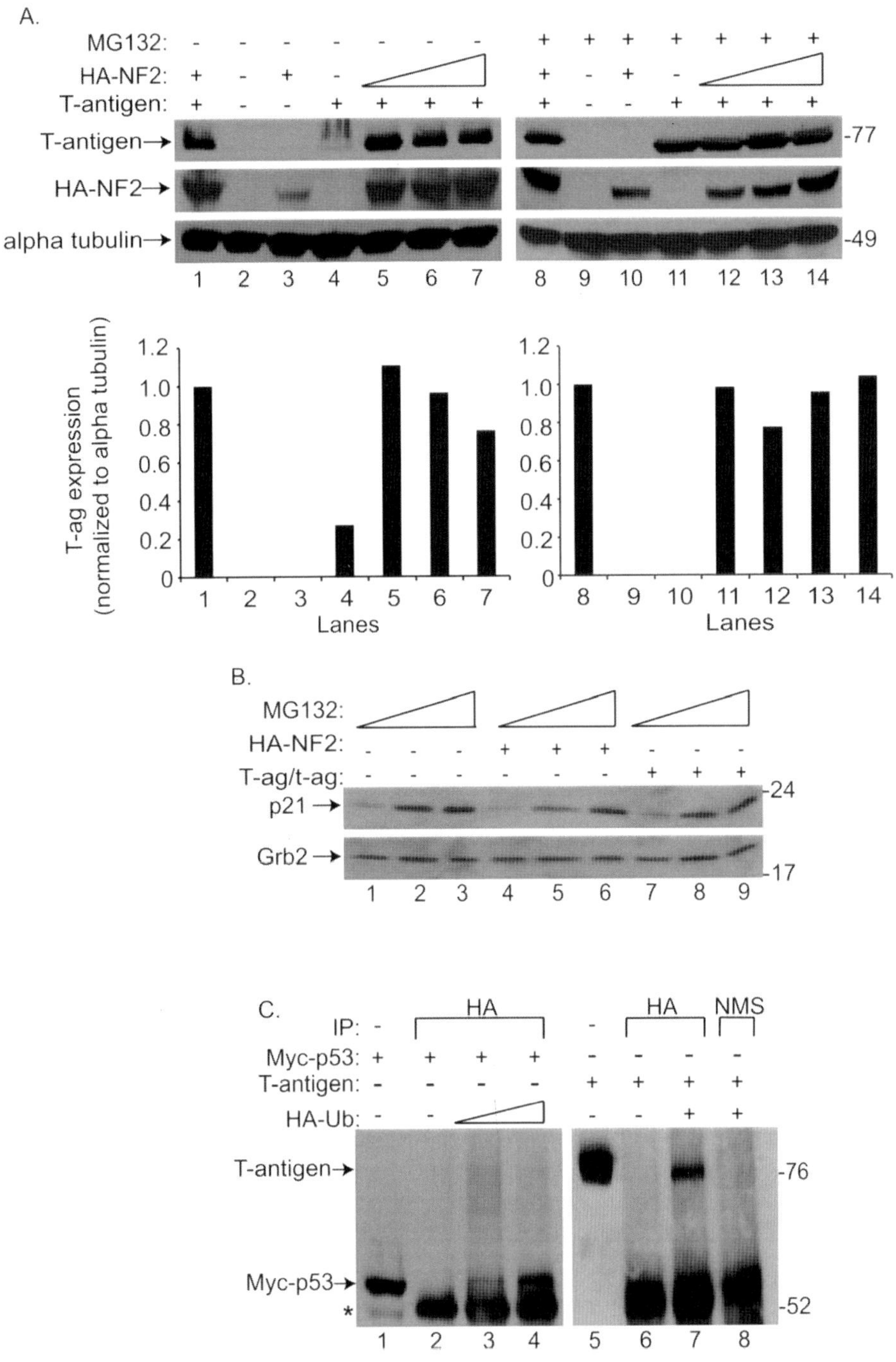

Figure 4. NF2 requires its FERM domain to bind and suppress T-antigen expression. To elucidate the domain of NF2 responsible for the downregulation of T-antigen protein expression, U-87 MG cells were cotransfected with T-antigen and increasing amounts of either HA-FERM or HA-ΔFERM NF2 truncation mutants (A). Immunoblotting revealed a dose-dependent decline in T-antigen expression in the presence of HA-FERM (A, lanes 1–3), but not HA-ΔFERM (A, lanes 4–6), indicating that the FERM domain is necessary for this mechanism. Band intensity representing T-antigen expression was quantified, normalized to its loading control (B). Lysates from U-87 MG cells co-transfected with T-antigen, HA-FERM, and HA-ΔFERM were utilized for Co-IP with T-antigen antibodies (C). In this assay, we demonstrate the ability of T-antigen to bind to the FERM (C, lane 5), but not ΔFERM (C, lane 10) region of NF2, further implicating FERM to be the necessary region facilitating the interaction among NF2 and T-antigen.

NF2's potential to regulate proteasome cargo or perhaps mRNA levels, as well as identifying its cellular target proteins, are the logical next steps.

Though NF2 is traditionally viewed as a cytoplasmic scaffold, it also has tumor suppressive roles in the nucleus. NF2 has not been shown to directly regulate the cell cycle; however its presence promotes cell cycle arrest in schwannoma, primary endothelial, mesothelioma, and patient-derived meningioma cells [14,22,48,49]. An intriguing protein of interest, which may link NF2 to the cell cycle, is the cyclin dependent kinase inhibitor, p21. Through its interactions with Mdm2, NF2 enhances the transcription of p21, a well established inhibitor of cell cycle

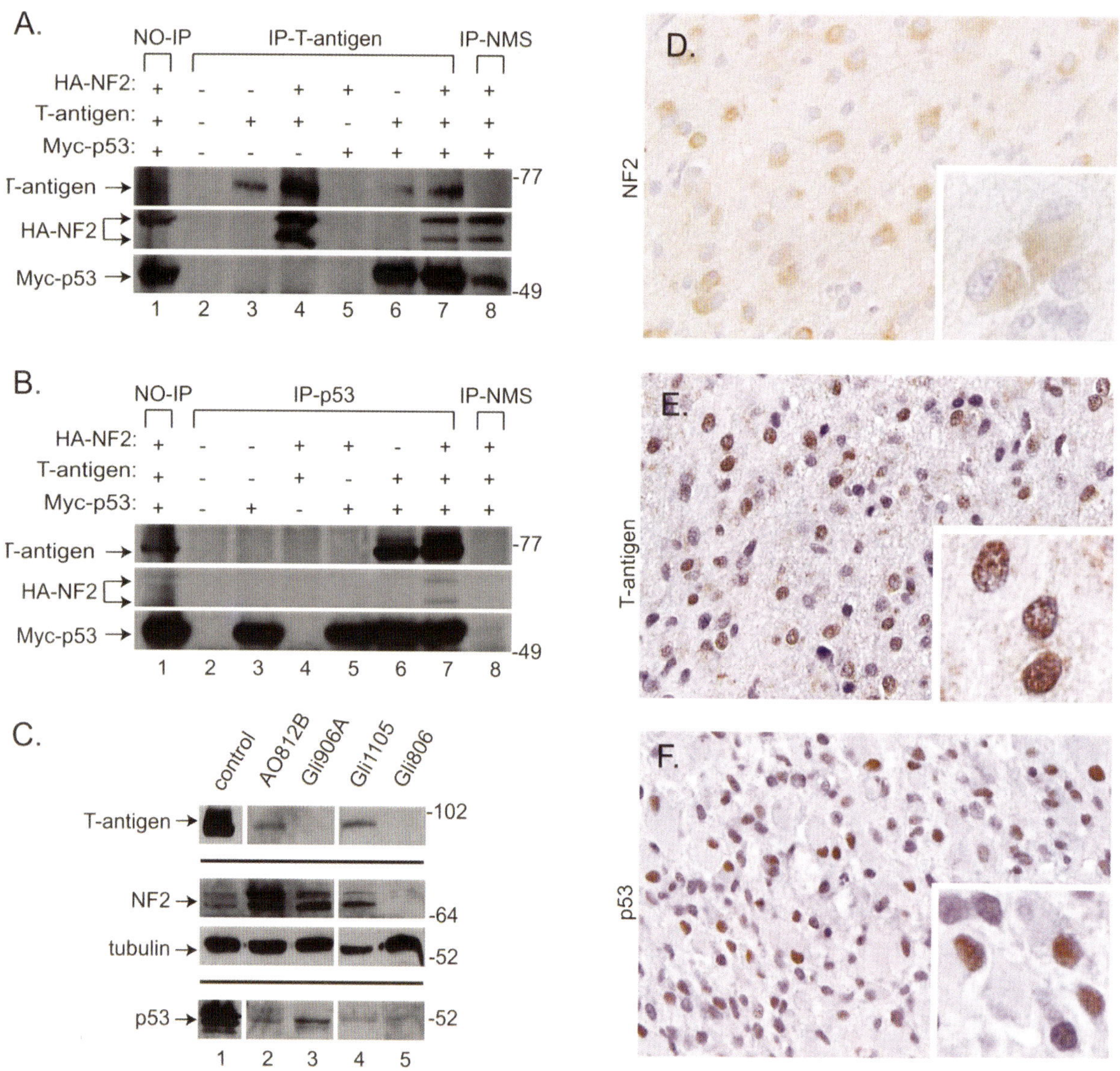

Figure 5. NF2, T-antigen, and p53 complex in human glioblastoma cells and are detected in high grade glioma samples. Immunoprecipitation of HA-NF2, T-antigen, and Myc-p53 proteins was performed using extracts from transiently transfected U-87 MG cells with antibodies against T-antigen (A), p53 antibody (B), or normal mouse serum as negative controls (A and B, lane 8), followed by immunoblotting to detect the presence of T-antigen, HA-NF2, or Myc-p53. As previously described, T-antigen binds NF2 (A, lane 4) and p53 (A and B, lane 6), individually. These proteins form a ternary complex (A and B, lane 7), however NF2 and p53 do not bind in the absence of T-antigen (B, lane 5). Protein lysates were prepared from fresh tissue specimens of surgically resected high grade gliomas utilized for immunoblotting revealed the presence of NF2 and p53 in an anaplastic oligodendroglioma (A, lane 2), as well as three glioblastomas (C, lanes 3–5). T- antigen was also detected in two of these tumor samples (C, lanes 2 and 4). Further, tumor tissue obtained from surgically resected high grade gliomas tumor, was paraffin embedded and used for immunohistochemistry. In the glioblastoma sample shown in Panel C, lane 4 (Gli1105), we detected cytoplasmic NF2 expression (Figure 5D). In comparable sections of the same glioblastoma sample T-antigen (E) and p53 (F) were localized to the nucleus. Panels D-F, original magnification x400; insets, original magnification, x1000; hematoxylin counterstain.

progression [42,50]. Furthermore, NF2 inhibits PAK2 from acting as a positive transcriptional regulator of the cell cycle enhancer, cyclin D1 [51]. Interestingly, T-antigen promotes the stabilization of Rac1, another cyclin D1 enhancer [52,53]. These studies have led some to speculate that NF2 may have a novel role as an upstream cell cycle regulator [22].

While NF2 is typically a cytoplasmic protein, we have previously shown its nuclear co-localization with T-antigen in tumors derived from JCV T-antigen transgenic mice. The pattern of NF2 localization in the human high grade gliomas we examined was predominantly cytoplasmic, though examination of a more extensive set of clinical samples would be informative. In any case, many prominent nuclear proteins are regulated within the cytoplasmic compartment, p53 regulation by MDM2 is one relevant example, and a portion of T-antigen can be detected within the cytoplasm as well as in the membrane fraction of cells. A direct interaction between NF2 and p53 was not observed in the absence of T-antigen, but previous studies have suggested significant overlap between these two pathways. Interestingly, NF2 and p53 were detected in one of our glioblastoma tissue samples (Gli906A) by immunoblotting, even in the absence of T-antigen (Figure 5C). The NF2 and p53 genes are linked in the mouse genome, and loss of both genes leads to the development of multiple highly metastatic tumors [4,44,54] and in meningiomas, the loss of functional NF2 and p53 correlate with enhanced tumor grade [43]. At the molecular level, NF2 was shown to upregulate transcription of the p53 gene, stabilize p53 protein, and sensitize cells to p53 induced apoptosis [42]. Since NF2 and p53 do not appear to directly bind together, other cellular mediators must facilitate their interactions. One such protein may include Mdm2, the p53 ubiquitin ligase, which has been shown to bind both p53 and NF2 in isolation [42].

In our limited analysis of patient derived gliomas, we have detected both nuclear and cytoplasmic interactions among NF2 and T-antigen. There are several possibilities as to the outcome of these interactions. Nuclear NF2, in its binding to T-antigen, may prevent it from sequestering p53 and Rb and overriding their control of the cell cycle. To explore this possibility, we will investigate if NF2 can aide T-antigen expressing gliomas in regaining control of the cell cycle. In light of our recent data on the proteasomal mediated degradation of T-antigen, perhaps cytoplasmic NF2 acts as a chaperone protein to guide ubiquitin-tagged T-antigen to the proteasome. In which case, the ubiquitin ligases known to interact with NF2, namely Mdm2 and DCAF1, would be attractive candidates to explore for their ability to degrade T-antigen. Further, we were not able to determine if the p53 we detected by either immunoblotting or immunohistochemistry is wild type or mutant in these glioma samples. Previously, we have observed wild-type p53 in nervous system tumors from T-antigen transgenic mice and have demonstrated that T-antigen only interacts with wild type and not mutant p53 [23,35,55]. We therefore hypothesize that T-antigen would associate with wild-type p53. However, immunohistochemical detection in formalin-fixed tissue does not allow the distinction between wild-type and mutant forms of p53, therefore other means, i.e. gene sequencing or immunoprecipitation analysis would be necessary to determine the p53 status of the human tumors.

Alteration of p53 remains one of the key genetic changes in human glioblastoma and its mutation or loss has been reported in some percentage of all subtypes of glioblastomas thus far described [56]. While NF2 inactivation has been linked to schwannomas and other tumors such as mesotheliomas, loss of NF2 expression appears to be infrequent in human glioblastoma, though it has been reported in up to one third of cases [10]. Indeed, we have observed high levels of NF2 expression in high grade gliomas. However, it is important to establish whether the presence of a tumor suppressor protein such as p53 or NF2 indicates a functional protein, as the pathway may be blocked downstream and thus unable to halt cell proliferation. Should the tumor suppressor pathway be intact, it may be possible to alter the blockage and thus restore cell cycle control. Visualizing the interactive nature of these proteins in human samples provides us with a better understanding of the complex interplay among tumor suppressors and oncoproteins that shape glioblastoma growth.

Materials and Methods

Ethics Statement - clinical Samples

Human brain tumor tissue was obtained from surgical resections or brain biopsy under the approval of the Temple University Institutional Review Board (IRB). Written informed consent for all samples was obtained and any clinical samples presented in this study have been coded and deidentified.

Plasmids and Cell Lines

The JCV_E and JCV_L promoter regions, from the Mad-4 strain of JC virus were cloned into separate pGL3 Basic Vectors, upstream of the *luc2P* reporter gene [57]. The expression constructs for JCV T-antigen and human p53, were created by PCR amplification and cloning into the KpnI and EcoRI sites, and the EcoRI and NotI sites of pcDNA6/myc-His vector (Invitrogen), respectively. The HA-tagged NF2 expression construct was created by cloning into the pcDNA3 vector as described previously [23]. The T7 tagged SF2 (T7-SF2) expression construct was a gift from Ilker Sariyer [36], and the HA-tagged ubiquitin plasmid (HA-Ub) was purchased (Addgene). The U-87 MG glioblastoma cell line was obtained from the ATCC and cultured in 1x DMEM-low glucose media (GIBCO), with 10% fetal bovine serum, and 0.5 µg/µl gentamicin. The JCV T-antigen positive cell line used in this study, BSB8, was derived from JCV T-antigen transgenic mice [35], and cultured in the same media.

Antibodies

Antibodies used for immunoblotting in this study included: HA-11 mouse monoclonal (clone 12CA5, Boehringer Mannheim), SV40 T-antigen Ab2 mouse monoclonal, which cross-reacts with JCV T-antigen, (clone pAb416, Oncogene Research Products), Myc mouse monoclonal (clone 9B11, Cell Signaling), p21 rabbit polyclonal (sc-756, Santa Cruz Biotechnologies) and alpha tubulin mouse monoclonal (clone B-5-1-2, Sigma Aldrich). For immunoprecipitation the following antibodies were utilized: SV40 T-antigen Ab2 mouse monoclonal, HA-11 mouse monoclonal, and p53 Ab-1 mouse monoclonal (clone pAb421, Wilex, Cambridge, MA). Immunohistochemistry was performed using NF2 rabbit polyclonal (C-18, Santa Cruz Biotechnologies), p53 mouse monoclonal (D07, Dako) and T-antigen mouse monoclonal (SV40 T-antigen Ab2). Patient samples were immunoblotted using NF2 rabbit polyclonal (C-18), T-antigen mouse monoclonal (SV40 T-antigen Ab2), and p53 sheep polyclonal (Ab-7, Millipore, Billerica, MA).

Luciferase Assay

U-87 MG cells were transfected in quadruplicate with increasing concentrations of expression plasmids for HA-NF2, T-antigen, and JCV_E or JCV_L reporter plasmids using Fugene 6 transfection reagent (Roche) in Optimem media (GIBCO) and total amounts of DNA were normalized with pcDNA3.1 (empty vector). Cells were harvested 48 hours post transfection in 1× passive lysis buffer (Promega) and luciferase activity was conducted with 10 µg of protein lysates using the Luciferase Assay System kit (Promega), measured with a Femtomaster FB 12 luminometer (Zylux Co.), and quantified to give a RLU/sec/10 µg of protein.

Immunoblotting

Whole cell extracts were prepared in 1x Promega passive lysis buffer or 0.5% NP-40, TNN buffer containing mammalian protease inhibitor cocktail (Sigma Aldrich). Proteins were separated by 9 or 12% SDS-PAGE, and transferred to nitrocellulose or PVDF membranes. Blots were blocked in 10% milk in 1× PBST, then incubated in primary antibodies for 2 hours at room temperature or overnight at 4°C. This was followed by washing, then incubation with secondary antibodies conjugated to horseradish peroxidase for detection with ECL chemiluminescence (GE Healthcare) or secondary antibodies conjugated to alkaline phosphatase for detection with CDP-Star (Perkin Elmer). Bands were quantified, using ImageJ software, and normalized to loading control.

Co-immunoprecipitation

U-87 MG cells were transfected with expression plasmids as described in their respective figures. Forty-eight hours after transfection, whole cell extracts were prepared in 0.5% NP-40, TNN buffer containing mammalian protease inhibitor cocktail (Sigma Aldrich) and 0.1 μg/μl DNaseI (Roche). 150 μg of protein lysates were incubated overnight at 4°C with 1 μg of antibodies against either p53 (Ab-1), HA-11 tag, or T-antigen (SV40 T-antigen Ab2). Immunocomplexes were isolated by incubation with Pansorbin cells (Calbiochem) in TNN buffer, at 4°C for 2 hours. Complexes were then washed 3–4 times in TNN buffer, eluted in 2× SDS-PAGE sample buffer and subjected to immunoblot analysis.

Proteasomal Inhibition Assay

U-87 MG cells were transfected with plasmids encoding T-antigen and increasing amounts of HA-NF2. Media was then supplemented with either 10 μM the proteasome inhibitor MG132 (Calbiochem) in DMSO or an equal amount of DMSO for 8 hours before harvesting. Whole cell extracts were prepared 48 h after transfection in TNN buffer and immunoblotted to detect T-antigen, HA-NF2, and alpha tubulin expression. In parallel, U-87 MG, untrasfected or transfected with either HA-NF2 or T-antigen plasmids, were exposed to DMSO or MG132 in DMSO (1 or 10 μM) for 8 hours. Prepared extracts were immunoblotted for the detection of p21 expression.

Alternative Splicing PCR and qRT-PCR

RNA was extracted from U-87 MG cells transfected with either HA-NF2, T-antigen, or T7-SF2 constructs alone, or in combination, using the RNeasy kit (Qiagen), following manufacturer's instructions. Samples were then treated with DNAse 1 (Roche) and RNAse inhibitor (Roche). Samples were subjected to PCR to verify absence of DNA contamination with primers specific for human GAPDH DNA: forward primer 5′ GAAGATGGTGATGGGATTTC 3′, reverse primer 5′ GAAGGTGAAGGTCGGAGTC 3′ at 50°C for 2 min (1×), 95°C for 10 min (1×), 95°C for 30 s/53°C for 30 s (45×), and 4°C for 1 min. When DNA was undetectable in these RNA samples, the reverse transcriptase enzyme from the Moloney Murine Leukemia Virus (Mo-MuLV RT), dNTPs, and random hexamers (Invitrogen) were used to synthesize cDNA. A portion of this cDNA was used for PCR reactions with primers to detect alternatively spliced forms of JCV T-antigen as described previously [36]: forward (4801–4780) 5′-CCTGATTTTGGTACATGGAA-3′, and reverse (4291–4313) 5′-GTGGGGTAGAGTGTTGGGATCCT-3′. The remaining cDNA was used for Q-PCR analysis of T-antigen mRNA copy number. The following primers (20 μM) and a FAM fluorophore labeled mRNA probe (10 μM) specific to JCV T-antigen were used in the PCR reaction: forward primer (4255–4274) 5′ AGTCTTTAGGGTCTTCTACC 3′, reverse primer (4408–4427) 5′ GTGCCAACCTATGGAACAG 3′, probe (4303–4327) 5′ FAM-AGTGTTGGGATCCTGTGTTTTCAT-CATC-BHQ1 3′. The PCR conditions for T-antigen amplification were 50°C for 2×min (1×), 95°C for 10×min (1×), 95°C for 15 s (45×), and 60°C for 1 min (1×). The standard mRNA copy number for each reaction was normalized to the average GAPDH copy number for those reaction conditions. The primers and probes used for the GAPDH PCR reactions 5′-HEX-CAAGCTTCCCGTTCTCAGCC-BHQ1–3′. All q-PCR reactions were performed in Universal Taq Man PCR Master Mix (Applied Biosystems) and amplified using the iCycler thermocycler (BioRad Laboratories).

Immunohistochemistry

Patient tumor resection samples were fixed in formalin for 24 hour, embedded in paraffin, and sectioned into 4μm slices using a Microm HM315 (Fisher Scientific). Paraffin was melted and slides were cleared in xylenes, and rehydrated in descending concentrations of ethanol. Antigen retrieval was conducted by warming slides in citrate buffer at 95°C for 30 min. Endogenous peroxidases were quenched in a solution of methanol and 30% peroxide for 20×min. Slides were blocked in normal goat or normal horse serum, for rabbit and mouse antibodies, respectively. Primary antibodies to NF2 (C-18), p53 (D-07) and T-antigen (SV40 T-antigen Ab2) were incubated on the slides overnight in a humidified chamber. For immunohistochemical analysis, slides were incubated with the appropriate biotinylated secondary antibody, followed avidin-biotin complexes for 1hr (Vector Laboratories). Slides were developed using DAB (Sigma Aldrich), dehydrated, counter stained with hematoxylin, mounted with Permount, and visualized by bright field microscopy.

Acknowledgments

The authors wish to thank past and present members of the Department of Neuroscience/Center for Neurovirology for their support and sharing of ideas and reagents. We would also like to thank the Temple University Neurosurgery Tumor Bank for providing clinical samples of glioblastoma.

Author Contributions

Conceived and designed the experiments: SB IS MW JG. Performed the experiments: SB EB JO. Analyzed the data: SB JG. Contributed reagents/materials/analysis tools: MW. Wrote the paper: SB JG.

References

1. Martuza RL, Eldridge R (1988) Neurofibromatosis 2 (bilateral acoustic neurofibromatosis). N Engl J Med 318(11): 684–8.
2. Evans DG, Huson SM, Donnai D, Neary W, Blair V, et al. (1992) A clinical study of type 2 neurofibromatosis. Q J Med 84(304): 603–18.
3. Sekido Y (2011) Inactivation of Merlin in malignant mesothelioma cells and the Hippo signaling cascade dysregulation. Pathol Int 61(6): 331–44.
4. McClatchey AI, Saotome I, Mercer K, Crowley D, Gusella JF, et al. (1998) Mice heterozygous for a mutation at the Nf2 tumor suppressor locus develop a range of highly metastatic tumors. Genes Dev 12(8): 1121–33.
5. Morrison H, Sperka T, Manent J, Giovannini M, Ponta H, et al. (2007) Merlin/neurofibromatosis type 2 suppresses growth by inhibiting the activation of Ras and Rac. Cancer Res 67(2): 520–7.
6. Johnson KC, Kissil JL, Fry JL, Jacks T (2002) Cellular transformation by a FERM domain mutant of the Nf2 tumor suppressor gene. Oncogene 21(39): 5990–7.
7. Houshmandi SS, Emnett RJ, Giovannini M, Gutmann DH (2009) The neurofibromatosis 2 protein, merlin, regulates glial cell growth in an ErbB2- and Src-dependent manner. Mol Cell Biol 29(6): 1472–86.
8. Lee H, Kim D, Dan HC, Wu EL, Gritsko TM, et al. (2007) Identification and characterization of putative tumor suppressor NGB, a GTP-binding protein that interacts with the neurofibromatosis 2 protein. Mol Cell Biol 27(6): 2103–19.
9. Lau YK, Murray LB, Houshmandi SS, Xu Y, Gutmann DH, et al. (2008) Merlin is a potent inhibitor of glioma growth. Cancer Res 68(14): 5733–42.
10. Morales FC, Molina JR, Hayashi Y, Georgescu MM (2010) Overexpression of ezrin inactivates NF2 tumor suppressor in glioblastoma. Neuro Oncol 12(6): 528–39.
11. Rouleau GA, Merel P, Lutchman M, Sanson M, Zucman J, et al. (1993) Alteration in a new gene encoding a putative membrane-organizing protein causes neurofibromatosis type 2. Nature 363(6429): 515–21.
12. Trofatter JA, MacCollin MM, Rutter JL, Murrell JR, Duyao MP, et al. (1993) A novel moesin-, ezrin-, radixin-like gene is a candidate for the neurofibromatosis 2 tumor suppressor. Cell 75(4): 826.
13. Tsukita S, Yonemura S (1997) ERM (ezrin/radixin/moesin) family: from cytoskeleton to signal transduction. Curr Opin Cell Biol 9(1): 70–5. 5.

14. Morrison H, Sherman LS, Legg J, Banine F, Isacke C, et al. (2001) The NF2 tumor suppressor gene product, merlin, mediates contact inhibition of growth through interactions with CD44. Genes Dev 15(8): 968–80.
15. Shaw RJ, Paez JG, Curto M, Yaktine A, Pruitt WM, et al. (2001) The NF2 tumor suppressor, merlin, functions in Rac-dependent signaling. Dev Cell 1(1): 63–72.
16. Grönholm M, Teesalu T, Tyynelä J, Piltti K, Böhling T, et al. (2005) Characterization of the NF2 protein merlin and the ERM protein ezrin in human, rat, and mouse central nervous system. Mol Cell Neurosci 28(4): 683–93.
17. McClatchey AI (2003) Merlin and ERM proteins: unappreciated roles in cancer development? Nat Rev Cancer 3(11): 877–83.
18. Bosco EE, Nakai Y, Hennigan RF, Ratner N, Zheng Y (2010) NF2-deficient cells depend on the Rac1-canonical Wnt signaling pathway to promote the loss of contact inhibition of proliferation. Oncogene 29(17): 2540–9.
19. McClatchey AI, Giovannini M (2005) Membrane organization and tumorigenesis–the NF2 tumor suppressor, Merlin. Genes Dev 19(19): 2265–77.
20. Kressel M, Schmucker B (2002) Nucleocytoplasmic transfer of the NF2 tumor suppressor protein merlin is regulated by exon 2 and a CRM1-dependent nuclear export signal in exon 15. Hum Mol Genet 11(19): 2269–78.
21. Muranen T, Grönholm M, Renkema GH, Carpén O (2005) Cell cycle-dependent nucleocytoplasmic shuttling of the neurofibromatosis 2 tumour suppressor merlin. Oncogene 24(7): 1150–8.
22. Li W, You L, Cooper J, Schiavon G, Pepe-Caprio A, et al. (2010) Merlin/NF2 suppresses tumorigenesis by inhibiting the E3 ubiquitin ligase CRL4(DCAF1) in the nucleus. Cell 140(4): 477–90.
23. Shollar D, Del Valle L, Khalili K, Otte J, Gordon J (2004) JCV T-antigen interacts with the neurofibromatosis type 2 gene product in a transgenic mouse model of malignant peripheral nerve sheath tumors. Oncogene 23(32): 5459–67.
24. Padgett BL, Walker DL, ZuRhein GM, Hodach AE, Chou SM (1976) JC Papovavirus in progressive multifocal leukoencephalopathy. J Infect Dis 133(6): 686–90.
25. White MK, Gordon J, Reiss K, Del Valle L, Croul S, et al. (2005) Human polyomaviruses and brain tumors. Brain Res Brain Res Rev 50(1): 69–85.
26. Krynska B, Gordon J, Otte J, Franks R, Knobler R, et al. (1997) Role of cell cycle regulators in tumor formation in transgenic mice expressing the human neurotropic virus, JCV, early protein. J Cell Biochem 67(2): 223–30.
27. Gan DD, Reiss K, Carrill T, Del Valle L, Croul S, et al. (2001) Involvement of Wnt signaling pathway in murine medulloblastoma induced by human neurotropic JC virus. Oncogene 20(35): 4864–70.
28. Lassak A, Del Valle L, Peruzzi F, Wang JY, Enam S, et al. (2002) Insulin receptor substrate 1 translocation to the nucleus by the human JC virus T-antigen. J Biol Chem 277(19): 17231–8.
29. Trojanek J, Croul S, Ho T, Wang JY, Darbinyan A, et al. (2006) T-antigen of the human polyomavirus JC attenuates faithful DNA repair by forcing nuclear interaction between IRS-1 and Rad51. J Cell Physiol 206(1): 35–46.
30. Seo GJ, Fink LH, O'Hara B, Atwood WJ, Sullivan CS (2008) Evolutionarily conserved function of a viral microRNA. J Virol 82(20): 9823–8.
31. Uleri E, Beltrami S, Gordon J, Dolei A, Sariyer IK (2011) Extinction of Tumor Antigen Expression by SF2/ASF in JCV-Transformed Cells. Genes Cancer 2(7): 728–36.
32. Shimazu T, Komatsu Y, Nakayama KI, Fukazawa H, Horinouchi S, et al. (2006) Regulation of SV40 large T-antigen stability by reversible acetylation. Oncogene 25(56): 7391–400.
33. Poulin DL, Kung AL, DeCaprio JA (2004) p53 targets simian virus 40 large T antigen for acetylation by CBP. J Virol 78(15): 8245–53.
34. Staib C, Pesch J, Gerwig R, Gerber JK, Brehm U, et al. (1996) p53 inhibits JC virus DNA replication in vivo and interacts with JC virus large T-antigen. Virology 219(1): 237–46.
35. Krynska B, Del Valle L, Gordon J, Otte J, Croul S, et al. (2000) Identification of a novel p53 mutation in JCV-induced mouse medulloblastoma. Virology 274(1): 65–74.
36. Sariyer IK, Khalili K (2011) Regulation of human neurotropic JC virus replication by alternative splicing factor SF2/ASF in glial cells. PLoS One 6(1): e14630.
37. Barret C, Roy C, Montcourrier P, Mangeat P, Niggli V (2000) Mutagenesis of the phosphatidylinositol 4,5-bisphosphate (PIP(2)) binding site in the NH(2)-terminal domain of ezrin correlates with its altered cellular distribution. J Cell Bio 151(5): 1067–80.
38. Cole BK, Curto M, Chan AW, McClatchey AI (2008) Localization to the cortical cytoskeleton is necessary for Nf2/merlin-dependent epidermal growth factor receptor silencing. Mol Cell Biol 28(4): 1274–84.
39. Mani T, Hennigan RF, Foster LA, Conrady DG, Herr AB, et al. (2011) FERM domain phosphoinositide binding targets merlin to the membrane and is essential for its growth suppressive function. Mol Cell Biol 31(10): 1983–96.
40. Kissil JL, Wilker EW, Johnson KC, Eckman MS, Yaffe MB, et al. (2003) Merlin, the product of the Nf2 tumor suppressor gene, is an inhibitor of the p21-activated kinase, Pak1. Mol Cell. 12(4): 841–9.
41. Scoles DR, Yong WH, Qin Y, Wawrowsky K, Pulst SM (2006) Schwannomin inhibits tumorigenesis through direct interaction with the eukaryotic initiation factor subunit c (eIF3c). Hum Mol Genet 15(7): 1059–70.
42. Kim H, Kwak NJ, Lee JY, Choi BH, Lim Y, et al. (2004) Merlin neutralizes the inhibitory effect of Mdm2 on p53. J Biol Chem 279(9): 7812–8.
43. Chang Z, Guo CL, Ahronowitz I, Stemmer-Rachamimov AO, MacCollin M, et al. (2009) A role for the p53 pathway in the pathology of meningiomas with NF2 loss. J Neurooncol 91(3): 265–70.
44. Kalamarides M, Acosta MT, Babovic-Vuksanovic D, Carpen O, Cichowski K, et al. (2011) Neurofibromatosis 2011: a report of the Children's Tumor Foundation Annual Meeting. Acta Neuropathol.123(3): 369–80.
45. Benkirane M, Neuveut C, Chun RF, Smith SM, Samuel CE, et al. (1997) Oncogenic potential of TAR RNA binding protein TRBP and its regulatory interaction with RNA-dependent protein kinase PKR. EMBO J 16(3): 611–24.
46. López-Lago MA, Okada T, Murillo MM, Socci N, Giancotti FG (2009) Loss of the tumor suppressor gene NF2, encoding merlin, constitutively activates integrin-dependent mTORC1 signaling. Mol Cell Biol 29(15): 4235–49.
47. Yu Y, Kudchodkar SB, Alwine JC (2005) Effects of simian virus 40 large and small tumor antigens on mammalian target of rapamycin signaling: small tumor antigen mediates hypophosphorylation of eIF4E-binding protein 1 late in infection. J Virol 79(11): 6882–9.
48. Ikeda K, Saeki Y, Gonzalez-Agosti C, Ramesh V, Chiocca EA (1999) Inhibition of NF2- negative and NF2-positive primary human meningioma cell proliferation by overexpression of merlin due to vector-mediated gene transfer. J Neurosurg 91(1): 85–92.
49. Okada T, Lopez-Lago M, Giancotti FG (2005) Merlin/NF-2 mediates contact inhibition of growth by suppressing recruitment of Rac to the plasma membrane. J Cell Biol 171(2): 361–71.
50. Lu Z, Hunter T (2010) Ubiquitylation and proteasomal degradation of the p21(Cip1), p27(Kip1) and p57(Kip2) CDK inhibitors. Cell Cycle 9(12): 2342–52.
51. Xiao GH, Gallagher R, Shetler J, Skele K, Altomare DA, et al. (2005) The NF2 tumor suppressor gene product, merlin, inhibits cell proliferation and cell cycle progression by repressing cyclin D1 expression. Mol Cell Biol 25(6): 2384–94.
52. Mamidipudi V, Zhang J, Lee KC, Cartwright CA (2004) RACK1 regulates G1/S progression by suppressing Src kinase activity. Mol Cell Biol 24(15): 6788–98.
53. Bhattacharyya R, Noch EK, Khalili K (2007) A novel role of Rac1 GTPase in JCV T-antigen mediated beta-catenin stabilization. Oncogene 26(55): 7628–36.
54. Altomare DA, Vaslet CA, Skele KL, De Rienzo A, Devarajan K, et al. (2005) A mouse model recapitulating molecular features of human mesothelioma. Cancer Res 65(18): 8090–5.
55. Gordon J, Del Valle L, Otte J, Khalili K (2000) Pituitary neoplasia induced by expression of human neurotropic polyomavirus, JCV, early genome in transgenic mice. Oncogene 19(42): 4840–6.
56. Riddick G, Fine HA (2011) Integration and analysis of genome-scale data from gliomas. Nat. Rev. Neurol 7: 439–450.
57. Stettner MR, Nance JA, Wright CA, Kinoshita Y, Kim WK, et al. (2009) SMAD proteins of oligodendroglial cells regulate transcription of JC virus early and late genes coordinately with the Tat protein of human immunodeficiency virus type 1. J Gen Virol 90(8): 2005–14.

Bevacizumab Treatment for Meningiomas in NF2: A Retrospective Analysis of 15 Patients

Fabio P. Nunes[1,2], Vanessa L. Merker[1,3], Dominique Jennings[4], Paul A. Caruso[5], Emmanuelle di Tomaso[6], Alona Muzikansky[7], Fred G. Barker II[8], Anat Stemmer-Rachamimov[6], Scott R. Plotkin[1,3]*

1 Neurology Department, Massachusetts General Hospital, Boston, Massachusetts, United States of America, **2** Genetics Department, Massachusetts General Hospital, Boston, Massachusetts, United States of America, **3** Stephen E. and Catherine Pappas Center for Neurooncology, Massachusetts General Hospital, Boston, Massachusetts, United States of America, **4** A.A. Martinos Center for Biomedical Imaging, Massachusetts General Hospital, Boston, Massachusetts, United States of America, **5** Department of Radiology, Massachusetts General Hospital, Boston, Massachusetts, United States of America, **6** Pathology Department, Massachusetts General Hospital, Boston, Massachusetts, United States of America, **7** Biostatistics Center, Massachusetts General Hospital, Boston, Massachusetts, United States of America, **8** Neurosurgical Service, Massachusetts General Hospital, Boston, Massachusetts, United States of America

Abstract

Bevacizumab treatment can result in tumor shrinkage of progressive vestibular schwannomas in some neurofibromatosis 2 (NF2) patients but its effect on meningiomas has not been defined. To determine the clinical activity of bevacizumab against NF2-related meningiomas, we measured changes in volume of meningiomas in NF2 patients who received bevacizumab for treatment of progressive vestibular schwannomas. A radiographic response was defined as a 20% decrease in tumor size by volumetric MRI analysis. In addition, we determined the expression pattern of growth factors associated with tumor angiogenesis in paraffin-embedded tissues from 26 unrelated meningiomas. A total of 48 meningiomas in 15 NF2 patients were included in this study with a median follow up time of 18 months. A volumetric radiographic response was seen in 29% of the meningiomas (14/48). Tumor shrinkage was not durable: the median duration of response was 3.7 months and the median time to progression was 15 months. There was no significant correlation between pre-treatment growth rate and meningioma response in regression models. Tissue analysis showed no correlation between tumor microvascular density and expression of VEGF pathway components. This data suggests that, in contrast to schwannomas, activation of VEGF pathway is not the primary driver of angiogenesis in meningiomas. Our results suggest that a minority of NF2-associated meningiomas shrink during bevacizumab therapy and that these responses were of short duration. These results are comparable to previous studies of bevacizumab in sporadic meningiomas.

Editor: Russell O. Pieper, University of California-San Francisco, United States of America

Funding: This work was supported by a United States National Institutes of Heath grant (5-T32-GM007748-32) to FPN. The funders had no role in study design, data collection and analysis, decision to publish, or preparation of the manuscript.

Competing Interests: The authors have declared that no competing interests exist.

* E-mail: splotkin@partners.org

Introduction

Meningiomas are the most common type of brain tumor, accounting for 34% of all central nervous system tumors.[1] Despite the high prevalence of meningiomas in the general population, there are currently no medical treatments available.[2,3] For sporadic meningiomas that require active treatment, surgery and radiation therapy are usually effective. Meningiomas are even more common in neurofibromatosis 2 (NF2) patients, with a cumulative incidence of 80% by age 70,[4] and are a major cause of morbidity and mortality in these patients.[5,6] The lack of effective medical therapy for meningiomas represents a significant challenge in the clinical management of NF2 patients. Unlike patients with sporadic tumors, NF2 patients often have multiple meningiomas, vestibular schwannomas, and ependymomas. The multiplicity of tumors make surgery and radiation therapy for all tumors impracticable.

Neovascularization is necessary for tumor growth beyond 2 – 3 mm,[3] the point at which diffusion alone becomes insufficient to meet basic tumor metabolic requirements,[7] and is driven by tumor produced angiogenic factors such as vascular endothelial growth factor (VEGF) that stimulate the growth of tumor capillaries. Bevacizumab is a humanized monoclonal antibody that neutralizes the activity of VEGF.[8] Bevacizumab prevents the binding of all VEGF isoforms to VEGF receptors, and is currently approved by the Food and Drug Administration (FDA) for clinical use in recurrent glioblastoma, metastatic colorectal cancer, advanced nonsquamous non-small cell lung cancer, and metastatic kidney cancer (www.fda.gov on 02/05/2012).

We have recently shown that treatment with bevacizumab can lead to hearing improvement and tumor shrinkage in some NF2 patients with progressive vestibular schwannomas.[9] Tissue analysis of schwannomas suggested activation of the VEGF pathway due to decreased expression of SEMA3, an angiogenesis inhibitor. The effects of bevacizumab on meningiomas are not clear. To date, two case reports and two case series have been published on bevacizumab use in intracranial meningiomas, with anecdotal reports of meningioma response to bevacizumab.[10–13] We present here a retrospective analysis of tumor response in 48 intracranial meningiomas from 15 NF2 patients treated with bevacizumab for progressive vestibular schwannoma.

Methods

Ethics Statement

This research study was approved by the Partners Human Research Committee Institutional Review Board. Requirement for informed consent was waived for this retrospective analysis of clinical data.

Patients

Between 2007 and 2011, a total of 31 NF2 patients were treated at our center using bevacizumab for progressive vestibular schwannomas. Of these 31 patients, 16 also had intracranial meningiomas (55%). Two patients were excluded from the study because of incompatibility between the MRI scan format performed at an outside facility and our volumetric analysis software. We included one additional NF2 patient who underwent surgical resection of bilateral vestibular schwannomas and was treated using bevacizumab for a single progressive meningioma. A total of 48 meningiomas and 18 vestibular schwannomas in 15 NF2 patients were included in the analysis. Patients received bevacizumab 5 mg/kg I.V. every 2 weeks as part of clinical care for their vestibular schwannoma. Higher doses used for malignant brain tumors (e.g., 10 mg/kg) were not used in order to minimize risk of toxicity. Brain MRI scans were performed within about 1 month prior to start of treatment, and approximately every 3 months after the start of treatment to monitor tumor response. Adverse events were classified according to the Common Terminology Criteria for Adverse Events, version 4.

Volumetric analysis

Commercial software (Alice; Hayden Image Processing Group/ Parexel International Corp, Waltham, MA) was used to create the volumetric measurements on contrast enhanced T1-weighted axial images. Once outlining was complete, actual volume measurements were calculated in Matlab (The MathWorks, Natick, MA) by counting the number of voxels in a given image and multiplying the count by the volume of a single voxel (as calculated using the in-plane and through-plane image resolution). A maximum number of eight tumors per patient can be measured using the Alice software. In patients with more than 8 tumors, volumetric analysis was first performed on vestibular schwannomas and then on meningiomas (from largest to smallest). Total intracranial tumor volume was defined as the sum of the volume of all intracranial meningiomas measured in a patient. We used clinically indicated MRIs performed prior to start of bevacizumab therapy to determine pre-treatment meningioma annual growth rate (AGR). Tumor growth rate was defined as (tumor volume – baseline tumor volume)/ baseline tumor volume.

Tumor contours for volumetric analysis were delineated by a single researcher (FN) who was blinded for patient identity, time of scan, and treatment status (pre- or post-bevacizumab). All tumor contours were performed using T1 post-contrast axial MRI scans. After contours were completed, a neuroradiologist (PC) with 10 years of post-fellowship academic experience reviewed the contours. For tumors with indistinct boundaries, the neuroradiologist reviewed axial, sagittal, and coronal slices of pre- and post-contrast T1-weighted, T2-weighted, diffusion-weighted images, FLAIR, susceptibility, FIESTA images, and CT scans when available. Details of the methodology used for determining tumor contours are available in the supplemental material (Text S1).

Definition of imaging response

A radiographic response was defined as a decrease in tumor volume of ≥20% at any time compared with baseline volume. Tumor progression was defined as an increase in volume of ≥ 20% when compared to baseline. Stable disease included all other responses. A sustained radiographic response was defined as a decrease in tumor volume of ≥ 20% when compared to baseline at the time of the last scan. Duration of response was determined as the time interval from the first and last scans showing a decrease in volume ≥ 20% from baseline, even if interim scans did not meet radiographic response criteria. Time to progression was defined as the time from first dose of bevacizumab to the first scan date in which the meningioma grew ≥ 20% in volume compared to baseline measurements.

Regression Analysis

We analyzed each outcome of interest on a per-tumor basis and on a per-patient basis. In the per-tumor analysis, each tumor was considered an independent event with no clustering effect for individual patients with multiple tumors. In the per-patient analysis, we accounted for the clustering effect of multiple tumors in individual patients by using a regression model that included a random effect. Details on the regression model used are available in the supplemental material. In both analyses, we calculated the tumor growth rate during the pre- and post-treatment periods using all scans available (up to 4 years before initiation of treatment). We also performed the analyses using only the scans in the 12 months immediately prior to initiation of therapy to determine pre-treatment annual tumor growth rate. We wanted to determine whether relative change in tumor volume (percent change from baseline) or absolute change in tumor volume would correlate with radiographic response to treatment. Therefore, tumor growth rate was represented as relative change in tumor volume from baseline (percentage response) and as absolute difference in tumor volume from baseline. We then correlated pre-treatment growth rates with post-treatment growth rates using patient demographic information (age at the start of treatment and gender), tumor size at baseline, and tumor location as covariates. Statistical analysis was performed with SAS software (version 9.2, SAS Institute Inc, NC, USA). A P value of <.05 was considered to be statistically significant.

Immunohistochemistry

In a parallel analysis, we determined the expression pattern of growth factors associated with tumor angiogenesis in paraffin-embedded tissues of 13 unrelated NF2-related meningiomas and 13 sporadic meningiomas from surgeries at Massachusetts General Hospital. A similar analysis for NF2-related and sporadic schwannomas was reported previously.[9]Five micron-thick sections were cut and immunostained with the following antibodies: CD31 (Dako, prediluted), αSMA (Sigma, 1:100), VEGF (Santa Cruz or Neomarker 1:100), VEGFR2, PDGFR-α, PDGFR-β (Cell Signaling; 1:250, 1:100 and 1:100 respectively), Neuropilin-1 (Chemicon, 1:40), Neuropilin-2 (R&D Biosystem, 1:500), Semaphorin 3A (Millipore, 1:100) and Semaphorin 3F (Chemicon 1:250). Semiquantitative analysis was performed by two authors who scored the intensity of staining of tumor cells and blood vessels on a scale from 0 (no staining) to 3 (strong staining). For calculation of microvascular density and diameter, CD31 labeling was used to highlight vessels. The quantification used at least 5 fields of confirmed tumor tissue at 200x magnification with an average of 100 vessels counted per section. A customized software analysis tool compatible with Image J (http://rsb.info.nih.gov/ij/) was then used to determine the number of vessels, perimeter, the minor axis of best-fitted ellipse (representative of the vessel diameter), and the total surface covered by vascular spaces. The same method was used substituting either VEGFR2 or NRP2 labeling to determine the percentage of vessels expressing these VEGF receptors. Consecutive sections were used to allow similar areas of the tumor to be quantified in all cases.

Results

A total of 48 meningiomas and 18 vestibular schwannomas from 15 NF2 patients (7 men, 8 women) were included in this study. Patient and tumor characteristics are listed in Table 1. The mean number of MRI scans per patient used for analysis of tumor response was 8 (range, 4 – 14). The median patient age at the start of treatment was 29.5 years (range, 16 – 63 years). The mean (median) volumes of meningiomas and vestibular schwannomas at the beginning of treatment were 6.2 cm^3 (1.9 cm^3), and 9.8 cm^3 (4.3 cm^3), respectively. The mean volumetric growth rate prior to treatment was 11.6% per year and median follow up time was 18 months (range 10 to 37 months). Bevacizumab was overall well tolerated, with only four grade 3 adverse events (hypertension, elevated liver enzymes, menorrhagia, irregular menses), and two grade 4 events (both associated with wound healing problems, including vascular access complications and tracheostomy wound healing delays).

A radiographic response was seen in 29% of tumors (14/48 tumors) using per-tumor analysis and was seen in 7% of patients (1/15 patients using a per-patient analysis) (Figure 1). Tumor shrinkage was not durable, with only 5/14 responding meningiomas maintaining a radiographic response at the last follow up. The median duration of meningioma response was 3.7 months (range 0 to 25 months), with six meningiomas having a single scan meeting criteria for radiographic response (decrease in meningioma volume ≥ 20%). Overall, 29/48 meningiomas (60%) progressed during the study. The median time to progression was 15 months on per-tumor analysis (Figure 2) and was 20 months on per-patient analysis. Progression–free survival at 6- and 12-months was 85% and 62%, respectively, on per-tumor basis. Progression-free survival at 6- and 12-months was 93% and 79%, respectively on per-patient basis.

The radiographic response rate for vestibular schwannomas in this cohort was 39% (7/18 tumors) when using whole brain MRI scans and was 44% (8/18 tumors) when using internal auditory

Table 1. Patient and tumor characteristics.

Characteristics	N (%)
Gender	
Female	8 (53%)
Male	7 (47%)
Age	
< 20y	2 (13%)
20 – 29y	7 (47%)
30 – 39y	2 (13%)
40 – 49y	3 (20%)
>50y	1 (7%)
Total meningiomas analyzed per patient	
1 – 2 meningiomas	8 (53%)
3 – 4 meningiomas	3 (20%)
>4 meningiomas	4 (27%)
Median meningioma baseline volume	1.9 cm^3
Distribution of meningioma volume at baseline (n = 48)	
< 2 cm^3	25 (52%)
2 – 10 cm^3	16 (34%)
10 – 20 cm^3	4 (8%)
> 20 cm^3	3 (6%)
Meningioma Pre-Treatment Annual Growth Rate	11.6% (range, -240% to 546%)
Meningioma location	
Orbital/Skull base	10 (21%)
Convexity/Falx	34 (71%)
Posterior fossa	4 (8%)
Median vestibular schwannoma volume at baseline	4.3 cm^3
Distribution of vestibular schwannoma volume at baseline (n = 18)	
< 2 cm^3	5 (27%)
2 – 10 cm^3	7 (39%)
10 – 20 cm^3	3 (17%)
> 20 cm^3	3 (17%)

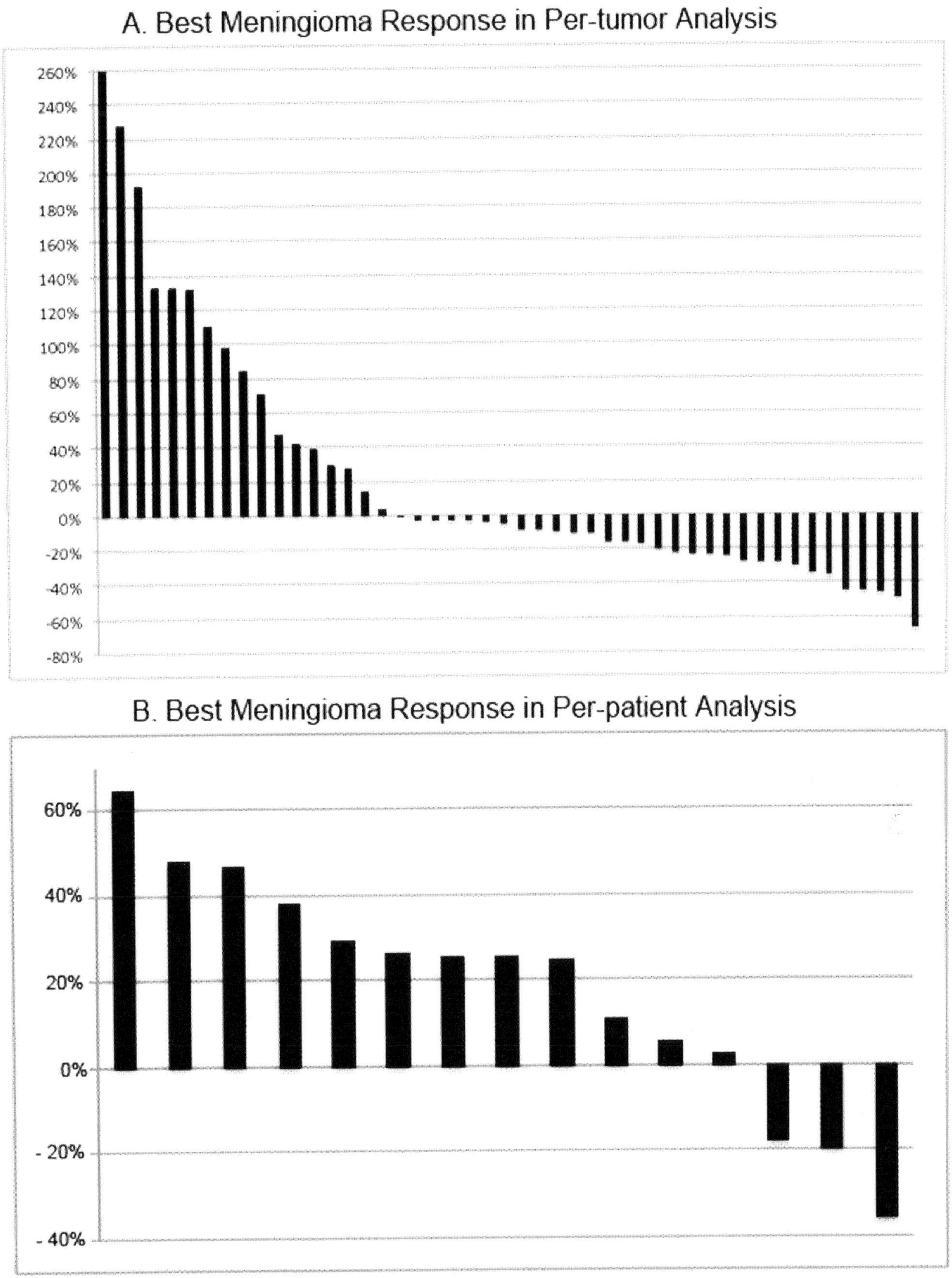

Figure 1. Radiographic Response of Meningiomas to Bevacizumab. Waterfall plot of best radiographic response for individual meningiomas (A) and for total meningioma volume in patients (B).

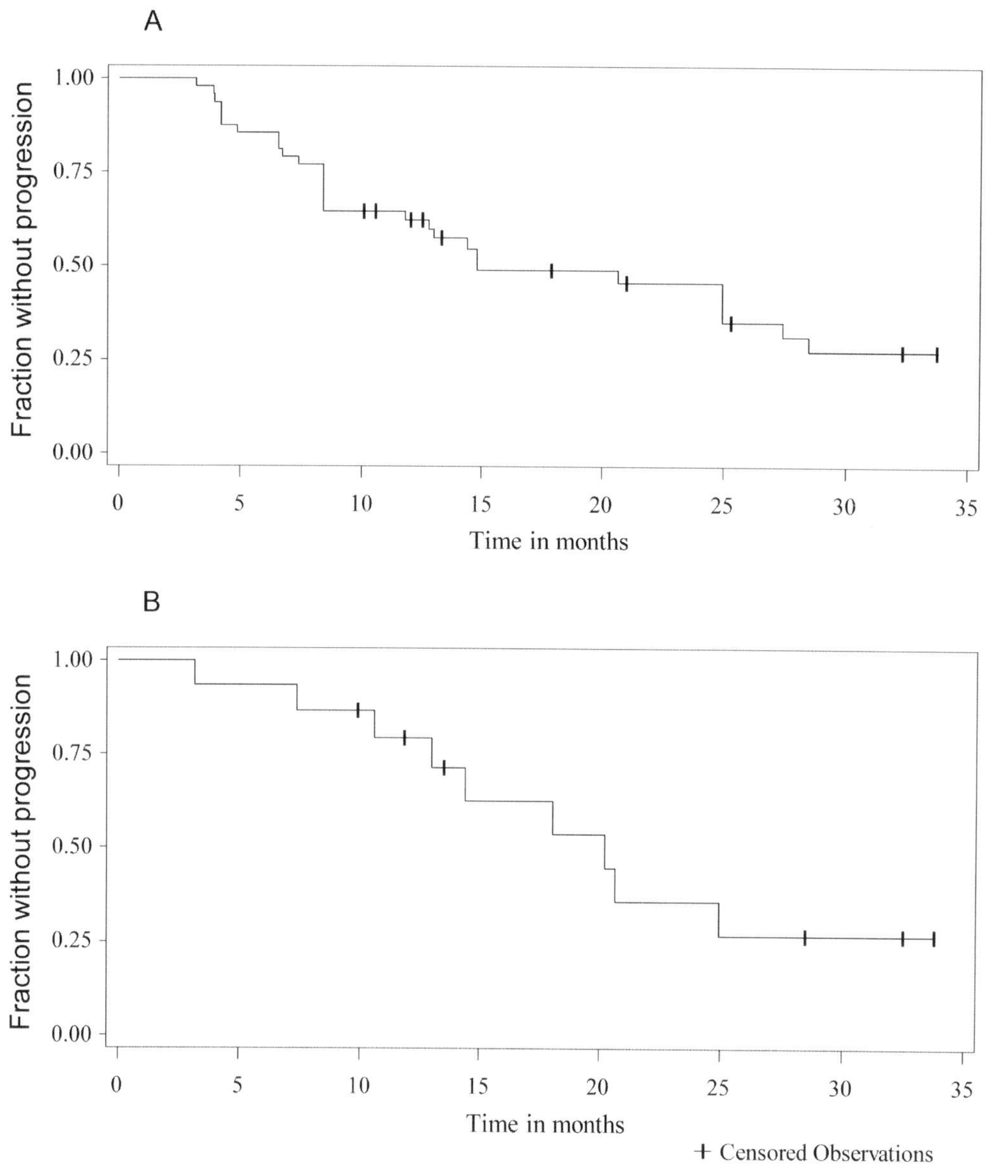

Figure 2. Time to Progression for Meningioma Treated with Bevacizumab. A. Kaplan-Meier curve for time to progression considering each meningioma as an independent event (per-tumor analysis). Progression was considered as an increase in tumor volume of 20% or more. B. Kaplan-Meier curve for time to progression using total intracranial meningioma volume for each patient as an independent event (per-patient analysis). Time to progression was 15 months for individual tumors and 20 months on per-patient analysis. Progression-free rate at six months was higher in the per-patient analysis at 93%, compared to 85% for the per-tumor analysis.

canal (3mm slices, no gap). The difference in response rate between the cohort of NF2 patients with meningiomas (44% response) and the entire treated NF2 cohort of 31 patients (55%, data not shown) was not statistically significant (Fisher exact two tail = .79).

A total of 47 meningiomas were included in regression analyses to identify clinical factors associated with post-treatment growth rate. For one meningioma, no pre-treatment scans were available for analysis. Growth rate estimates and statistical results are summarized on Table 2. There was no significant correlation between pre-treatment and post-treatment growth rates for individual meningiomas using per-tumor analysis (p = .33). This finding persisted when pre-treatment growth was calculated using only the 12 months immediately prior to treatment (p = .79). There was no significant difference in the results when tumor response was calculated using absolute change in tumor volume or percent change in tumor volume (p = 0.72). When only meningiomas with a pre-treamtent growth rate $\geq$ 20% and with baseline volume $\geq$ 1 cm^3 were included in the analysis, radiographic response was seen in only one out of five meningiomas (20% of tumors). Figure 3 shows the correlation between meningioma best response and pre-treatment growth rate.

In the per-patient analyses, there was no significant association between pre-treatment tumor growth and tumor response when using percentage change in tumor volume (p = .23), or absolute change in tumor volume (p = .37). There was no difference in the results when pre-treatment period included only the 12 months immediately prior to start of therapy. Interestingly, there was a

Table 2. Summary of Regression Analysis Results for Growth Rate Estimates in Per-Tumor and Per-Patient Models.

Factor	Per-tumor Analysis				Per-patient Analysis			
	Percentage Change in Tumor Volume		Absolute Change in Tumor Volume		Percentage Change in Tumor Volume		Absolute Change in Tumor Volume	
	Parameter Estimate	*p-value*	*Parameter Estimate*	*p-value*	*Parameter Estimate*	*p-value*	*Parameter Estimate*	*p-value*
Tumor Growth by Month Using All Scans	−0.053	0.33	−0.011	0.72	−0.066	0.23	−0.025	0.37
Tumor Growth by Month Using last 12 months	−0.014	0.79	0.002	0.94	−0.016	0.56	−0.04	0.43
Male Gender	N/A	N/A	N/A	N/A	−0.015	0.07	−0.06	0.33
Age	N/A	N/A	N/A	N/A	−0.0007	0.04	−0.004	0.09

correlation between increased post-treatment growth rate and male gender ($p = .07$), and older age ($p = .04$).

Immunohistochemical analysis of meningiomas showed no significant difference in the expression of components of the VEGF angiogenesis pathway (VEGF, VEGFR2, PDGFR-α, PDGFR-β, neuropilin-1, neuropilin-2, semaphorin 3A, and semaphorin 3F) between sporadic meningiomas and NF2-associated meningiomas. Microvascular density was significantly greater in sporadic meningiomas compared to NF2-related meningiomas (52 vessels/mm2 vs. 32 vessels/mm2; t-test $p = .01$). There was no significant difference of average perimeter or diameter between the two groups.

Discussion

Medical treatments for meningiomas are desperately needed for patients with meningiomas that cannot be adequately treated with surgery and radiation. The list of drugs without a clear benefit for these tumors continues to grow and includes tamoxifen,[14] irinotecan,[15] temozolomide,[16] octreotide,[17,18] mifepristone,[19] erlotinib,[20] gefitinib,[20] imatinib,[21] and alpha-interferon.[22,23] Although initial results with hydroxyurea were promising,[24] further studies showed that radiographic response to hydroxyurea in meningiomas is uncommon.[25,26]

Our results for NF2-related meningiomas are comparable to case series of sporadic meningiomas treated with bevacizumab [12,13]. These studies, which included all grades of meningiomas, reported median PFS of 18−26 months and radiographic response rates of 0−7%. Because multiple meningiomas are common in NF2 patients, we analyzed our data on a per-tumor basis and on a per-patient basis. Using per-tumor analysis, the median PFS was 15 months; using per-patient analysis, the PFS was 20 months. The per-tumor radiographic response rate was 29% in our series and exceeded the rate in previous reports; however, the durability of response was short. This contrasts with the durability of response in schwannoma.[9] These results suggest that the clinical benefit of tumor shrinkage in our patients was minimal.

Analysis of tumor growth rate can be determined as a relative change (percentage) in tumor volume from baseline, or as an absolute volume change from baseline measurement. The use of relative change is the standard method used for radiographic response to treatment, whether linear measurements or volumetric analysis methods are used in the study.[27] We analyzed our data in both ways to account for potential bias in the determination of response rate based on tumor size at baseline. Relative changes in tumor volume are usually larger in small tumors, leading to bias in the statistical analysis when smaller and likely asymptomatic tumors are included in the study. Instead, larger tumors are more likely to have larger absolute volume changes than small tumors, even if only a small percentage change in total volume has occurred. Due to the biology of VEGF inhibitors, such as bevacizumab, we decided to determined response rate using both relative change in tumor volume, as well as absolute changes in volume from baseline for comparison. In this retrospective analysis, neither measurement of pre-treatment growth rate was found to be significantly associated with treatment response. This may be due to poor response to treatment seen in this study, small sample size, or selection bias from this retrospective study. Although there was a statistical association between older patients and meningioma response to treatment, the relative effect on response was small, and likely not clinically relevant.

We have previously shown that treatment with bevacizumab can lead to tumor shrinkage of vestibular schwannomas in patients

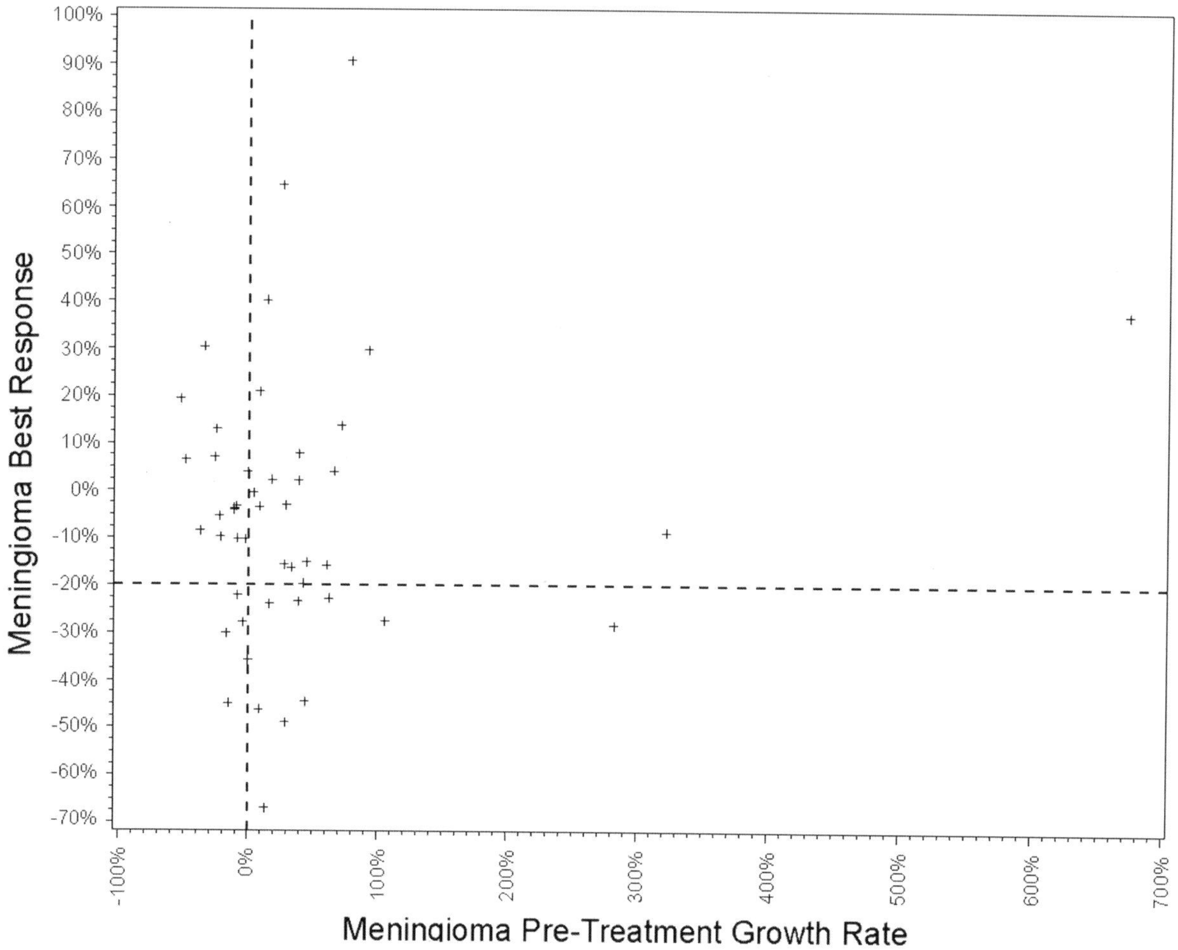

Figure 3. Meningioma Best Response Compared to Pre-treatment Growth Rate. Scatter-plot of meningioma best response vs. relative change in tumor volume prior to treatment. Horizontal dashed lines show threshold for radiographic response at 20% decrease in tumor volume post treatment, and vertical dashed line separates tumors with positive growth prior to therapy.

with NF2,[9] with follow up study showing radiographic response in 55% of vestibular schwannomas, and hearing improvement in 57% in our cohort of 31 patients.[28] In these same patients, radiographic responses for meningiomas were seen in only 29% of meningiomas and were short-lived.. The difference in response rate between vestibular schwannomas and meningiomas does not seem to correlate with degree of angiogenesis, since expression of VEGF in the tumor, expression of VEGFR2 in tumor blood vessels, and microvascular density are greater in meningiomas than in vestibular schwannomas.[9] However, immunohistochemical analysis of expression of the VEGF pathway components shows different patterns in schwannomas and meningiomas. In our previous study, analysis of the VEGF angiogenesis pathway in schwannomas showed very low expression of SEMA3 (angiogenesis inhibitor) and a positive correlation between VEGF/SEMA3 expression ratio and tumor microvascular density; consistent with the hypothesis that the angiogenesis in schwannomas was driven by activation of the VEGF pathway. In contrast, in this study, we found a robust expression of SEMA3 in meningiomas (NF2 associated and sporadic) and furthermore; there was no correlation between expression of VEGF pathway components and tumor microvascular density. These findings suggest that the VEGF pathway may not be an important driving force of angiogenesis in meningiomas and may explain the different response rates observed for the two types of tumors. Currently, prospective studies of bevacizumab (NCT01125046) and combination of bevacizumab and everolimus (NCT00972335) are underway for patients with sporadic recurrent or progressive meningiomas.

Conclusion

NF2-related meningiomas were not effectively treated by bevacizumab in this analysis of NF2 patients treated for their progressive vestibular schwannomas. We did not identify any predictors of tumor response to bevacizumab in our cohort. Pathologic analysis of components of the VEGF angiogenesis pathway and of tumor microvascular density in meningiomas showed robust expression of SEMA3 (an angiogenesis inhibitor that was not expressed in schwannomas) and in contrast of our findings in schwannomas, there was no correlation between expression of VEGF pathway components and tumor microvascular density in meningiomas. These findings suggest that the VEGF pathway may not be a driving force in angiogenesis in meningiomas and may explain limited clinical response in meningiomas.

Acknowledgments

The authors would like to thank Drs. Robert Martuza and Steven Greenberg for their guidance and critical review of this manuscript.

Author Contributions

Imaging analysis: FPN PAC DJ. Conceived and designed the experiments: FPN EdT SRP FGB ASR. Performed the experiments: FPN VLM DJ PAC EdT. Analyzed the data: FPN AM DJ ASR SRP. Contributed reagents/materials/analysis tools: EdT AM. Wrote the paper: FPN SRP FGB ASR.

References

1. CBTRUS (2012 March) CBTRUS Statistical Report: Primary Brain and Central Nervous System Tumors Diagnosed in the United States in 2004–22008.
2. Bria C, Wegner RE, Clump DA, Vargo JA, Mintz AH, et al. (2011) Fractionated stereotactic radiosurgery for the treatment of meningiomas. J Cancer Res Ther 7: 52–57.
3. Norden AD, Drappatz J, Wen PY (2009) Advances in meningioma therapy. Curr Neurol Neurosci Rep 9: 231–240.
4. Smith MJ, Higgs JE, Bowers NL, Halliday D, Paterson J, et al. (2011) Cranial meningiomas in 411 neurofibromatosis type 2 (NF2) patients with proven gene mutations: clear positional effect of mutations, but absence of female severity effect on age at onset. J Med Genet 48: 261–265.
5. Baser ME, Friedman JM, Aeschliman D, Joe H, Wallace AJ, et al. (2002) Predictors of the risk of mortality in neurofibromatosis 2. Am J Hum Genet 71: 715–723.
6. Nunes F, MacCollin M (2003) Neurofibromatosis 2 in the pediatric population. J Child Neurol 18: 718–724.
7. Rosen LS (2002) Clinical experience with angiogenesis signaling inhibitors: focus on vascular endothelial growth factor (VEGF) blockers. Cancer Control 9: 36–44.
8. Ferrara N, Hillan KJ, Gerber HP, Novotny W (2004) Discovery and development of bevacizumab, an anti-VEGF antibody for treating cancer. Nat Rev Drug Discov 3: 391–400.
9. Plotkin SR, Stemmer-Rachamimov AO, Barker FG, Halpin C, Padera TP, et al. (2009) Hearing improvement after bevacizumab in patients with neurofibromatosis type 2. N Engl J Med 361: 358–367.
10. Goutagny S, Raymond E, Sterkers O, Colombani JM, Kalamarides M (2011) Radiographic regression of cranial meningioma in a NF2 patient treated by bevacizumab. Ann Oncol 22: 990–991.
11. Puchner MJ, Hans VH, Harati A, Lohmann F, Glas M, et al. (2010) Bevacizumab-induced regression of anaplastic meningioma. Ann Oncol 21: 2445–2446.
12. Lou E, Sumrall AL, Turner S, Peters KB, Desjardins A, et al. (2012) Bevacizumab therapy for adults with recurrent/progressive meningioma: a retrospective series. J Neurooncol 109: 63–70.
13. Nayak L, Iwamoto FM, Rudnick JD, Norden AD, Lee EQ, et al. (2012) Atypical and anaplastic meningiomas treated with bevacizumab. J Neurooncol 109: 187–193.
14. Goodwin JW, Crowley J, Eyre HJ, Stafford B, Jaeckle KA, et al. (1993) A phase II evaluation of tamoxifen in unresectable or refractory meningiomas: a Southwest Oncology Group study. J Neurooncol 15: 75–77.
15. Chamberlain MC, Tsao-Wei DD, Groshen S (2006) Salvage chemotherapy with CPT-11 for recurrent meningioma. J Neurooncol 78: 271–276.
16. Chamberlain MC, Tsao-Wei DD, Groshen S (2004) Temozolomide for treatment-resistant recurrent meningioma. Neurology 62: 1210–1212.
17. Johnson DR, Kimmel DW, Burch PA, Cascino TL, Giannini C, et al. (2011) Phase II study of subcutaneous octreotide in adults with recurrent or progressive meningioma and meningeal hemangiopericytoma. Neuro Oncol 13: 530–535.
18. Schulz C, Mathieu R, Kunz U, Mauer UM (2011) Treatment of unresectable skull base meningiomas with somatostatin analogs. Neurosurg Focus 30: E11.
19. Grunberg SM, Weiss MH, Russell CA, Spitz IM, Ahmadi J, et al. (2006) Long-term administration of mifepristone (RU486): clinical tolerance during extended treatment of meningioma. Cancer Invest 24: 727–733.
20. Norden AD, Raizer JJ, Abrey LE, Lamborn KR, Lassman AB, et al. (2009) Phase II trials of erlotinib or gefitinib in patients with recurrent meningioma. J Neurooncol.
21. Wen PY, Yung WK, Lamborn KR, Norden AD, Cloughesy TF, et al. (2009) Phase II study of imatinib mesylate for recurrent meningiomas (North American Brain Tumor Consortium study 01–08). Neuro Oncol 11: 853–860.
22. Chamberlain MC, Glantz MJ (2008) Interferon-alpha for recurrent World Health Organization grade 1 intracranial meningiomas. Cancer 113: 2146–2151.
23. Kaba SE, DeMonte F, Bruner JM, Kyritsis AP, Jaeckle KA, et al. (1997) The treatment of recurrent unresectable and malignant meningiomas with interferon alpha-2B. Neurosurgery 40: 271–275.
24. Schrell UM, Rittig MG, Anders M, Koch UH, Marschalek R, et al. (1997) Hydroxyurea for treatment of unresectable and recurrent meningiomas. II. Decrease in the size of meningiomas in patients treated with hydroxyurea. J Neurosurg 86: 840–844.
25. Loven D, Hardoff R, Sever ZB, Steinmetz AP, Gornish M, et al. (2004) Non-resectable slow-growing meningiomas treated by hydroxyurea. J Neurooncol 67: 221–226.
26. Mason WP, Gentili F, Macdonald DR, Hariharan S, Cruz CR, et al. (2002) Stabilization of disease progression by hydroxyurea in patients with recurrent or unresectable meningioma. J Neurosurg 97: 341–346.
27. Eisenhauer EA, Therasse P, Bogaerts J, Schwartz LH, Sargent D, et al. (2009) New response evaluation criteria in solid tumours: revised RECIST guideline (version 1.1). Eur J Cancer 45: 228–247.
28. Plotkin SR, Merker VL, Halpin C, Jennings D, McKenna MJ, et al. (2012) Bevacizumab for progressive vestibular schwannoma in neurofibromatosis type 2: a retrospective review of 31 patients. Otol Neurotol 33: 1046–1052.

Stratified Whole Genome Linkage Analysis of Chiari Type I Malformation Implicates Known Klippel-Feil Syndrome Genes as Putative Disease Candidates

Christina A. Markunas[1], Karen Soldano[1], Kaitlyn Dunlap[1], Heidi Cope[1], Edgar Asiimwe[1], Jeffrey Stajich[1], David Enterline[2], Gerald Grant[3], Herbert Fuchs[3], Simon G. Gregory[1¶], Allison E. Ashley-Koch[1*¶]

1 Department of Medicine, Duke University Medical Center, Durham, North Carolina, United States of America, **2** Department of Radiology, Duke University Medical Center, Durham, North Carolina, United States of America, **3** Department of Surgery, Duke University Medical Center, Durham, North Carolina, United States of America

Abstract

Chiari Type I Malformation (CMI) is characterized by displacement of the cerebellar tonsils below the base of the skull, resulting in significant neurologic morbidity. Although multiple lines of evidence support a genetic contribution to disease, no genes have been identified. We therefore conducted the largest whole genome linkage screen to date using 367 individuals from 66 families with at least two individuals presenting with nonsyndromic CMI with or without syringomyelia. Initial findings across all 66 families showed minimal evidence for linkage due to suspected genetic heterogeneity. In order to improve power to localize susceptibility genes, stratified linkage analyses were performed using clinical criteria to differentiate families based on etiologic factors. Families were stratified on the presence or absence of clinical features associated with connective tissue disorders (CTDs) since CMI and CTDs frequently co-occur and it has been proposed that CMI patients with CTDs represent a distinct class of patients with a different underlying disease mechanism. Stratified linkage analyses resulted in a marked increase in evidence of linkage to multiple genomic regions consistent with reduced genetic heterogeneity. Of particular interest were two regions (Chr8, Max LOD = 3.04; Chr12, Max LOD = 2.09) identified within the subset of "CTD-negative" families, both of which harbor growth differentiation factors (GDF6, GDF3) implicated in the development of Klippel-Feil syndrome (KFS). Interestingly, roughly 3–5% of CMI patients are diagnosed with KFS. In order to investigate the possibility that CMI and KFS are allelic, GDF3 and GDF6 were sequenced leading to the identification of a previously known KFS missense mutation and potential regulatory variants in GDF6. This study has demonstrated the value of reducing genetic heterogeneity by clinical stratification implicating several convincing biological candidates and further supporting the hypothesis that multiple, distinct mechanisms are responsible for CMI.

Editor: Ralf Krahe, University of Texas MD Anderson Cancer Center, United States of America

Funding: Financial support for this study was generously provided by the National Institutes of Health (http://www.nih.gov/, NS063273, AAK and SGG), American Syringomyelia and Chiari Alliance Project (http://www.asap.org/, AAK), and Chiari and Syringomyelia Foundation (http://www.csfinfo.org/, CAM). The funders had no role in study design, data collection and analysis, decision to publish, or preparation of the manuscript.

Competing Interests: 1) Financial: An invention disclosure form (IDF) has been submitted for the invention titled "Genes Involved in Chiari Type I Malformation". It was received by the Duke Office of Licensing and Ventures and assigned the IDF#3930 (CAM, SGG, and AAK), and 2) Professional: Dr. Allison Ashley-Koch is chair of the Chiari and Syringomyelia Foundation (CSF) scientific, education, and advisory board. CSF provided partial funding for this study, as well as salary support for Ms. Christina Markunas. This does not alter the authors' adherence to all the PLOS ONE policies on sharing data and materials.

* E-mail: allison.ashleykoch@duke.edu

¶ These authors contributed equally to this work.

Introduction

Chiari Type I Malformation (CMI) is characterized by displacement of the cerebellar tonsils below the base of the skull and occurs with an estimated prevalence of less than one percent in the United States [1,2]. Although magnetic resonance imaging (MRI) is considered the gold standard for diagnosis, no universally accepted diagnostic criteria exist. Patients are usually considered affected if one cerebellar tonsil is herniated 5 mm or more [3] or both tonsils are herniated 3 mm or more [4]. CMI patients exhibit a wide range of neurologic symptoms, including headaches, dizziness, difficulty sleeping, numbness/tingling of an upper extremity, fatigue, nausea, shortness of breath, blurred vision, among others [5]. Currently, the only treatment to alleviate symptoms for CMI is suboccipital decompression surgery to both expand the cranial base and re-establish normal cerebrospinal fluid (CSF) flow.

Although multiple mechanisms have been proposed for cerebellar tonsillar herniation, including cranial constriction, cranial settling, spinal cord tethering, intracranial hypertension, and intraspinal hypotension [6], "classical" CMI is generally hypothesized to occur through the "cranial constriction" mechanism. More specifically, "classical" CMI is thought to be caused by an underdeveloped occipital bone, resulting in a posterior fossa (PF) which is too small and shallow to accommodate the normal sized cerebellum [7,8]. Herniation of the cerebellar tonsils and an upward shift of the tentorium are thought to occur secondarily [8]. In addition to the "cranial constriction" mechanism, accumulating evidence supports an association between connective tissue disorders (CTDs) and some occurrences of CMI [9]. Importantly,

CMI patients diagnosed with CTDs may represent a distinct class of patients that can be grouped under the "cranial settling" mechanism where both the occipital bone and posterior cranial fossa volume are normal in size but occipitoatlantoaxial joint instability exists [6].

While no disease gene has been identified for CMI to date, several lines of evidence support a genetic contribution to disease in at least a subset of nonsyndromic cases. These include twin studies [1,10,11,12,13,14,15,16], familial clustering [10,14,15,17,18,19,20,21,22,23,24,25,26,27,28,29,30], and co-segregation with known genetic syndromes or conditions commonly found as part of a genetic syndrome, including Ehlers-Danlos syndrome [9,31,32,33], Marfan syndrome [9,34,35,36], Klippel-Feil syndrome [23,37,38,39,40,41,42,43,44,45,46,47,48], growth hormone deficiency [45,46,49,50,51,52,53,54,55], craniosynostosis [56,57], and Neurofibromatosis type I [58,59]. Furthermore, in a study conducted by Milhorat and colleagues, it was reported that out of a cohort of 364 symptomatic patients, 43 (12%) had at least one close relative with CMI with or without syringomyelia or idiopathic syringomyelia [23]. Additionally, 72 patients (20%) were reported as having at least one close relative with a similar symptomology without an official CMI diagnosis. Despite evidence for a genetic component, genetic studies for CMI have been limited. Ascertainment for family studies has been hindered due to a relatively rare disease prevalence together with the small proportion of cases that are familial [23]. In addition, the ability to obtain MRIs on a large series of individuals for diagnostic purposes and lack of consistent disease criteria has led to increased phenotypic variability across patients resulting in phenotyping challenges. Only one whole genome linkage screen, but no genome wide association studies, has been published for CMI. Using 23 Caucasian multiplex families containing 67 sampled individuals affected with CMI with or without syringomyelia, Boyles, et al. conducted a whole genome linkage screen and identified significant evidence for linkage to regions on chromosomes 9 and 15 [17]. While this study took an important first step in trying to elucidate the genetic basis of CMI, the genetics of CMI is still very much unknown. Our limited understanding of the biological mechanism, lack of consistent diagnostic criteria, and complex etiology pose exciting challenges for studying the genetics of CMI.

One major challenge is the variability of clinical presentation within the CMI patient population. This clinical heterogeneity presents as differences with respect to the pattern and severity of symptoms, response to surgery, presence of associated conditions, age of onset, and the extent of tonsillar herniation. As CMI is thought to be influenced by multiple genetic and environmental factors, this clinical heterogeneity likely reflects in part an underlying genetic heterogeneity. While this can have substantial implications during the design stage of a genetic study, the selection of families that are genetically homogeneous is not straight forward. One approach is to stratify families using clinical features that may identify groups of families that share similar genetic risk factors. In other words, reducing phenotypic variability may lead to a reduction in genetic variability. Although the pool of candidate clinical features to use for stratification can be quite large, previous clinical associations observed with the disorder provide some insight into which features to select.

To address these issues, we performed the largest whole genome linkage screen to date using 367 individuals from 66 nonsyndromic CMI multiplex families. Based on the limited evidence for linkage using the complete collection of families, we performed a stratified whole genome linkage analysis using the presence or absence of CTD related conditions and successfully identified putative CMI susceptibility genes in the genetically more homogeneous strata.

Materials and Methods

Ethics Statement

All participating family members provided written informed consent for this study. If participants were minors, written consent was obtained from a parent or legal guardian for participants younger than 18 years of age. Participants between 12 and 17 years of age were asked to provide written assent. Written informed consent and assent, when applicable, were obtained by approved clinical staff. Consent forms were either discussed in person or were mailed and then discussed over the telephone. All participant interactions were logged in Progeny 8 (Delray Beach, FL), our clinical data collection software program. The original signed consent is maintained by the study and a copy was provided to participants. The consent form, procedure described above, and this study were specifically approved by the institutional review board of Duke University Medical Center.

Study Population

Participants were ascertained across the United States primarily through self-referral in response to advertisements on the web (e.g. Duke Center for Human Genetics and GeneTests), mailings and/or presentations to patient support groups and physician referral. Families were enrolled in the current study if at least two sampled individuals were diagnosed with CMI with or without syringomyelia. Exclusion criteria included the following: 1) families with a positive family history of a known genetic syndrome (e.g. Ehlers-Danlos syndrome, Marfan syndrome, Klippel-Feil syndrome, Crouzon syndrome, Neurofibromatosis), 2) family history of spina bifida or tethered cord syndrome, and 3) individuals thought to have a secondary form of CMI, such as occurring due to a brain tumor. Although syndromic families formally diagnosed with hereditary CTDs were excluded from our genetic screen, many family members exhibited conditions such as hypermobility, mitral valve prolapse and scoliosis which are often associated with CTDs as described in further detail below. Blood samples were collected from affected individuals and all available connecting family members, regardless of affection status. Additionally, study participants completed a family and medical history telephone interview, responded to a detailed clinical questionnaire, and submitted release forms for medical records and pre-surgical MRIs. When possible, a diagnosis of CMI was determined based on MRI measurements in which affection status was defined as cerebellar tonsillar herniation of 3 mm or more for both tonsils or herniation of 5 mm or more for either tonsil (refer to Table 1 for MRI availability). MRI measurements were taken from pre-surgical T1-weighted brain MRIs. Herniation of the left and right tonsils was measured linearly from the tip of the cerebellar tonsils perpendicularly to the foramen magnum on a sagittal image to the left and right of the midline, respectively. All measurements were reviewed by a board certified neuroradiologist (D.E). In the event that appropriate pre-surgical MRIs were not available, affection status was based on medical records or patient report when that was the only source available. Detailed population characteristics are provided in Table 1.

Genotyping and Quality Control

Blood samples were collected from study participants in EDTA tubes and DNA was extracted using the AutoPure LS® DNA extraction kit with Puregene® system reagents (Qiagen, Valencia, CA). A small amount of DNA (0.3 µg) was run on a 0.8% agarose

Table 1. Population characteristics.

Description	No. Individuals	No. Families
Total	**367[a]**	**66**
Number of affected individuals/family	**2.77±0.99 [2–6][b]**	
Sex		
Female	223	65
Male	144	61
CMI		
Affected	183	66
Female	124	60
Male	59	44
Unaffected/Uncertain	184	61
Female	99	51
Male	85	53
Syringomyelia		
Affected	50	41
CMI-Affected	47	40
Female	26	24
Male	21	19
CMI-Unaffected/Uncertain	3	3
Female	2	2
Male	1	1
Unaffected/Uncertain	317[a]	65
CMI-Affected	136	62
Female	98	53
Male	38	32
CMI-Unaffected/Uncertain	181	60
Female	97	50
Male	84	53
Posterior fossa decompression surgery[c]		
Yes	91	57
No	53	38
Unknown	39	24
MRI data		
Available	126	50
CMI-Affected	95	49
CMI-Unaffected/Uncertain	31	21
Unavailable	241	65
CMI-Affected	88	52
CMI-Unaffected/Uncertain	153	54

[a]Only considered genotyped individuals after exclusions were applied (See Methods section for details).
[b]Mean +/− standard deviation [range].
[c]Only considered affected individuals.
Abbreviations: CMI: Chiari Malformation Type I; No.: number.

gel in order to assess quality and each sample was quantified using the Nanodrop (Wilmington, DE). In total, 436 individuals from 75 families were genotyped using Illumina Human610-Quad BeadChips (San Diego, CA) per the manufacturer's instructions and chips were scanned using the Illumina iScan system (San Diego, CA). Due to the duration of ascertainment for this study, genotyping was performed in two separate batches (Batch 1:234 individuals from 40 families; Batch 2:202 individuals from 41 families). In addition to samples from study participants, replicate samples were included across sample plates and checked for mismatches. Specifically, two CMI family (1 male, 1 female) and two Centre d'Etude du Polymorphism Humain (CEPH) (1 male, 1 female) samples were included across three 96-well sample plates per batch in an alternating pattern.

Quality control (QC) procedures were performed to ensure high quality data were used for analysis. Initial quality assessment was performed separately for each batch using the Illumina GenomeStudio genotyping module (San Diego, CA). Single nucleotide polymorphism (SNP) data (N = 585497 combined across batches 1 and 2) quality were further assessed using PLINK v1.07 [60] to detect deviations from Hardy-Weinberg equilibrium (HWE; calculated using unaffected founders), estimate minor allele frequency (MAF; calculated using unaffected founders), and identify Mendelian errors (Parent-Parent-Child (P-P-C)). Parent-Child (P-C) errors were identified separately using custom scripts since PLINK does not examine trios with missing parents. Additional sample quality checks in PLINK included estimating pairwise identity by descent (IBD) in order to verify known relationships and check for cryptic relatedness (–genome; markers were pruned first), identifying Mendelian errors as described previously, calculating inbreeding coefficients (–het; markers were pruned first), performing a multidimensional scaling analysis in order to detect population stratification as different ethnicities could alter MAF estimates thus affecting the linkage analysis (1 individual per family used; –cluster –ppc 1e-4–mds-plot 2; markers were pruned first), and checking for sex discrepancies (–check-sex).

Whole Genome Linkage Analysis

Power for the whole genome linkage study was determined using SIMLINK [61]. Family structures, disease and sample statuses were based on the CMI multiplex linkage families used in the screen and provided as input for the simulations ($N_{replicates}$ = 1,000). Additional model parameters used for the simulations included: disease MAF of 0.001, marker MAF of 0.30, and an affecteds-only, low penetrance function (0, 0.001, 0.001).

All linkage analyses were performed using MERLIN 1.1.2 and MINX (MERLIN in X) [62] and allele frequencies were estimated using founders only for all analyses subsequently described. Since the underlying genetic model for CMI is unknown, both parametric (model dependent) and nonparametric (model free) linkage analyses were performed. For the parametric linkage analysis, an "affecteds only" low penetrance function was used (0, 0.001, 0.001) and a rare disease allele frequency of 0.001 was assumed. We performed an "affecteds-only" analysis because unaffected/unknown individuals will only contribute genotypic information, while affected individuals will contribute both phenotypic and genotypic information to the analysis. This approach protects against misclassification of non-penetrant individuals within the families. In addition to the standard LOD score analysis, MERLIN also provides estimates of the proportion of linked families (α) and the maximum heterogeneity LOD score (HLOD) which was used to detect linkage allowing for heterogeneity for the parametric analysis [62]. For the nonparametric linkage (NPL) analysis, the S_{all} scoring function was used which assesses IBD sharing across subsets of affected individuals [63]. In addition, both the Kong and Cox linear and exponential model were applied in order to evaluate statistical significance [64].

For both the parametric and nonparametric linkage analysis, two-point and multipoint analyses were performed. In order to maintain the correct type I error rate when conducting a multipoint analysis in families when one or both parents are missing, the option, "–rsq", in MERLIN was implemented which allows for the modeling of inter-marker linkage disequilibrium (LD) between SNPs [62]. An r^2 threshold of 0.16 [65] was selected to group SNPs into clusters.

Prior to whole genome linkage analysis, MERLIN's error detection option was used to identify possible genotyping errors, such as unlikely double recombinants [62]. All genotypes flagged as potentially problematic were set as missing for the linkage analysis.

Stratified Whole Genome Linkage Analysis

Families (N = 66) were stratified based on medical record documentation or self-reported family history of any of the following CTD related conditions: hypermobility (N = 4), kyphosis (N = 2), aneurysm (N = 11), mitral valve prolapse (N = 9), pectus excavatum (N = 1), scoliosis (N = 15), orthostatic hypotension (N = 1), supraventricular tachycardia (N = 2), heart valve disease (N = 12), and/or heart murmur (N = 6). In total, 34 families were grouped as "CTD-positive" and the remaining 32 families were "CTD-negative". CTD-positive families had a significant history for one (47.1%), two (32.4%), three (14.7%), or five (5.9%) of the CTD-related conditions described above.

Permutation Tests

A series of permutation tests were performed using custom scripts in order to determine genome-wide and chromosome-wide empirically derived significance levels for the stratified analyses conditional on the prior evidence for linkage. This was used to assess the relationship between the increased evidence for linkage and clinical criteria used to stratify families. For both the parametric (two-point and multipoint) and nonparametric (linear and exponential model; two-point and multipoint) analyses the following was performed: 1) The dataset was randomly split in half creating two datasets each containing 33 families, 2) Linkage analyses were conducted using MERLIN 1.1.2 and MINX for the X chromosome [62] as previously described in each set of families separately, 3) For each analysis (N = 6), the maximum LOD score was retained for each chromosome as well as genome-wide, and 4) Steps 1 through 3 were repeated 500 times in order to construct an empirical distribution (N_{total} = 1000).

Candidate Gene Sequencing

Candidate gene selection for *de novo* sequencing was based on results from the CTD stratified whole genome linkage analysis described below. All affected individuals from any of the 66 linkage families that showed a positive family specific LOD score for the peak marker on chromosome 8 (rs2446871) or chromosome 12 (rs10505755) were selected for Sanger sequencing of growth differentiation factors, GDF6 and GDF3. In total, 96 affected individuals from 39 families and 75 affected individuals from 28 families were initially screened for mutations in GDF6 and GDF3, respectively. Seventeen GDF6 primer sets were designed to cover the exons (including intron-exon boundaries), 5′ and 3′ untranslated regions (UTR), as well as three intronic regions with high conservation (UCSC genome browser: Placental Mammal Basewise Conservation by PhyloP). Three GDF3 primer sets were designed to cover exons (including intron-exon boundaries) and 5′ and 3′ UTRs. Primer sequences, PCR conditions and kits are described in detail (Tables S1–S2). PCR amplicons and primers were sent off to Agencourt (Danvers, MA) and GeneWiz (South Plainfield, NJ) for Sanger sequencing. SNPs, as well as insertions and deletions (indels) were identified using Sequencher 5.0 (Ann Arbor, MI) and all sequences were manually inspected for each variant and indel called. Additionally, all individuals were checked for sufficient sequencing coverage for each amplicon. The nomenclature used to describe novel variants was based on recommendations by den Dunnen and Antonarakis [66]. Bi-directional sequencing in affected as well as unaffected family members was performed in order to follow-up eight identified variants that met subsequent criteria: 1) 1000 Genomes European MAF <0.05 (Integrated Phase 1 Release v3), 2) Identified in more than one affected individual (except two novel variants that were identified within the same family), and 3) 1000 Genomes European MAF was less than the study population MAF which was roughly estimated using all affected family members. Sequence data for novel variants were submitted to GenBank under accession numbers KC174775-KC174780.

Results

Genotyping Quality

Out of the 592532 SNPs genotyped on the Illumina Human610-Quad BeadChips (San Diego, CA), 7544 (1.3%) and 6835 (1.2%) SNPs were excluded from batches 1 and 2, respectively, due to call rates <98%, presence on chromosomes 24–26, high replicate error rate, as well as Illumina specific quality metrics including AB T Mean, AB R Mean, cluster separation, among others. Within each batch, replicate reproducibility rates exceeded 99.999% and all samples, except for one of the CEPH samples in batch 2, had a call rate >99%. Additional SNPs were excluded with Mendelian errors in >4% families (N = 220), MAF <0.05 (N = 66355), HWE p<0.001 (N = 275), identical physical location (Human genome build GRCh37/hg19; N = 2), no genetic distance available from deCODE (N = 948), call present in only batch 1 (N = 2445), call present in only batch 2 (N = 2991), and identical genetic position (based on two decimal places; N = 290918). Genotypes for all SNPs showing non-Mendelian inheritance were set as missing for the entire family. A total of 221343 SNPs remained after filtering and were used to construct the two-point linkage map. From those remaining SNPs, 12056 were selected for use in the multipoint linkage analysis using criteria such as genetic distance in order to create an evenly spaced map and high MAF estimates resulting in increased marker heterozygosity (Mean distance (cM) between SNPs: 0.31±0.008; Mean MAF: 0.42±0.09). In addition to SNP exclusions, three individuals were excluded due to large genomic duplications and/or regions of loss of heterozygosity detected from log R ratio and B allele frequency plots in Illumina GenomeStudio. This ultimately resulted in a total loss of 14 individuals due to two families that were no longer useful for linkage analysis. After additional sample exclusions were applied, 367 individuals from 66 families remained for analysis. Detailed sample exclusions are provided, along with the multidimensional scaling analysis used to identify sample outliers (Table S3 and Figure S1).

Whole Genome Linkage Screen: Primary Analysis

SIMLINK [61] was used to estimate power for our whole genome linkage screen. Assuming homogeneity and a low recombination fraction ($\Theta = 0.01$), the probability of obtaining a LOD score exceeding 3 was 0.94 using all 66 families collectively suggesting that we had adequate power to conduct the whole genome screen.

Following data quality assessment, both two-point and multipoint parametric and nonparametric linkage analyses were conducted. Initial findings across all 66 families showed minimal evidence for linkage, with no multipoint maximum LOD scores exceeding 2 although several two-point LOD scores exceeded 3 across the various models (See Table S4 for summary). Although no multipoint LOD scores exceeded 2, maximum multipoint LOD scores between 1.25 and 2 were found on 2q37.3 (Max LOD = 1.40, exponential model), 8q21.3–q22.2 (Max LOD = 1.38, linear model), 9p22.3–p21.3 (Max HLOD = 1.96, $\alpha = 0.28$), 9q21.31–q22.33 (Max LOD = 1.32, linear model), 12p13.31–p13.2 (Max HLOD = 1.54, $\alpha = 0.25$), and 18q21.33–q22.3 (Max HLOD = 1.78, $\alpha = 0.22$). Based on the limited significance of these results, stratified analyses using clinical criteria were conducted in order to reduce potential genetic heterogeneity thus improving power to localize CMI susceptibility genes.

Stratified Whole Genome Linkage Screen

Families were stratified based on a family history of CTD related conditions and two-point and multipoint nonparametric and parametric whole genome linkage analyses were performed within the CTD-negative and CTD-positive group of families separately. Genome-wide results from the two-point analyses are shown in Figure 1 and the most significant two-point results are included in Table 2. As expected, different regions of the genome exhibit evidence for linkage depending on the subset of families examined. No two-point LOD scores under a linear model exceeded 3 within either family subset and were therefore not included in Figure 1 or Table 2. Maximum multipoint LOD scores exceeding 2 within either set of families are summarized in Figure 2 and Table 2. While no multipoint LOD scores exceeding 2 were previously obtained when all 66 families were analyzed collectively, multiple genomic regions now exhibit maximum LOD scores exceeding 2 and in one case exceeding 3 on chromosome 8. Notably, the most significant two-point LOD scores are found within the 1 LOD down supporting intervals for regions on chromosomes 8, 9, and 12 within the CTD-negative group of families and regions on chromosome 1 within the CTD-positive group of families (Table 2).

Permutation Tests

In order to assess the relationship between the CTD stratification criteria and evidence for linkage, both genome-wide (GW) and chromosome-wide (CW) empirical p-values were obtained for both multipoint and two-point analyses under the three linkage models. Although no marker met GW significance, the peak marker for 8q21.3–q22.1 had a GW empirical p-value of 0.07 with a highly significant CW empirical p-value of 0.008. Additionally, several markers from the two-point and multipoint analyses had CW empirical p-values less than 0.05 as shown in Table 2. It is important to note that the empirical p-values derived from the permutation tests are approximate due to the fact that these families are of different sizes and structures.

Candidate Gene Sequencing

Sanger sequencing was performed on all affected individuals from families with a positive LOD score for the linkage peak marker in the chromosome 8 or 12 linkage regions. The primary focus was on the most significant multipoint linkage peak found on chromosome 8 within the CTD-negative group of families (8q21.3–q22.1; Max LOD = 3.04, linear model). The 1 LOD down supporting interval contained 49 candidate RefSeq genes (Chr8:91334498–98960813, GRCh37/hg19). Of those, one of particular interest was Growth differentiation factor 6 (GDF6) which is a member of the bone morphogenetic protein (BMP) subfamily and has been previously associated with a wide range of phenotypes including ocular, such as microphthalmia and coloboma, as well as skeletal, such as Klippel-Feil syndrome (KFS) which is characterized by fusion of any two of the seven cervical vertebrae [67,68]. The candidate interval on chromosome 12p13.31–p13.2 (Max HLOD = 2.09, 1 LOD down interval: Chr12:7794736–12721298, GRCh37/hg19) identified within a clinically similar subset of families (CTD-negative) also harbored a growth differentiation factor (GDF3), mutations in which have been previously associated with KFS [69]. As CMI and KFS may be allelic disorders, both GDF6 and GDF3 were selected for candidate gene sequencing in order to identify mutations and/or rare variants that increase susceptibility for disease.

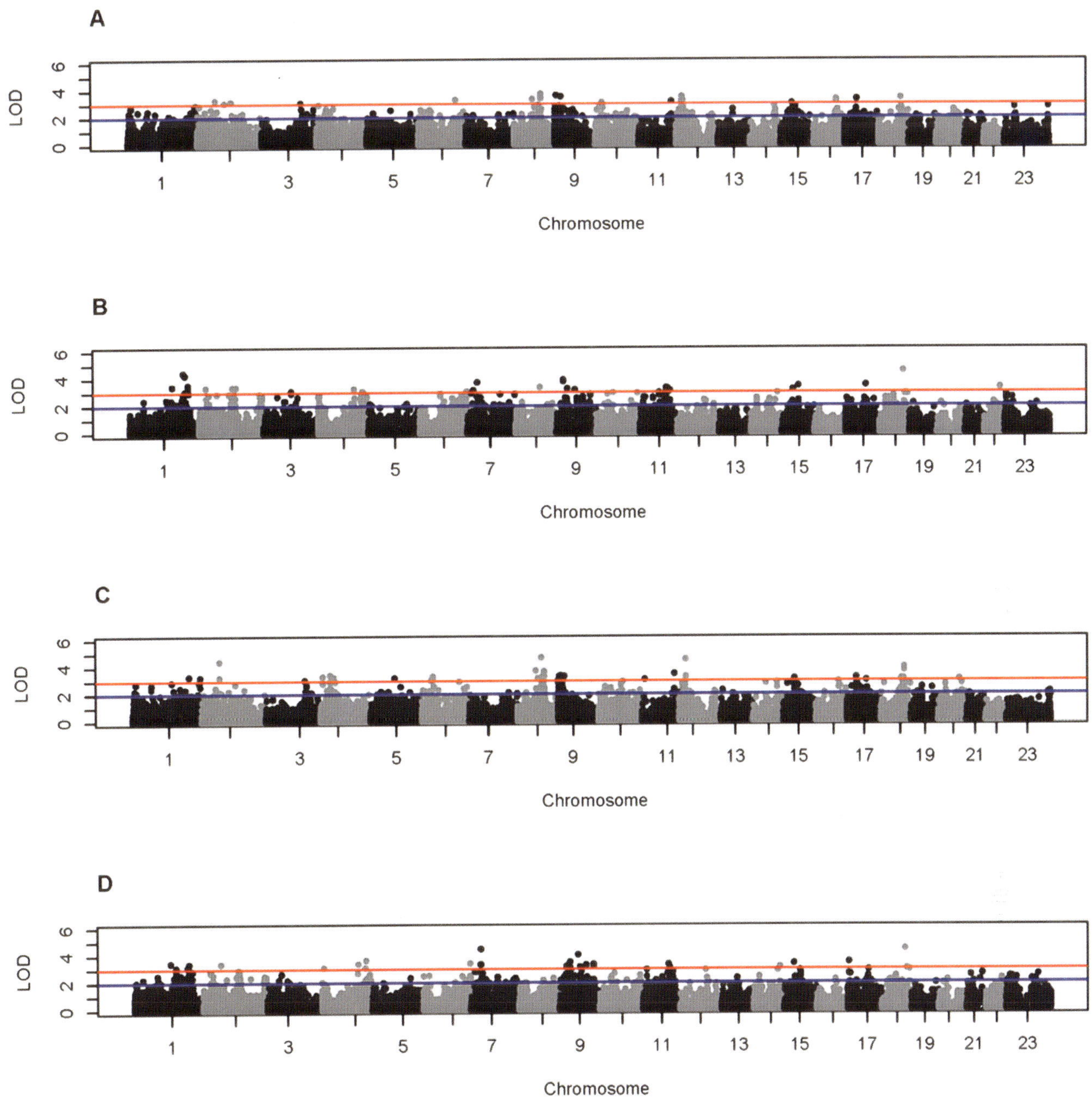

Figure 1. Whole genome two-point LOD scores obtained from stratified analysis. LOD score thresholds of 2 and 3 are indicated by the blue and red lines, respectively. HLOD scores for CTD-negative (A) and CTD-positive family subsets (B), and LOD scores under an exponential model for CTD-negative (C) and CTD-positive family subsets (D). LOD scores under a linear model are not shown as no two-point LOD scores exceeded 3. Negative two-point LOD scores are set to zero. Manhattan plots were created in R 2.15.0 using modified code obtained from "Getting Genetics Done" (http://gettinggeneticsdone.blogspot.com/).

In total, 22 SNPs, 2 insertions, and 1 deletion were found in GDF6 and 3 SNPs were found in GDF3 (Table S5). Of these, 6 were novel and 12 were rare (1000 Genomes European MAF <0.05) in GDF6 and 1 was rare in GDF3. In order to validate and establish segregation for a subset of these variants, 8 variants (7 in GDF6 and 1 in GDF3) were selected for follow-up sequencing (Table 3; see Methods under the candidate gene sequencing section for selection criteria). Within this subset of rare and novel variants, complete sharing across affected family members was observed with only two of the variants: 1) Novel SNP, g.406+2780C>T and 2) rs140757891. Reduced penetrance was observed for all variants of interest, except for rs121909352 although this is likely due to the fact that DNA samples were not available for all family members. Of particular interest is the missense variant, rs121909352 (A249E), which is a heterozygous mutation previously identified in KFS patients [67,68] as well as patients with microphthalmia and coloboma [68,70,71]. Pedigrees showing segregation of this mutation with affection status are shown in Figure 3. Within family 9453, all individuals presenting with CMI and syringomyelia, except for individual 2002, were

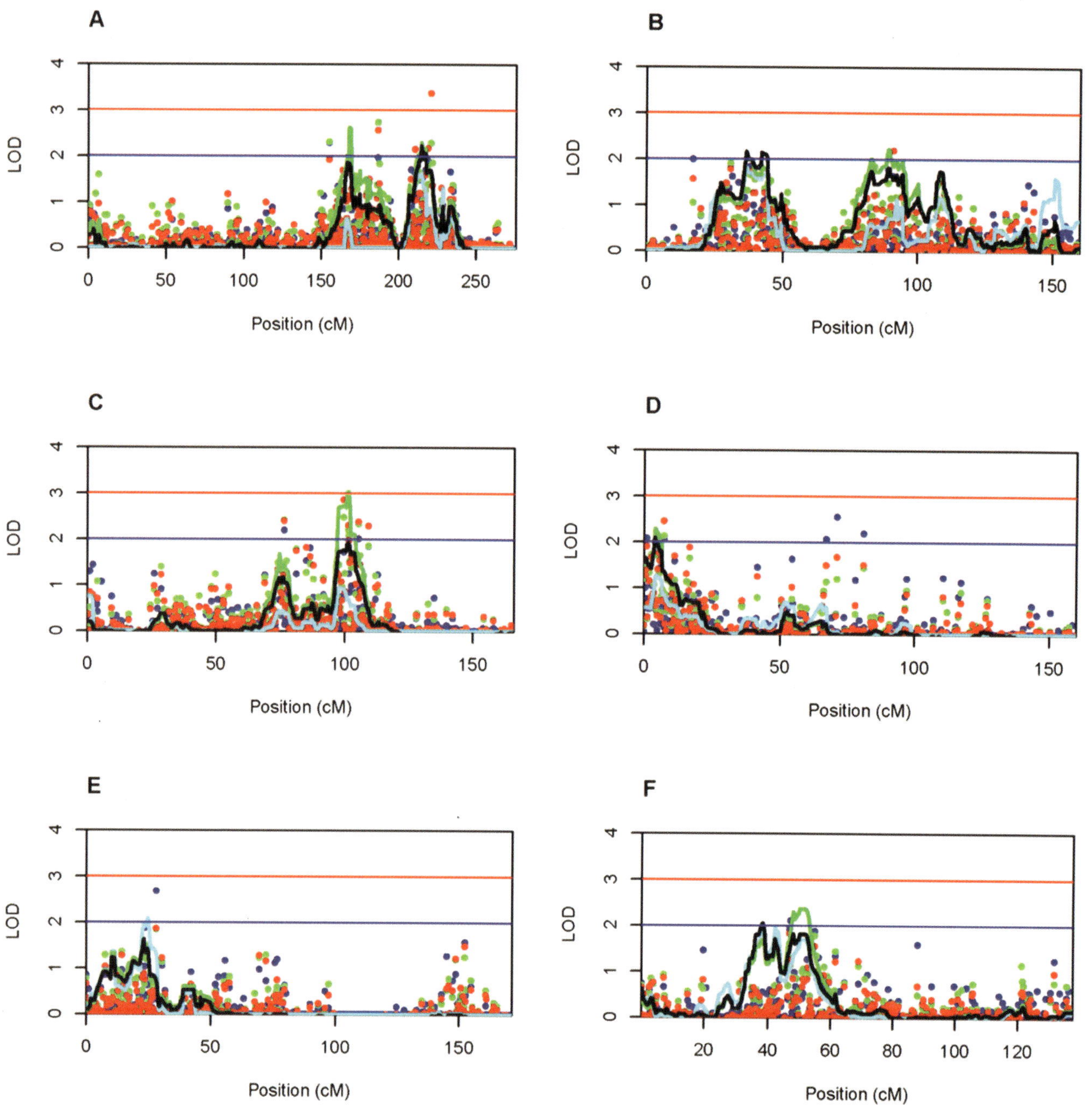

Figure 2. Two-point and multipoint LOD scores obtained from stratified analysis. Only chromosomes with a maximum multipoint LOD score >2 are shown. LOD score thresholds of 2 and 3 are indicated by the blue and red lines, respectively. Green points and lines represent LOD scores under a linear model, blue points and lines represent HLOD scores, and red points and black lines represent LOD scores under an exponential model. CTD-positive families: Chr1 (A), CTD-positive families: Chr9 (B), CTD-negative families: Chr8 (C), CTD-negative families: Chr9 (D), CTD-negative families: Chr12 (E), and CTD-negative families: Chr17 (F). Negative two-point and multipoint LOD scores are set to zero. Plots were created in R 2.15.0.

heterozygous for the mutation. Individual 2002 was found to have increased homozygosity as determined by an F inbreeding coefficient >4 standard deviations away from the mean and had been previously removed from the linkage analysis. In addition, one individual presenting with a suspected Chiari Malformation Type 0 (CM0) in family 9453 was heterozygous for the mutation; a detailed clinical description of this individual has been provided previously [72]. CM0 patients present with syringomyelia without tonsillar herniation that improves following posterior fossa decompression surgery. In family 9476, only one individual diagnosed with CMI and syringomyelia was heterozygous for the mutation (Figure 3); one additional individual with CMI and syringomyelia (1004) and one individual with tonsillar ectopia (1001) did not have the mutation.

In addition, the two intronic variants (Novel SNP, g.406+2780C>T and rs140757891) that are shared across all affected family members are located within potential regulatory regions (Table 3). The novel intronic SNP (g.406+2780C>T) is located within a predicted regulatory region for the protein, Suppressor of zeste 12 homolog (SUZ12), based on chromatin

Table 2. Most significant two-point and multipoint LOD scores.[a]

Family description	Linkage model	Location (markers)[b]	Two-point LOD[c]	Emp p-value (CW/GW)[d]	Multipoint LOD[c]	Emp p-value (CW/GW)[d]
CTD-positive	Parametric: dominant	18q22.1 (rs17079623, rs574539)	***4.53***	**0.027**/0.150	0.71	0.787/1
		1q32.3 (rs2165993, rs3862952)	***4.42***	0.053/0.208	1.63	0.131/0.834
	NPL: exponential	7p15.3 (rs1476697, rs4719814)	***4.46***	**0.025**/0.553	0.57	0.601/1
		18q22.1 (rs17079623, rs2048329)	***4.44***	0.059/0.573	0.42	0.856/1
	NPL: linear	1q23.3-q24.2 (rs10494474)	0.87	1/1	**2.63**	**0.032**/0.184
		1q32.2-q41(rs3862952)	0.35	1/1	**2.3**	0.053/0.356
		9q21.31-q22.31 (rs10746837)	1.49	1/1	**2.22**	0.112/0.423
		9p22.3-p21.31 (rs2840790)	0.27	1/1	**2.15**	0.133/0.484
CTD-negative	Parametric: dominant	8q22.3 (rs12545537, rs544821)	***3.72***	0.156/0.871	0.01	1/1
		9p24.2 (rs2181829, rs7024139)	***3.62***	0.316/0.928	1.26	0.596/0.990
		12p13.31-p13.2 (rs6488255)	0.63	1/1	**2.09**	0.066/0.439
	NPL: exponential	8q22.1(rs1597301, rs6989464)	***4.69***	**0.031**/0.394	1.73	0.066/0.768
		12p13.2 (rs7312834, rs205534)	***4.54***	**0.014**/0.498	0.85	0.414/1
		17p12 (rs6502282)	0.08	1/1	**2.06**	**0.044**/0.491
	NPL: linear	8q21.3-q22.1 (rs7013599)	**2.21**	0.700/1	***3.04***	**0.008**/0.070
		17p12-q11.2 (rs7406339)	0.6	1/1	**2.37**	**0.027**/0.309
		9p24.3-p24.2 (rs1416621)	1.72	1/1	**2.29**	0.097/0.366

[a]The top two most significant two-point results within each model and family subset as well as any maximum multipoint LOD score exceeding 2 are included.
[b]When two markers are listed, the first corresponds to the marker used for the two-point result shown. The second corresponds to the closest marker included in the multipoint analysis.
[c]LOD scores exceeding 2 are bold and LOD scores exceeding 3 are bold and italicized. For the parametric model, HLOD scores are shown.
[d]Empirical p-values less than 0.05 are bold.
Abbreviations: CTD: connective tissue disorder, NPL: nonparametric linkage, LOD: logarithm of the odds, Emp: empirical, CW: chromosome-wide, GW: genome-wide, N/A: not applicable.

immunoprecipitation sequencing (ChIP-seq) data from the Encyclopedia of DNA Elements Consortium (ENCODE) (UCSC Genome browser: GRCh37/hg19 human assembly). The rare intronic SNP, rs140757891, is also located within a predicted regulatory region for SUZ12 as well as the GATA binding protein 2 (GATA2) based on ChIP-seq data from ENCODE (UCSC Genome browser: GRCh37/hg19 human assembly). In addition, rs140757891 is part of a CpG dinucleotide located within a predicted CpG island spanning 701 base pairs (UCSC Genome browser: GRCh37/hg19 human assembly). When the variant allele is present the guanine (G) becomes an adenine (A) (reverse strand). Segregation of these two intronic variants, along with two additional novel variants (g.18328T>G and g.15169-59T>A) found in one of these families are provided in Figure S2.

Discussion

In order to gain a better understanding of the genetic architecture of CMI, we conducted a whole genome linkage screen using a collection of 66 nonsyndromic families with at least two sampled individuals presenting with CMI with or without syringomyelia. It was hypothesized that the limited evidence for linkage across all 66 families collectively was due to genetic heterogeneity and may be associated with the phenotypic variability observed. Based on the co-occurrence of CMI and CTDs, families were stratified by CTD related conditions in order to identify phenotypically and potentially genetically more homogeneous groups of families for linkage analysis. Stratified analyses identified multiple genomic regions showing increased evidence for linkage consistent with reduced genetic heterogeneity across families as a result of the CTD related stratification criteria. Furthermore, several plausible disease genes were identified as discussed in detail below.

Prior to describing our most significant results, it is important to relate our findings to the only other whole genome linkage screen conducted to date which implicated regions on chromosomes 9 and 15 [17]. We only identified suggestive evidence for linkage to the region on chromosome 9 within our CTD-positive group of families. Importantly, 12/66 of our total families and 7/34 CTD-positive families overlap with the families used in the initial screen conducted by Boyles and colleagues; therefore, these results do not provide independent replication for this region. Lack of replication for chromosome 15 could be due to the use of: 1) different genotyping chips (Illumina Human610-Quad BeadChips versus Affymetrix 10K SNP Chip) and marker quality control procedures, 2) different linkage software packages (Merlin versus Allegro; e.g. different with respect to an error detection option and accounting for inter-marker LD) and genetic models (penetrance function and S scoring function), 3) additional families which are likely genetically heterogeneous, and/or 4) different analytical approaches (stratified analyses). While the original finding could be a false positive, it is equally possible that as additional families are collected and other approaches to reduce genetic heterogeneity are applied to the data this region may present again as a promising candidate genomic interval warranting follow-up.

While we presented linkage results within the subsets of both CTD-positive and CTD-negative families, the focus of the current paper has been on the CTD-negative families as these are thought to represent more "classical" CMI due to cranial constriction and

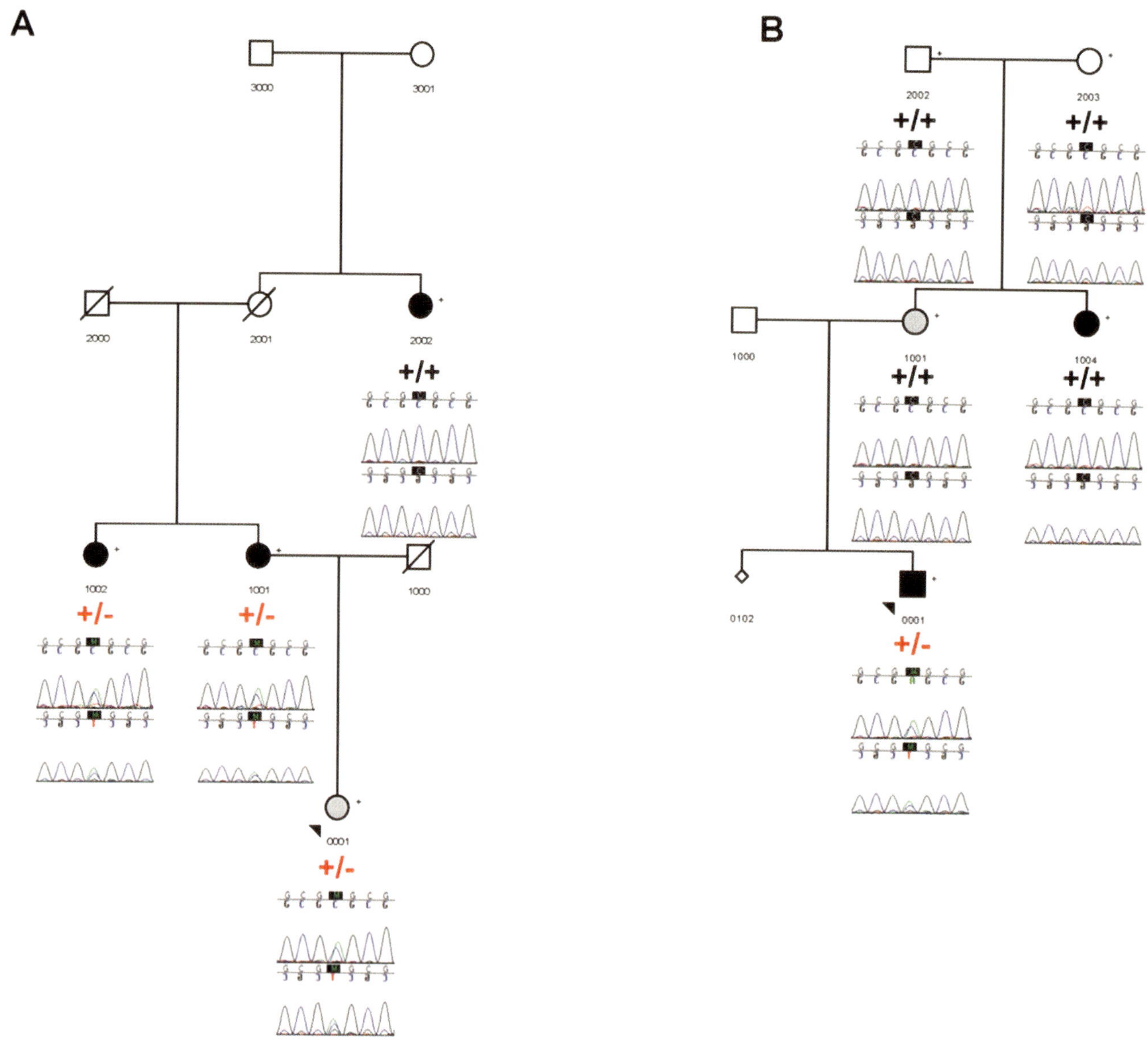

Figure 3. Segregation of the missense mutation, rs121909352 (A249E), in two CMI pedigrees. Family 9453 (A) and Family 9476 (B). Symbols shaded in black indicate a diagnosis of CMI with or without syringomyelia, small diamonds represent a miscarriage, and symbols shaded in grey indicate an uncertain diagnosis. 9453-0001 has been diagnosed with a suspected Chiari Malformation Type 0 and 9476-1001 has been diagnosed with tonsillar ectopia. "+/+" indicates homozygous for the reference allele; "+/−" indicates heterozygous for the variant allele. Sequences were generated in both the forward and reverse direction and are shown below each sampled individual. Progeny 8 (Delray Beach, FL) was used to construct the pedigrees and Sequencher 5.0 (Ann Arbor, MI) was used to create the chromatograms.

also resulted in the identification of the only genomic region with a maximum LOD score exceeding 3. The most significant of our findings implicated the growth differentiation factors, GDF6 and GDF3, both of which had been previously implicated in KFS [67,68,69] which is characterized by cervical vertebral fusion and may be associated with a wide range of conditions including renal abnormalities, cardiovascular abnormalities, orthopedic anomalies, pulmonary problems, deafness, and synkinesia [73]. Interestingly, roughly 3–5% of CMI patients are diagnosed with KFS [23,45], suggesting a shared genetic etiology between these disorders. Further, it has been proposed that KFS and CMI should be classified as post-otic neural crest syndromes, thus sharing a common cellular etiology [74]. Although the exact relationship between these disorders is unknown, one possibility is that CMI and KFS may be allelic disorders. In order to investigate this possibility, GDF3 and GDF6 were sequenced in a collection of CMI patients from our linkage families. While GDF3 still presents as an intriguing biological candidate and additional sequencing of potential regulatory elements may yield putative disease variants, no variants of obvious significance were identified in this study. However, several interesting variants were identified in GDF6. A previously identified KFS mutation, A249E (rs121909352), was found in two of our CMI families. The functional effect of this mutation has been determined previously *in-vitro*. Asai-Coakwell and colleagues evaluated changes to bone morphogenetic protein (BMP) signaling by co-transfecting an expression construct with the A249E mutation and a Sex determining region Y-box 9 (SOX-9)-responsive reporter gene into primary limb mesenchymal cells

Table 3. GDF6 and GDF3 selected sequence variants.[a]

Gene	Chr	Location[b]	Variant ID[c]	Alleles[d]	Variant Class	CMI/1KG MAF[e]	All Affs[f,g]	Reduced Pen[g]
GDF6	8	97154593	g.18328T>G	T/G	3′ UTR	0.005/NA	No (1/2)	Yes (1/2)
GDF6	8	97154813	rs112542818	C/T	3′ UTR	0.026/0.003	No (5/8)	Yes (2/4)
GDF6	8	97157223	rs148861809	C/G	Coding-syn	0.036/0.028	No (7/10)	Yes (3/8)
GDF6	8	97157413	rs121909352	G/T	Missense	0.016/0.003[h]	No (4/6)[i]	Unknown (0/3)
GDF6	8	97157811	g.15169-59T>A	T/A	Intronic	0.005/NA	No (1/2)	Yes (1/2)
GDF6	8	97169735	g.406+2780C>T	C/T	Intronic	0.010/NA	Yes (2/2)	Yes (1/2)
GDF6	8	97170374	rs140757891	C/T	Intronic	0.021/0.013	Yes (4/4)	Yes (2/10)
GDF3	12	7842587	rs2302516	C/G	Missense	0.047/0.024	No (7/11)	Yes (1/14)

[a]Only variants which were followed-up are shown here (See Methods section); Variants were validated by bidirectional sequencing and all sampled affected and unaffected individuals within each identified family were sequenced.
[b]Base pair positions based on human genome build GRCh37/hg19.
[c]The nomenclature used to describe novel variants was based on recommendations by the Human Genome Variation Society (den Dunnen and Antonarakis 2001). Nucleotide numbering was based on the GDF6 RefSeq genomic sequence, NG_008981.1, and intron-exon boundaries were defined based on the GDF6 mRNA sequence, NM_001001557.
[d]Alleles: Reference allele/Alternate allele.
[e]CMI MAF estimate based on all affected family members initially screened; 1KG MAF: Based on 1000 Genomes Integrated Phase 1 Release v3: European population.
[f]Is sharing observed across all affected individuals within each family?
[g]Numbers in parentheses: Numerator: number of sampled individuals carrying the variant, Denominator: total number of sampled individuals. Only affecteds were considered for "All affecteds" and only unaffecteds/uncertains were considered for "Reduced penetrance".
[h]MAF estimate was not available from 1000 Genomes; MAF estimate based on the Exome sequencing project: European population.
[i]Individual suspected to have Chiari Malformation Type 0 is counted as "affected" for the purposes of this table.

and assessed SOX-9 reporter activity [68]. Reduced activation of the reporter was observed ($p<0.034$), suggesting altered chondrogenic potential [68]. In addition, a 23% reduction in secreted mature GDF6 protein expression was observed for the mutant as determined by Western blot analysis [68].

Although there is evidence for a functional effect, the expression of A249E is complex with previous evidence of pleiotropy (ocular versus skeletal phenotypes), variable expressivity (e.g. coloboma versus microphthalmia), and reduced penetrance [68]. Consistent with these reports, we also observe variable expressivity within our CMI families (CMI with syringomyelia versus CM0). In fact, the identification of A249E in both CMI and a suspected CM0 individual within the same family (9453) further supports the hypothesis that these disorders share an underlying genetic basis and represent part of a continuum of Chiari phenotypes [72,75,76,77,78]. Although A249E is not necessary to cause disease in either of these families, it still likely contributes to disease presentation together with additional genetic and potentially environmental factors.

Additional variants of interest from our study include two intronic GDF6 variants, rs140757891 and a novel SNP, g.406+2780C>T. ChIP-seq data from a small number of cell lines indicate that both variants are located within predicted targets of SUZ12, a polycomb protein involved in epigenetic silencing of developmental genes. Interestingly, haploinsufficient SUZ12 mice exhibit cerebellar herniation, as well as spina bifida, an enlarged brainstem, and occipital cortical changes [79]. Although these clinical features appear to be due to an enlarged tectum and only demonstrate partial clinical similarity with CMI, Miro and colleagues suggest that an additional link between SUZ12 and central nervous system disorders may come from neurofibromatosis 1 (NF1), a disorder characterized by the development of neurofibromas and the presence of café-au-lait spots [79]. SUZ12 and NF1 are located within 560 kb of each other on chromosome 17 and while most NF1 patients have point mutations in NF1 some harbor larger genomic deletions that encompass NF1 as well as other genes, including SUZ12 resulting in a more severe clinical presentation [79]. Roughly 5% of CMI patients present with NF1 [45] and it has been previously suggested that these two disorders may share an underlying genetic basis [58]. Remarkably, within the same group of families that showed increased evidence for linkage to the region containing GDF6 (CTD-negative) we also observed suggestive evidence for linkage to 17p12–q11.2 (Max LOD = 2.37, CW emp p-val = 0.03) which contains both SUZ12 and NF1 providing further support for a potential role in disease development.

While encouraged by our findings, we acknowledge several limitations of this study. First, because we enforced strict eligibility criteria (exclusion of syndromic cases) and required families to have multiple affected individuals, the total number of families eligible for the study was low and likely contributed to reduced power. However, despite the relatively small sample size, the number of families examined was almost three times as large as the collection of families used in the only other whole genome linkage screen published to date [17]. Second, MRIs were not available for all study participants thus misclassification of affection status cannot be ruled out. Importantly, none of our analyses used phenotype information from "unaffected" family members (i.e. affecteds-only analysis), thus the greatest impact of potential misclassification would be if individuals were incorrectly classified as affected. Furthermore, clinical information used for the stratified analysis was mostly ascertained through a general medical interview upon enrollment in the study; therefore, misclassification of families as CTD-positive or CTD-negative is possible. Nevertheless, our data suggest that the increased evidence for linkage observed for the stratified analysis based on CTD related conditions is non-random (e.g. 8q21.3–q22.1: GW emp p-val = 0.07, CW emp p-val = 0.008). This observation would seem unlikely if a high degree of misclassification existed.

Future work will include functional follow-up of variants of interest as well as sequencing GDF3 and GDF6 in a larger cohort of sporadic and familial CMI cases. Furthermore, the distant regulatory elements previously identified for GDF6 [80,81,82] represent excellent candidate regions for future *de novo* variant detection. Other candidate genes, such as low density lipoprotein receptor-related protein 6 (LRP6) present within the chromosome 12 candidate interval could also be investigated as LRP6, when specifically deleted from early mesenchyme, causes a slight delay in mouse skull ossification [83]. In addition, rather than simply taking a candidate gene approach, targeted capture and next generation sequencing of candidate genomic intervals defined by linkage analysis or whole genome sequencing would be an obvious next step to comprehensively follow-up these findings. Finally, taking a more quantitative approach to disease, for example by focusing on cranial base morphometrics, may yield greater insight into the genetic etiology due to increased statistical power and reduced misclassification rates among individuals.

Conclusion

The current study demonstrates the utility of using clinical stratification to reduce genetic heterogeneity in CMI by identifying genomic regions showing increased evidence for linkage with maximum LOD scores exceeding 2 and even 3, as well as having implicated credible candidate genes in CMI susceptibility. Although further work is necessary to confirm the involvement of these genes and individual sequence variants in the development of CMI, this work makes several important contributions to the field of CMI research: 1) We conducted the largest whole genome linkage screen to date providing multiple candidate intervals for future investigation and replication, 2) Our results suggest a relationship between CTD related conditions and genetic etiology which is consistent with the hypothesis that CMI with CTDs versus CMI without CTDs occur through different mechanisms ("cranial settling" versus "cranial constriction"), 3) Multiple biological candidates were implicated from the analysis, including the only two GDFs currently known to be associated with KFS suggesting a shared genetic etiology between CMI and KFS. This is consistent with the fact that KFS is known to co-occur with CMI and share a common cellular etiology, 4) Identified a known KFS missense mutation in two of our families that is not necessary for disease but likely contributes to the phenotype due to its rare frequency in the general population, known functional effect *in vitro*, and the fact that it has been identified in multiple skeletal and ocular disease cohorts, and 5) Identified two potential regulatory variants (one novel, one rare) shared across all affected individuals in the families they were identified in and located within predicted regulatory regions for SUZ12 which itself is an excellent candidate gene for CMI. Further investigation of GDF3 and GDF6, other plausible biological candidates such as SUZ12, NF1, and LRP6, as well as the genetic relationship between CMI and KFS is warranted.

Supporting Information

Figure S1 Multidimensional scaling (MDS) analysis. This was performed using a pruned marker dataset and only one representative individual from each family. The red and black colors correspond to different clusters (PLINK's pairwise population concordance test: –ppc 1e-4). Individuals shown in red represent families that are self-reported Caucasian, Hispanic. MDS plot was created in R 2.15.0.

Figure S2 Segregation of select variants in three CMI pedigrees. Family 9772 (A), Family 9496 (B), and Family 9432 (C). Alleles "A" and "a" represent a novel SNP at Chr8:97154593, Alleles "B" and "b" represent a novel SNP at Chr8:97157811, alleles "C" and "c" represent RS140757891, and alleles "D" and "d" represent a novel SNP at Chr8:97169735. Individual 108 from family 9496 has previously had brain surgery and a shunt; no additional information is known. Symbols shaded in black indicate a diagnosis of CMI with or without syringomyelia and small diamonds represent miscarriages. Lower case letters shown in red indicate the variant allele. Genotype calls are based on bi-directional sequencing. Progeny 8 (Delray Beach, FL) was used to construct the pedigrees.

Table S1 PCR primer sequences and conditions.

Table S2 PCR primer kits and thermocycler conditions.

Table S3 Quality control of sample data.

Table S4 Most significant two-point and multipoint LOD scores.

Table S5 GDF6 and GDF3 identified sequence variants.

Acknowledgments

We would like to thank all family members for participating in the Chiari genetics study. In addition, we acknowledge the technical assistance received from Carol Haynes, Colette Blach, and Blair Chesnut at the Duke Center for Human Genetics.

Author Contributions

Conceived and designed the experiments: CAM SGG AAK. Performed the experiments: CAM KS KD HC EA JS. Analyzed the data: CAM. Contributed reagents/materials/analysis tools: DE GG HF SGG AAK. Wrote the paper: CAM KS KD HC EA JS DE GG HF SGG AAK.

References

1. Speer MC, Enterline DS, Mehltretter L, Hammock P, Joseph J, et al. (2003) Chiari type I malformation with or without syringomyelia: Prevalence and genetics. Journal of Genetic Counseling 12: 297–311.
2. Meadows J, Kraut M, Guarnieri M, Haroun RI, Carson BS (2000) Asymptomatic Chiari Type I malformations identified on magnetic resonance imaging. J Neurosurg 92: 920–926.
3. Aboulezz AO, Sartor K, Geyer CA, Gado MH (1985) Position of cerebellar tonsils in the normal population and in patients with Chiari malformation: a quantitative approach with MR imaging. J Comput Assist Tomogr 9: 1033–1036.
4. Barkovich AJ, Wippold FJ, Sherman JL, Citrin CM (1986) Significance of cerebellar tonsillar position on MR. AJNR Am J Neuroradiol 7: 795–799.
5. Mueller DM, Oro JJ (2004) Prospective analysis of presenting symptoms among 265 patients with radiographic evidence of Chiari malformation type I with or without syringomyelia. J Am Acad Nurse Pract 16: 134–138.
6. Milhorat TH, Nishikawa M, Kula RW, Dlugacz YD (2010) Mechanisms of cerebellar tonsil herniation in patients with Chiari malformations as guide to clinical management. Acta Neurochir (Wien) 152: 1117–1127.
7. Marin-Padilla M, Marin-Padilla TM (1981) Morphogenesis of experimentally induced Arnold–Chiari malformation. J Neurol Sci 50: 29–55.
8. Nishikawa M, Sakamoto H, Hakuba A, Nakanishi N, Inoue Y (1997) Pathogenesis of Chiari malformation: a morphometric study of the posterior cranial fossa. J Neurosurg 86: 40–47.
9. Milhorat TH, Bolognese PA, Nishikawa M, McDonnell NB, Francomano CA (2007) Syndrome of occipitoatlantoaxial hypermobility, cranial settling, and chiari malformation type I in patients with hereditary disorders of connective tissue. J Neurosurg Spine 7: 601–609.
10. Atkinson JL, Kokmen E, Miller GM (1998) Evidence of posterior fossa hypoplasia in the familial variant of adult Chiari I malformation: case report. Neurosurgery 42: 401–403; discussion 404.

11. Cavender RK, Schmidt JH 3rd (1995) Tonsillar ectopia and Chiari malformations: monozygotic triplets. Case report. J Neurosurg 82: 497–500.
12. Iwasaki Y, Hida K, Onishi K, Nanba R (2000) Chiari malformation and syringomyelia in monozygotic twins: birth injury as a possible cause of syringomyelia–case report. Neurol Med Chir (Tokyo) 40: 176–178.
13. Solth A, Barrett C, Holliman D, Mitchell P (2010) Chiari malformation in female monozygotic twins. Br J Neurosurg 24: 607–608.
14. Stovner LJ, Cappelen J, Nilsen G, Sjaastad O (1992) The Chiari type I malformation in two monozygotic twins and first-degree relatives. Ann Neurol 31: 220–222.
15. Szewka AJ, Walsh LE, Boaz JC, Carvalho KS, Golomb MR (2006) Chiari in the family: inheritance of the Chiari I malformation. Pediatr Neurol 34: 481–485.
16. Turgut M (2001) Chiari type I malformation in two monozygotic twins. Br J Neurosurg 15: 279–280.
17. Boyles AL, Enterline DS, Hammock PH, Siegel DG, Slifer SH, et al. (2006) Phenotypic definition of Chiari type I malformation coupled with high-density SNP genome screen shows significant evidence for linkage to regions on chromosomes 9 and 15. Am J Med Genet A 140: 2776–2785.
18. Coria F, Quintana F, Rebollo M, Combarros O, Berciano J (1983) Occipital dysplasia and Chiari type I deformity in a family. Clinical and radiological study of three generations. J Neurol Sci 62: 147–158.
19. George S, Page AB (2006) Familial Arnold-Chiari Type I malformation. Eye (Lond) 20: 400–402.
20. Gimenez-Roldan S, Benito C, Mateo D (1978) Familial communicating syringomyelia. J Neurol Sci 36: 135–146.
21. Herman MD, Cheek WR, Storrs BB (1990) Two siblings with the Chiari I malformation. Pediatr Neurosurg 16: 183–184.
22. Mavinkurve GG, Sciubba D, Amundson E, Jallo GI (2005) Familial Chiari type I malformation with syringomyelia in two siblings: case report and review of the literature. Childs Nerv Syst 21: 955–959.
23. Milhorat TH, Chou MW, Trinidad EM, Kula RW, Mandell M, et al. (1999) Chiari I malformation redefined: clinical and radiographic findings for 364 symptomatic patients. Neurosurgery 44: 1005–1017.
24. Schanker BD, Walcott BP, Nahed BV, Kahle KT, Li YM, et al. (2011) Familial Chiari malformation: case series. Neurosurg Focus 31: E1.
25. Speer MC, George TM, Enterline DS, Franklin A, Wolpert CM, et al. (2000) A genetic hypothesis for Chiari I malformation with or without syringomyelia. Neurosurg Focus 8: E12.
26. Stovner LJ, Sjaastad O (1995) Segmental hyperhidrosis in two siblings with Chiari type I malformation. Eur Neurol 35: 149–155.
27. Tubbs RS, Hill M, Loukas M, Shoja MM, Oakes WJ (2008) Volumetric analysis of the posterior cranial fossa in a family with four generations of the Chiari malformation Type I. J Neurosurg Pediatr 1: 21–24.
28. Weisfeld-Adams JD, Carter MR, Likeman MJ, Rankin J (2007) Three sisters with Chiari I malformation with and without associated syringomyelia. Pediatr Neurosurg 43: 533–538.
29. Yabe I, Kikuchi S, Tashiro K (2002) Familial syringomyelia: the first Japanese case and review of the literature. Clin Neurol Neurosurg 105: 69–71.
30. Zakeri A, Glasauer FE, Egnatchik JG (1995) Familial syringomyelia: case report and review of the literature. Surg Neurol 44: 48–53.
31. Castori M, Camerota F, Celletti C, Danese C, Santilli V, et al. (2010) Natural history and manifestations of the hypermobility type Ehlers-Danlos syndrome: a pilot study on 21 patients. Am J Med Genet A 152A: 556–564.
32. Jacome DE (2001) Blepharoclonus and Arnold-Chiari malformation. Acta Neurol Scand 104: 113–117.
33. Jacome DE (1999) Headache in Ehlers-Danlos syndrome. Cephalalgia 19: 791–796.
34. Puget S, Kondageski C, Wray A, Boddaert N, Roujeau T, et al. (2007) Chiari-like tonsillar herniation associated with intracranial hypotension in Marfan syndrome. Case report. J Neurosurg 106: 48–52.
35. Braca J, Hornyak M, Murali R (2005) Hemifacial spasm in a patient with Marfan syndrome and Chiari I malformation. Case report. J Neurosurg 103: 552–554.
36. Owler BK, Halmagyi GM, Brennan J, Besser M (2004) Syringomyelia with Chiari malformation; 3 unusual cases with implications for pathogenesis. Acta Neurochir (Wien) 146: 1137–1143; discussion 1143.
37. Abel TJ, Chowdhary A, Gabikian P, Ellenbogen RG, Avellino AM (2006) Acquired chiari malformation type I associated with a fatty terminal filum. Case report. J Neurosurg 105: 329–332.
38. Cakmakkaya OS, Kaya G, Altintas F, Bakan M, Yildirim A (2006) Anesthetic management of a child with Arnold-Chiari malformation and Klippel-Feil syndrome. Paediatr Anaesth 16: 355–356.
39. Kagawa M, Jinnai T, Matsumoto Y, Kawai N, Kunishio K, et al. (2006) Chiari I malformation accompanied by assimilation of the atlas, Klippel-Feil syndrome, and syringomyelia: case report. Surg Neurol 65: 497–502; discussion 502.
40. Khan AA, Bhatti SN, Khan G, Ahmed E, Aurangzeb A, et al. (2010) Clinical and radiological findings in Arnold Chiari malformation. J Ayub Med Coll Abbottabad 22: 75–78.
41. Konstantinou DT, Chroni E, Constantoyiannis C, Dougenis D (2004) Klippel-Feil syndrome presenting with bilateral thoracic outlet syndrome. Spine (Phila Pa 1976) 29: E189–192.
42. Perrini P, Rawlinson A, Cowie RA, King AT (2008) Acute external hydrocephalus complicating craniocervical decompression for syringomyelia-Chiari I complex: case report and review of the literature. Neurosurg Rev 31: 331–335.
43. Ritterbusch JF, McGinty LD, Spar J, Orrison WW (1991) Magnetic resonance imaging for stenosis and subluxation in Klippel-Feil syndrome. Spine (Phila Pa 1976) 16: S539–541.
44. Samartzis D, Shen FH, Herman J, Mardjetko SM (2010) Atlantoaxial rotatory fixation in the setting of associated congenital malformations: a modified classification system. Spine (Phila Pa 1976) 35: E119–127.
45. Tubbs RS, Beckman J, Naftel RP, Chern JJ, Wellons JC 3rd, et al. (2011) Institutional experience with 500 cases of surgically treated pediatric Chiari malformation Type I. J Neurosurg Pediatr 7: 248–256.
46. Tubbs RS, McGirt MJ, Oakes WJ (2003) Surgical experience in 130 pediatric patients with Chiari I malformations. J Neurosurg 99: 291–296.
47. Ulmer JL, Elster AD, Ginsberg LE, Williams DW 3rd (1993) Klippel-Feil syndrome: CT and MR of acquired and congenital abnormalities of cervical spine and cord. J Comput Assist Tomogr 17: 215–224.
48. Woosley RE, Whaley RA (1982) Use of metrizamide in computerized tomography to diagnose the Chiari I malformation. J Neurosurg 56: 373–376.
49. Gupta A, Vitali AM, Rothstein R, Cochrane DD (2008) Resolution of syringomyelia and Chiari malformation after growth hormone therapy. Childs Nerv Syst 24: 1345–1348.
50. Hamilton J, Blaser S, Daneman D (1998) MR imaging in idiopathic growth hormone deficiency. AJNR Am J Neuroradiol 19: 1609–1615.
51. Hamilton J, Chitayat D, Blaser S, Cohen LE, Phillips JA 3rd, et al. (1998) Familial growth hormone deficiency associated with MRI abnormalities. Am J Med Genet 80: 128–132.
52. Hilal L, Hajaji Y, Vie-Luton MP, Ajaltouni Z, Benazzouz B, et al. (2008) Unusual phenotypic features in a patient with a novel splice mutation in the GHRHR gene. Mol Med 14: 286–292.
53. Marwaha R, Menon PS, Jena A, Pant C, Sethi AK, et al. (1992) Hypothalamo-pituitary axis by magnetic resonance imaging in isolated growth hormone deficiency patients born by normal delivery. J Clin Endocrinol Metab 74: 654–659.
54. Murphy RL, Tubbs RS, Grabb PA, Oakes WJ (2007) Chiari I malformation and idiopathic growth hormone deficiency in siblings: report of three cases. Childs Nerv Syst 23: 1221–1223.
55. Tubbs RS, Wellons JC 3rd, Smyth MD, Bartolucci AA, Blount JP, et al. (2003) Children with growth hormone deficiency and Chiari I malformation: a morphometric analysis of the posterior cranial fossa. Pediatr Neurosurg 38: 324–328.
56. Sandberg DI, Navarro R, Blanch J, Ragheb J (2007) Anomalous venous drainage preventing safe posterior fossa decompression in patients with chiari malformation type I and multisutural craniosynostosis. Report of two cases and review of the literature. J Neurosurg 106: 490–494.
57. Strahle J, Muraszko KM, Buchman SR, Kapurch J, Garton HJ, et al. (2011) Chiari malformation associated with craniosynostosis. Neurosurg Focus 31: E2.
58. Tubbs RS, Rutledge SL, Kosentka A, Bartolucci AA, Oakes WJ (2004) Chiari I malformation and neurofibromatosis type 1. Pediatr Neurol 30: 278–280.
59. Hara H, Arakawa H (2005) Coexistence of neurofibromatosis 1 and chiari type I malformation: an unusual association. J Dermatol 32: 34–37.
60. Purcell S, Neale B, Todd-Brown K, Thomas L, Ferreira MA, et al. (2007) PLINK: a tool set for whole-genome association and population-based linkage analyses. American Journal of Human Genetics 81: 559–575.
61. Boehnke M (1986) Estimating the power of a proposed linkage study: a practical computer simulation approach. Am J Hum Genet 39: 513–527.
62. Abecasis GR, Cherny SS, Cookson WO, Cardon LR (2002) Merlin–rapid analysis of dense genetic maps using sparse gene flow trees. Nat Genet 30: 97–101.
63. Whittemore AS, Halpern J (1994) A class of tests for linkage using affected pedigree members. Biometrics 50: 118–127.
64. Kong A, Cox NJ (1997) Allele-sharing models: LOD scores and accurate linkage tests. American Journal of Human Genetics 61: 1179–1188.
65. Boyles AL, Scott WK, Martin ER, Schmidt S, Li YJ, et al. (2005) Linkage disequilibrium inflates type I error rates in multipoint linkage analysis when parental genotypes are missing. Hum Hered 59: 220–227.
66. den Dunnen JT, Antonarakis SE (2001) Nomenclature for the description of human sequence variations. Hum Genet 109: 121–124.
67. Tassabehji M, Fang ZM, Hilton EN, McGaughran J, Zhao Z, et al. (2008) Mutations in GDF6 are associated with vertebral segmentation defects in Klippel-Feil syndrome. Hum Mutat 29: 1017–1027.
68. Asai-Coakwell M, French CR, Ye M, Garcha K, Bigot K, et al. (2009) Incomplete penetrance and phenotypic variability characterize Gdf6-attributable oculo-skeletal phenotypes. Hum Mol Genet 18: 1110–1121.
69. Ye M, Berry-Wynne KM, Asai-Coakwell M, Sundaresan P, Footz T, et al. (2010) Mutation of the bone morphogenetic protein GDF3 causes ocular and skeletal anomalies. Hum Mol Genet 19: 287–298.
70. den Hollander AI, Biyanwila J, Kovach P, Bardakjian T, Traboulsi EI, et al. (2010) Genetic defects of GDF6 in the zebrafish out of sight mutant and in human eye developmental anomalies. BMC Genet 11: 102.
71. Gonzalez-Rodriguez J, Pelcastre EL, Tovilla-Canales JL, Garcia-Ortiz JE, Amato-Almanza M, et al. (2010) Mutational screening of CHX10, GDF6, OTX2, RAX and SOX2 genes in 50 unrelated microphthalmia-anophthalmia-coloboma (MAC) spectrum cases. Br J Ophthalmol 94: 1100–1104.

72. Markunas CA, Tubbs RS, Moftakhar R, Ashley-Koch AE, Gregory SG, et al. (2012) Clinical, radiological, and genetic similarities between patients with Chiari Type I and Type 0 malformations. J Neurosurg Pediatr 9: 372–378.
73. Kim SH, Lim BC, Chae JH, Kim KJ, Hwang YS (2010) A case of Rubinstein-Taybi Syndrome with a CREB-binding protein gene mutation. Korean J Pediatr 53: 718–721.
74. Matsuoka T, Ahlberg PE, Kessaris N, Iannarelli P, Dennehy U, et al. (2005) Neural crest origins of the neck and shoulder. Nature 436: 347–355.
75. Bogdanov EI, Heiss JD, Mendelevich EG, Mikhaylov IM, Haass A (2004) Clinical and neuroimaging features of "idiopathic" syringomyelia. Neurology 62: 791–794.
76. Iskandar BJ, Hedlund GL, Grabb PA, Oakes WJ (1998) The resolution of syringohydromyelia without hindbrain herniation after posterior fossa decompression. J Neurosurg 89: 212–216.
77. Tubbs RS, Elton S, Grabb P, Dockery SE, Bartolucci AA, et al. (2001) Analysis of the posterior fossa in children with the Chiari 0 malformation. Neurosurgery 48: 1050–1054; discussion 1054–1055.
78. Tubbs RS, Wellons JC 3rd, Blount JP, Oakes WJ (2004) Syringomyelia in twin brothers discordant for Chiari I malformation: case report. J Child Neurol 19: 459–462.
79. Miro X, Zhou X, Boretius S, Michaelis T, Kubisch C, et al. (2009) Haploinsufficiency of the murine polycomb gene Suz12 results in diverse malformations of the brain and neural tube. Dis Model Mech 2: 412–418.
80. Mortlock DP, Guenther C, Kingsley DM (2003) A general approach for identifying distant regulatory elements applied to the Gdf6 gene. Genome Res 13: 2069–2081.
81. Portnoy ME, McDermott KJ, Antonellis A, Margulies EH, Prasad AB, et al. (2005) Detection of potential GDF6 regulatory elements by multispecies sequence comparisons and identification of a skeletal joint enhancer. Genomics 86: 295–305.
82. Reed NP, Mortlock DP (2010) Identification of a distant cis-regulatory element controlling pharyngeal arch-specific expression of zebrafish gdf6a/radar. Dev Dyn 239: 1047–1060.
83. Joeng KS, Schumacher CA, Zylstra-Diegel CR, Long F, Williams BO (2011) Lrp5 and Lrp6 redundantly control skeletal development in the mouse embryo. Dev Biol 359: 222–229.

Permissions

All chapters in this book were first published in PLOS ONE, by The Public Library of Science; hereby published with permission under the Creative Commons Attribution License or equivalent. Every chapter published in this book has been scrutinized by our experts. Their significance has been extensively debated. The topics covered herein carry significant findings which will fuel the growth of the discipline. They may even be implemented as practical applications or may be referred to as a beginning point for another development.

The contributors of this book come from diverse backgrounds, making this book a truly international effort. This book will bring forth new frontiers with its revolutionizing research information and detailed analysis of the nascent developments around the world.

We would like to thank all the contributing authors for lending their expertise to make the book truly unique. They have played a crucial role in the development of this book. Without their invaluable contributions this book wouldn't have been possible. They have made vital efforts to compile up to date information on the varied aspects of this subject to make this book a valuable addition to the collection of many professionals and students.

This book was conceptualized with the vision of imparting up-to-date information and advanced data in this field. To ensure the same, a matchless editorial board was set up. Every individual on the board went through rigorous rounds of assessment to prove their worth. After which they invested a large part of their time researching and compiling the most relevant data for our readers.

The editorial board has been involved in producing this book since its inception. They have spent rigorous hours researching and exploring the diverse topics which have resulted in the successful publishing of this book. They have passed on their knowledge of decades through this book. To expedite this challenging task, the publisher supported the team at every step. A small team of assistant editors was also appointed to further simplify the editing procedure and attain best results for the readers.

Apart from the editorial board, the designing team has also invested a significant amount of their time in understanding the subject and creating the most relevant covers. They scrutinized every image to scout for the most suitable representation of the subject and create an appropriate cover for the book.

The publishing team has been an ardent support to the editorial, designing and production team. Their endless efforts to recruit the best for this project, has resulted in the accomplishment of this book. They are a veteran in the field of academics and their pool of knowledge is as vast as their experience in printing. Their expertise and guidance has proved useful at every step. Their uncompromising quality standards have made this book an exceptional effort. Their encouragement from time to time has been an inspiration for everyone.

The publisher and the editorial board hope that this book will prove to be a valuable piece of knowledge for researchers, students, practitioners and scholars across the globe.

List of Contributors

Lara Moumne and Gillian P. Bates
Department of Medical and Molecular Genetics, King's College London, London, United Kingdom

Ken Campbell and Yingbin Ouyang
Taconic, Cranbury, New Jersey, United States of America

David Howland
CHDI Management/CHDI Foundation, Princeton, New Jersey, United States of America

Ashok R. Asthagiri, Raul A. Vasquez, Keaton Morgan and Russell R. Lonser
Surgical Neurology Branch, National Institute of Neurological Disorders and Stroke, National Institutes of Health, Bethesda, Maryland, United States of America

Raul A. Vasquez
Department of Neurological Surgery, University of Florida, Gainesville, Gainesville, Florida, United States of America

John A. Butman
Radiology and Imaging Sciences, The Clinical Center at the National Institutes of Health, National Institutes of Health, Bethesda, Maryland, United States of America

Tianxia Wu
Clinical Neurosciences Program, National Institute of Neurological Disorders and Stroke, National Institutes of Health, Bethesda, Maryland, United States of America

Carmen C. Brewer, Kelly King and Chris Zalewski
Audiology Unit, Otolaryngology Branch, National Institute on Deafness and Other Communication Disorders, National Institutes of Health, Bethesda, Maryland, United States of America

H. Jeffrey Kim
Office of the Clinical Director, National Institute on Deafness and Other Communication Disorders, National Institutes of Health, Bethesda, Maryland, United States of America

Inês Bernardino, Susana Mouga, Marieke van Asselen, Guiomar Oliveira and Miguel Castelo-Branco
Visual Neuroscience Laboratory, IBILI, Faculty of Medicine, Coimbra, Portugal

Susana Mouga, Joana Almeida and Guiomar Oliveira
Neurodevelopment and Autism Department from Child Center of Pediatric Hospital of Coimbra, Coimbra, Portugal

Guiomar Oliveira
Research and Clinical Training Department from Pediatric Hospital of Coimbra, Coimbra, Portugal

Karen N. McFarland, Ting Ting Sun, Eva Xia, Gavin R. Sangrey, Ghazaleh Sadri-Vakili and Jang-Ho J. Cha
Department of Neurology, MassGeneral Institute for Neurodegenerative Disease, massachusetts General Hospital, Charlestown, Massachusetts, United States of America

Sudeshna Das, Dmitri Leyfer and Timothy W. Clark
MIND Informatics, MassGeneral Institute for Neurodegenerative Disease, Massachusetts General Hospital, Cambridge, Massachusetts, United States of America

Alexandre Kuhn and Ruth Luthi-Carter
Brain Mind Institute, Ecole Polytechnique Fédérale de Lausanne, Lausanne, Switzerland

David Marcellin, Dorothee Abramowski, Douglas Young, Jens Richter, Andreas Weiss, Audrey Marcel, Julia Maassen, Muriel Kauffmann, Miriam Bibel, Derya R. Shimshek, Rainer R. Kuhn, P. Herman Van der Putten, Peter Schmid and Gregor P. Lotz
Novartis Institutes for BioMedical Research, Novartis Pharma AG, Basel, Switzerland

Richard L. M. Faull
Centre for Brain Research, Auckland University, Auckland, New Zealand

Gillian P. Bates
Department of Medical and Molecular Genetics, King's College London, London, United Kingdom

Koichi Suenaga, Yoshiki Tatsumi, Hiroo Yoshikawa and Takashi Kimura
Division of Neurology, Department of Internal Medicine, Hyogo College of Medicine, Nishinomiya, Hyogo, Japan

Kuang-Yung Lee and Maurice S. Swanson
Department of Molecular Genetics and Microbiology, College of Medicine, University of Florida, Gainesville, Florida, United States of America

Kuang-Yung Lee
Department of Neurology, Chang Gung Memorial Hospital, Keelung, Taiwan

Masayuki Nakamori and Masanori P. Takahashi
Department of Neurology, Osaka University Graduate School of Medicine, Suita, Osaka, Japan

Harutoshi Fujimura
Department of Neurology, National Hospital Organization Toneyama Hospital, Toyonaka, Osaka, Japan

Kenji Jinnai
Department of Neurology, National Hospital Organization Hyogo-Chuo Hospital, Ohara, Hyogo, Japan

Hongqing Du and Manuel Ares Jr.
Department of Molecular, Cell and Developmental Biology, RNA Center, Sinsheimer Labs, University of California Santa Cruz, Santa Cruz, California, United States of America

Maria Paschou and Epaminondas Doxakis
Molecular and Cellular Neurobiology Lab, Center of Neurosciences and Social Psychiatry, Biomedical Research Foundation, Academy of Athens, Athens, Greece

Belvin Gong, Catherine Kielar and A. Jennifer Morton
Department of Pharmacology, University of Cambridge, Cambridge, United Kingdom

Belvin Gong
UC Davis/NIH NeuroMab Facility, Department of Neurobiology, Physiology and Behavior, University of California Davis, Davis, California, United States of America

Wei-na Cong, Huan Cai, Rui Wang, Caitlin M. Daimon and Bronwen Martin
Metabolism Unit, National Institute on Aging, National Institutes of Health, Baltimore, Maryland, United States of America

Stuart Maudsley
Receptor Pharmacology Unit, National Institute on Aging, National Institutes of Health, Baltimore, Maryland, United States of America

Kerstin Raber, Fabio Canneva and Stephan von Hörsten
Department for Experimental Therapy, Friedrich-Alexander-Universität Erlangen-Nürnberg, Erlangen, Germany

Nesrin Sabha, Karolyn Au, Sameer Agnihotri, Sanjay Singh, Rupinder Mangat, Abhijit Guha and Gelareh Zadeh
Arthur and Sonia Labatt Brain Tumour Research Centre, Hospital for Sick Children Research Institute, University of Toronto, Toronto, Canada

Abhijit Guha and Gelareh Zadeh
Department of Surgery (Neurosurgery), Western Hospital, University of Toronto, Toronto, Canada

Shashwath A. Meda and Tricia A. Thornton-Wells
Department of Molecular Physiology and Biophysics, Center for Human Genetics and Research, Vanderbilt University, Nashville, Tennessee, United States of America

Jennifer R. Pryweller
Interdisciplinary Studies in Neuroimaging of Neurodevelopmental Disorders, The Graduate School, Vanderbilt University, Nashville, Tennessee, United States of America

Katherine H. Karlsgodt, Tyrone D. Cannon, Alcino Silva and Carrie E. Bearden
Semel Institute for Neuroscience and Behavior, University of California Los Angeles, Los Angeles, California, United States of America

Katherine H. Karlsgodt, Tyrone D. Cannon and Carrie E. Bearden
Center for Cognitive Neuroscience, University of California Los Angeles, Los Angeles, California, United States of America

Evan S. Lutkenhoff, Tyrone D. Cannon, Alcino Silva and Carrie E. Bearden
Department of Psychology, University of California Los Angeles, Los Angeles, California, United States of America

Tena Rosser
Children's Hospital Los Angeles, Los Angeles, California, United States of America

Alcino Silva
Department of Neurobiology, University of California Los Angeles, Los Angeles, California, United States of America

Patricia Gervan, Ferenc Gombos and Ilona Kovacs
Department of Cognitive Science, Budapest University of Technology and Economics, Budapest, Hungary

Inês R. Violante, Maria J. Ribeiro, Gil Cunha, Inês Bernardino, João V. Duarte and Miguel Castelo-Branco
Visual Neuroscience Laboratory, Institute of Biomedical Research in Light and Image, Faculty of Medicine, University of Coimbra, Coimbra, Portugal

Fabiana Ramos and Jorge Saraiva
Medical Genetic Department, Pediatric Hospital of Coimbra, Coimbra, Portugal

Eduardo Silva
Centre for Hereditary Eye Diseases, Department of Ophthalmology, University Hospital of Coimbra, Coimbra, Portugal

Aviv Cohen, Liron Ross, Iftach Nachman and Shoshana Bar-Nun
Department of Biochemistry and Molecular Biology, George S. Wise Faculty of Life Sciences, Tel Aviv University, Tel Aviv, Israel

Yi-Chao Lee
Ph.D. Program for Neural Regenerative Medicine, College of Medical Science and Technology, Taipei Medical University, Taipei, Taiwan, Republic of China

Ying-Chen Yang and Tsun-Yung Kuo
Department of Animal Science, National Ilan University, Ilan, Taiwan, Republic of China

Chuen-Lin Huang
Medical Research Center, Cardinal Tien Hospital, Hsintien, New Taipei City, Taiwan, Republic of China
Graduate Institute of Physiology and Department of Physiology and Biophysics, National Defense Medical Center, Taipei, Taiwan, Republic of China

Tsun-Yung Kuo
Institute of Biotechnology, National Ilan University, Ilan, Taiwan, Republic of China

Jung-Hsin Lin
School of Pharmacy, National Taiwan University, Taipei, Taiwan, Republic of China
Division of Mechanics, Research Center for Applied Sciences, Academia Sinica, Taipei, Taiwan, Republic of China
Institute of Biomedical Sciences, Academia Sinica, Nankang, Taipei, Taiwan, Republic of China

Ming Yang
Department of Medical Research and Education, Taipei Veterans General Hospital, Taipei, Taiwan, Republic of China
Institute of Biophotonics, National Yang-Ming University, Taipei, Taiwan, Republic of China

Nai-Kuei Huang
Institute of Biophotonics, National Yang-Ming University, Taipei, Taiwan, Republic of China
National Research Institute of Chinese Medicine, Taipei, Taiwan, Republic of China

Liliana B. Menalled, Andrea E. Kudwa, Sam Miller, Jon Fitzpatrick, Judy Watson-Johnson, Nicole Keating, Melinda Ruiz, Richard Mushlin, William Alosio, Kristi McConnell, David Connor, Carol Murphy, Steve Oakeshott, Mei Kwan, Jose Beltran, Afshin Ghavami, Dani Brunner and Sylvie Ramboz
PsychoGenics Inc., Tarrytown, New York, United States of America

Larry C. Park and David Howland
CHDI Management/CHDI Foundation, Princeton, New Jersey, United States of America

Fumiko Hoeft, Brian W. Haas, Kristen Sheau and Allan L. Reiss
Center for Interdisciplinary Brain Sciences Research (CIBSR), Stanford University School of Medicine, Stanford, CA, United States of America

Fumiko Hoeft and Masaru Mimura
Department of Neuropsychiatry, Keio University, School of Medicine, Tokyo, Japan

Li Dai and Julie R. Korenberg
Department of Pediatrics and The Center for Integrated Neuroscience and Human Behavior, The Brain Institute, University of Utah, Salt Lake City, UT, United States of America

Brian W. Haas
Department of Psychology, University of Georgia, Athens, GA, United States of America

Debra Mills
School of Psychology, Bangor University, Gwynedd, United Kingdom

Albert Galaburda
Department of Neurology, Beth Israel-Deaconess Medical Center, Harvard Medical School, Cambridge, MA, United States of America

Ursula Bellugi
Laboratory for Cognitive Neuroscience, Salk Institute for Biological Studies, La Jolla, CA, United States of America

Allan L. Reiss
Departments of Radiology and Pediatrics, Stanford University School of Medicine, Stanford, CA, United States of America

Sarah Beltrami, Emanuela Branchetti, Ilker K. Sariyer, Jessica Otte and Jennifer Gordon
Department of Neuroscience and Center for Neurovirology, Temple University School of Medicine, Philadelphia, Pennsylvania, United States of America

Sarah Beltrami
Biomedical Neuroscience Graduate Program, Temple University School of Medicine, Philadelphia, Pennsylvania, United States of America

Michael Weaver
Department of Neurosurgery, Temple University School of Medicine, Philadelphia, Pennsylvania, United States of America

Fabio P. Nunes, Vanessa L. Merker and Scott R. Plotkin
Neurology Department, Massachusetts General Hospital, Boston, Massachusetts, United States of America

Fabio P. Nunes
Genetics Department, Massachusetts General Hospital, Boston, Massachusetts, United States of America

Vanessa L. Merker and Scott R. Plotkin
Stephen E. and Catherine Pappas Center for Neurooncology, Massachusetts General Hospital, Boston, Massachusetts, United States of America

Dominique Jennings
A.A. Martinos Center for Biomedical Imaging, Massachusetts General Hospital, Boston, Massachusetts, United States of America

Paul A. Caruso
Department of Radiology, Massachusetts General Hospital, Boston, Massachusetts, United States of America

Emmanuelle di Tomaso and Anat Stemmer-Rachamimov
Pathology Department, Massachusetts General Hospital, Boston, Massachusetts, United States of America

Alona Muzikansky
Biostatistics Center, Massachusetts General Hospital, Boston, Massachusetts, United States of America

Fred G. Barker II
Neurosurgical Service, Massachusetts General Hospital, Boston, Massachusetts, United States of America

Christina A. Markunas, Karen Soldano, Kaitlyn Dunlap, Heidi Cope, Edgar Asiimwe, Jeffrey Stajich, Simon G. Gregory and Allison E. Ashley-Koch
Department of Medicine, Duke University Medical Center, Durham, North Carolina, United States of America

David Enterline
Department of Radiology, Duke University Medical Center, Durham, North Carolina, United States of America

Gerald Grant and Herbert Fuchs
Department of Surgery, Duke University Medical Center, Durham, North Carolina, United States of America

Index